**FOR REFERENCE**

Do Not Take From This Room

# ENCYCLOPEDIA OF
# BIOETHICS

# ENCYCLOPEDIA OF
# BIOETHICS

## REVISED EDITION

## Warren Thomas Reich

*EDITOR IN CHIEF*

Georgetown University

**Volume 5**

MACMILLAN LIBRARY REFERENCE USA

SIMON & SCHUSTER MACMILLAN

NEW YORK

SIMON & SCHUSTER AND PRENTICE HALL INTERNATIONAL

LONDON   MEXICO CITY   NEW DELHI   SINGAPORE   SYDNEY   TORONTO

ENCYCLOPEDIA OF BIOETHICS

Simon & Schuster Macmillan
866 Third Avenue, New York, NY 10022

PRINTED IN THE UNITED STATES OF AMERICA

printing number
  2   3   4   5   6   7   8   9   10

LIBRARY OF CONGRESS CATALOG-IN-PUBLICATION DATA
Encyclopedia of bioethics / Warren T. Reich, editor in chief. — Rev.
  ed.
    p. cm.
    Includes bibliographical references and index.
    ISBN 0-02-897355-0 (set)
    1. Bioethics—Encyclopedias.   2. Medical ethics—Encyclopedias.
  I. Reich, Warren T.
  QH332.E52   1995
  174'.2'03—dc20                                    94-38743
                                                       CIP

Lines from the poem "The Scarred Girl" by James Dickey, quoted in the entry on "Interpretation," originally appeared in *Poems, 1957–1967,* © 1978 by James Dickey, Wesleyan University Press, and have been reprinted here by permission of the University Press of New England.

The paper used in this publication meets the minimum requirements of American National Standard for Information Sciences—Permanence of Paper for Printed Library Materials, ANSI Z39.48-1984.

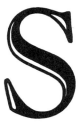

# SANCTITY OF LIFE

*See* LIFE; *and* LIFE, QUALITY OF.

# SAUDI ARABIA

*See* MEDICAL ETHICS, HISTORY OF, *section on* NEAR AND MIDDLE EAST, *article on* CONTEMPORARY ARAB WORLD.

---

# SCIENCE, PHILOSOPHY OF

Philosophy of science as an autonomous subject is a product of the twentieth century. Its development stemmed from the great intellectual challenges of quantum and relativity theory, but philosophical issues surrounding such theories as psychoanalysis, evolutionary theory, Marxist and capitalist economics, the ethics of human experimentation, and the enormously increased importance of science as an intellectual endeavor led to a great expansion of the field. Work within philosophy of science tends to fall into two approaches. The first sees science as a testing ground for traditional philosophical problems. Chief among these traditional problems is this: Can we have any knowledge that is certain and in terms of which all other knowledge in the area can be justified (*foundationalism*), or are all claims to knowledge uncertain (*fallibilism*)? Within the realm of things that can be known by empirical investigation it would seem that science has the best claim to secure knowledge. Philosophers of science have thus devoted a considerable amount of time to what kinds of scientific methods are effective in producing such reliable knowledge. On the other hand, many philosophers, especially in recent times, have denied that science actually produces a privileged body of knowledge, and have argued that all scientific knowledge is a product of its historical and social context.

The second principal area in philosophy of science focuses on issues that are peculiar to individual sciences. Of particular interest here is the possibility of reducing biology to chemistry or physics, and of reducing some of the social sciences, especially psychology, to biology. If these reductionist projects were to be successful, then issues that appear to be peculiarly biological, such as the question of what makes something a living organism, would turn out to be merely a question of degrees of complexity, and not specifically biological at all. In addition, the moral issues that pertain to humans and animals because of their psychological characteristics would be approached very differently if psychological properties were unreal or merely disguised biological properties. These differences in the sciences are obviously crucial. A great deal of medical research cannot enjoy the unlimited freedom of laboratory experimentation that is characteristic of physics simply because of the ethical constraints its subjects require. Moreover, the variability of its subjects makes universal laws hard to formulate, in distinction to, for example, astronomy.

## Predecessors to contemporary viewpoints

It was the logical positivists and logical empiricists of the Vienna Circle (1923–1936) and the Berlin School

(1928–1933) who succeeded in placing scientific issues near the heart of the philosophical enterprise. (A classic, albeit sententious, presentation of the logical positivists' views can be found in A. J. Ayer's *Language, Truth and Logic*, 1946.) For philosophers such as Moritz Schlick, Rudolf Carnap, Hans Reichenbach, and Carl Hempel, all of whom had a scientific education, the task was to provide a foundation for genuine knowledge, and this foundation was to be as secure as the best science of the time. The logical positivists were squarely within the empiricist tradition, which holds that all genuine knowledge must be reducible in principle to knowledge obtainable by empirical methods, and ultimately to that obtainable through the human sensory apparatus. To this empiricist view they added a deep concern with language resulting from developments in logic in the late nineteenth and early twentieth centuries. Although the most famous manifestation of their approach was the attempt to eliminate metaphysical claims through the verificationist criterion of meaning (which asserts that a sentence is factually significant to a given individual if and only if he knows what observations would lead him to accept that proposition as true or to reject it as false), their true legacy has been the view that it is by means of logical analyses of philosophical concepts that genuine understanding is achieved. It is no exaggeration to say that philosophy of science since 1950 has been primarily engaged in a struggle to decide which elements of the positivist monolith to retain, and what should be the replacement approaches for those parts that have been rejected.

## Falsificationism

An important alternative to the positivist program has been the falsificationist approach of Karl Popper. Although his *Logik der Forschung* was published in 1934, its impact was muted until the expanded English translation appeared in 1959 as *The Logic of Scientific Discovery*. Popper set himself the task of providing a criterion that would distinguish between genuine scientific hypotheses and pseudoscientific statements. A key reason driving Popper's views was his view that the traditional problem of induction could not be solved. Most generally, inductive inference involves reasoning from what has been observed to what has not been observed, a characterization that covers inferences from the past to the future, from observed data to the existence of unobservable microentities, and from finite data sets to the universal hypotheses that represent scientific laws and general theories. The case of induction was a serious problem for logical positivism, because the verificationist criterion ruled out all universal scientific theories and laws as meaningless, simply because no amount of finite

data could conclusively verify these general claims. Popper proposed instead the demarcation criterion that a statement or theory was scientific only if it was falsifiable; that is, it must be possible to state in advance a set of possible observations which, if observed, would result in the statement or theory being rejected. Theories such as astrology and psychoanalysis were, according to Popper, branded as pseudoscientific on the basis of this criterion because they traditionally accommodated themselves to fit any observations whatsoever. To refuse to relinquish a theory in the face of recalcitrant data is a characteristic feature of scientific irrationality. Popper's brand of falsificationism is comprehensive, for it requires that even reports of observations be falsifiable. Thus, in contrast to the positivists' foundationalism, which is grounded in an empirical base that is certain, falsificationism is a deeply fallibilist position, within which claims to certainty are relinquished at all levels of generality.

Popper was well aware of a point often made by the French philosopher Pierre Duhem, to the effect that in order to draw out testable predictions from scientific hypotheses, we ordinarily need to assume the truth of various background assumptions and theories (Duhem, 1962). Thus, if the prediction turns out to be false, the force of the falsification could be deflected away from the principal hypothesis on to the background assumptions. Hence the need in the above specification of falsificationism to state *in advance* what would result in the hypothesis being rejected.

Although this strategy removes the force of Duhem's criticism that there are no crucial experiments that can conclusively decide between competing theories, it moves the emphasis away from a method of testing that is based only on logic and empirical data to one where a (human) decision plays a central role, and this once again introduces a characteristically conventional element into the picture. Popper's views have been elaborated by Imre Lakatos, but it as well to clear up a continuing confusion about the status of falsificationism. Falsificationism is primarily a normative methodology, for it prescribes and proscribes courses of action with respect to scientific hypotheses. As historical and sociological studies of science have become increasingly influential, there has been a concomitant emphasis on the need for methodological theories to be descriptively accurate of what scientists do and have done. It is easy to find cases where historically important episodes of science do not fit the falsificationist model, where scientists refused to abandon theories in the face of clear counter evidence. The difficult task is to articulate when this furthers broad scientific ends, rather than just narrow personal motives. But to reject falsificationism merely because it is not descriptively accurate of everything done in the name of science would be as misguided as the attempt to turn ethics into a purely descriptive enterprise.

## Thomas Kuhn's work

One of the best known alternatives to the positivist approach is Thomas Kuhn's. Ironically, Kuhn's seminal work *The Structure of Scientific Revolutions* (1970) was originally published in the positivists' *International Encyclopedia of Unified Science* (Kuhn, 1955). Kuhn's strategy was to bring the history of science as a proving ground for methodological positions in the philosophy of science. This history, Kuhn claimed, could be divided into two distinct types of periods. There were long stretches of normal science punctuated by brief periods of revolutionary science. To illuminate both kinds of science, Kuhn introduced the concept of a scientific paradigm. This concept, in its mature characterization, consists of four components. First, there are the symbolic generalizations, those fundamental laws and principles of a science that underpin all theoretical work in the field, such as the laws of genetic replication or the principle of natural selection of species. Second, is the metaphysical component of the paradigm, within which the fundamental kinds of things constituting the subject matter of the science are specified, such as atomistic or field-theoretic assumptions in physics, or a commitment to specifically mental properties, as opposed to material properties, in psychology. Third, we have the value commitments. These not only concern what constitutes an acceptable piece of evidence in the science, but what the appropriate goals for a science are, and what the ethical standards to which one should adhere are. Thus, double-blind studies will be considered the standard methodology for drug trials. Fourth, there are the exemplars, those quintessential successes that a scientific field can point to as evidence for the fruitfulness of the first three elements, as, for instance, Newtonian mechanics could point to its success in predicting the existence of the planet Neptune.

Normal science, then, is science conducted entirely within the framework of a single paradigm, whereas revolutionary science consists in the development of a competing paradigm and the process of a scientific community's transfer of allegiance to the new paradigm. A seemingly inescapable consequence of paradigm change in periods of revolutionary science, and one that is deeply disturbing to many, is that the process of change is determined by neither rational argument nor empirical evidence. Because a change in paradigm necessarily involves a change in at least one of the four components already described, there will inevitably be fundamental differences of opinion about whether the old or the new

component is preferable, and the remaining three components will frequently not provide a large enough common ground to resolve the dispute in an impartial way. In this way, paradigms are, to use Kuhn's term, incommensurable. There is then a deep difference here between Kuhn and both Popper and the positivists.

Equally important is the distinction between internal and external descriptions of science. Within both the positivists' and Popper's approaches, the way in which science proceeds ought to be appraised in terms only of influences that are purely internal to the science at hand, including the construction of theories, the invention of new experimental apparatus, and the verification or falsification of hypotheses by empirical data. Any interference by nonscientific factors, such as economic considerations, political pressure, and religious prohibitions are to be condemned as illegitimate influences to be resisted in practice, and ignored in writing the history of the science. In contrast, Kuhn holds that not only are influences usually present and causally effective in propelling or impeding the elaboration of a paradigm, but they are frequently important in fixing the values component of a paradigm. Thus, the religious opposition to research on fetal tissue derived from deliberate abortions, the political pressure to direct funds in molecular biology toward acquired immunodeficiency syndrome (AIDS) research, and the decision to allocate significant financial resources to the Human Genome Project are all part of an externalist appraisal of the scientific research concerned. Inseparable from this externalist approach is the shift in emphasis from scientific theories as logical entities whose existence and appraisal are objective matters, and the truth or falsity of which is something to be discovered, to a position where the opinions of a community of scientists are primary, and acceptance of a paradigm is determined by a consensus in that community rather than by the paradigm's truth or falsity. Coupled with the inclusion of externalist factors, this leads naturally toward a focus on the sociology of science, rather than its philosophy as traditionally conceived.

Some further consequences of the Kuhnian approach are worth mentioning. Because of the incommensurability of paradigms, revolutions lead to schisms in the path of science, with a resulting loss of the notion of scientific progress. Comparative judgments of the kind "Paradigm A is superior to Paradigm B" can no longer be made on a uniform scale of comparison, and what remains is technological progress without any necessary concomitant progress toward the truth. Consequently, what has come to be known as the Whig view of the history of science, which sees the development of science as an uninterrupted triumphal march up to the peak of contemporary success, has to be abandoned in favor of a contextually sympathetic interpretation of previous theoretical traditions. Finally, there is no longer anything peculiarly privileged in the scientific enterprise if Kuhn is correct. The development of art, architecture, music, and so forth can all be characterized in terms of paradigms, normal practice, and revolutionary changes, a feature that has not escaped Kuhn's critics.

## Feyerabend, Lakatos, and Hacking

The early views of Paul Feyerabend played an important role in undermining the plausibility of falsificationism and verificationism, especially when supported by detailed historical case studies. His influential arguments favored an extreme incommensurability of theories, based on the view that theoretical concepts gained their content from the entire theoretical structure within which they were embedded, and so even slight changes in that structure lead to changes in the meaning of the concepts involved. Feyerabend's later writings exerted little influence on the field and seemed designed more to provoke than to inform. He advocated epistemological anarchism in the form of allowing all methodologies into science, thereby making no distinctions between charlatans and experts.

Two more figures merit mention. Imre Lakatos's work may be viewed both as a partially successful attempt to save falsificationism from its conventionalist components and as a way of making precise some of the vaguer elements of Kuhn's approach (although it must be emphasized that Lakatos's empiricism is explicitly at odds with Kuhn's conventionalism). Rather than taking single theories or hypotheses as the unit of scientific appraisal, Lakatos suggested that science takes place in the context of theoretical research programs, within which elementary theories are sequentially elaborated, eliminating known false consequences while widening their scope. If this sequence of theories generates new predictions that are borne out by experience, then the research program is progressing; if not, then it is degenerating, and must be abandoned if a suitable replacement program is available. The internal progress of the research program is guided by the requirement that the so-called "hard core" of commitments that provide the identity of the program (these are similar to the first three components of a Kuhnian paradigm) must not be subject to falsification. A good example of a progressive research program is that of molecular biology (Lakatos, 1970). Starting in 1953 with the discovery of the basic structure of deoxyribonucleic acid (DNA), the fundamental tenets of this approach have produced spectacular results. A clear case of a degenerating research program is that of homeopathy which, despite its popular following, has never produced a significant scientific advance. A signal advantage of Lakatos's approach is that one can determine from within a research program whether it is degenerating or progressing; a disadvantage is that a program may temporarily go into a degenerating phase and be prematurely rejected before it reaches full flower.

The work of Ian Hacking is less easy to describe briefly. Under the influence of the French philosopher Michel Foucault, Hacking (1975) has attempted to show, especially in the history of probability and statistics, that the traditional boundaries between scientific disciplines obscure important formative and developmental influences on scientific subjects. This is deeply external history and philosophy of science that trades on the kind of holism espoused by W. V. Quine (1951) and Kuhn. In addition, Hacking and others have tried to account for the role played by experimentation in science in such a way that it provides a kind of direct access to reality that bypasses the incommensurability problems stressed by Kuhn and by Feyerabend.

## Other contemporary work in the field

Perhaps the most important consequence of the collapse of the positivists' domination in the philosophy of science has been the splintering of the field into subdisciplines. Broadly speaking, these fall into two types. The first type continues to explore issues that were important to the logical empiricists but often uses methods different from those endorsed by those philosophers. A selective list, which is representative but inevitably incomplete, includes the following: Foundational studies, within which axiomatic formulations of specific sciences play a key role, continue to be important in clarifying the nature and structure of specific scientific theories such as rational choice theory and quantum mechanics. An influential attempt to recapture part of the lost empiricist territory can be found in The Scientific Image by Bas van Fraassen (1980). The nature of scientific explanation is a topic of perennial interest, with a variety of causal, pragmatic, and unification approaches replacing Carl Hempel's (1966) logical model (Salmon, 1990). Issues regarding the autonomy of particular sciences have replaced the positivists' view of unified science, within which all genuine science was presumed to employ the same method of testing and confirmation that physics employs. The traditional differences between the natural and the social sciences no longer mark a dichotomy. There is now a "philosophy of X" for almost every science X, from economics to geology. In particular, the philosophy of biology and the philosophy of medicine are well established subfields with their own problems and subjects.

A new and vital field comprises the intersection of philosophical psychology, cognitive science, and artificial intelligence, wherein traditional philosophical answers concerning the nature of free will, language use, consciousness, and other properties characteristic of complex organisms have been supplemented by novel insights. These investigations relate directly to the issue of what it is to be human. Computer-assisted diagnostic procedures in medicine form a small but important proving ground for inference procedures. An elementary, albeit argumentative, discussion of some basic issues in cognitive science can be found in John Searle's *Minds, Brains, and Science* (1984).

The second type of subdiscipline results from a radical rejection of traditional a priori methods in philosophy of science, that is, a rejection of methods that do not rely on empirical investigations to achieve their goals. An influential program here involves what are called naturalistic approaches to philosophical problems, within which scientific methods replace philosophical methods. This can take many forms, depending on the topic of interest. For example, instead of specifying a priori the inferences that an ideal reasoner should make in deciding which course of action is appropriate in some clinical setting, a naturalist will investigate the actual psychological processes that underlie reasoning used in clinical practice (Osherson and Smith, 1990). In its extreme form, naturalism turns into "the science of science," wherein science itself is treated as the object of a scientific study, bringing to bear whatever sociological, anthropological, economic, and other techniques are suited to the task (Hull, 1988). Of course, without some antecedent idea of what counts as an acceptable scientific method, it is hard to see how the science of science could know what its subject matter is and what would be an appropriate method to use in investigating it. Hence the field of science studies, which is a continuation of the holistic and externalist trends described earlier, combines the philosophy of science, the history of science, and some aspects of social science to illuminate various facets of the scientific enterprise.

## Summary

Philosophy of science and bioethics share a common concern. Each must draw a line between the prescriptive and the descriptive, between what is rational and justified on the one hand, and what is merely popular opinion and prejudice on the other. Both Galileo and Ignaz Semmelweiss were victims of such antiscientific attacks, the first for advocating the correct theory of the solar system, the second for discovering the mode of transmission of childbed fever. It is thus essential to have some clear distinction between fact and opinion, between the rational evaluation of a hypothesis or ethical view and its mere acceptance, between what is ethically justified and the way individuals happen to act, and to use a specific example, between what science can do to allow premature babies to survive and how we can evaluate the quality of life they might expect. This, if nothing else, is why the apparently dry and abstract issues of the foundations of knowledge, of internal and external influences on science, and of fact versus convention bear directly upon matters of more immediate concern.

PAUL W. HUMPHREYS

*Directly related to this entry is the entry* BIOLOGY, PHILOSOPHY OF. *For a further discussion of topics mentioned in this entry, see the entries* RESEARCH BIAS; *and* RESEARCH METHODOLOGY. *This entry will find application in the entry* ANIMAL RESEARCH. *For a discussion of related ideas, see the entries* INTERPRETATION; *and* VALUE AND VALUATION.

## Bibliography

AYER, A. J. 1946. *Language, Truth, and Logic.* 2d ed. London: Gollancz.

BOYD, RICHARD; GASPER, PHILIP; and TROUT, J. D., eds. 1991. *The Philosophy of Science.* Cambridge, Mass.: MIT Press.

BRODY, BARUCH A., and GRANDY, RICHARD E., eds. 1989. *Readings in the Philosophy of Science.* 2d ed. Englewood Cliffs, N.J.: Prentice Hall.

DUHEM, PIERRE. 1962. [1906]. *The Aim and Structure of Physical Theory.* New York: Atheneum.

FEYERABEND, PAUL K. 1981. *Philosophical Papers.* Vols. 1–2. Cambridge: At the University Press.

———. 1988. *Against Method.* Rev. ed. London: Verso.

HACKING, IAN. 1975. *The Emergence of Probability.* Cambridge: At the University Press.

———. 1983. *Representing and Intervening: Introductory Topics in the Philosophy of Natural Science.* Cambridge: At the University Press.

HEMPEL, CARL G. 1966. *Philosophy of Natural Science.* Englewood Cliffs, N.J.: Prentice Hall.

HOLLIS, MARTIN, and LUKES, STEVEN, eds. 1982. *Rationality and Relativism.* Cambridge, Mass.: MIT Press.

HULL, DAVID L. 1988. *Science as Process: An Evolutionary Account of the Social & Conceptual Development of Science.* Chicago: University of Chicago Press.

KOURANY, JANET A., ed. 1987. *Scientific Knowledge: Basic Issues in the Philosophy of Science.* Belmont, Calif.: Wadsworth.

KUHN, THOMAS S. 1955. *The Structure of Scientific Revolutions.* Vol. 2, no. 2 of *The International Encyclopedia of Unified Science.* Edited by Otto Neurath. Chicago: University of Chicago Press.

———. 1970. *The Structure of Scientific Revolutions.* 2d ed. Chicago: University of Chicago Press.

LAKATOS, IMRE. 1970. "Falsification and the Methodology of Scientific Research Programmers." In *Criticism and the Growth of Knowledge,* pp. 91–195. Edited by Imre Lakatos and Alan Musgrave. Cambridge: At the University Press.

OSHERSON, DANIEL N., and SMITH, EDWARD E., eds. 1990. *Thinking*. Vol. 3 of their *An Invitation to Cognitive Science*. Cambridge, Mass.: MIT Press.

POPPER, KARL R. *Logik der Forschung*. 1935. Vienna: Julius Springer. Translated by Karl Popper, Julius Freed, and Lan Freed under the title *The Logic of Scientific Discovery*. London: Hutchinson, 1959.

QUINE, W. V. 1951. "Two Dogmas of Empiricism." *Philosophical Review* 60, no. 1:20–43.

SALMON, WESLEY C. 1990. *Four Decades of Scientific Explanation*. Minneapolis: University of Minnesota Press.

SEARLE, JOHN. 1984. *Minds, Brains, and Science*. Cambridge, Mass.: Harvard University Press.

VAN FRAASEN, BAS C. 1980. *The Scientific Image*. Oxford: At the Clarendon Press.

# SCIENTIFIC MISCONDUCT

See FRAUD, THEFT, AND PLAGIARISM; *and* RESEARCH, UNETHICAL.

# SELF-HELP

The term "self-help" is an elastic and imprecise term often used differently by physicians, social workers, booksellers, and the lay public. Its most common meanings include (1) mutual aid groups for addictions, disabilities, bereavement, and scores of other health concerns; and (2) popularized psychology and health care as presented through mass media, such as, for example, self-help books. This is a broad and powerful social movement, now a robust influence on medical care. According to pollster George Gallup, "one American in three belongs to some kind of small support or self-help group" (White and Madara, 1992, p. 114), and many of these people will invest considerable time, money, and hope in self-help resources. Self-help has several bioethical implications, concerning such issues as its relationship to standard medical care (as adjunct, alternative, or even antagonist); its notions of healing, notably mind-body interactions; and its availability, often only to those who can afford it.

"Self-help" is not a scientific term like "radiotherapy," but a popular one, and therefore continually evolving. For this entry, self-help means health care chosen by an individual and managed, completely or in large part, by that individual, often within a group of individuals with similar concerns. Self-help may or may not have any connection with standard medical care. Indeed, self-help may or may not be helpful, since some forms of self-help can cause harm. It is difficult to formulate generalizations concerning the term because it has been applied to topics as diverse as self-care, self-

medication, and aftercare; to alternative therapies such as crystals, imagery, and herbalism; to astrology, yoga, acupuncture, and self-hypnosis; and to a large and commercially successful range of so-called personal growth materials, including books, videos, and tapes. Because of the success of such groups as Alcoholics Anonymous (the oldest and largest self-help group), the wide use of the mass media, and the enormous appetite of the public, the notion of self-help is, for better and for worse, a major force in contemporary health care.

## Historical background

In English, the phrase "self-help" dates from the middle of the nineteenth century, when the meaning was either general (providing for oneself), economic, or legal, but not medical. To a poet's ear, the two words are a near rhyme, perhaps an aesthetic reason for the phrase's survival. In 1859 Samuel Smiles, a Scotsman, wrote *Self-Help: With Illustrations of Conduct and Perseverance* (Smiles, 1958). He may have appropriated the concept from Ralph Waldo Emerson's "self-reliance," but for him the argument was primarily economic: that young men—and men only—should make fortunes by dint of individual worth and effort. In France, pharmacist René Coué championed "autosuggestion" at the turn of the century ("Every day, in every way, I am getting better and better"). In America, Dale Carnegie wrote *How to Win Friends and Influence People* in 1936; 15 million copies have now been sold; more recently, Norman Cousins symbolized mind-over-matter healing with his *Anatomy of an Illness* (1979). But the general concept of self-care and mind–body interaction is much older.

A verse in Proverbs (ca. 500 B.C.E.) runs, "A cheerful heart is a good medicine, but a downcast spirit dries up the bones," suggesting the relationship between personal consciousness and health (17:22). In the Renaissance (1598), Francis Bacon wrote: "There is a wisdom beyond the rules of physic: a man's own observation, what he finds good of, and what he finds hurt of, is the best physic to preserve health" (see his "Of Regimen of Health," 1979). The Enlightenment suggested the notion of infinite progress, illustrated by Benjamin Franklin's aggressive self-help plan to improve his virtues and precepts (*Autobiography*, entry of 1784; see Franklin, 1961). With the rise of high-tech medicine in the twentieth century, economics has also become a powerful force: Some persons stay home to treat themselves because they cannot afford care, cannot travel to medical centers, or cannot imagine themselves in the architectural and bureaucratic labyrinths that modern medical care has become.

Indeed it might be argued that for many early peoples, self-care was the only care available, through folk medicine, tribal rituals, and what we would now call "home remedies." Even care by priests, shamans, or midwives may have elicited from the patient a more active role in healing along with participation at more levels of consciousness than are typical today. Many of the poor (whether in the Third World or rural or urban subcultures within the First World) exclusively practice versions of self-help because standard care is simply not available. The advent of scientific and professional medicine contributed to a split of Western medical care into two streams: the standard care provided by physicians, hospitals, and pharmacies, and the huge range of alternative medicine, including self-help.

Many political and economic issues have emerged regarding the medical care of women, who have seen neighborhood midwifery replaced by male-dominated hospital care. In 1971 *Our Bodies, Ourselves* became a landmark in feminist self-help (Boston Women's Health Collective, 1971). Indeed, one recent definition of self-help appears in the *New A–Z of Women's Health:* "Routine gynecologic care, involving breast and pelvic examination, simple laboratory tests, fitting and insertion of birth control devices, and similar procedures, carried on in a group setting where women are encouraged to participate in their own health care. The development of the movement in North America began in the late 1960s, when a small but growing number of women rebelled against the male-dominated profession of gynecology" (Ammer, 1989, p. 387).

Self-help is a notion particular to societies of the Western world, where there is a great emphasis on the self, the individual, freedom, personal rights, and the power of persons to "control their own destiny." (In many Eastern traditions, the concept of self is less important, particularly when transcended by higher realities.) In the United States, for example, people can take college courses in personal finance, earn Boy Scout merit badges for personal fitness, and hire personal trainers. Not only is the self a favored concept, but the notion of "help" is much cherished. Help is understood not only as aid and assistance, sometimes even a religious duty, but also as improving, making, or doing in the traditions of Enlightenment progress, nineteenth-century "muscular Christianity," "Yankee ingenuity," or just plain old "can do." A 1989 bestseller, *The Seven Habits of Highly Effective People,* lists first the quality of being "proactive," or "taking the initiative" (Covey, 1989).

In sum, a large number of historical and social values inform the concept of self-help, making it central to contemporary Western popular culture. Entrepreneurs have sought to reach this market through books, magazines, tapes, videos, workshops, and inspirational lectures. Self-help, like many areas of medicine, is now big business, but because self-help is at once an adjunct to and a competitor with medicine, related bioethical issues are numerous.

## Bioethical implications

**Autonomy and empowerment.** The English phrase "self-help" is one possible translation of the word "autonomy" (literally "self-rule"). Philosophers, theologians, artists, and others have given much attention to the self, especially in the West. Patients in particular often cherish autonomy as a right. In many Western nations, a compelling interest in personal freedom and choice motivates people toward self-care, especially when a person's health is threatened. The movie *Lorenzo's Oil* (1992) celebrates parents who find—on their own—a cure for the rare disease afflicting their son. Other stories of folk cures for cancer or AIDS do not, however, have such happy endings, since autonomy is an ideal created by humans, not an absolute principle; forces of biology, economics, and death limit us all.

If the self is not (and cannot be) an absolute, neither is the concept of rule. However much people may wish for the power to direct the health of their bodies, they simply do not have absolute power over them. The urge for knowledge and control has been critiqued in classic narratives from *Oedipus Rex* to *Frankenstein,* but still human beings persist in wishing to control their natural environment, outer space, and their bodies. A 1960 book—*Psycho-Cybernetics,* by Maxwell Maltz—promoted "the self-image," "the habit of happiness," and "that winning feeling," all by mind control; the book still sells well in the 1990s. Modern advertising often suggests our regrettable lack of control over a cough, diet, or tooth color in order to present the "perfect" product for gaining such control.

Another problem arises when the concept of autonomy becomes a form of narcissism, an anti-social urge of greed and self-absorption. Imagine, for example, the case of a young man who spends most of his free time attempting to perfect his physical body, at the cost of friendships, family, and his own economic welfare. At what point does a model of health become a model of disease, and motivate an individual toward self-harm?

And yet, when self-help is kept within reasonable limits, it is surely better to have persons take responsibility for self-care than to take no responsibility or even to cause self-injury. Self-help, when thoughtfully used and placed in the contexts of social knowledge and cooperation, can be a worthy adjunct to standard care. Medical personnel have long promoted patient responsibility, whether in the older, more paternalistic term "compliance," or in the more recent terms of "cooperation" and "collaboration"; but with increasing evidence of the power of the mind to heal or maintain the body, the patient's active role takes on greater significance. Anecdotes abound of patients who choose to live until some date (the New Year, a birthday, the arrival of a relative), then promptly die. Athletes have used imaging techniques with much success: "Mind over matter," they say, and their personal and collective records keep improving. The work of David Spiegel and others suggests that psychosocial interventions can have a strong, positive impact on the treatment of cancer patients (Spiegel, 1985–1986, 1991, 1992). From these and other observations, it seems clear that personal attitudes can have a powerful impact on physiology, although Western science has far to go in completely understanding this relationship.

Wise health-care personnel—physicians, nurses, therapists, and others—have long recognized the value of patient participation in medical care, whether in the form of prevention, long-term care, or psychological health. It is now arguable that standard care should include referral to appropriate self-help resources, much as providers routinely refer patients to a pharmacy for a prescription. Increased self-care also means less reliance on health-care personnel, money, office time, and other resources.

**Benefits.**    At its best, self-help offers several advantages: (1) attitudes of empowerment, affective stability, increased confidence and self-esteem; (2) increased motivation for changing or maintaining long-term behaviors in regard to exercise, smoking, physical therapy, and the like; (3) information about health, through books, magazines, and tapes; and (4) social structures, such as groups that promote validation from others, social support, and progress checks (Borkman, 1990).

Millions of people benefit from published information and various forms of self-help groups: The *Harvard Mental Health Letter* estimates that six million people participate in groups each year, 12–15 million at some point in their lifetimes ("Self-Help Groups," 1993). The help may be measurable ("sober for one year") or not. There may be discernible progress, or simply a maintenance of the status quo—sometimes a victory in itself. Some benefits may be attributable to the placebo effect (Connelly, 1991). For families dealing with a terminal illness, such as Alzheimer's disease, a support group may guide members to realize that the help or progress lies in accepting dying and death. (For theories of group efficacy, see Stewart, 1990.)

Surveying lists of groups, whether national or local, reveals an enormous range of illnesses, psychological states, and behaviors that groups focus on. Barbara J. White and Edward J. Madara (1992) list 277 topics, organized as follows: addictions/dependencies (9); bereavement (5); disabilities (11); health (189); mental health (6); parenting/family (11); physical/emotional

abuse (3); and forty-three other or miscellaneous groups. Groups deal with subjects as diverse as gambling, fetal loss, autism, AIDS, breast implants, infertility, Tourette syndrome, depression, adoption, rape, and near-death experience. That there are scores of groups, meeting year after year, suggests that some participants are getting some amount of help. But degrees of success are hard to determine, given the relative independence of group members and the total independence of consumers of books, videos, and tapes. Further, enthusiastic self-helpers may claim success that might have occurred anyway or by other means. Nor is the generic placebo effect that elicits healing responses from the patient completely understood. Even given such difficulties, however, there appear to be large numbers of group participants and media consumers who are happy with their experience and who, in their repeated involvement, perceive significant benefits.

**Harms.**    The very phrase "self-help" rhetorically influences our perception: certainly anything labeled "self-help" must be, ipso facto, helpful. Unfortunately, this is not always the case. Self-help can do harm indirectly, by replacing or delaying standard care. A person treating a tumor, a wound, or abdominal pain at home with prayer and aspirin may not be causing immediate harm but may delay proper diagnosis and access to medical treatment, allowing the condition to worsen, perhaps even to threaten life. This dilemma can be frustrating and saddening to medical personnel, who may shake their heads and think, "If only this patient had come in sooner. . . ."

Another tragic version of self-help is inappropriate care given by parents to children, who typically accept parental authority. Sometimes subcultural or religious values, more or less tolerated within a free society, influence home care. Emergency room workers may find an herbal poultice applied to the chest of a child with a readily treatable pneumonia. In some cases they may seek a court order to provide for standard treatment or, in cases of outright abuse, turn to a child-protection team.

Highly personal versions of self-help may lead to harm. In one case, relatives brought a patient to the hospital; he was emaciated, with gums bleeding, owing to an exclusive diet of rice over several weeks. This extreme version of self-help reduced not only his weight but also his general health through malnutrition. Without treatment and counseling, this person might have died. Even standard medical care has side effects and risks, and sometimes results in iatrogenic illness; but self-help—without controls, observation, and standards of care—can be particularly dangerous, especially when notions become idiosyncratic and obsessive. A misguided belief may overlap with pathology. The area of diet has many dramatic examples. One young woman institutionalized for anorexia lost weight even on a high-calorie diet until she was discovered running in place much of the night, on a folded blanket.

A particularly controversial area of self-help includes diseases, such as AIDS, for which there is no highly effective standard care. *Borrowed Time: An AIDS Memoir,* by Paul Monette, shows AIDS patients trying every standard medical therapy and reading voraciously about current research, but also visiting Mexico for unapproved drugs:

> The pharmacy was in a dusty town across from a bull-ring. . . . We bought all the ribavirin and isoprinosine they had, chatting amiably with a couple from San Francisco who were buying cancer drugs. I realized then we weren't the only ones being driven underground by the FDA [Food and Drug Administration]. We were part of the nether world of the sick, trying to get some control, taking risks the government wouldn't sanction, and all in the same boat. (Monette, 1988, p. 175)

Monette makes clear the various moods (desperation, abandonment, a fellowship of the dispossessed) that can lead to high-risk versions of self-help.

Indeed, some self-help groups have been criticized for their tendencies toward self-isolation or even a quasi-religious cult status. This point is controversial, of course, since the ultimate benefit–harm ratio to group members may be hard to judge. Once again, medical personnel should counsel patients about the realistic potentials and limits of both standard medical care and forms of self-help as an adjunct or alternative.

A subtle dilemma faces patients who have followed doctor-approved, appropriate self-help regimens but have become sicker. The harms here can be guilt ("I did something wrong") or depression ("I'm no good; everything I do fails"). Here again, a professional's counsel can put self-help into reasonable perspective, especially when the disease appears to be intractable. Sometimes a medical caregiver, aiming to be positive or compassionate, denies patients a frank discussion about morbidity and death; the upbeat discussions that ensue may seem unrealistic to patients, who may turn to self-help as more practical. But self-help can be misleading as well, suggesting healing where none is possible. At its worst, self-help can become faddism, quackery, or commercial exploitation of a market that is hurting, needy, or desperate.

Booksellers know that most self-help literature is purchased by women. There may be two underlying reasons for such market concentration: (1) the nature of women's bodies often makes them more aware of their health and more responsible for it; men, less aware and more stoic, may not buy such books; (2) women are no sicker than men, but they are more often told of their inadequacies and therefore doubt themselves, becoming more vulnerable to the marketing of products claiming solutions or cures. Social psychologist Carol Tavris (1993) argues that incest-survivor books, for example, encourage feelings of victimization. Another reason women purchase self-help literature may be that they yearn for an intimacy that busy husbands and friends—even society at large—cannot or will not offer.

## Critique of standard medicine

Whether consciously or not, self-help often provides a theoretical critique of standard medical care. Many forms of self-help suggest or even emphasize a holistic approach that integrates mind, body, and sometimes spirit (Dossey, 1982). Standard medicine often seems—and sometimes is—highly technical, specialized, rationalistic, mechanistic, and fraught with the Cartesian dualism that divides mind from body. At its root, self-help means that healing happens within a body and largely because of that body, not because of the physician, drugs, or other externalities. Mike Samuels, a physician, and Hal Bennett write, "Your body is a three-million-year-old healer" (1973, p. 1), and counsel understanding the body's powers to heal itself, although not to the exclusion of "your doctor as a resource" (1973, p. 299).

Sometimes self-help's critique is political, as in the women's movement; sometimes it is economic, as in care for the poor and uninsured; sometimes it is legal and cultural, as in the efforts of the Hemlock Society to provide information about death and dying and to reshape public attitudes about death.

The conversation between medicine and self-help runs the risk of caricature and parody. Self-help, in its myriad forms, may be presented as frivolous, misguided, and dangerous; standard medicine, as monolithic, heartless, and ineffectual. Neither portrayal is adequate.

## Justice

As suggested above, poor persons may practice self-help by necessity and on a limited basis, while others may seek benefits through more costly and elaborate means, such as videotapes and workshops. As forms of self-help multiply (through faxes, computer links, and expanding home-treatment technology), the gap between self-help for the rich and the poor will probably widen.

## Forms of self-help

While the term "self-help" is most frequently used to describe groups and published materials it can refer more generally to a range of human behavior and attitudes, and even to the self-healing capacity of the human body (Samuels and Bennett, 1973); this capacity, including mind–body interactions, may underlie all forms of self-help and is an area for imaginative research: Some yogis are documented to have stopped and restarted their own hearts. The following review of varieties of self-help is organized from the most individual (and often the most idiosyncratic) to the most social and, typically, the most controlled.

At its widest level of definition, self-help could describe personal rituals, routine but symbolic acts that order people's lives: how people bathe, dress, eat, travel, work, socialize, worship, experience the arts, and relax. These rituals are an unavoidable part of being human; when war or other catastrophe makes them impossible, modern concepts of human identity are threatened and people are reduced to conditions of mere animal survival. Such activities of daily living (ADL, to occupational therapists) are often, like gravity, invisible. When individuals are sick or injured, however, they become monumentally obvious: Walking to a bathroom can be a victory to a postoperative patient. At one basic level, all people are self-helpers.

A second grouping includes individual action, but with the guidance of published materials and/or mentors. Here the individual is free to interpret (or misinterpret) information, and the information itself may or may not be valid or appropriate to the person. "I was using Bill Rogers' workouts until I got injured," a runner said, having severely strained his Achilles tendons. And yet, in the marketplace consumers select and use the books they like, books they believe are helpful. Some persons say they "live by" particular popular psychology books. It is likely that they would keep on living without them, of course, but somehow the insights afforded by the terminology, the images, and the narratives seem so clarifying and compelling that readers give much credit to such guides.

There are well over a thousand self-help books on sale in the United States alone. Some, like George Bach and Peter Wyden's *The Intimate Enemy* (1969), deal with marriage. Some, like Robert Bly's *Iron John* (1990), deal with men's roles, while others, like Clarissa Pinkola Estes' *Women Who Run with the Wolves* (1992), deal with women's issues. Thomas A. Harris popularized transactional psychology in *I'm OK—You're OK* (1969). John Bradshaw (1990) writes about family influence and the inner child. M. Scott Peck (1988) is much read for the spiritual implications of self-growth. Edward Charlesworth and Ronald Nathan (1985) tell us how to avoid stress. Many more books could be named in this widely variable and commercially successful subgenre.

Critic Wendy Kaminer makes fun of all such books, TV shows, workshops, support groups, and pop theology in her book, *I'm Dysfunctional, You're Dysfunctional: The Recovery Movement and Other Self-Help Fashions* (1992). She argues that such promotion of individualism actually encourages mass conformity and denies real personal thinking, while accruing wealth for the purveyors. Gerald M. Rosen (1987) says that many books make exaggerated claims, cannot monitor compliance, have no follow-up, and lack professional guidance.

Among magazines, *Self* is typical. This magazine targets young women and presents short articles on diet, health, psychology, personal success, careers, beauty tips, longevity, and the like. Articles are by journalists, frequently citing M.D.s and Ph.D.s. The advertising (for cosmetics, exercise, retail outlets) appeals to health, sexuality, and glamour. A more specialized publication, the *University of California at Berkeley Wellness Letter*, is written by physicians and researchers who use current findings. A typical issue may touch on diet, smoking, athletics, episiotomies, Vitamin E, and other topics.

Among self-help groups, a variety of styles characterizes the relationship of leaders and their followers. Some groups have no leaders whatsoever, relying on the cooperation of peers. Leaders may draw support through personal charisma and level (or lack) of training; at worst, they may even be deranged personalities exploiting unmet emotional needs of their followers. Some leaders are professionals who do not themselves have the illness or concern their followers do—and this is a point of controversy. Is there special knowledge or added credibility in the afflicted or wounded healer? In *The Self-Help Sourcebook* (1992, p. 37), Barbara White and Edward Madara quote Thomas Jefferson: "Who then can so softly bind up the wound of another as he who has felt the same wound himself?"

While groups that meet weekly and monthly are widespread, there is great variety in the format of self-help. It ranges from talk shows providing a mass-market confessional to one-time workshops, or from informal and formal counseling sessions to conversations with co-workers, family members, and neighbors.

Groups for self-help vary from an informal neighborhood group (sometimes called a "model group") to a worldwide organization such as Alcoholics Anonymous. Some start with two persons—through a newspaper ad, a phone call, or a computer link—and spread and grow to national or global status, sometimes with a large bureaucracy of fundraisers, marketers, trainers, and leaders. Some critics feel that groups do best when they are close to the grass-roots and that the members should plan or lead the groups themselves (although some commentators urge cooperation between lay leaders and professionals). In the words of the *Merck Manual*, "Psychiatrists can help group leaders to avoid the risks of unrealistic goals or excessive hope and also to learn more about the essential psychological mechanisms of inspiration and hope inherent in the movement" (Berkow et al., 1992, pp. 1533–1534).

With the advent of computer technology, a new form of self-help has emerged. Individuals can meet and communicate by linking their computers with national on-line databases (see "Mutual Help Via Your Personal Computer" in White and Madara, 1992).

## Self-help as narrative

Self-help exists for several reasons. One pervasive reason is that self-help generally implies an exemplary story at its base that offers followers a model they can live out. "Exercise and help your heart"; "Stop drinking and gain control of your life"; "Wear this crystal; it will attune you." The first two mottoes (or potential stories) would find support in contemporary medicine; the third, in most medical practice, would not. However, self-helpers may find all three not only credible but compelling. These mottoes suggest a potential narrative for patients to follow, a paradigm of order and a comforting promise to patients for whom other stories have broken down (Brody, 1987).

For those who are sick, stories of personal well-being have often come to ruin; many yearn for a story that offers healing and return to power. Often the medical stories of therapeutic technology, differential diagnoses, pharmaceutical side effects, and the like may be unintelligible, unattractive, or simply unavailable. For persons living in a fragmented world, with neither religious nor intellectual models as guides, stories of self-help may seem like oases of meaning; whether they are sources of life or merely mirages is another question.

While many have written about effective doctor–patient communication, self-help may further emphasize the continuous rhetorical challenge to reach patients with clarifying and enabling stories, stories that speak to individual patients' own values and backgrounds. A physician can explain a lesion to an eight-year-old, but can he or she also tell this patient one or more stories of possible healing, even when the healing may be death?

Self-help is a given: We all practice it. Whether we are middle-class persons, millionaires, or one of the homeless, we all take care of our daily food, sleep, and personal hygiene, drawing on the folkways of our cultures or subcultures. It makes moral and practical sense for the medical establishment to enroll self-help as an ally and adjunct by encouraging patient responsibility, by criticizing errant self-help, by promoting education, by training and guiding leaders, and by developing the narrative clarity that is one of the resources of self-help.

A richer dialectic between standard medicine and self-help may bring together the strengths from each camp. Self-help could benefit from standard medicine through scientific scrutiny, professional supervision, institutional sponsorship, and wider research and commentary. Standard medicine could benefit from fuller patient involvement, more adequate models of personhood, and better definitions of health, handicap, and death. Society at large could benefit through a higher level of health and economic savings afforded by the resources of self-help, including patient-directed care and improved preventive medicine.

ALBERT HOWARD CARTER III

*For a further discussion of topics mentioned in this entry, see the entries* ALTERNATIVE THERAPIES; HARM; HEALING; HUMAN NATURE; JUSTICE; LIFESTYLES AND PUBLIC HEALTH; *and* NARRATIVE. *For a discussion of related ideas, see the entries* AUTONOMY; RESPONSIBILITY; RIGHTS, *article on* RIGHTS IN BIOETHICS; *and* VALUE AND VALUATION. *Other relevant material may be found under the entries* BEHAVIOR MODIFICATION THERAPIES; HEALTH PROMOTION AND HEALTH EDUCATION; *and* MENTAL-HEALTH THERAPIES.

## Bibliography

*Alcoholics Anonymous: The Story of the Many Thousands of Men and Women Who Have Recovered from Alcoholism.* 1976. 3d ed. New York: Alcoholics Anonymous World Services.

AMMER, CHRISTINE. 1989. *The New A-to-Z of Women's Health: A Concise Encyclopedia.* Rev. ed. New York: Facts on File.

BACH, GEORGE R., and WYDEN, PETER. 1969. *The Intimate Enemy.* New York: Avon.

BACON, FRANCIS. 1979. [1598]. "Of Regimen of Health." In *Bacon's Essays.* New York: W. W. Norton.

BERKOW, ROBERT; FLETCHER, ANDREW J.; and CHIR, B., eds. 1992. *The Merck Manual of Diagnosis and Therapy.* 16th ed. Rahway, N. J.: Merck Research Laboratories.

BLY, ROBERT. 1990. *Iron John: A Book About Men.* New York: Vintage.

BORKMAN, THOMASINA. 1990. "Self-Help Groups at the Turning Point: Emerging Egalitarian Alliances with the Formal Health Care System?" *American Journal of Community Psychology* 18, no. 2:321–332.

BOSTON WOMEN'S HEALTH COLLECTIVE. 1971. *Our Bodies, Ourselves: A Book by and for Women.* Boston: Author.

———. 1984. *The New Our Bodies, Ourselves.* 2d ed., rev. New York: Simon and Schuster.

BRADSHAW, JOHN. 1990. *Homecoming: Reclaiming and Championing Your Inner Child.* New York: Bantam.

BRODY, HOWARD. 1987. *Stories of Sickness.* New Haven, Conn.: Yale University Press.

CARNEGIE, DALE. 1981. [1936]. *How to Win Friends and Influence People.* Rev. ed. New York: Pocket Books.

CHARLESWORTH, EDWARD A., and NATHAN, RONALD G. 1985. *Stress Management: A Comprehensive Guide to Wellness.* Rev. ed. New York: Ballantine.

CONNELLY, ROBERT J. 1991. "Nursing Responsibility for the Placebo Effect." *Journal of Medicine and Philosophy* 16, no. 3:325–341.

COUSINS, NORMAN. 1979. *Anatomy of an Illness as Perceived by the Patient: Reflections on Healing and Regeneration.* New York: W. W. Norton.

COVEY, STEPHEN R. 1989. *The Seven Habits of Highly Effective People*. New York: Simon and Schuster.

DOSSEY, LARRY. 1982. *Space, Time, and Medicine*. Boulder, Colo.: Shambhala.

ESTES, CLARISSA PINKOLA. 1992. *Women Who Run With the Wolves: Myths and Stories of the Wild Woman Archetype*. New York: Ballantine.

FRANKLIN, BENJAMIN. 1961. *Autobiography*. Reprinted in *The Autobiography and Other Writings*. New York: Signet.

FRIEDMAN, MEYER, and ROSENMAN, RAY H. 1974. *Type A Behavior and Your Heart*. New York: Fawcett Crest.

HARRIS, THOMAS A. 1969. *I'm OK—You're OK*. New York: Avon.

KAMINER, WENDY. 1992. *I'm Dysfunctional, You're Dysfunctional: The Recovery Movement and Other Self-Help Fashions*. Reading, Mass.: Addison-Wesley.

MALTZ, MAXWELL. 1960. *Psycho-Cybernetics*. New York: Pocket Books.

MONETTE, PAUL. 1988. *Borrowed Time: An AIDS Memoir*. New York: Avon.

PECK, M. SCOTT. 1988. *The Road Less Traveled*. New York: Simon and Schuster.

ROSEN, GERALD M. 1987. "Self-Help Treatment Books and the Commercialization of Psychotherapy." *American Psychologist* 42, no. 1:46–51.

SAMUELS, MIKE, and BENNETT, HAL Z. 1973. *The Well Body Book*. New York: Random House.

"Self-Help Groups." 1993. *Harvard Mental Health Letter* 9, no. 9:1–3 (pt. 1), no. 10:1–4 (pt. 2).

SMILES, SAMUEL. 1958. [1859]. *Self-Help: With Illustrations of Conduct & Perseverance*. London: John Murray.

SPIEGEL, DAVID. 1985–86. "Psychosocial Interventions with Cancer Patients." *Journal of Psychosocial Oncology* 3, no. 4:83–95.

———. 1990. "Facilitating Emotional Coping During Treatment." *Cancer* 15, no. 66 (suppl. 6):1422–1426.

———. 1991. "Psychosocial Aspects of Cancer." *Current Opinion in Psychiatry* 4:889–897.

———. 1992. "Effects of Psychosocial Support on Patients with Metastatic Breast Cancer." *Journal of Psychosocial Oncology* 10, no. 2:113–120.

STEWART, MIRIAM J. 1990. "Expanding Theoretical Conceptualizations of Self-Help Groups." *Social Science and Medicine* 31, no. 9:1057–1066.

*Surgeon General's Workshop on Self-Help and Public Health*. 1988. Washington, D.C.: U.S. Government Printing Office.

TAVRIS, CAROL. 1993. "Beware the Incest-Survivor Machine." *New York Times Book Review*, January 3, pp. 1, 16–17.

WHITE, BARBARA J., and MADARA, EDWARD J., eds. 1992. *The Self-Help Sourcebook: Finding and Forming Mutual Aid Self-Help Groups*. 4th ed. Denville, N.J.: American Self-Help Clearinghouse, Saint Clares-Riverside Medical Center.

# SEVENTH-DAY ADVENTISTS

*See* ALTERNATIVE THERAPIES; *and* PROTESTANTISM.

# SEX-CHANGE SURGERY

*See* GENDER IDENTITY AND GENDER-IDENTITY DISORDERS; *and* SEXUAL IDENTITY.

---

# SEXISM

Sexism is both the belief that one sex is superior to the other and the many consequences of this belief. The term "sexism" almost always refers to men's claimed or perceived superiority over women; the occasionally expressed belief that women are superior to men is referred to as female chauvinism and does not affect men's economic or social status in the way that male sexism affects women's status. Feminists coined the term "sexism" in the mid-1960s as a way to characterize the condition they sought to remedy (hooks, 1984). Given its origin as a political term, sexism has been more a rhetorical device than an analytic tool, and the term often conflates discrimination against women and the oppression of women. By distinguishing between discrimination and oppression, we can fully appreciate the scope, nature, origins, and effects of sexism, and its importance as a category in ethical thought and in bioethics.

Discrimination and oppression are analytically distinct (Young, 1990). To discriminate means to distinguish. Hence, not all discrimination is a concern for ethicists, but only those discriminations that raise ethical issues, such as those based on prejudices and considered unjust or unfair or disrespectful. To oppress means to thwart, to use force or other means to control and to hold down. Oppression is necessarily wrong from the standpoint of fairness, justice, and equality. Not all forms of discrimination, then, are oppressive, and not all forms of oppression are discriminatory: Oppression can be indiscriminate, directed at everyone. By distinguishing between discrimination and oppression, we can clarify four different senses of sexism. Depending on which definition is used, the nature, origins, effects, and remedies for sexism are different.

## Sexism as natural

Opponents of feminism view sexism as an ideological construction put forth by misguided feminists. According to this approach, discrimination by sex is a result of the natural differences between men and women, especially in reproduction and physical strength. Hence, while discrimination exists between women and men, the sex-based distinctions that exist in societies are not discriminatory in any pejorative sense but necessary for the proper functioning of human society. Hence, "sexism" is ideological, in the sense of being a false belief, because it is an attempt by women to change the natural order. Those who view sex differences as natural can agree with feminists that women and men have different roles, and that women have largely been excluded from some spheres of life, but believe that these differences do not constitute oppression. To try to remedy such discriminations, such thinkers argue, will cause more harm than good (Goldberg, 1973; Schlafly, 1977).

## Classic sexism

This most common account of sexism posits that discrimination between men and women leads to women's oppression. Classic sexism presumes that when the biological distinction of sex, between male and female, becomes the cultural distinction of gender, which marks men and women, then biological differences are changed into a cultural category that oppresses women. Feminists thus point to the existence of prejudices or practices that constrict women's opportunities and restrict their lives, and conclude that discriminations affecting women are wrong.

Most feminists believe that sexism is ubiquitous. Feminist historians argue that all known cultures engage in gender distinctions, and in virtually all historical societies, men have dominated in spiritual, public, economic, and cultural life. Archaeologists and anthropologists argue that some prehistoric and nonindustrial societies were and are more egalitarian than most societies recorded in Western history (Sanday, 1981; Anderson and Zinsser, 1988).

In Western societies, feminist scholars can point to many instances of sexism directed against women, from the story of the creation of humans in the Old Testament (where God created Adam first) to current social conditions of women. Aristotle doubted women's rationality; Roman law made the father the head of the household. Contemporary institutions continue to reflect the exclusion of women from some spheres of life: Women hold relatively few public offices, are excluded from the ranks of the clergy in many religions, remain largely excluded from the military, are less educated and hold fewer academic appointments than men, are rarely included among the highest ranks of corporation officers, and are generally more marginal members of the working force. Few women are economically independent, and women remain largely responsible for family life and domestic work, even in societies that boast of greater equality in these realms (United Nations, 1991). Violence against women is at epidemic levels (Radford and Russell, 1992). Culturally, women have been excluded throughout most of Western history from central roles in the cultural production, and are often treated as inferiors in cultural work.

Feminists have argued against sexism throughout the world in the nineteenth and twentieth centuries (Jayawardena, 1986). Many cultures have practiced ways of controlling women and their sexuality. The dislocations caused by changing patterns of employment and consumption in an increasingly globalized economy seem to have particularly harmful effects on women (Joekes, 1987). Amartya K. Sen, a development economist, has argued that at present the numbers of women and men in the world are unbalanced: As he describes it, this fact means that millions of women are "missing" from the world's population. To Sen, this demographic imbalance points to systematic devaluation of women's lives: Women receive less food, education, and medical attention (Sen, 1990).

Within this account of classic sexism, different views exist of the origin and nature of the oppression embodied in sexism. Some liberal feminists see this oppression as a sum total of individual discriminatory acts. They view sexism as a result of continued prejudice; because the distinctions between men and women played a larger role in earlier human societies, they persist. The continuation of sexism is the result of the inability of societies to discard some of their outmoded traditional habits. Hence, the fact that sexism has deep historical roots does not mean that it cannot be eliminated through careful reconstruction of social institutions (Okin, 1989).

Another strand of liberal feminism posits that sexism originates primarily from Western practices of child-rearing. Children's psychological development, including their senses of gender and of identity, depend on how they interact with caregivers in the first years of life. Because women do most of the caregiving to infants, boys and girls have different patterns of psychological relationship to these primary caregivers; boys learn to separate from others while girls learn to remain connected. These gender differences in "object relations" continue to inform the differing psychology of men and women. By this theory, eliminating the gendered division of parenting that predominates in Western society would eliminate sexism (see Chodorow, 1978).

Other feminists view the discrimination against women and the resulting oppression of women as deeply embedded in social institutions, so that merely changing individuals' prejudiced attitudes and practices will not alleviate sexism. Some of these feminists are influenced by Marxist ideas and view sexism as a concomitant of private property. As long as it is necessary to ensure the proper inheritance of private property, men must regulate women's sexual activities (Engels, 1972). Friedrich Engels argued that since the systematic exploitation of women began with property, women's oppression would end with the Communist revolution. A number of socialists have challenged the simplicity of this argument, and the treatment of women under so-called socialist regimes has not been encouraging (Hansen and Philipson, 1990).

Thus, a point of contention about the nature of classic sexism is whether it is a matter of prejudice and discriminatory attitudes, beliefs, and practices that are expressed by individuals or groups; or whether sexism is a systemic form of discrimination that permeates social, political, and economic institutions. A parallel exists with the study of racism, where racism often appears to be only a matter of individual attitudes rather than a quality inherent in social institutions. Those who believe racism is a more intractable problem often refer to this phenomenon as "institutional racism"; there is a parallel understanding of institutional sexism (see, e.g., Hall and Sandler 1982; Rothenberg, 1992).

This split within the understanding of classic sexism matters greatly for the study of ethics on two levels. First, the tasks involved in solving an attitudinal and a behavioral problem are different from those involved in changing institutions fundamentally. Second, responsibility for sexism is quite different depending upon whether it is simply a matter of prejudice or a more deeply rooted social phenomenon. If sexism is simply a matter of prejudice, then those who believe that they no longer harbor prejudiced attitudes are no longer sexist. On the other hand, if sexism is a part of the social structure, then simply changing one's attitudes does not equal a solution to the problem. In recent years in the United States, some attitudes expressed toward women have become more favorable, but no equal transformation in women's economic, political, and social standing has occurred (see Faludi, 1991). This fact suggests that seeing sexism as institutionalized is more plausible.

## Androcentrism

Androcentrism argues that sexism does not begin from a conscious act of discriminating between men and women; it begins from the assumption that men's experiences are universal, and that women's experiences are essentially similar to men's. Androcentrism is the view that men's lives and experiences, their bodies, behaviors, activities, and beliefs, should serve as the normal starting point when thinking about humans (MacKinnon, 1987). Those who argue that androcentrism describes sexism contend that in defining the male experience as normal, women's experiences, lives, bodies, and so forth are necessarily viewed as lacking, as a departure from the normal. Androcentrism grows from the recognition that while discriminations may not even be stated as such, they may still have oppressive consequences (MacKinnon, 1987).

An example of androcentrism is the medical practice of considering male bodies as normal, and excluding women from clinical trials because female hormones make medical observations more complicated. As a result, women may receive less medical attention, and less may be known about how diseases such as heart disease affect women. Another example of androcentrism is the sexism implicit in language, where linguistic practices shape conceptions—for example, that an unmarked reference to "doctor" is not the same as the marked category "woman doctor" (Miller and Swift, 1988; Tannen, 1990). Hence, androcentrism does not highlight overt discrimination as connected to oppression but explores how the assumption of the male as normal gives rise to women's oppression.

## Masculinism

Masculinism raises the possibility of oppression arising without any prior discrimination—indeed, of oppression arising out of categories presumed to be universal and nondiscriminatory. Critics of masculinism argue that many categories that seem not to distinguish gender have the effect of discriminating among men and women and leading to women's oppression because they contain hidden assumptions about the superiority of men and an implicit preference for masculinity over femininity. For example, Susan Bordo has argued that Descartes's mind–body distinction, while ostensibly not about men and women at all, results in the denigration of women because it implicitly associates mind with masculinity and body with femininity and posits the superiority of mind over body (Bordo, 1987).

## Conclusion

These different accounts of the nature of sexism obviously have a profound effect on how bioethicists might address the problem of sexism. Adopting the first understanding, sexism is not even a problem. Among the other three definitions, which are not necessarily mutually exclusive, the depth to which investigators must go to try to understand and to remove the effects of sexism vary. If one adopts a classic, liberal view, then removing one's own prejudice is enough. If sexism is also deeply rooted in social institutions, then one must be cognizant of its effects throughout those institutions: For example, economic oppression may affect access to medical services. If sexism is androcentrism, then thinkers and practitioners must constantly be on their guard to make certain that categories, practices, and experiments do not presume the male as normal even though they are not overtly discriminatory. If sexism is understood as masculinism, then all of the categories and practices used by bioethicists must be explored to determine if they contain a hidden gendered dimension.

The existence of sexism raises problems of social justice and challenges notions of basic equality (see, e.g., Okin, 1989). It also raises questions about related forms of discrimination and oppression, and about whether the elimination of sexism requires the recognition of multiple oppressions. To admit, for example, that discrimination on the basis of gender roles is wrong raises the question of whether it is proper to discriminate against gay men and lesbians on the basis of their sexual orientation, a form of discrimination called heterosexism. To admit that sexism is wrong because discrimination leads to oppression raises questions among feminists about how to cope with racism among women. Those feminists who see sexism as a form of androcentrism or masculinism will argue that eliminating sexism will result in much more broad-reaching social changes. For example, some feminists argue that because women are less warlike than men, eliminating sexism requires a commitment to pacifism (Ruddick, 1989). Others suggest that sexism is a discrete phenomenon and that to broaden it to include other forms of discrimination or undesirable social practices weakens the focus on gender.

"Sexism" is a term of disapprobation; it raises fundamental ethical questions because if sexism exists, it challenges our ability to treat everyone fairly and equally, and with respect. By pointing to the existence of sexism, feminists have raised the centrality of asking about gender in all areas of ethical inquiry.

JOAN C. TRONTO

*Directly related to this entry are the entries* FEMINISM; *and* WOMEN. *For a further discussion of topics mentioned in this entry, see the entries* ABUSE, INTERPERSONAL, *article on* ABUSE BETWEEN DOMESTIC PARTNERS; FAMILY; JUSTICE; MARRIAGE AND OTHER DOMESTIC PARTNERSHIPS; PATERNALISM; *and* RIGHTS. *This entry will find application in the entries* ABORTION; ADVERTISING; CIRCUMCISION, *article on* FEMALE CIRCUMCISION; FERTILITY CONTROL; HEALTH-CARE DELIVERY; HEALTH-CARE RESOURCES, ALLOCATION OF; HOMOSEXUALITY; MATERNAL–FETAL RELATIONSHIP; MEDICAL EDUCATION; MEDICINE AS A PROFESSION; NURSING AS A PROFESSION; POPULATION ETHICS; POPULATION POLICIES; PROFESSIONAL–PATIENT RELATIONSHIP; PROSTITUTION; REPRODUCTIVE TECHNOLOGIES; RESEARCH METHODOLOGY; RESEARCH POLICY; SEXUAL ETHICS; SEXUAL ETHICS AND PROFESSIONAL STANDARDS; SEXUAL IDENTITY; *and* SEXUALITY IN SOCIETY. *For a discussion of related ideas, see the entry* RACE AND RACISM. *Other relevant material may be found under the entries* CARE; HEALTH POLICY, *article on* POLITICS AND HEALTH CARE; HUMAN NATURE; LOVE; *and* NATURE.

## Bibliography

ANDERSON, BONNIE S., and ZINSSER, JUDITH P. 1988. *A History of Their Own: Women in Europe from Prehistory to the Present.* 2 vols. New York: Harper & Row.

BEAUVOIR, SIMONE DE. 1952. *The Second Sex.* Translated and edited by Howard Madison Parshley. New York: Alfred A. Knopf.

BORDO, SUSAN. 1987. *The Flight to Objectivity: Essays on Cartesianism and Culture.* Albany: State University of New York Press.

CARD, CLAUDIA, ed. 1991. *Feminist Ethics.* Lawrence: University Press of Kansas.

CHODOROW, NANCY. 1978. *The Reproduction of Mothering: Psychoanalysis and the Sociology of Gender.* Berkeley: University of California Press.

ENGELS, FRIEDRICH. 1972. [1884]. *The Origin of the Family, Private Property, and the State.* Edited by Eleanor Burke Leacock. New York: International Publishers.

FALUDI, SUSAN. 1991. *Backlash: The Undeclared War Against American Women.* New York: Crown.

GILLIGAN, CAROL. 1982. *In a Different Voice: Psychological Theory and Women's Development.* Cambridge, Mass.: Harvard University Press.

GOLDBERG, STEVEN. 1973. *The Inevitability of Patriarchy.* New York: William Morrow.

HALL, ROBERTA M., and SANDLER, BERNICE R. 1982. *The Classroom Climate: A Chilly One for Women?* Washington, D.C.: Project on the Status and Education of Women, Association of American Colleges.

HANSEN, KAREN V., and PHILIPSON, ILENE J., eds. 1990. *Women, Class and the Feminist Imagination: A Socialist–Feminist Reader.* Philadelphia: Temple University Press.

HOOKS, BELL. 1984. *Feminist Theory from Margin to Center.* Boston: South End Press.

JAGGAR, ALISON M. 1983. *Feminist Politics and Human Nature.* Totowa, N.J.: Rowman & Littlefield.

JAYAWARDENA, KUMARI. 1986. *Feminism and Nationalism in the Third World.* London: Zed Books.

JOEKES, SUSAN P. 1987. *Women in the World Economy: An INSTRAW Study.* New York: Oxford University Press.

MACKINNON, CATHARINE A. 1987. *Feminism Unmodified: Discourses on Life and Law.* Cambridge, Mass.: Harvard University Press.

MILLER, CASEY, and SWIFT, KATE. 1988. *The Handbook of Nonsexist Writing.* 2d ed. New York: Harper & Row.

MILLETT, KATE. 1970. *Sexual Politics.* Garden City, N.Y.: Doubleday.

OKIN, SUSAN MOLLER. 1989. *Justice, Gender and the Family.* New York: Basic Books.

RADFORD, JILL, and RUSSELL, DIANA E. H. 1992. *Femicide: The Politics of Woman Killing.* New York: Macmillan.

ROTHENBERG, PAUL S., ed. 1992. *Race, Class, and Gender in the United States: An Integrated Study.* 2d ed. New York: St. Martin's Press.

RUDDICK, SARA. 1989. *Maternal Thinking: Toward a Politics of Peace.* Boston: Beacon Press.

RUETHER, ROSEMARY RADFORD. 1983. *Sexism and God-Talk: Toward a Feminist Theology.* Boston: Beacon Press.

SANDAY, PEGGY REEVES. 1981. *Female Power and Male Dominance: On the Origins of Sexual Inequality.* Cambridge: At the University Press.

SCHLAFLY, PHYLLIS. 1977. *The Power of Positive Woman.* New York: Arlington House.

SEN, AMARTYA K. 1990. "More Than 100 Million Women Are Missing." *New York Review of Books,* December 20, pp. 61–66.

TANNEN, DEBORAH. 1990. *You Just Don't Understand: Women and Men in Conversation.* New York: William Morrow.

UNITED NATIONS. 1991. *The World's Women, 1970–1990: Trends and Statistics.* Social Statistics and Indicators, ser. K. no. 8. New York: Author.

YOUNG, IRIS M. 1990. *Justice and the Politics of Difference.* Princeton: Princeton University Press.

# SEX SELECTION

*See* REPRODUCTIVE TECHNOLOGIES, *article on* SEX SELECTION.

---

# SEX THERAPY AND SEX RESEARCH

I. Scientific and Clinical Perspectives
   *Sharon K. Turnbull*
II. Ethical Issues
   *Sharon K. Turnbull*

## I. SCIENTIFIC AND CLINICAL PERSPECTIVES

Sex has many varied functions—allowing procreation, providing reassurance of desirability and worth, and forging bonds between individuals. Human beings have not been content to view sex as a natural physical experience. Instead, they invest it with additional significance, seeing it as a special gift conveying the message of love and affection, a means to dominate and control, or even an evil requiring punishment. Beliefs and attitudes about what is normal, about what is right and ideal, establish the boundaries of sexual expression within a given culture. Beliefs and behaviors vary widely among different times and places. It is not surprising, then, that the fields of sex therapy and sex research are laden with paradox and with issues of value and ethics. This article describes the current status of sex therapy and research, highlighting those aspects that give rise to these issues.

## Sex research

Scientific and clinical interest in human sexuality is ancient. One of the earliest records of medical thinking, the Hunan Papyrus, demonstrates a clear awareness of the sexual transmission of certain diseases. Writings from China, India, Persia, and other ancient cultures reflect an avid interest in descriptive research, categorizing and classifying both sexual behavior and techniques designed to increase erotic pleasure and to overcome certain conditions which we now refer to as sexual dysfunctions. Several therapeutic techniques that were developed in the United States in the 1980s for the treatment of sexual dysfunctions have been described, with minor differences, in Taoist manuals attributed to Master Tung-hsuan, who is believed to have been a physician living in seventh-century China.

Henry Havelock Ellis is generally considered the "father" of modern sex therapy and research. His multivolume *Studies in the Psychology of Sex* (1896–1928) established an enduring framework for the conceptualization of sexuality. His work challenged the nineteenth-century pseudoscientific theories that linked nonreproductive sexual activity with insanity and disease. Unlike Ellis, whose work focused exclusively on sexuality, Sigmund Freud (1856–1939) included sexuality as a central aspect of a comprehensive theory of personality. Overcoming the barriers of intolerance and prudery that had silenced public and scientific discussion, Ellis and Freud ensured the subject would remain a legitimate focus for scientific inquiry.

Until the 1930s, however, knowledge about sex had been based largely on the systematic observation of what Donn Byrne (1977) referred to as "animal sex, native sex, or crazy sex," that is, studies of the behavior of other species, other (nonindustrialized, non-Western, "primitive") cultures, or people seeking psychotherapy for emotional disturbances. In 1938, Alfred Kinsey and his colleagues (Pomeroy, 1972) began a series of studies that lasted two decades, using questionnaires and conducting interviews with thousands of Americans about their sexual experience and behaviors, providing a rich description of the behavior of "normal" Americans. Kinsey's work provided the foundation for the first studies of human sexual response based on direct observation and physiological measurements. Beginning in the 1950s, studies by William Masters and Virginia Johnson (1966, 1970, 1976, 1977) dispelled many prevalent myths about normal sexual response and provided valuable information about the mechanisms and treatment of various sexual problems.

The public outcry against the landmark research of Masters and Johnson (1966) on the anatomy and physiology of human sexual function spoke volumes about society's acute discomfort that sex, heretofore shrouded in privacy, should enter the public domain of scientific inquiry. Although the study's contribution to the creation of a social climate more conducive to the scientific study of sexual behavior was profound, it was Masters and Johnson's publication of *Human Sexual Inadequacy* (1970) that led to the emergence of sex therapy as a distinct professional entity.

Just as earlier sex researchers had faced loss of membership in their professional organizations and even excommunication from their churches, twentieth-century scientists have faced social, personal, and political resistance. Vern Bullough (cited in Allgeier and Allgeier, 1988) suggested that, given "this kind of mindset," contemporary researchers are implicitly encouraged to limit their attention to those aspects of sexuality that are relevant to the solution of social problems such as divorce, teen pregnancy, venereal disease, prostitution, homosexuality, and "other forms of stigmatized activity" (p. 39). Although the concerns raised by the AIDS epidemic heighten the need for understanding, many governments and foundations remain reticent about supporting basic research on sexual behavior ("Ethics and Research," 1990).

Notwithstanding these handicaps and its infant status, contemporary sex research is a broad and active field that ranges from theological analyses of the sexuality of Jesus to the bioengineering of devices to measure the intensity of uterine contractions during orgasm. Generally, the domain of research topics can be classified as studies of sexual attitudes, knowledge, and beliefs; sexual orientation and gender identity; sexual function (anatomy and physiology); sexual fantasies and feelings, such as attraction and bonding; and sexual behaviors, ranging from courtship behavior to the paraphilias (sexual deviations, characterized by preference for non-human objects in achieving arousal, imposition of humiliation or suffering, or coercion of nonconsenting partners).

Research methods include psychological testing, surveys, interviews, case histories, direct observation, and biochemical and physiological measurement. Maneuvering in an area shrouded by considerable sensitivity and secrecy, the inherent necessity to draw samples from volunteer and/or patient populations often limits the generalizability of research results. Such constraints highlight the need to replicate studies with a variety of samples, situations, and cultures.

## Sex counseling and therapy

Sex counseling is primarily educative. It tends to focus entirely on the presenting sexual concern, and usually requires only a few (one to three) visits. Many sexual problems, however, are complex and require a more extensive approach to diagnosis and management. Sex therapy is distinguished by its effort to place the sexual problem within the broader context of personality and relationship. While education is part of the therapy process, a variety of treatment approaches are used.

The goal of sex therapy is to resolve sexual problems. Most often the term "sex therapy" is used to refer to the treatment of the psychosexual dysfunctions characterized by interference with normal physiological sexual response (desire, excitement, orgasm) or function. For the purpose of this article it will also include the treatment of those disorders that involve sexual expression in manners that do not have social approval, such as exhibitionism and coercive sex. Problems of gender identity and sexual orientation are discussed elsewhere. Many different dissatisfactions and worries bring people to seek the services of sex therapists. Consequently, the practice of sex therapy is characterized by its diversity.

**Sex counseling.**    Some clients need only information—or more frequently, the correction of misinformation. Some need only reassurance, perhaps an expert's permission to abandon unrealistic "standards" for beauty and behavior promulgated by the media, for example. Others come as part of a couple, seeking an intermediary who will help them communicate their desires and expectations when they are without an adequate vocabulary, or burdened by embarrassment or fear of wounding the partner. Many seek encouragement and practical advice in sorting out the day-to-day problems of a stressful life that leaves little time or energy for sex. Some need help in adapting to physical limitations imposed by arthritis or a recent heart attack. Still others want to learn new positions and techniques to enrich sex that has become predictable and stale.

The sex education component may attempt to modify emotional and attitudinal factors that elicit the patient's anxiety about sex. The most common model (Bjorkstein, 1976) is the Sexual Attitude Restructuring Process (SAR), a workshop developed by the National Sex Forum, which involves exposure to sexually explicit media accompanied by group discussions in which reactions are explored.

**Sex therapy: Conceptual foundations.**    The techniques and formats used in sex therapy are largely derived from three intellectual traditions: the psychotherapeutic approach, the behavioral, and the medical. Some sex therapy programs offer an eclectic approach, making use of all three.

Psychotherapeutic approaches are based on the assumption that sexual difficulties arise from psychological factors. Adherents of psychoanalytic theory, especially that based on the work of Freud, trace the origin of dysfunction to unresolved conflicts that arise in childhood. Treatment is directed toward the search for, and resolution of, these conflicts, focusing on the integration of the total personality rather than the immediate sexual symptom. Treatment tends to be lengthy and expensive, and its effectiveness in alleviating sexual symptoms is largely subjective and hence unmeasurable. Other psychotherapeutic approaches, derived from a variety of conceptual frameworks, place greater emphasis on sexual experiences occurring later in life, including communication difficulties, injurious relationships, and the incorporation of faulty attitudes and beliefs into the personality structure.

Behavioral approaches are characterized by the assumption that sexual responses, including behavior, are learned, and can therefore be unlearned and/or replaced by more desirable responses. Anxiety is seen as the predominant mechanism that mediates sexual problems, whether the problem is largely cognitive (e.g., concern over strength of erection) or emotional (e.g., a phobia that blocks arousal). Without extensive probing into the client's past, personality, or relationships, behavioral approaches deal directly with the sexual problem by using conditioning techniques designed to overcome anxiety or to lessen sensitivity to stimuli that provoke anxiety. The most commonly used techniques are based on systematic desensitization, but others, ranging from aversive conditioning to sexual fantasy alteration, supplement the therapists' arsenal of useful behavioral techniques.

Cognitive-behavioral approaches, which combine elements of both behavioral and cognitive psychologies, have also proved useful in treating many disorders. An excellent overview of these approaches is found in an article describing their use in treating victims of sexual abuse for their psychological distress and the sexual problems that have occurred as a result of their victimization (Talmadge and Wallace, 1991).

Medical approaches focus on the contribution of organic factors to the development of sexual dysfunction. Helen Singer Kaplan (1974) describes five major categories that affect sexual functioning: neurological, vascular, and endocrine disorders; debilitating diseases; and drugs (illicit, prescription, and over-the-counter). Systematic inquiry into the physiological mechanisms that govern the sexual system is a recent phenomenon and has focused mostly on male populations. This gender bias can be attributed to several factors, one being the preponderance of male researchers in the field. Others include the female's ability to hide sexual dysfunction by "faking" satisfaction, the reluctance of many women to discuss sexual matters, and a lack of concern by some women about the loss of sexual function as long as their affectional needs are being met. Much remains to be learned, especially about the effects of various medications and illnesses on female sexual functioning.

**Sex therapy: Professional practice.** The specific approaches used in the process of sex therapy vary considerably, depending on the nature of the sexual complaints and, of course, the theoretical bent of the therapist. The classic approach, originally developed by Masters and Johnson for use with heterosexual couples, involves a two-week program of daily therapy with the couple removed from their usual family and work environment. The couple is assigned two therapists (one male, one female), so that each will have a "friend in court," and the couple is treated as a unit. Since this approach is impractical for many patients, other therapists use modifications including the use of one therapist, willingness to treat those with homosexual and bisexual orientations, provision of treatment to individuals as well as couples, use of group therapy (Barbach, 1980), and the inclusion of traditional psychotherapy, especially when behavioral therapies are not working (Kaplan, 1979).

However, certain components are shared by most treatment programs. A first step is an assessment of the sexual problem, which may include a consultation visit to identify the problem and discuss approaches to treatment; a detailed sexual history, which may be accompanied by an assigned autobiography describing sexual attitudes, experiences, and feelings; paper-and-pencil tests of sexual knowledge, attitudes, and beliefs; and a medical history and physical examination, including a guided sexological exam designed to educate patients about their sexual organs.

Specific behavioral exercises appropriate to the diagnosed disorder are then assigned for practice. Sex education is provided, and the therapist(s) and patient(s) meet to share feedback from the assignments, discuss concerns and plans, and facilitate the couple's communication. Joseph LoPiccolo and his colleagues, for example, offer a treatment program for women with inhibited orgasm, which includes masturbation training, role-playing exaggerated orgasmic responses to reduce her anxiety about the sensation of loss of control that may occur with orgasm, and the practice of orgasmic behaviors such as breath-holding during arousal. In addition the woman and her partner undertake skill training, using sensate focus homework exercises that include exploration, touching, and caressing the partner's body while genital touching and intercourse are initially prohibited, thereby learning to give and receive pleasure while freed from the pressure to "perform" (Lo-Piccolo, 1978).

**Advances in sex therapy.** The field of sex therapy has witnessed dramatic shifts in its base of knowledge and theory that have affected profoundly the ways in which care should be provided. Following the pioneering research of Masters and Johnson in the 1960s, behavioral therapies derived from those developed by Joseph Wolpe and his associates formed the central element in sex therapy (Wolpe, 1958; Lazarus and Rosen, 1976; Masters and Johnson, 1976). Prior to this time sexual problems had been viewed largely as the result of emotional conflict, and sex therapy was primarily the domain of the psychotherapist. While anxiety—seen either as a learned response or as the result of intrapsychic or intrapersonal forces—was previously viewed as the predominant factor in virtually all cases of sexual dysfunction, it became clear in the 1970s that illnesses and drugs caused a substantial proportion of sexual disorders. Consequently, an evaluation by a physician with sufficient expertise in sexual medicine is often necessary before therapy is undertaken.

Two conceptual advances resulting from research and extensive clinical experience over the past three decades have revolutionized the field of sex therapy. The first was the recognition of separate, but interlocking, phases of the sexual response cycle (excitement, plateau, orgasm, and resolution, as originally conceptualized by Masters and Johnson, 1966). The second was the understanding that a multiplicity of psychological and physical factors act in very specific ways to "produce a variety of disorders that are responsive to specific and rational treatment strategies" (Kaplan, 1979, p. 4). These advances led to clinical developments that address the immediate and specific determinants, greatly improving treatment outcomes.

To a considerable extent, the effectiveness of any therapeutic approach depends on two factors. The nature of the problem heavily influences outcome; for example, successful treatment of the inability to experience orgasm is much more likely than alleviating low sexual desire (libido). Effectiveness also varies with the precision in the selection of treatment strategies and the extent to which they are based on accurate and complete diagnoses. Brief behavioral approaches, for example, are replaced by or supplemented with psychotherapy when a history of incest or childhood sexual abuse emerges during the course of treatment. Brief sex therapy methods have proved remarkably effective when used with appropriately selected patients. Treatment failures rise considerably in the presence of substantial medical and psychological problems or serious marital conflict.

In addition to being questionable ethically, therapies used to change sexual orientation have not been very effective, and their use has declined in recent years. Instead, most therapists now focus on helping their homosexual patients adapt to the stress of living in a disapproving society (Diamant, 1977).

The escalation of sexual aggression over the past several decades has been accompanied by the development of numerous treatment programs for sex offenders, generally for those who are incarcerated. "Conspicuous by its absence from the vast literature on offender typologies and treatment approaches is any general claim of treatment efficacy" (Dvoskin, 1991, p. 229). The few programs whose outcomes have been carefully evaluated yielded only modest results, discouraging research and program development in an area of acute need.

**Qualifications for professional practice of sex therapy.** One of the crucial issues facing any emerging discipline is that of professionalization. Who should be allowed to practice the specialty? What knowledge, skills, and attitudes should they possess, and who should certify their competency to practice? How does the discipline police itself to prevent exploitation of the public by the unscrupulous and the incompetent? These questions have been widely debated since the emergence of sex therapy as a profession in the 1970s, but they remain unresolved. Without doubt, the area is susceptible to charlatans seeking profit or outright sexual exploitation. Referral by physicians who are aware of the credentials and practices of therapists provides some protection from the unscrupulous. Many professional sex therapy organizations also provide patient referrals to practitioners. Most have developed codes of ethical behavior that prohibit sexual contact between therapists and clients and establish procedures to discipline or terminate membership of those who violate them.

Sex therapy treatment ranges from hypnosis and biofeedback to implants and microsurgical procedures to increase penile blood flow and depends on a variety of practitioners. Especially problematic are health professionals who, protected by the licensing of their primary professions, may undertake to do therapy with insufficient training in the specialized evaluation and treatment of sexual disorders. Attention given to sexuality and sex therapy in the professional training of physicians, nurses, psychologists, and social workers has increased considerably since the 1960s. But complete answers to the question of which disciplines can ethically practice sex therapy, and how much and what sort of specialized training should be required, await the maturing of the profession.

SHARON K. TURNBULL

*Directly related to this article is the companion article in this entry:* ETHICAL ISSUES. *For a further discussion of topics mentioned in this article, see the entries* HOMOSEXUALITY; PROFESSIONAL–PATIENT RELATIONSHIP; PROFESSION AND PROFESSIONAL ETHICS; PSYCHOANALYSIS AND DYNAMIC THERAPIES; SEXUAL DEVELOPMENT; SEXUAL ETHICS; SEXUAL ETHICS AND PROFESSIONAL STANDARDS; SEXUAL IDENTITY; *and* SEXUALITY IN SOCIETY. *For a discussion of related ideas, see the entries* FREEDOM AND COERCION; *and* VALUE AND VALUATION. *Other relevant material may be found under the entries* BEHAVIOR MODIFICATION THERAPIES; MENTAL-HEALTH THERAPIES; RESEARCH, UNETHICAL; RESEARCH METHODOLOGY; *and* RESEARCH POLICY.

## Bibliography

*[The bibliography for this article and its companion article can be found following the companion article.]*

## II. ETHICAL ISSUES

Simply defined, sex is a physical act, a biological drive. Sexuality is a broader term, encompassing sexual orientation, beliefs and attitudes, morality, and personal identity with its attendant concepts of femininity and masculinity.

Sexual expression, and consequently sex therapy and research, are heavily dependent upon the culture within which they occur. Beliefs and attitudes about what is normal, what is desirable, and what is moral vary widely across time and place. For example, the Judaeo-Christian belief, influential for many centuries, that procreation is the primary or even sole legitimate purpose of sex leads to a view in which nonreproductive activities such as masturbation and homosexuality are seen as a threat to health and morality.

The concept of romantic love, with its origins in the harems of early Arabic culture, was not adopted by Western cultures until the sixteenth century, when romantic love and intimacy (as opposed to economic and political interests) became accepted as the basis for an enduring sexual bond such as marriage (Tannahill, 1992). This linkage of sex and such personal, intrinsic factors as romantic love introduces numerous ethical issues and concerns about relationship, alienation, and commitment (Allgeier and Allgeier, 1988).

Sexuality is central to one's personal identity, and its expression is inextricably intertwined with the experiences of a given culture and its history, religion, and politics. The way sexuality is defined by that culture greatly influences the goals and the means of therapy and research. The possibility of a truly unbiased, value-free endeavor is greatly strained. While sex research and therapy share the same ethical precepts as other disciplines, the special factors surrounding the subject of sex make this domain somewhat different.

The further sex therapy and research move from a purely biological model to embrace the richer concerns of sexual psychology, sociology, and politics, the greater the risk of introducing moral conflict and bias. This is the basis of many of the dilemmas facing the widening field.

### The nature of sex

The ethical therapist or researcher must be sensitive to the special vulnerabilites created by the nature of sex itself. Sex concerns are often cloaked in privacy and occasionally even in secrecy. The experience of fusion, a transitory dissolution of interpersonal boundaries, ob-

tained in sexual union satisfies a great libidinal hunger for attachment, for merger with an other. The intimate connection between sex, attachment, and identity magnifies the obligation of the therapist toward the patient, particularly to do no harm.

Given that sexual expression is often one of the deepest and most personal experiences, what unknown dangers await the client who enters therapy for a sexual problem? Since sex may be merely one troubled area of an overall relational system, tinkering with just the genital system often causes underlying emotional and relational problems to surface. Should therapists, like the maps of old, warn clients of possible consequences before assigning exercises that quite commonly evoke unexpected feelings that themselves demand therapeutic attention?

### The social construction of sex

What unquestioned values and presuppositions are embedded in sex therapy and research because their development occurred largely within the context of the predominantly white, middle-class North American scientific establishment? How appropriate are therapeutic modalities designed originally for the treatment of heterosexual married couples, for example, in treating the sexual problems of a gay couple or a bisexual individual? Do members of ethnic minority groups encounter barriers to therapy because they are likely to be judged by standards which are not their own?

Cultural expectations, shared beliefs, and definitions about what is normal can influence the professional as well as public labeling of sexual behaviors, thoughts, and feelings (Szasz, 1980). It was not until 1973 that the American Psychiatric Association, in recognition of the absence of any direct correspondence between sexual preference and mental disorder, acted to remove homosexuality from its list of recognized mental disorders.

A sizable literature speaks to the inherent risks that attend the social construction of sexuality, suggesting that the power politics of sexuality have profoundly influenced the way in which it has been defined. Culturally influenced beliefs about female sexuality, for example, have both reflected and determined the treatment of women throughout history (Laqueur, 1990). In the absence of reliable data to the contrary, various societies (and the scientific communities of their times) have felt free to speculate widely about the very nature of female sexuality. At times societies have believed women to be insatiable or, at other times, incapable of desire; insisted that she could conceive only if she experienced orgasm; and judged her as less psychologically mature if she experienced clitoral orgasms to be as satisfying as vaginal ones, which presumably were produced by intercourse with a male partner. The work of Phyllis Chesler (1972) and others suggests that women, especially those who deviate from the predominant cultural expectations regarding sexuality and gender role, are particularly vulnerable to being described by the medical establishment as neurotic, or at best, as incompliant with care.

The controversy surrounding infibulation provides a dramatic example of the collision of cultures. Infibulation, also called "female circumcision," is widely practiced in large parts of Africa and the Middle East. The practice entails amputation of the clitoris and sometimes, as well, sewing the vaginal lips together or excising them. Feminists and health officials plead for the enforcement of laws prohibiting the practice, which mutilates large numbers of young girls, rendering intercourse an unsatisfying if not painful experience and resulting in the deaths of many. Governments have been slow to respond, defending their inaction by noting that intervention would be tantamount to criminalizing ethnicity, restricting the individual's right to practice the usual behaviors of the culture. They point to the reluctance of the women themselves to abandon this ancient rite of passage designed to confer femininity, while critics argue that this is yet another example of the conditioning of women to allow a male-dominated culture to define the nature of woman's sexuality.

A growing rift in the women's movement that accompanies the emergence of "sexual agency" feminism brings additional challenges to the issue of who defines a woman's sexuality. Confronting the notion that sex is fraught with male dominance and female submission, the "sexual agency" movement challenges the predominant assumption of female victimhood (Brownmiller, 1975; Dworkin, 1991; Faludi, 1991) and calls for an assertion of an aggressive sexual liberation and equality—demanding a return of sex from the political realm to the personal (Roiphe, 1993; Wolf, 1993).

## Values of the therapist

What of the therapists themselves? What attitudes, values, and longings do they bring to the therapeutic relationship? Whether they practice sex therapy as specialists or as other health-care professionals who address patients' sexual problems, therapists themselves often experience powerful emotional reactions that affect their ethical decisions. The therapist's automatic investment in keeping marriages together, abhorrence of abuse (physical, emotional, or financial), or strong preference for egalitarian relationships can profoundly influence therapy. It is assumed that the therapist must have a positive attitude about sexuality as a creative, life-enhancing force, and be conflict-free and tolerant. Recognizing that these virtues may be rare, therapists have

an obligation to disclose any personal values or preferences that might hinder their ability to respond to the needs of the patient. The first and least controversial duty of patient care is to provide care. Ironically, it is the most frequently violated. Physicians, who are in an ideal position to detect and treat sexual problems, often neglect to inquire about the development of sexual problems known to be related to various medical illnesses and the medications they prescribe. The obligation to evaluate and treat reversible sexual dysfunction is not diminished by the professional's own personal level of discomfort with the subject.

Many of the ethical dilemmas therapists face place them squarely in a double-bind situation, where any action taken can evoke guilt or a sense of helplessness in the therapist. Take, for example, the principle of confidentiality. Patients and research subjects must be assured that the information they provide will be kept private. Any breach of confidentiality raises the specter that the patient's relationship with others could be harmed. Without the guarantee of confidentiality, many persons would be reluctant to disclose sensitive information, even if it meant forgoing a solution to their sexual problems. Knowing this, what would constitute the most ethical action by a couple's therapist following a patient's disclosure of a homosexual affair of which his partner is unaware? Balanced against the obligation for truth-telling to the spouse, a bind is inevitable. Ultimately, every therapist has an obligation to analyze carefully the principles that must guide care, explore his or her own moral boundaries, and respectfully consider the impact of choices on the patient as an individual and in relationship to family and the broader community.

Little is known of the psychological mechanisms that those who do sex therapy use to manage their own feelings in these difficult situations. Undoubtedly, many health professionals and sex therapists wrestle with the difficult issues, while others cling rigidly to the rules of professional conduct embodied in the various codes of ethics endorsed by their professional organizations, blind to and poorly defended against the ordinary human needs and passions that may draw them and their colleagues into liaisons that prove dangerous to both themselves and their patients.

## Special issues in therapy

**Sexual contact between therapist and patient.** Although there are a very few therapists who openly advocate sexual therapist–patient intimacy as a part of sex therapy, it is generally considered unethical, destructive to the therapeutic relationship, and charged with the potential for doing great psychological harm to the patient (Charlton, 1993; Lebacqz and Barton, 1991; Rutter, 1991).

Even though the discussions with the therapist, reading and viewing materials, and homework assignments are explicitly sexual, overt sexual activities do not occur in the therapist's presence. With the exception of the conduct of a complete physical exam by a physician or nurse practitioner, the patient will not be asked to disrobe.

By virtue of role and expertise, therapists hold a position of greater power, not only with power over the patient's emotional state but with the authority to define the nature of the relationship. The factors of power, trust, and dependency raise the possibility that the patient cannot freely give consent to sexual contact, that is, that the dynamics of the relationship render the patient unable to withhold consent. Consequently, external controls on the sexual exploitation of trust have been encoded in the standards of professional conduct of virtually all licensing bodies and professional associations in the United States that represent specialists in sex therapy or others who practice sex therapy as one component of their helping professions. Although these codes may vary in detail (e.g., as to whether they proscribe sexual contact with *former* clients and patients), they generally hold that no matter how provocative or consenting the patient, the therapist, by virtue of the unequal power in the relationship, always bears the burden of blame and liability.

There is no evidence to suggest that sex therapists are any more likely than those in other disciplines to violate the boundaries that prohibit sexual contact within professional relationships of trust. Indeed, the considerable attention devoted to this issue by the young discipline (and the inclusion of prohibitions in the codes of ethics of most professional organizations) may have afforded some level of protection against the risk and has encouraged some training programs to devote significantly more attention to the issue of the attraction that can arise in the course of therapy, helping clinicians to develop appropriate mechanisms for managing their reactions and feelings.

**Sexual surrogates.**    In North America, the use of sexual surrogates has been extremely contentious and is not widely practiced. Sexual surrogates are, however, often utilized in other countries. In Japan, for example, people without partners can attend "sex school" (Allgeier and Allgeier, p. 258), trying various positions and techniques with clothed models under an instructor's supervision.

Most sexual therapies involve exercises that require a partner. Some therapists, attempting to help clients who do not have a partner, provide sexual surrogates (paraprofessionals working under the supervision of the therapist) to engage in private sexual activity with the patient. Critics contend that the use of surrogates differs little from prostitution, and that the use of surrogates provides only "technical" training, failing to evoke and

address the interpersonal and emotional issues often involved in sexual dysfunction. Defenders of the practice cite the screening, training, and supervision that surrogates undergo and argue that it is not ethical to deprive those without cooperative partners of the care they need. It seems unlikely that the controversy surrounding this issue will end until the effectiveness of this approach is clarified.

## Professionalization

The sheer magnitude of the need for services suggests that efforts to limit the practice of sex counseling and therapy to those with specialized training may be doomed from the outset. Masters and Johnson (1970) estimate that approximately 50 percent of all married couples will develop a sexual dysfunction that would benefit from therapy. Does the pressure to create a speciality with elevated standards of training and care risk raising the public's expectations of care while placing it beyond their reach?

Prior to the professionalization of sex therapy, the work fell to others—beauticians and bartenders, priests and courtesans. More recently, these resources have been augmented by a flood of self-help manuals, articles in the popular press, and "family life" classes in schools and churches. Assuming that nonprofessionals will continue to play a role for some time to come, how should professional sex therapists work with them to ensure that appropriate information and care is provided, helping them to provide accurate information and advice and to make referrals for professional treatment of sexual dysfunction in cases where it is needed?

With little forethought a system comprising various levels of care is emerging. School programs, community agencies, and the popular press have increased the knowledge of the general population. Many health-care providers have accepted a larger role in basic counseling and brief therapy, and there has been a tremendous increase in the availability of multidisciplinary programs that specialize in the treatment of complex or difficult cases. Professional ethics requires that coordination of the various components of the system become a priority in an effort to conserve scarce resources and to see to it that patients find the appropriate level of care. In addition, there is a twofold implication of the exclusion of coverage for sex therapy in most health insurance programs: those without sufficient wealth seldom receive treatment, and, consequently, our ability to generalize about the effectiveness of therapy may be limited.

## The research endeavor

Numerous ethical issues emerge from research into sexual response, dysfunction, and behavior. As in other fields, most research projects are scrutinized in advance by review boards to safeguard subjects by protecting them from physical or psychological harm, securing their informed consent, and ensuring their freedom from coercion.

Subjects are usually guaranteed anonymity and confidentiality. Beyond these concerns, research procedures must minimize the risk that the study might negatively affect the subject's emotional state, sexual adjustment, or relationships. A study might involve exposure to erotic material some prefer to avoid or require that the subject divulge highly personal information. Another study might involve the observation or measurement of physiological responses during sexual activity. The principle of informed consent requires that subjects be informed of all the procedures they will undergo, including any aspects that might be embarrassing or damaging to them, before they consent to participate.

A troublesome research issue is the use of children as research subjects. Answers to many fundamental questions about human sexuality reside in childhood, among them the emergence of sexual orientation, the formation of beliefs and attitudes, and the development of paraphilias (sexual deviations, characterized by preference for nonhuman objects in achieving arousal, imposition of humiliation or suffering, or coercion of nonconsenting partners). In the interest of protecting children from sexual stimulation, or from the emotional distress that would presumably follow, research about sexual attitudes and behaviors has generally depended on retrospective reports by adult subjects, or where children have been involved, limited to rather innocuous topics.

Several ethical issues surround research into strategies designed to treat the paraphilias that may result in incarceration (e.g., rape or pedophilia). First is the ethical obligation to avoid coercion of the subject's participation in the research—for example, by raising the hope of early release. Another issue relates to the type of treatment approaches that have been used. Allgeier and Allgeier (1988) note that although other techniques, for example, cognitive behavioral approaches and heterosexual skills training, have been increasingly used, the previous reliance on painful approaches, such as castration and aversion therapies that pair arousing stimuli for deviant behavior with unpleasant events such as electric shocks or chemicals that induce nausea or vomiting, seen aimed more at punishing than curing. Questions regarding the efficacy of treatment programs abound (Schwartz and Cellini, 1988)—suggesting that ineffective programs that accelerate the release of unsuccessfully treated inmates could actually increase the incidence of sexual offenses by providing a false sense of security. Unfortunately, few resources are available to those who are not incarcerated. Treatment programs are unavailable to the "many . . . on parole [who] request treatment" (Dvoskin, 1991). The growing public concern about the incidence of crime, short sentences, and

the early return of offenders to the community heightens the need for increasing both the effectiveness and availability of these programs.

Setting the priorities for research in a field where much awaits exploration is an ethical dilemma in itself. What choices should be made about the allocation of scarce resources? What role should researchers play in informing public policy? For example, should the paucity of research concerning the sexual functioning of women in response to various medical disorders and treatments be rapidly redressed? What of the special needs of those in populations long neglected—those with physical or emotional disabilities? What priority should be given to the investigation of pedophilia, incest, and the realms of the psyche where sex and violence merge? If we neglect these areas, we do so at great social cost.

Alternatively, should the fundamental questions have priority? What causes a person to be heterosexual? Or homosexual? What are the connections between sex and eating, sex and pain, danger, or profound grief? What is the biochemistry of sexual attraction and arousal? And ultimately, what does sex have to do with love?

SHARON K. TURNBULL

*Directly related to this article is the companion article in this entry:* SCIENTIFIC AND CLINICAL PERSPECTIVES. *For a further discussion of topics mentioned in this article, see the entries* CHILDREN, *article on* HEALTH-CARE AND RESEARCH ISSUES; CIRCUMCISION, *article on* FEMALE CIRCUMCISION; ETHICS, *article on* RELIGION AND MORALITY; GENDER IDENTITY AND GENDER-IDENTITY DISORDERS; HOMOSEXUALITY; INFORMED CONSENT, *article on* CONSENT ISSUES IN HUMAN RESEARCH; LOVE; MEDICAL CODES AND OATHS; PROFESSIONAL–PATIENT RELATIONSHIP; PROFESSION AND PROFESSIONAL ETHICS; SEXISM; SEXUAL DEVELOPMENT; SEXUAL ETHICS; SEXUAL ETHICS AND PROFESSIONAL STANDARDS; SEXUAL IDENTITY; SEXUALITY IN SOCIETY; *and* WOMEN. *For a discussion of related ideas, see the entries* FREEDOM AND COERCION; HUMAN NATURE; INTERPRETATION; TRUST; *and* VALUE AND VALUATION. *Other relevant material may be found under the entries* BEHAVIOR MODIFICATION THERAPIES; MENTAL-HEALTH THERAPIES; RESEARCH, UNETHICAL; RESEARCH METHODOLOGY; *and* RESEARCH POLICY.

## Bibliography

ALLGEIER, ALBERT R., and ALLGEIER, ELIZABETH R. 1988. *Sexual Interactions.* Lexington, Mass.: D.C. Heath.

ANDREASEN, NANCY C., and BLACK, DONALD. 1991. "Sexual Disorders." In their *Introductory Textbook of Psychiatry,* pp. 335–373. Washington, D.C.: American Psychiatric Press.

BARBACH, LONNIE B. 1980. "Group Treatment of Anorgasmic Women." In *Principles and Practice of Sex Therapy*, pp. 107–146. Edited by Sandra R. Leiblum and Lawrence A. Pervine. New York: Guilford Press.

BJORKSTEIN, OLIVER J. W. 1976. "Sexually Graphic Material in the Treatment of Sexual Disorders." In *Clinical Management of Sexual Disorders*, pp. 161–194. Edited by Jon K. Meyer. Baltimore: Williams and Wilkins.

BRECHER, EDWARD M., and BRECHER, JEREMY. 1986. "Extracting Valid Sexological Findings from Severely Flawed and Biased Populations." *Journal of Sex Research* 22:6–20.

BRODY, HOWARD. 1990. "Ethical Aspects of the Physician–Patient Relationship." In *Behavior and Medicine*, pp. 199–207. Edited by Danny Wedding. St. Louis, Mo.: Mosby Year Book.

BROWNMILLER, SUSAN. 1975. *Against Our Will: Men, Women, and Rape.* New York: Simon and Schuster.

BYRNE, DONN. 1977. "Social Psychology and the Study of Sexual Behavior." *Personality and Social Psychology Bulletin* 3, no. 1:3–30.

CHARLTON, BRUCE G. 1993. "Sexual Ethics in Psychiatry." *Current Opinion in Psychiatry* 6, no. 5:713–716.

CHESLER, PHYLLIS. 1972. *Women and Madness.* Garden City, N.Y.: Doubleday.

COURTOIS, CHRISTINE A. 1988. *Healing the Incest Wound: Adult Survivors in Therapy.* New York: W. W. Norton.

DIAMANT, LOUIS. 1977. "The Therapies." In *Male and Female Homosexuality: Psychological Approaches*, pp. 199–217. Edited by Louis Diamant. New York: Hemisphere.

DONNERSTEIN, EDWARD, and LINZ, DANIEL G. 1986. "Mass Media, Sexual Violence and Media Violence." *American Behavioral Scientist* 29, no. 5:601–618.

DVOSKIN, JOEL A. 1991. "Allocating Treatment Resources for Sex Offenders." *Hospital and Community Psychiatry* 42, no. 3:229.

DWORKIN, ANDREA. 1991. [1981]. *Pornography: Men Possessing Women.* New York: NAL/Dutton.

"Ethics and Research: Sex, Hearts, and Brains." 1990. *Nature* 343, no. 6253:8–9.

FALUDI, SUSAN. 1991. *Backlash: The Undeclared War Against American Women.* New York: Crown.

KAPLAN, HELEN SINGER. 1974. *The New Sex Therapy: Active Treatment for Sexual Dysfunctions.* New York: Bruner/Mazel.

———. 1979. *Disorders of Sexual Desire and Other New Concepts and Techniques.* New York: Bruner/Mazel.

KINSEY, ALFRED C.; POMEROY, WARDELL B.; and MARTIN, CLYDE E. 1948. *Sexual Behavior in the Human Male.* Philadelphia: W. B. Saunders.

KINSEY, ALFRED C.; POMEROY, WARDELL B.; MARTIN, CLYDE E.; and GEBHARD, PAUL H. 1953. *Sexual Behavior in the Human Female.* Philadelphia: W. B. Saunders.

LAQUEUR, THOMAS. 1990. *Making Sex: Body and Gender from the Greeks to Freud.* Cambridge, Mass.: Harvard University Press.

LAZARUS, ARNOLD A., and ROSEN, RAYMOND C. 1976. "Behavior Therapy Techniques in the Treatment of Sexual Disorders." In *Clinical Management of Sexual Disorders*, pp. 148–160. Edited by Jon K. Meyer. Baltimore: Williams and Wilkins.

LEBACQZ, KAREN, and BARTON, RONALD G. 1991. *Sex in the Parish.* Louisville, Ky.: Westminster/John Knox Press.

LOPICCOLO, JOSEPH. 1978. "Direct Treatment of Sexual Dysfunction." In *Handbook of Sex Therapy*, pp. 1–17. Edited by Joseph LoPiccolo and Leslie LoPiccolo. New York: Plenum.

MARKS, ISAAC M. 1986. *Behavioural Psychotherapy: Maudsley Pocket Book of Clinical Management.* Bristol, England: John Wright.

MARQUES, JANICE K.; HAYNES, ROBERT L.; and NELSON, CRAIG. 1991. "Forensic Treatment in the United States: A Survey of Selected Forensic Hospitals." *International Journal of Law and Psychiatry* 16, nos. 1–2:57–70.

MASTERS, WILLIAM H., and JOHNSON, VIRGINIA E. 1966. *Human Sexual Response.* Boston: Little, Brown.

———. 1970. *Human Sexual Inadequacy.* Boston: Little, Brown.

———. 1976. "Principles of the New Sex Therapy." *American Journal of Psychiatry* 133, no. 5:548–554.

MASTERS, WILLIAM H.; JOHNSON, VIRGINIA, E.; and KOLODNY, ROBERT C., eds. 1977. *Ethical Issues in Sex Therapy and Research.* Boston: Little, Brown.

McCARTHY, BARRY W. 1986. "A Cognitive-Behavioral Approach to Understanding and Treating Sexual Trauma." *Journal of Sex and Marital Therapy* 12, no. 4:322–329.

POMEROY, WARDELL B. 1972. *Dr. Kinsey and the Institute for Sex Research.* New York: Harper & Row.

ROIPHE, KATIE. 1993. *The Morning After: Sex, Fear, and Feminism on Campus.* Boston: Little, Brown.

RUTTER, PETER. 1991. *Sex in the Forbidden Zone: When Men in Power—Therapists, Doctors, Clergy, Teachers, and Others—Betray Women's Trust.* Los Angeles: Jeremy P. Tarcher.

SCHWARTZ, BARBARA K., and CELLINI, H. R. 1988. *A Practitioner's Guide to Treating the Incarcerated Male Sex Offender.* Washington, D.C.: U.S. Department of Justice, National Institute of Corrections.

SHELP, EARL E., ed. 1987. *Sexuality and Medicine.* 2 vols. Dordrecht, Netherlands: Reidel.

SZASZ, THOMAS. 1980. *Sex by Prescription.* New York: Penguin.

TALMADGE, LYNDA D., and WALLACE, SHARON C. 1991. "Reclaiming Sexuality in Female Incest Survivors." *Journal of Sex and Marital Therapy* 17, no. 3:163–182.

TANNAHILL, REAY. 1992. *Sex in History.* Rev. ed. New York: Scarborough House.

WOLF, NAOMI. 1993. *Fire with Fire: The New Female Power and How It Will Change the Twenty-first Century.* New York: Random House.

WOLPE, JOSEPH. 1958. *Psychotherapy by Reciprocal Inhibition.* Stanford, Calif.: Stanford University Press.

# SEXUAL DEVELOPMENT

Anatomy is not destiny. Even biology in its broadest sense does not strictly determine psychosexual identity. Sexual development, like other facets of human development, does have biological foundations that help in orienting the growing and enculturating individual. A genetically encoded "blueprint" is provided that normally orchestrates sexual developmental events according to a more or less predictable timetable. This biological impetus is not, however, sufficiently determinative to account for the end product. Children are taught along the way how to be (or not to be) sexual beings in their sociocultural time and place in history. Nature and nurture interweave in sexual development; we sometimes refer to the "nature" part of growing up as "maturation," to differentiate its stages and processes from those that are more directly the result of "nurture"—socioenvironmental influences, especially learning and behavioral shaping. "Biopsychosocial" is the term used in medicine and psychiatry for an integrative model of human development, health, and disease.

Social and moral issues arise around the events encountered at each stage of the development of human sexuality—and follow from them, as well. Sexual attitudes, customs, and practices, all historically and culturally variable, interact in complex ways with chromosomal, hormonal, and anatomical influences. An analysis of the ethics of sexual development must therefore include issues of individual, embodied sexuality and also of sexual relationships, understood using concepts of biology, psychology, and culture.

Ethical analysis is complicated by the varying answer to the question, "Whose ethics?" Sometimes ethical questions confront the growing child, but infants have little if any capacity for moral reasoning, and children after the age of five are just developing their moral and ethical sense. More often, therefore, the issues of sexual development perplex the child's caregivers and teachers, who seem to young people to be overburdened with exhortations. And always there are crucial social issues. Fundamental concepts—the nature of bodies, of pleasure and its limitations or dangers, of sin and shame, and of the human identities of men and of women—shape social values on gender and sexuality; these in turn shape individual ethics and practices, and what we teach our children. Religion and government have always concerned themselves with human sexuality, including gender roles and reproductive practices; and family values centrally define positions on sex roles, sexual choices and behaviors, and reproduction. At issue when others influence children is the tension between respecting and caring for their individual development of desires and choices, versus attempting to "socialize" them—that is, to protect them from the dangers of impulsive and ignorant choices, and to teach them the values of their culture's adult society.

The result is a fully developed and personalized sexuality, reflecting an amalgamated complex of idiosyncratic and sociocultural meanings, symbols, and associations. Sexual fantasy and behaviors, or quiet reflection about one's sexuality and its interpersonal impact, are ethical and spiritual matters, with a heavier freight of ethics and aesthetics than of logic. Still, specific sexuality is experienced as an unscripted communion and dyadic meditation in a rare, precious zone of interpersonal ecstasy, spontaneity, and enthusiasm that becomes increasingly important in postindustrial bureaucratized societies.

## Defining "sexual"

We use the adjective "sexual" in describing many things: maleness or femaleness, behaviors surrounding intercourse, fantasies that excite. Confusing simple efforts at definition, "sexual" may point to biological aspects of being male or female, to social roles and behaviors, or to psychological phenomena.

**Biological sex.** This seemingly simple concept becomes complicated under the close inspection of sex researchers, who distinguish six categories of biological maleness or femaleness (Reinisch, 1990): chromosomal sex (the XX-female or XY-male chromosome pattern); gonadal sex (ovaries or testicles); hormonal sex (having more androgenic hormones than estrogens and progestins yields male characteristics); anatomical sex, internal (uterus or prostate gland); anatomical sex, external (clitoris and labia, or penis and scrotum); and brain sex (female and male brains show some differences in structure and levels of chemicals; their significance is not yet clear).

**Gender.** "Biology" ("sex") refers to male and female, "gender" to masculinity and femininity.

*Core gender identity.* "I am a girl" or "I am a boy": This vital part of identity begins with the sex assignment made at birth, usually by an authority (doctor or midwife) based on the appearance of the external genitals. "It's a girl!" or "It's a boy!" answers the question often asked even before "Is it healthy?" (The rare doubtful assignment of "I'm not sure, it isn't exactly a boy *or* a girl" reflects those accidents of nature in which hermaphroditism or some other sexual abnormality has occurred.) Everyone in the infant's environment confirms the assigned sex in the name given, the way it is held or played with, the color and kind of clothing provided, and innumerable other ways, deliberate and otherwise. As the child grows, messages become more explicit; for example, certain ways of acting or dressing are forbidden or encouraged for little girls, others for little boys. All of this is absorbed into the deepest levels of the child's sense of who he or she "is." Between the ages of eighteen months and three years, the child will normally have acquired an abiding core gender identity. Even in cases where the biological sex was not apparent at birth, core gender identity has been established in accordance with the gender assignment if it was unambiguously made by the parents; it has been found to be virtually immutable after 30 months of age (Money and Ehrhardt, 1972; Stoller, 1979).

*Gender role.* Usually congruent with gender identity, gender role refers to the way a person enacts femininity or masculinity—what one does to suggest to others that one is a boy or girl, a man or woman. This evolves and is refined throughout life but is largely built through learning acquired (consciously and unconsciously) in childhood.

*Sexual orientation.* This is based on one's attraction to and falling in love with partners of either the same or the opposite sex, or both.

*Reproductive role.* This refers to one's becoming or not becoming (choosing not to be, or being unable to be) a parent.

## The stages of sexual development

**Prenatal sexuality.** By the time we are born we have (in most cases) come to have a distinct biological sex under the absent or present influence of the Y-chromosome on the bipotential gonad of the fetus. If Y is present, testes differentiate and produce androgens so that a male develops; if not, a female develops. Thus, the basic template of the embryo (the "default" that will develop unless hormones intervene) is female—a relatively late scientific discovery, contradicting the metaphor of woman as created from Adam's rib. Other intrauterine factors, notably maternal hormones, may complement or interfere with chromosomally destined gender development.

There are ethical issues even at this stage. Individuals and cultures frequently value male babies over females, a gender preference that has been expressed after birth by female infanticide. This is a contemporary as well as a historical practice, documented in large numbers in (for one example) China under the pressure of government-mandated limits on family size (Tannahill, 1992). Technologies of prenatal testing now make it possible to select the desired sex before birth via abortion. Available statistics, like those showing a preponderance of abortions of female fetuses in certain cultures, suggest that where the choice is available, social and individual values of caring for gender equality are tested against the pervasive legacy of discrimination against females.

We may soon be able to manipulate the hormonal environment of the developing fetus to "fine-tune" its sexuality—to ensure, let us say, that a boy will be more aggressive, or a girl less so. Although the origins of sexual orientation are not yet clear and are probably complex, many researchers believe that there is a genetic component. If so, it may become possible to detect and "correct" or abort homosexually destined infants prenatally. When there is no actual abnormality (excessive

maternal hormones, or drug-generated chromosomal defects, for example), such interventions would reveal a value for personal or cultural preferences more than for human diversity.

**Infantile sexuality.** When Sigmund Freud made infantile sexuality a cornerstone of his psychoanalytic theory of psychosexual development, he caused great and continuing controversy. Yet it is observably true that by the time of birth the baby girl is capable of physiological sexual readiness, showing clitoral turgor and vaginal lubrication cyclically in the initial neonatal hours; the baby boy shows penile erections that may have been observed prenatally by ultrasound imaging, and sometimes at the moment of birth (Rutter, 1980). Such readiness seems to be species-specific and phylogenetically programmed. It is perhaps the first indication of a way in which humans are unique from other mammals: We have sexual desires, urges, and acts that know no oestrus, no season.

We vaunt our kinship with mammals, however, by our mouthy behavior, particularly sucking. Freud believed that this "oral activity" was the first manifestation of the sexual instinct (libido), defining the oral stage as that when pleasurable excitation of the mucosal membranes of the mouth and lips is at center stage for the infant.

Mothers with suckling babies hold creatures of great dependency in their arms. As the mother initiates and responds in her attachment to the baby, the baby senses times of maternal tension and relaxation, and learns a human style in reciprocal interaction. Homilies are delivered while caregiving: "Be nice, don't be so lazy, can you really be hungry already? Don't you dare fall asleep on me and wake me up in half an hour," and so on. The baby is nourished on values along with milk.

Until about two years old the infant functions cognitively in a sensorimotor way (Piaget, 1956) that is regained for many, even when old, at times of sexual delight.

The enormous vulnerability and dependency of human babies confer ethical responsibilities on their caregivers. Powerful messages about bodies, sensual pleasures, gender, and desire are conveyed in these early, mostly nonverbal communications; these will contribute to the foundations of the child's developing sexuality. Early attachments are not meant to be delibidinized or intellectualized, for that risks minimizing their earthy and sexy qualities; life itself for the infant is derived from, and made pleasurable by, the body of another. Infantile attachment is a good groundwork for developing tenderness, trust, and sexuality. The later capacity for skin eroticism, so invaluable to sensual and sexual pleasure, probably depends on the infant's having enjoyed skin-to-skin contact with the body of another who enjoys this contact too.

Infants are avid social learners in many more ways than previously thought. They smile, gaze, recognize; they live within relatedness to others. Sensorimotor infants thrive in durable and reliable relationships of great dependency. Later, they can grow up to be not independent but interdependent and reliable. The dilemmas of infancy—trust versus mistrust, autonomy versus shame and doubt (Erikson, 1963), merger versus separation-individuation (Rank, 1936; Mahler and Furer, 1968)—are existential issues in being human that recur in all stages of the life cycle and do not disappear after one phase-specific hassle. During the first years of life, security must be consumed by an infant, and the more adults who can dispense parental security and sensual holding, the better.

**Toddlers and small children.**    By 30 months of age a host of establishments of selfhood have emerged—the body image, the core gender identity, the nuclear self concept—as confluences of nature and nurture. Girls and boys both are made mainly under the care of women. Both sexes thus form their primary identifications originally with the mother. Freud hypothesized that this gave boys a surer path to adult (hetero) sexuality, as girls had to switch to men for their objects of sexual desire. Later theorists pointed to a different complication for boys, who must differentiate their gender identity from that of the mother (Greenson, 1978). Yet again, girls' sense of separateness may suffer from the lack of such a contrapuntal sounding board (Chodorow, 1978).

The extent to which body image includes an accurate knowledge and a valuing of clitoris and labia or penis and scrotum depends on the willingness of caregivers to name and value these parts. Often, vague or coy nicknames or the ominous "down there" substitute for accuracy. The body ego can then remain hazy or, worse, become devalued; this blurring of self-knowledge may threaten an individual's trust in bodily sensations and perceptions as important sources of information about either self or external reality. Gender role may then depend more upon generic self-labeling based on messages about gender-assignment from others (Fast, 1984). Worse, the child may associate his or her genitals (girls are more vulnerable because their anatomy is less available for their own inspection) with the "dirty" and embarrassing experiences that too often mar toilet training.

After age two and up to about seven years, the typical child functions cognitively on a "preoperational" level (Piaget, 1956), preparing for "concrete" operations that usually occur from ages seven to eleven. Selfhood and attitudes of self-regard, as well as sexual self-definition, develop on these early cognitive levels. Children will candidly express curiosity about sex, as about everything around them, if they are not inhibited from doing so. "Where did I come from?" demands an accurate yet uncomplicated answer, suitable for the nonabstract cognitions of the curious child, and uncontaminated by the mist of anxiety and shame that can confuse and frighten.

Only toward the end of this age range do sex-role differentiation and strong structuring of masculine or feminine gender roles, and other sociocultural aspects of sex development, take root. A child's capacity to learn societal preferences in sexual matters depends on cognitive level; hence, bright children may more easily be both enculturated and made skeptical (Kohlberg, 1966). Studies in the United States of children three and four years old show 80 percent of them to have marriage as a goal, although they seldom emphasize the sexual aspects of marriage at their age; interestingly, by the time they are thirty, 80 percent are married. Sociocultural construction of heterosexism (thinking and acting as though only heterosexuality were normal, often leading to unfair treatment of bisexual or homosexual individuals) is pervasive.

Consistently boyish or girlish behavior is not well established and distributed to the socially appropriate gender group until kindergarten; and even then, and thereafter, rigid stereotyping may not occur if it is not enforced. Conversely, "tomboyishness" (girls) and "sissiness" (boys) need not predict adult sexual orientation or preference. Even cross-dressing in childhood does not foretell homosexuality later, since over half of heterosexual adults recall such dressing in childhood and many homosexuals do not. Homosexual adults seldom have any uncertainty about their core gender identity, even when males are effeminate or females are "butch."

Feminist theorists have undertaken considerable reassessment of historically taken-for-granted social arrangements and gender-restricted roles and have raised serious questions about the price paid in pain and gender- and sexual-identity disturbances or constrictions. Humanity can ill afford to force individuals to suppress parts of their potential talents and human qualities as the "ticket of admission" to social affirmation of their sexual or gender identity.

Caregivers and educators often face the dilemma of how to transcend their own life experience. How can one accurately satisfy the innocent curiosity of children if one's own upbringing transformed simple questions into something different, fascinating but forbidden, embarrassing, even "nasty"?

Even young children can reflect on how they treat others who are "different"; in this as in many things, they take cues from grown-ups. Cruelty toward "sissies" has emotionally scarred many boys whose temperament and play preferences did not fit the "macho" mold. Girls have it easier, for a change, in that so-called tomboys are generally better tolerated—at least before puberty. But the question of "gender nonconformity" troubles many caregivers. Should a child whose behavior does not meet societal gender rules be taken to a doctor or religious leader to be "fixed"? Are marriage and parenting the only sexual roles to which children should aspire? Unfortunately, experts do not agree on how to distinguish children whose gender identity is seriously troubled, and who may benefit from professional help, from those whose unconventionally unfolding selves need only loving support and acceptance. For parents, caregivers, and counselors, the ethical imperatives are competence, respect, and care (Young, 1966).

**Children (7 to 11 years).** Long called "latency," these years for most children are not devoid of sexual desire and experience. Masturbation may be the most common sexual activity, but the highest rate of sex play among children occurs between the ages of six and ten years; boys often masturbate in groups. Children often shift from generalized sex play to deliberate pursuit of erotic arousal by the age of eight or nine. An increasing percentage of children under thirteen have had coitus, some of them homosexual anal intercourse, or oral-genital sexual experiences (Reinisch, 1990).

These sexual experiences are not always with age-mates, which may be harmless, but sometimes with much older persons, which is harmful and exploitative. As a clinical rule of thumb, child sexual abuse is assumed when there is an age discrepancy of more than five years between the older perpetrator and the younger victim. Moralists and social reformers have returned to Freud's original "seduction theory," focusing on actual adult molestation of children, rather than attributing such reports to fantasies or the unconscious desires of children. The women's movement has had a vital role to play in this rediscovery of childhood sexual abuse.

Curiously, masturbation has historically received more public attention as a moral issue. In the United States as recently as the nineteenth century, common devices to discourage and punish children's masturbation included straitjackets, or metal mittens, "genital cages," and special spike-lined tubes to prevent erections. Doctors actually advised parents to wrap cold, wet sheets around persistent masturbators, or to tie their hands to bedposts; more drastic prescriptions included applying leeches, electric current, or hot irons to genitals, or even castration and clitoridectomy (surgical removal of the clitoris) (Reinisch, 1990). Children appear not to be naturally ashamed when they discover the pleasure of genital self-stimulation, but they are easily made to feel shame and guilt, thus producing anguished questions: "Should I masturbate at all? Only when no suitable sexual partner is available? How often? How?"

For parents and educators, the parallel issues involve reacting to the child's sex play (with self or others), and teaching her or him about privacy, modesty, and what is good or bad, permitted or forbidden. Contrast the typical advice of twentieth-century counselors in the West—that when children reach the ages of two or three years, parents can begin to teach them that self-touching is appropriate in private—with the reaffirmation in the Roman Catholic catechism that sex for any purpose other than procreation is wrong. Clearly this is not a settled question, despite advances since the days when medical texts solemnly declared that idiocy could result from "self-abuse."

**Preadolescence.** In late latency, even before the pubertal onslaught has appeared, many preadolescents become sexually active. Many of these youngsters engage in what some have called a normal homosexual phase. A first love experience outside the family with someone who is so much like oneself may provide validation of one's worth naturally and gracefully in a loving homoerotic interchange (Sullivan, 1953). That loving crush dispels loneliness for many a preadolescent, confirms his or her value, and may sometimes (but not always) give some opportunity for homosexual involvement.

Whether or not one is ethically troubled by these activities will depend on one's views about premarital sex in general, and about homosexuality in particular. "Compulsory heterosexuality" (Rich, 1982) has been held by many, but not all, cultures to be the only acceptable goal of childhood sexual socialization. Many families hold religious beliefs that characterize homosexuality as sinful and unacceptable. Even parents who tolerate in principle the concept of normal homosexuality may fear that their child will be unhappy, subject to discrimination and danger, and unable to enjoy family and parenting if he or she shows signs of same-sex love.

**Adolescence.** By age fourteen a conscience is established, so all sexuality thenceforth is expressed with some degree of ethical sensitivity and illumination. Also, by age eleven to fifteen years, the reasoning powers of the youth with normal IQ have matured to the adult level of formal operations (Piaget, 1956). Pubarche occurs mainly in the same years, so body and brain are ready to handle mature tasks and pleasures. Readiness for adult sexuality is present. In the United States, about two-thirds of boys and almost half of girls will have had sexual intercourse by the age of eighteen (Rutter, 1980).

Adolescent sexuality is always recognized as a potent force, but it often faces a societal moratorium of sorts, especially in societies that prize virginity and chastity. This is the age for moralistic questions about sexuality and sexual ethics, which have never been more keenly debated than they are today. In epochs with a high incidence of sexually transmitted diseases, a backlash routinely emerges to curb sexual freedom for adolescents. HIV infection and AIDS certainly impede the sexual freedom of today's adolescents; indeed, they erect a prospect of safe sexuality only with multiple barriers in place, diminishing intimacy and shared moistures. Public-health warnings and education appear to be ineffective among many adolescents, who are generally depicted as feeling invulnerable and immortal.

Still, from ages twelve to eighteen years, the sexual repertoire enlarges: For a large percentage of adolescents, coitus occurs before age eighteen; for many, orogenital experimentation occurs; for many, pregnancy has occurred; for some, offspring have been born. But age alone is not the only telling marker of sexuality, for we are sexually programmed to be like all other human beings in only a few traits. Gender, class, and race also have an impact; we tend to resemble our ethnic, economic, and cultural subgroupings, sexually speaking. Hence, by adolescence one's sexual activities and choices are quite similar to others with whom we feel identified. Lower-class males, for example, show earlier coitus than do their middle-class counterparts. Poor adolescents seem to use sexuality as a property substitute, as a medium of exchange, and as a source of prestige, entertainment, and selfhood consolidation (Rutter, 1980).

Then again, there are some ways in which each of us is like no others on the planet; we feel "first" or "unique" proudly, and that our individuality is laden with enormous value. Our developing sexual behavior, usually held private and secret, during all the phases of our lifetime provides for the psychologist a shorthand notation on our emerging personality. Most believe today that character, or personality, determines sexuality: We are as we use our genitals with and without others. (That consensus did not reign in periods when some experts held that sexuality determined character rather than being determined by it [Fromm, 1948].)

## Adult sexuality

Although development need not and should not stop after adolescence, and psychological theory has increasingly explicated the various stages of adult development, most of the ethical debates surrounding adult sexuality have been elaborated under such topics of scholarship as sexuality and homosexuality per se. The following sections will therefore touch more briefly on some specifically developmental aspects of the ethics of adult sexuality.

**Young adulthood.** From eighteen to twenty-five years, sexuality becomes more patterned, heterosexism and machismo more rigidly established, and marriage and childbearing much more common. Gays come out. Sexual careers are carved out, typecast, settled into, and sometimes show ossification during young adulthood. One's own way of being sexual gets settled for many. Some embrace the option of chastity during this age period; some embrace a homosexual orientation; others choose the bisexual option.

Most adults remember their first sexual encounter with another person, or at least remember their first orgasm when awake. It is not always a delightful milestone. But if it was not strictly an exercise in power or exploitation, every sexual interaction is usually remembered and cherished. Many who are heterosexual virtuosi turn in their dreams mainly to the face-to-face missionary position, which, though occasionally denigrated, is also characterized (Comfort, 1972) as providing supremely close, intimate, and egalitarian loving. Often we harbor fantasies of new sexual possibilities still unattained. Human sexuality, not bound to times of oestrus, thrives on fantasy. The human neural organization of hand-eye-mouth and the integrating cerebral cortex enable us to live symbolically, to "play brain" and to attain arousal simply by imagining a desired partner or other sufficiently stimulating images, thus sliding us from everyday into erotic reality (Davis, 1983). Sexual arousal brings us joyful interludes from the tedium of the workaday world.

**Mid-life.** Parenthood has become a central focus of daily life and personal identity for many between the ages of twenty-five and forty-five years. Libidinized caregiving to mate and children can create a more fulfilled sexual being. If previous developmental issues have not been resolved, however, becoming a parent may activate old conflicts and inhibitions, to the detriment of sexual pleasure. The struggle to redeem sexuality from what has been called the "wet-blanket" pattern may produce a push toward extramarital affairs, raising ethical issues about monogamy and fidelity versus "self-actualization" and passion as a need or even a right. Jealousy forces reexamination of the ethics of commitment: When is the promise of exclusivity mature, when is it the product of a childish and illusory sense of ownership? Tempted, some may question whether to deny lustful yearnings for the sake of the partner who would be hurt, or to shun such self-denial as a form of bondage. To talk about such issues as a couple or to decide them privately is also an issue in many marriages. As children pass through the lively stages of sexual development, their parents can hardly avoid being touched by resonances of unfinished business in their own psychosexual history.

Some eschew pairing and childbearing with a measure of cynicism in their decision; others may be fully generative without reproducing biologically and devote their lives to altruistic caring for the young of the species.

**Late life.** Sexual desire and activity continue throughout life for most people. They are intimate aspects of one's moral career and are not readily disclaimed, even when health is failing. Widowhood or single status after age 50, when women in particular are sometimes judged "old" even today, can crimp sexuality. If confidence in sexual attractiveness is not undermined, however, this life stage often brings an opportunity for new bonding and a new lease on life and love. The empty nest may facilitate the sexuality of a man and woman, or may unhinge them radically. The old person who has lived with one mate for forty years or more (Young, 1966) may well ask, if our sexuality when young was to be called love, what superlative word do we have in English for a fidelity of love and sex that has weathered a long span, in sickness and health and with a delight in sexuality, the nurturing of offspring, and growing old together?

JOAN A. LANG
PAUL L. ADAMS

*Directly related to this entry are the entries* GENDER IDENTITY AND GENDER-IDENTITY DISORDERS; HOMOSEXUALITY, *article on* CLINICAL AND BEHAVIORAL ASPECTS; SEX THERAPY AND SEX RESEARCH, *article on* SCIENTIFIC AND CLINICAL PERSPECTIVES; SEXUAL ETHICS; SEXUAL IDENTITY; *and* SEXUALITY IN SOCIETY, *article on* SOCIAL CONTROL OF SEXUAL BEHAVIOR. *For a discussion of theories of female sexuality, see the entries* FEMINISM; HUMAN NATURE; SEXISM; *and* WOMEN, *article on* HISTORICAL AND CROSS-CULTURAL PERSPECTIVES. *Other relevant material may be found under the entries* BEHAVIOR MODIFICATION THERAPIES; BODY, *article on* SOCIAL THEORIES; FAMILY; FERTILITY CONTROL; HOMOSEXUALITY, *article on* ETHICAL ISSUES; LOVE; MARRIAGE AND OTHER DOMESTIC PARTNERSHIPS; MENTAL ILLNESS, *article on* CONCEPTIONS OF MENTAL ILLNESS; SEX THERAPY AND SEX RESEARCH, *article on* ETHICAL ISSUES; *and* SEXUALITY IN SOCIETY, *article on* LEGAL APPROACHES TO SEXUALITY.

## Bibliography

BALINT, MICHAEL. 1956. *Problems of Human Pleasure and Behavior.* New York: Liveright.

BOSTON WOMEN'S HEALTH COLLECTIVE. 1992. *The New Our Bodies, Ourselves: A Book by and for Women. Updated and Expanded for the 1990s.* New York: Simon & Schuster.

CHODOROW, NANCY. 1978. *The Reproduction of Mothering: Psychoanalysis and the Sociology of Gender.* Berkeley: University of California Press.

COMFORT, ALEX, ed. 1972. *The Joy of Sex: A Gourmet Guide to Lovemaking.* New York: Crown.

DAVIS, MURRAY S. 1983. *Smut: Erotic Reality/Obscene Ideology.* Chicago: University of Chicago Press.

ERIKSON, ERIK. 1963. *Childhood and Society.* 2d ed. New York: W. W. Norton.

FAST, IRENE. 1984. *Gender Identity: A Differentiation Model.* Hillsdale, N.J.: Analytic Press.

FREUD, SIGMUND. 1955. "Three Essays on the Theory of Sexuality (1905)." In vol. 7 of *The Standard Edition of the Complete Psychological Works of Sigmund Freud,* pp. 123–243. Translated by James Strachey. London: Hogarth.

FROMM, ERICH. 1948. "Sex and Character: The Kinsey Report Viewed from the Standpoint of Psychoanalysis." In *About the Kinsey Report: Observations by Eleven Experts on "Sexual Behavior in the Human Male,"* pp. 47–58. Edited by Donald Porter. New York: New American Library.

GREENSON, RALPH R. 1978. "Disidentifying from Mother: Its Special Importance for the Boy (1968)." In his *Explorations in Psychoanalysis,* pp. 305–312. New York: International Universities Press.

KOHLBERG, LAWRENCE. 1966. "A Cognitive-Developmental Analysis of Children's Sex-Role Concepts and Attitudes." In *The Development of Sex Differences,* pp. 82–173. Edited by Eleanor E. Maccoby. Stanford, Calif.: Stanford University Press.

LAPLANCHE, JEAN, and PONTALIS, J. B. 1973. *The Language of Psycho-Analysis.* Translated by Donald Nicholson-Smith. New York: W. W. Norton.

LAQUEUR, THOMAS W. 1990. *Making Sex: Body and Gender from the Greeks to Freud.* Cambridge, Mass.: Harvard University Press.

MAHLER, MARGARET S. and FURER, MANUEL. 1968. *Infantile Psychosis.* Vol. I of their *On Human Symbiosis and the Vicissitudes of Individuation.* New York: International Universities Press.

MONEY, JOHN, and EHRHARDT, ANKE. 1972. *Man and Woman, Boy and Girl: Differentiation and Dimorphism of Gender Identity from Conception to Maturity.* New York: New American Library.

NATHANSON, DONALD L. 1992. *Shame and Pride: Affect, Sex, and the Birth of the Self.* New York: W. W. Norton.

PIAGET, JEAN. 1956. "Les stades du developpement intellectuel de l'enfant et de l'adolescent." In *Le Problème des Stades en Psychologie de l'Enfant,* pp. 33–42. Edited by P. Osterrieth et al. Paris: Presses universitaires de France.

RANK, OTTO. 1936. *Will Therapy: An Analysis of the Therapeutic Process in Terms of Relationship.* New York: Alfred A. Knopf.

REINISCH, JUNE M. 1990. *The Kinsey Institute New Report on Sex: What You Must Know to Be Sexually Literate.* New York: St. Martin's Press.

RICH, ADRIENNE C. 1982. *Compulsory Heterosexuality and Lesbian Existence.* Denver, Colo.: Antelope Press.

RUTTER, MICHAEL. 1980. "Psychosexual Development." In *Developmental Psychiatry,* pp. 322–339. Edited by Michael Rutter. Washington, D.C.: American Psychiatric Press.

RUTTER, MICHAEL, and RUTTER, MARJORIE. 1993. *Developing Minds: Challenge and Continuity Across the Life Span.* New York: Basic Books.

STOLLER, ROBERT J. 1979. *Sexual Excitement: Dynamics of Erotic Life.* New York: Pantheon.

SULLIVAN, HARRY STACK. 1953. *Conceptions of Modern Psychiatry.* New York: W. W. Norton.

TANNAHILL, REAY. 1992. *Sex in History.* Lanham, Md.: Scarborough House.

VANCE, CAROLE S. 1992. *Pleasure and Danger: Exploring Female Sexuality.* London: Pandora Press.

YOUNG, WAYLAND H. 1966. *Eros Denied: Sex in Western History.* New York: Grove Press.

# SEXUAL ETHICS

Insofar as bioethics is concerned with human bodily health, it has an interest in the way health is influenced by and contributes to sexual functioning. There is a sense, then, in which bioethics includes sexual ethics, or at least some of the key questions of sexual ethics, such as the meaning of human sexuality and the causes and effects of sexual attitudes, orientations, and activities. Concepts of the human person—of desire and obligation, disease and dysfunction, even of justice and purity—can be found overlapping in various bioethical and sexual ethical theories. Like bioethics generally, sexual ethics considers standards for intervention in physical processes, rights of individuals to self-determination, ideals for human flourishing, and the importance of social context for the interpretation and regulation of sexual behavior. Bioethics specifically incorporates issues surrounding contraception and abortion, artificial reproduction, sexually transmitted diseases, sexual paraphilias, gendered roles and sexual conduct of the medical professionals, and sex research, counseling, and therapy. All of these issues are importantly shaped by moral traditions, so that health professionals frequently find themselves called upon to deal with questions of sexual ethics.

Historically, medicine has interacted with philosophy and religion in shaping and rationalizing the sexual ethical norms of a given culture. Medical opinion often simply reflects and conserves the accepted beliefs and mores of a society, but sometimes it is also a force for change. In either case, its influence can be powerful. For example, from the Hippocratic corpus in ancient Greece to the writings of the physician Galen in the second century c.e., medical recommendations regarding sexual discipline echoed and reinforced the ambivalence of Greek and Roman philosophers regarding human sexual activity. Galen's theories retained considerable power all the way into the European Renaissance. The interpretation of syphilis as a disease rather than a divine punishment came in the fifteenth century as the result of medical writings in response to a high incidence of the disease among the socially powerful. In nineteenth-century western Europe and North America, medical writers were enormously influential in shaping norms regarding such matters as masturbation (physicians believed it would lead to insanity), homosexuality (newly identified with perversions that medicine must diagnose and treat), contraception (considered unhealthy because it fostered sexual excess and loss of physical power), and gender roles (promoted on the basis of medical assessments of women's capacity for sexual desire). Today sex counseling and therapy communicate, however implic-

itly, normative ethical assumptions. Indeed, so great has been the influence of the medical profession on moral attitudes toward sexual options that critics warn of the "tyranny of experts," referring not to moral philosophers or religious teachers but to scientists and physicians.

The history of sexual ethics provides a helpful perspective for understanding current ethical questions regarding human sexuality. This article focuses on Western philosophical, scientific-medical, and religious traditions of sexual ethics and on the contemporary issues that trouble the heirs of these traditions. A historical overview of sexual ethics is not without its difficulties, however, as critical studies have shown (Brown, 1988; Foucault, 1978; Fout, 1992; Plaskow, 1990).

First of all, while it is possible to find a recorded history of laws, codes, and other guides to moral action regarding sexual behavior, it is almost impossible to determine what real people actually believed and did in the distant past. Or at least the historical research has barely begun. Second, ethical theory regarding sex (e.g., what is to be valued, what goals are worth pursuing, what reasons justify certain sexual attitudes, activities, and relationships) is predominantly theory formulated by an elite group of men. Women's experiences, beliefs, and values are largely unrecorded and, until recently, have been almost wholly inaccessible. The same is true of men who do not belong to a dominant class. Third, what we do find through historical research is necessarily subject to interpretation. It makes a difference, for example, whether one is looking for historical evaluations of human sexual desire or historical silences about sexual abuse of women. Finally, if one takes seriously the social construction of gender and sexuality, it is not clear that any kind of coherent historical narrative is possible. All of these difficulties notwithstanding, it is possible to survey (with appropriate caution) a Western normative and theoretical history regarding sex and to gain from the richness of varying contemporary interpretations. Central strands of this history can be traced to classical Greek and Roman antiquity, Judaism, and early and later developments in Christianity.

## Ancient Greece and Rome

**General attitudes and practice.** Ancient Greece and Rome shared a general acceptance of sex as a natural part of life. Both were permissive regarding the sexual behavior of men. In Athens, for example, the only clear proscriptions applicable to citizen-class men were in incest, bigamy, and adultery (insofar as it violated the property of another man). The focus of sexual concern in the two cultures was significantly different, however. For the Greeks, adult male love of adolescent boys occupied a great deal of public attention, whereas the Romans focused public concern on heterosexual marriage as the foundation of social life.

Marriage for both Greeks and Romans was monogamous. In Greece, however, no sexual ethic confined sex to marriage. Marriage as the expected pattern for citizen-class individuals was based not on the affective bond between husband and wife but on what were considered natural gender roles regarding procreation and service to the city. Male human nature was generally assumed to be bisexual, and the polyerotic needs of men were taken for granted. Concubinage, male and female prostitution, and the sexual use of slaves were commonly accepted. In practice, much of this was true in ancient Rome as well, even though ideals of marital fidelity became much more important. The development of marriage as a social institution was, however, considered a central achievement of Roman civilization. This included a growing appreciation of the importance of affective ties between wives and husbands.

Greece and Rome were male-dominated societies, and for citizens a gendered double standard prevailed in regard to sexual morality. Both Greek and Roman brides, but not bridegrooms, were expected to be virgins. In Greece, the only women who were given some equal status with men were a special class of artistically and educationally sophisticated prostitutes, the hetaerae. Generally women were considered intellectually inferior to men. In addition, Greek husbands and wives were unequal in age (wives were much younger) and in education. Wives had no public life, though they were given the power and responsibility of managing the home. In the Roman household, on the contrary, the husband retained power and could rule with an entirely free hand. Here the ideal of the patria potestas reached fulfillment. Mutual fidelity was much praised, but in fact absolute fidelity was required of wives while husbands could consort freely with slaves or prostitutes. Although by the first century C.E., women in Rome had achieved considerable economic and political freedom, they could not practice the sexual freedom traditionally granted to men.

Homosexuality was accepted in both Greek and Roman antiquity. Especially for the Greeks, however, it was less a matter of some men being sexually attracted only to men (or, more likely, boys) than a matter of men generally being attracted to beautiful individuals, whether male or female. Desire was of greater interest, as both possibility and problem, than its object; and desire was not essentially differentiated according to the gender of its object. Greek men were expected to marry, in order to produce an heir. Yet love and friendship, and sometimes sex, between men could be of a higher order than anything possible within marriage (for gender equality obtained between men, despite differences in age). Same-sex relations were not thereby wholly un-

problematic, however, as cultural cautions against male passivity attested. Moreover, the ethos tended not to support a positive evaluation of sexual relationships between women. Lesbian relations were often judged negatively because they counted as adultery (since women belonged to their husbands) or because a cultural preoccupation with male sexual desire made sex between women appear unnatural.

In both Greece and Rome, abortion and infanticide were common. Concern about the need to limit population influenced Greek sexual practices at various times, whereas efforts to improve a low birthrate in imperial Rome led to legal incentives to marry and to procreate. Divorce was more readily available in ancient Greece than in Rome, but eventually both cultures provided for it and for the resulting economic needs of divorced women; in Greece, husbands continued to administer their former wives' dowries, while in Rome a woman took her dowry with her.

Scholars today tend to dispute the belief that the last years of the Roman Empire saw a great weakening of sexual norms, a sexual dissipation at the heart of a general moral decline. The favored historical reading is now the opposite: that general suspicion of sexuality grew, and normative restrictions of sexual activity increased. In part, this was the result of the gradual influence of philosophical theories that questioned the value of sexual activity and emphasized the dangers in its consequences.

**Greek and Roman philosophical appraisals.** Michel Foucault's influential history of Graeco-Roman theory regarding sex identifies two problems that preoccupied philosophers: the natural force of sexual desire, with its consequent tendency to excess, and the power relations involved in the seemingly necessary active/passive roles in sexual activity (Foucault, 1986, 1988). The first problem contributed to the formulation of an ideal of self-mastery within an aesthetics of existence. Self-mastery could be achieved through a regimen that included diet, exercise, and various practices of self-discipline. The second problem yielded criteria for love and sex between men and boys. Active and passive roles were not a problem in adult male relations with women or with slaves, for the inferior passive role was considered natural to women, including wives, and to servants or slaves. This was a problem, however, for citizen-class boys, who must come to be equal with men. The solution, according to some philosophers (e.g., Demosthenes), was to regulate the age of boy lovers and the circumstances and goals of their liaisons with men. Others (e.g., Plato) preferred transcending and eliminating physical sex in erotic relations between men and boys.

The aspects of Greek and Roman thought about sex that were to have the most influence on subsequent Western theory included a distrust of sexual desire and a judgment of the inferior status of sexual pleasure, along with the inferior status of the body in relation to the soul. While sex was not considered evil, it was considered dangerous—not only in its excess but also in its natural violence (orgasm was sometimes described as a form of epileptic seizure); in its expenditure of virile energy (it was thought to have a weakening effect); and in its association with death (nature's provision for immortality through procreation made sex a reminder of mortality) (Foucault, 1986).

The Pythagoreans in the sixth century B.C.E. advocated purity of the body for the sake of cultivating the soul. The force of their position was felt in the later thinking of Socrates and Plato. Although Plato moved away from a general hostility to bodily pleasure, he made a careful distinction between lower and higher pleasures (in, for example, the *Republic, Phaedo, Symposium,* and *Philebus*): Sexual pleasure was a lower form of pleasure, and self-mastery required domination over its demands. Plato advocated unleashing, not restraining, the power of eros for the sake of uniting the human spirit with the highest truth, goodness, and beauty. Insofar as bodily pleasures could be taken into this pursuit, there was no objection to them. But Plato thought that sexual intercourse diminished the power of eros for the contemplation and love of higher realities and that it even compromised the possibility of tenderness and respect in individual relationships of love (*Phaedrus*).

Aristotle, too, distinguished lower and higher pleasures, placing pleasures of touch at the bottom of the scale, characteristic as they are of the animal part of human nature (*Nicomachean Ethics*). Aristotle, more thisworldly than Plato, advocated moderation rather than transcendence. However, for Aristotle the highest forms of friendship and love, and of happiness in the contemplation of the life of one's friend, seemed to have no room for the incorporation of sexual activity or even for Platonic eros. Aristotle never conceived of the possibility of equality or mutuality in relationships between women and men, and he opposed the design for this that Plato had offered in the *Republic* and *Laws*.

Of all Graeco-Roman philosophies, Stoicism probably had the greatest impact on later developments in Western thought about sex. Musonius Rufus, Epictetus, Seneca, and Marcus Aurelius, for example, taught strong doctrines of the power of the human will to regulate emotion and of the desirability of such regulation for the sake of inner peace. Sexual desire, like the passions of fear and anger, was in itself irrational, disruptive, liable to excess. It needed to be moderated if not eliminated. It ought never to be indulged in for its own sake but only insofar as it served a rational purpose. Procreation was that purpose. Hence, even in marriage sexual intercourse was considered morally good only when engaged in for the sake of procreation.

With the later Stoics came what Foucault calls the "conjugalization" of sexual relations (1988, p. 166). That is, the norm governing sexual activity was now "no sex outside of marriage," derived from what others have called the "procreative" norm. Marriage was considered a natural duty, excused only in special circumstances such as when an individual undertook the responsibilities of life as a philosopher. The good effects of marriage included progeny and the companionship of husband and wife. It became the context for self-control and the fashioning of the virtuous life. Plutarch (in *Dialogue on Love*) took the position that marriage, not homosexual relationships, was the primary locus for erotic love and for friendship.

Overall, the Graeco-Roman legacy to Western sexual ethics holds little of the sexual permissiveness that characterized ancient Greece. The dominant themes carried through to later traditions were skepticism and control. This may have been due to the failure of almost all Greek and Roman thinkers to integrate sexuality into their best insights into human relationships. Whether such an integration is possible in principle has been at least a tacit question for other traditions.

## The Jewish tradition

Earliest Jewish moral codes were simple and without systematic theological underpinnings. Like other ancient Near Eastern legislation, they prescribed marriage laws and prohibited rape, adultery, and certain forms of prostitution. In contrast with neighboring religions, the Jews believed in a God who is beyond sexuality but whose plan for creation makes marriage and fertility holy and the subject of a religious duty (Gen. 2:24). At the heart of Judaism's tradition of sexual morality is a religious injunction to marry. The command to marry holds within it a command to procreate, and it assumes a patriarchal model for marriage and family. These two aspects of the tradition—the duty to procreate and its patriarchal context—account for many of its specific sexual regulations.

While the core of the imperative to marry is the command to procreate, marriage was considered a duty also because it conduced to the holiness of the partners. Holiness referred to more than the channeling of sexual desire, though it meant that also; it included the companionship and mutual fulfillment of spouses. In fact, monogamous lifelong marriage was considered the ideal context for sexuality, and in time it became the custom and not only an ideal. Yet the command to procreate historically stood in tension with the value given to the marriage relationship. Thus while the laws of *onah*, of marital rights and duties, aimed to make sex a nurturant of love (Lamm, 1980), polygamy, concubinage, and divorce and remarriage were long accepted as solutions to a childless marriage. Only in the eleventh century C.E.

was polygamy finally banned (much later in the East), and it was only in the twelfth century that Maimonides explicitly condemned concubinage (Novak, 1992).

Judaism has traditionally shown a concern for the "improper emission of seed" (appealing to interpretations of Gen. 38:9). Included in this concern have been proscriptions of masturbation and homosexual acts. The latter in particular have been considered unnatural (Lev. 18:22, 20:13), failing in responsibility for procreation, beneath the dignity of humanly meaningful sexual intercourse, indicative of uncontrolled (and hence morally evil) sexual desire, and a threat to the stability of heterosexual marriage and the patriarchal family. Lesbian relations were not regulated by biblical law, and in rabbinic literature were treated far less seriously than male homosexuality.

Throughout the Jewish tradition there has been a marked difference in the treatment of women's and men's sexuality (Plaskow, 1990). In part, this was because of women's subordinate role in the family and in society. The regulation and control of women's sexuality was considered necessary to the stability and the continuity of the family. Premarital sex, extramarital sex, and even rape were legally different for women than for men. In the biblical period, husbands but not wives could initiate divorce (Deut. 24:1–4), although later rabbinic law made it possible for either to do so. Adultery was understood as violating the property rights of a husband and could be punished by the death of both parties. Women's actions and dress were regulated in order to restrict their potential for luring men into illicit sex. The laws of *onah* required men to respect the sexual needs of their wives; but the laws of *niddah* (menstrual purity) had the symbolic consequence, however unintended, of associating women with defilement.

The perspective on sex, in all the branches of Judaism, has been an enduringly positive one, yet not without ambivalence. The sexual instinct was considered a gift from God, but it could still be called by the rabbis the "evil impulse" (*yetzer hara*) (Plaskow, 1990). The tradition was not immune from the suspicion regarding sex that, with the rise of Stoic philosophies and the advent of certain religious movements from the East, permeated all Middle Eastern cultures. Interpretations of the relation between sexuality and the sacred have not been univocal, as evidenced in differences between mainstream Jewish thinking and kabbalistic mysticism. Hence, some issues of sexual ethics have not been resolved once and for all. Contemporary developments in the Jewish tradition include growing pluralism regarding questions of premarital sex, contraception, abortion, gender equality, and homosexuality (Borowitz, 1969; Feldman, 1974; Plaskow, 1990; Biale, 1992; Posner, 1992). Current conflicts involve the interpretation of traditional values, the analysis of contemporary situa-

tions, and the incorporation of hitherto unrepresented perspectives, in particular those of heterosexual women and of gays and lesbians.

## Christian traditions

Like other religious and cultural traditions, the teachings of Christianity regarding sex are complex and subject to multiple influences, and they have changed and developed through succeeding generations. Christianity does not begin with a systematic code of ethics. The teachings of Jesus and his followers, as recorded in the New Testament, provide a central focus for the moral life of Christians in the command to love God and neighbor. Beyond that, the New Testament offers grounds for a sexual ethic that (1) values marriage and procreation on the one hand, and singleness and celibacy on the other; (2) gives as much or more importance to internal attitudes and thoughts as to external actions; and (3) affirms a sacred symbolic meaning for sexual intercourse, yet both subordinates it to other human values and finds in it a possibility for evil. As for unanimity on more specific sexual rules, this is difficult to find in the beginnings of a religion whose founder taught as an itinerant prophet and whose sacred texts were formulated in "the more tense world" of particular disciples, a group of wandering preachers (Brown, 1988, pp. 42–43).

**Early influences on Christian understandings of sex.** Christianity emerged in the late Hellenistic age, when even Judaism was influenced by the dualistic anthropologies of Stoic philosophy and Gnostic religions. Unlike the Greek and Roman philosophies of the time, Christianity's main concern was not the art of self-mastery and not the preservation of the city or the empire. Unlike major strands of Judaism at the time, its focus was less on the solidarity and continuity of life in this world than on the continuity between this world and a life to come. Yet early Christian writers were profoundly influenced both by Judaism and by Graeco-Roman philosophy. With Judaism they shared a theistic approach to morality, an affirmation of creation as the context of marriage and procreation, and an ideal of single-hearted love. With the Stoics they shared a suspicion of bodily passion and a respect for reason as a guide to the moral life. With the Greeks, Romans, and Jews, Christian thinkers assumed and reinforced views of women as inferior to men (despite some signs of commitment to gender equality in the beginnings of Christianity as a movement). As Christianity struggled for its own identity, issues of sexual conduct were important, but there was no immediate agreement on how they should be resolved.

Gnosticism was a series of religious movements that deeply affected formulations of Christian sexual ethics for the first three centuries c.e. (Noonan, 1986). For example, some Gnostics taught that marriage was evil or at least useless, primarily because the procreation of children was a vehicle for forces of evil. This belief led to two extreme positions—one in opposition to all sexual intercourse, and hence in favor of celibacy, and the other in favor of any form of sexual intercourse so long as it was not procreative. Neither of these positions prevailed in what became orthodox Christianity.

What did prevail in Christian moral teaching was a doctrine that incorporated an affirmation of sex as good (because part of creation) but seriously flawed (because the force of sexual passion as such cannot be controlled by reason). The Stoic position that sexual intercourse can be brought under the rule of reason not by subduing it but by giving it a rational purpose (procreation) made great sense to early Christian thinkers. The connection made between sexual intercourse and procreation was not the same as the Jewish affirmation of the importance of fecundity, but it was in harmony with it. Christian teaching could thus both affirm procreation as the central rationale for sexual union and advocate celibacy as a praiseworthy option (indeed, the ideal) for Christians who could choose it.

With the adoption of the Stoic norm for sexual intercourse, the direction of Christian sexual ethics was set for centuries to come. A sexual ethic that concerned itself primarily with affirming the good of procreation, and thereby the good of otherwise evil tendencies, was reinforced by the continued appearance of antagonists who played the same role the Gnostics had played. No sooner had Gnosticism begun to wane than, in the third century, Manichaeanism emerged. It was largely in response to Manichaeanism that Saint Augustine formulated his sexual ethic, an ethic that continued and went beyond the Stoic elements incorporated by Clement of Alexandria, Origen, Ambrose, and Jerome.

**The sexual ethics of Saint Augustine and its legacy.** Against the Manichaeans Augustine argued in favor of the goodness of marriage and procreation, though he shared with them a negative view of sexual desire as in itself an evil passion. Because evil was for Augustine, however, a privation of right order (something missing in what was otherwise basically good), he thought at first that it was possible to reorder sexual desire according to right reason, to integrate its meaning into a right and whole love of God and neighbor. This reordering could be done only when sexual intercourse was within heterosexual marriage and for the purpose of procreation (On the Good of Marriage, 6). Intercourse within marriage but without a procreative purpose was, according to Augustine, sinful, though not necessarily mortally so. Marriage, on the other hand, had a threefold purpose: not only the good of children but also the goods of fidelity between spouses (as opposed to adul-

tery) and the indissolubility of the union (as opposed to divorce).

In his later writings against the Pelagians (Marriage and Concupiscence), Augustine tried to clarify the place of disordered sexual desire in a theology of original sin. Although for Augustine the original sin of Adam and Eve was a sin of the spirit (a sin of prideful disobedience), its effects were most acutely present in the conflict between sexual desire and reasoned love of higher goods. Moreover, this loss of integrity in affectivity was passed from one generation to another through the mode of procreation—sexual intercourse. In this debate Augustine argued that there is some evil in all sexual intercourse, even when it is within marriage and for the sake of procreation. Most of those who followed Augustine disagreed with this, but his basic formulation of a procreative ethic held sway in Christian moral teaching for centuries.

Some early Christian writers (e.g., John Chrysostom) emphasized the Pauline purpose for marriage—marriage as a remedy for incontinence. Such a position hardly served to foster a more optimistic view of sex, but it did offer a possibility for moral goodness in sexual intercourse without a direct relation to procreation. However, from the sixth to the eleventh century, it was Augustine's rationale that was codified in penitentials (manuals for confessors, providing lists of sins and their prescribed penances) with detailed prohibitions against adultery, fornication, oral and anal sex, contraception, and even certain positions for sexual intercourse if they were thought to be departures from the procreative norm. Gratian's great collection of canon law in the twelfth century contained rigorous regulations based on the principle that all sexual activity is evil unless it is between husband and wife and for the sake of procreation. A few voices (e.g., Abelard and John Damascene) maintained that concupiscence (sexual passionate desire) does not make sexual pleasure evil in itself, and that intercourse in marriage can be justified by the simple intention to avoid fornication.

Overall, the Christian tradition in the first half of its history developed a consistently negative view of sex, despite the fact that Augustine and most of those who followed him were neither anti-body nor anti-marriage. The statement that this tradition was negative must be a qualified claim, of course, for it was silent or vacillating on many questions of sexuality (e.g., on the question of homosexuality); and there is little evidence that Christians in general were influenced by the more severe sexual attitudes of their leaders (Boswell, 1980). The direction and tone that the early centuries gave to the tradition's future, however, were unmistakable. What these leaders were concerned about was freedom from bondage to desires that seemingly could not in themselves lead to God. In a quest for transformation of the body along with the spirit, even procreation did not appear very important. Hence, regulation of sexual activity and even the importance of the family were often overshadowed by the ideal of celibacy. As Peter Brown's massive study has shown, sexual renunciation served both eros and unselfish love, and it suited a worldview that broke boundaries with this world without rejecting it as evil (Brown, 1988).

**The teaching of Aquinas.**    Thomas Aquinas wrote in the thirteenth century, when rigorism already prevailed in Christian teaching and church discipline. His remarkable synthesis of Christian theology did not offer much that was innovative in the area of sexual ethics. Yet the clarity of what he brought forward made his contribution significant for the generations that followed. He taught that sexual desire is not intrinsically evil, since no spontaneous bodily or emotional inclination is evil in itself; only when there is an evil moral choice is an action morally evil. Consequent upon original sin, however, there is in human nature a certain loss of order among natural human inclinations. Sexual passion is marked by this disorder, but it is not morally evil except insofar as its disorder is freely chosen.

Aquinas offered two rationales for the procreative norm the tradition had so far affirmed. One was the Augustinian argument that sexual pleasure, in the fallen human person, hinders the best working of the mind. It must be brought into some accord with reason by having an overriding value as its goal. No less an end than procreation can justify it (*Summa theologiae*, I–II.34.1, ad 1). But second, reason does not merely provide a good purpose for sexual pleasure. It discovers this purpose through the anatomy and biological function of sexual organs (*Summa theologiae* II–II.154.11; *Summa contra Gentiles* III.122.4, 5). Hence, the norm of reason in sexual behavior requires not only the conscious intention to procreate but also the accurate and unimpeded (i.e., noncontraceptive) physical process whereby procreation is possible.

From the procreative norm there followed other specific moral rules. Many of them were aimed at the well-being of offspring that could result from sexual intercourse. For example, Aquinas argued against fornication, adultery, and divorce on the grounds that children would be deprived of a good context for their rearing. He considered sexual acts other than heterosexual intercourse to be immoral because they could not be procreative. Aquinas's treatment of marriage contained only hints of new insight regarding the relation of sexual intercourse to marital love. He offered a theory of love that had room for a positive incorporation of sexual union (*Summa theologiae* II–II.26.11), and he suggested that marriage might be the basis of a maximum form of friendship (*Summa contra Gentiles* III.123).

Though what had crystallized in the Middle Ages canonically and theologically would continue to influence Christian moral teaching into the indefinite future, the fifteenth century marked the beginning of significant change. Finding some grounds for opposing the prevailing Augustinian sexual ethic in both Albert the Great and in the general (if not the specifically sexual) ethics of Aquinas, writers (e.g., Denis the Carthusian and Martin LeMaistre) began to talk of the integration of spiritual love and sexual pleasure, and the intrinsic good of sexual pleasure as the opposite of the pain of its lack. This did not reverse the Augustinian tradition, but it weakened it. The effects of these new theories were felt in the controversies of the Reformation.

**Protestant teachings on sex.**    Questions of sexual behavior played an important role in the Protestant Reformation beginning in the sixteenth century. Clerical celibacy, for example, was challenged not just in its scandalous nonobservance but also as a Christian ideal. Marriage and family replaced it among the reformers as the center of sexual gravity in the Christian life. Martin Luther and John Calvin were both deeply influenced by the Augustinian tradition regarding original sin and its consequences for human sexuality. Yet both developed a position on marriage that was not dependent on a procreative ethic. Like most of the Christian tradition, they affirmed marriage and human sexuality as part of the divine plan for creation, and therefore good. But they shared Augustine's pessimistic view of fallen human nature and its disordered sex drive. Luther was convinced, however, that the necessary remedy for disordered desire was marriage (*On the Estate of Marriage*). And so the issue was joined over a key element in Christian sexual ethics. Luther, of course, was not the first to advocate marriage as the cure for unruly sexual desire, but he took on the whole of the tradition in a way that no one else had. He challenged theory and practice, offering not only an alternative justification for marriage but also a view of the human person that demanded marriage for almost all Christians.

According to Luther, sexual pleasure itself in one sense needed no justification. The desire for it was simply a fact of life. It remained, like all the givens in creation, a good so long as it was channeled through marriage into the meaningful whole of life, which included the good of offspring. What there was in sex that detracted from the knowledge and worship of God was sinful, but it had simply to be forgiven, as did the inevitable sinful elements in all human activity. After 1523, Luther shifted his emphasis from marriage as a "hospital for the incurables" to marriage as a school for character. It was within the secular, nonsacramental institution of marriage and family that individuals learned obedience to God and developed the important human virtues.

The structure of the family was hierarchical, husband having authority over wife, parents over children.

Calvin, too, saw marriage as a corrective to otherwise disordered desires. He expanded the notion of marriage as the context for human flourishing by maintaining that the greatest good of marriage and sex was the society that is formed between husband and wife (*Commentary on Genesis*). Calvin was more optimistic than Luther about the possibility of controlling sexual desire, though he, too, believed that whatever fault remained in it was "covered over" by marriage and forgiven by God (*Institutes of the Christian Religion*, 2.8.44). Like earlier writers, he worried that marriage as a remedy for incontinence could nonetheless in itself offer provocation to uncontrolled passion.

As part of their teaching on marriage, Luther and Calvin opposed premarital and extramarital sex and homosexual relations. So concerned was Luther to provide some institutionally tempering form to sexual desire that he once voiced an opinion favoring bigamy over adultery. Both Luther and Calvin were opposed to divorce, though its possibility was admitted in a situation of adultery or impotence.

**Modern Roman Catholic developments.**  During and after the Roman Catholic Counterreformation, from the late sixteenth century on, new developments alternated with the reassertion of the Augustinian ethic. The Council of Trent (1545–1563) was the first ecumenical council to address the role of love in marriage, but it also reaffirmed the primacy of procreation and reemphasized the superiority of celibacy. In the seventeenth century, Jansenism, a morally austere and ultimately heretical movement, reacted against what it considered a dangerous lowering of sexual standards and brought back the Augustinian connection between sex, concupiscence, and original sin. Alphonsus Liguori in the eighteenth century gave impetus to a manualist tradition (the development and proliferation of moral manuals designed primarily to assist confessors) that attempted to integrate the Pauline purpose of marriage (as a remedy for incontinence) with the procreative purpose. Nineteenth-century moral manuals focused on "sins of impurity," choices of any sexual pleasure apart from procreative marital intercourse. Then came the twentieth century, with the rise of Catholic theological interest in personalism and the move by the Protestant churches to accept birth control.

In 1930, Pope Pius XI responded to the Anglican approval of contraception by reaffirming the procreative ethic (*Casti connubii*). But he also gave approval to the use of the rhythm method for restricting procreation. Moral theologians began to move cautiously in the direction of allowing sexual intercourse in marriage without a procreative intent and for the purpose of fostering

marital union. The change in Roman Catholic moral theology from the 1950s to the 1970s was dramatic. The wedge introduced between procreation and sexual intercourse by the acceptance of the rhythm method joined with new understandings of the totality of the human person to support a radically new concern for sex as an expression and cause of married love. The effects of this theological reflection were striking in the 1965 Second Vatican Council teaching that the love essential to marriage is uniquely expressed and perfected in the act of sexual intercourse (*Gaudium et spes*, 49). Although the Council still held that marriage is by its very nature ordered to the procreation of children, it no longer ranked what the tradition considered the basic ends of marriage, offspring and spousal union, as primary and secondary.

In 1968, Pope Paul VI insisted that contraception is immoral (*Humanae vitae*). Rather than settling the issue for Roman Catholics, however, this occasioned intense conflict. The majority of moral theologians disagreed with the papal teaching, even though a distinction between nonprocreative and antiprocreative behavior mediated the dispute for some. Since then, many of the specific moral rules governing sexuality in the Catholic tradition have come under serious question. Official teachings have sustained past injunctions, though some modifications have been made in order to accommodate pastoral responses to second marriages, homosexual orientation (but not sexual activity), and individual conscience decisions regarding contraception. Among moral theologians there has been serious debate (and by the 1990s, marked pluralism) regarding premarital sex, homosexual acts, remarriage after divorce, infertility therapies, gender roles, and clerical celibacy (Curran and McCormick, 1993).

**Post-Reformation Protestantism.**  Twentieth-century Protestant sexual ethics developed even more dramatically than Roman Catholic sexual ethics. After the Reformation, Protestant theologians and church leaders continued to affirm heterosexual marriage as the only acceptable context for sexual activity. Except for the differences regarding celibacy and divorce, sexual norms in Protestantism looked much the same as those in the Catholic tradition. Nineteenth-century Protestantism shared and contributed to the cultural pressures of Victorianism. But in the twentieth century, Protestant thinking was deeply affected by biblical and historical studies that questioned the foundations of Christian sexual ethics, by psychological theories that challenged traditional views, and by the voiced experience of church members.

It is difficult to trace one clear line of development in twentieth-century Protestant sexual ethics, or even as clear a dialectic as may be found in Roman Catholicism. The fact that Protestantism in general was from the beginning less dependent on a procreative ethic allowed it almost unanimously to accept contraception as a means to responsible parenting. Overall, Protestant sexual ethics has moved to integrate an understanding of the human person, male and female, into a theology of marriage that no longer deprecates sexual desire as self-centered and dangerous. It continues to struggle with issues of gendered hierarchy in the family, and with what are often called "alternative lifestyles," such as the cohabitation of unmarried heterosexuals and the sexual partnerships of gays and lesbians. For the most part, the ideal context for sexual intercourse is still seen to be heterosexual marriage, but many Protestant theologians accept premarital sex and homosexual partnerships with general norms of noncoercion, basic equality, and so on. Every mainline Protestant church in the 1990s has task forces working particularly on questions of homosexuality, professional (including clergy) sexual ethics, and sex education. Traditional positions have either changed or are open and conflicted.

## Modern sexology: Philosophical, medical, social scientific

The contemporary shaking of the foundations of Western sexual ethics, religious and secular, is traceable to many factors. These quite obviously include the rapid development of reproductive technologies, none more important than the many forms of contraception. But there have been other factors as well, such as changes in economic structures under capitalism and in social structures following major shifts of population to urban centers. Of important influence, too, has been the rise of the modern women's movement and of movements for gay and lesbian civil rights. Along with these developments, as both cause and effect, there have been significant contributions from disciplines such as history, psychology, anthropology, sociology, and medicine. Philosophy has generally followed these changes, though in the late twentieth century it, too, has contributed to cultural alterations in perspectives on sex.

**Philosophical developments.** As surveyors of the history of philosophy note, philosophers have not paid much attention to sex. They have written a great deal on love but have left sexual behavior largely to religion, poetry, medicine, or the law (Baker and Elliston, 1975; Soble, 1991). After the Greeks and Romans, and medieval thinkers such as Thomas Aquinas whose work is philosophical as well as theological, there is not much to be found in the field regarding sexuality until the twentieth century. Some exceptions to this are the sparse eighteenth-century writings on sex and gender by David Hume, Jean-Jacques Rousseau, Immanuel Kant, Mary Wollstonecraft, and Johann Gottlieb Fichte, and the nineteenth-century writings of Arthur Schopen-

hauer, Karl Marx, Friedrich Engels, John Stuart Mill, and Friedrich Nietzsche. Most of these writers reinforced the norm of heterosexual procreative sex within marriage. Hume, for example, in his "Of Polygamy and Divorce" (1742), insisted that all arguments finally lead to a recommendation of "our present European practices with regard to marriage." Rousseau's La Nouvelle Héloïse (1761) deplored the faults of conventional marriage but strongly opposed divorce and marital infidelity. Kant defended traditional sexual mores, although in his Lectures on Ethics (1781) he introduced a justification for marriage not in terms of procreation but of altruistic love, arguing that only a mutual commitment in marriage can save sexual desire from making a sexual partner into a mere means to one's own pleasure. Schopenhauer viewed sexual love as subjectively for pleasure, though objectively for procreation; his strong naturalism paved the way for a more radical theory of sex as an instinct without ethical norms (The Metaphysics of Sexual Love, 1844).

Philosophers in these centuries came down on both sides of the question of gender equality. Fichte, for example, asserted an essentially passive nature for women, who, if they were to be equal with men, would have to renounce their femininity (The Science of Rights, 1796). But Mary Wollstonecraft in her A Vindication of the Rights of Women (1792), and Mill in his "The Subjection of Women" (1869), offered strong challenges to the traditional inequality of gender roles in society. Marx and Engels critiqued bourgeois marriage as a relationship of economic domination (e.g., in their The Origin of the Family, Private Property and the State, first published by Engels in 1884). Schopenhauer, reacting to feminist agendas, advocated polygamy on the basis of a theory of male needs and female instrumental response (On Women, 1848). Nietzsche, like Schopenhauer, moved away from traditional ethical norms but also reinforced a view of the solely procreative value of women (Thus Spake Zarathustra, 1892).

Twentieth-century European philosophers attempted to construct new meanings for human sexuality in the light of new philosophical theories of freedom and interpersonal love. Jean-Paul Sartre analyzed sexuality as an ontological paradigm for human conflict (Being and Nothingness, 1943); Maurice Merleau-Ponty tried to challenge this and to go beyond it (The Phenomenology of Perception, 1945); Simone de Beauvoir fueled a feminist movement with a stark and revealing analysis of sexism and its influence on the meaning of both gender and sex (The Second Sex, 1949). With the exception of Bertrand Russell (Marriage and Morals, 1929), it was not until the late 1960s that British and American philosophers began to turn their attention to sexual ethics. Then, however, key essays by analytic philosophers began to appear on issues such as sexual desire, gender, marriage, adultery, homosexuality, abortion, sexual perversion, rape, pornography, and sexual abuse (Baker and Elliston, 1975; Shelp, 1987; Soble, 1991). All of these efforts were profoundly influenced by nineteenth- and twentieth-century contributions from other disciplines.

**Freud and psychoanalysis.** The emergence of psychoanalytic theory brought with it new perceptions of the meaning and role of sexuality in the life of individuals. Whatever the final validity of Sigmund Freud's insights, they burst upon the world with a force that all but swept away the foundations of traditional sexual morality. Augustine's and Luther's assertions about the indomitability of sexual desire found support in Freud's theory, but now the power of sexual need was not the result of sin but a natural drive, centrally constitutive of the human personality (*Three Essays on the Theory of Sexuality*, 1905). Past efforts to order sexuality according to rational purposes could now be understood as repression. After Freud, when sex went awry, it was a matter of psychological illness, not moral evil. Taboos needed demythologizing, and freedom might be attained not through forgiveness but through medical treatment.

Yet psychoanalytic theory raised as many questions as it answered. Freud argued for liberation from sexual taboos and from the hypocrisy and sickness they caused, but he nonetheless maintained the need for sexual restraint. His theory of sublimation called for a discipline and channeling of the sexual instinct if the individual and society were to progress (*Civilization and Its Discontents*, 1930). The concern for sexual norms therefore remained, and Freud's own recommendations were in many ways quite traditional. But new work had clearly been cut out for thinkers in both secular and religious traditions.

**Science, social science, and medicine.** Freud was not the only force in nineteenth- and twentieth-century scientific and social thought that shaped changes in Western sexual mores. Biological studies of the human reproductive process offered new perspectives on male and female roles in sex and procreation. Animal research showed that higher forms of animals masturbate, perform sexual acts with members of the same sex, and generally engage in many sexual behaviors that were previously assumed to be unnatural for humans because they were unnatural for animals. Anthropologists found significant variations in the sexual behavior of human cultural groups, so that traditional notions of human nature seemed even more questionable. Surveys of sexual activities in Western society revealed massive discrepancies between accepted sexual norms and actual behavior, undercutting consequential arguments for some of the norms (e.g., the fact that 95% of the male population in the United States engaged in autoerotic acts made it difficult to support a prohibition against masturbation on grounds that it leads to insanity).

Modern sexology, then, has incorporated the work not only of sexual psychology but also of biology, anthropology, ethnology, and sociology—the research and the theories of individuals like Richard von Krafft-Ebing, Havelock Ellis, Magnus Hirschfield, Alfred Kinsey, Margaret Mead, William Masters, and Virginia Johnson. The results have not all been toward greater liberty in sexual behavior, but they have shared a tendency to secularize and medicalize human sexuality. In theory, sex has become less an ethical or even an aesthetic problem than a health problem. In practice, experts of all kinds—physicians, counselors, psychiatrists, social workers, teachers—provide guidance; and the guidance can at least appear to carry moral weight. An example of the intertwining of science, the medical professions, and morality is clear in the long efforts to define and identify sexual deviance or perversion—from Krafft-Ebing in the nineteenth century to the debates in the American Psychiatric Association in the 1970s and 1980s over the classification of homosexuality as a disease.

**Lessons of history.** Historians, too, have played an important role in the weakening of traditional sexual ethical norms. The very disclosure that sexual prescriptions have a history has revealed the contingency of their sources and foundations. To see, for example, that a procreative ethic rose as much from Stoic philosophies as from the Bible has allowed many Christians to question its validity. Feminist retrievals of elements in the Western tradition have led to critiques of taboo moralities and a consequent need for reconstruction. In an effort to make sense of present beliefs, historians have searched for the roots and developments of these beliefs, and the result has seldom been a reinforcement of the original rationales (Foucault, 1978; Boswell, 1980).

But it is not only the history of ideas that has had an impact on contemporary sexual ethics. It is also the historical excavation of the moral attitudes and actual practices of peoples of the past, and an identification of the shifting centers of influence on the sexual mores of different times and places (D'Emilio and Freedman, 1988; Peiss and Simmons, 1989; Fout, 1992). Sometimes referred to as a history of sexuality rather than a history of theories about sexuality or of institutionalized norms for sexuality, this is a task that is barely under way, and it has strong critics. Yet it has already had an impact on, for example, understandings of homosexuality and what can be called the politics of sex. This kind of history also attempts to provide narratives, describing shifts like the one in the United States from family-centered procreative sexual mores to romantic notions of emotional intimacy to a commercialization of sex and its idealization as the central source of human happiness (D'Emilio and Freedman, 1988). The history of sexuality and of sexual ethics, no less than the analysis of contemporary sexual norms, thus becomes subject to interpretation.

## Interpretive theories: Sex, morality, and history

No one may have been more influential in determining current questions about the history of sexuality and sexual ethics than the French philosopher Michel Foucault. His ideas permeate much of the work of other sexual historians as well as philosophers and theologians. Yet his is not the only formative study in the history of sexual ethics, and his conclusions have provoked both positive and negative responses.

**Michel Foucault: A history of desire.** Foucault originally planned to write a history of what he called "the experience of sexuality" in modern Western culture. In the course of his work, he became convinced that what was needed was a history of desire, or of the desiring subject. At the heart of this conviction was the premise that sexuality is not an ahistorical constant. Neither is sex a natural given, a biological referent that simply expresses itself in different experiences of sexuality shaped historically by changing moral norms. Sexuality is, rather, a transfer point for relations of power—between women and men, parents and children, teachers and students, clergy and laity, and so forth. Power in this sense is diffused through a field of multiple "force relations immanent in the sphere in which they operate" (Foucault, 1978, p. 92). In other words, sex is not a "stubborn drive" that requires the control of power. Power produces and constitutes sexual desire much more than it ever represses it. Power determines, shapes, and deploys sexuality, and sexuality determines the meaning of sex (Foucault, 1978).

Foucault denied, then, the "repressive hypothesis" as an explanation of the eighteenth- and nineteenth-century Western experience of sexuality. That is, he denied that the Victorian era had been an era of sexual repression and socially enforced silence about sex. He argued, rather, that it had been a time of an expanding deployment of sexuality and a veritable explosion of discourse about sexuality. The questions that interested him were not "Why are we repressed?" but "Why do we say that we are repressed?" and within this, not "Why was sex associated with sin for such a long time?" but "Why do we burden ourselves today with so much guilt for having made sex a sin?" (Foucault, 1978, pp. 8–9). Since the key to these questions was, Foucault thought, to be found in a study of discourse, he began with an examination of what he considered a Western impulse to discover the "truth" about sex. This, in his view, included a striking Western compulsion to self-examination and self-reporting regarding sexual experience, whether in the discourses of religion, medicine, psychiatry, or criminal justice.

To make sense of the connections between power, sexuality, and truth in the modern period, Foucault revised his project to include a study of the variations on sexual themes in other historical periods. His move to the past began with his thesis that a forerunner of modern discourse on sex was the seventeenth-century Christian ecclesiastical emphasis on confession. To put this in perspective, he undertook studies of pagan antiquity and of Christianity prior to the seventeenth century. Thus, volumes 2 and 3 of his *History of Sexuality* address the sexual mores of the fourth-century B.C.E. Greeks and the first- and second-century C.E. Romans (1990 and 1988, respectively). His unpublished fourth volume (*The Confessions of the Flesh*) examine developments within Christianity. The contrasts (and, as it turned out, the continuities) between the different historical periods shed some light on each period and on the overall Western pursuit of the kind of knowledge that promised power in relation to sex, what Foucault called the *scientia sexualis*.

Foucault came to the conclusion that the sexual morality of the Greeks and Romans did not differ essentially from Christian sexual morality in terms of specific prescriptions. He rejected the commonly held view that the essential contrast between sexual ethics in antiquity and in early Christianity lies in the permissiveness of Graeco-Roman societies as distinguished from the strict sexual rules of the Christians, or in an ancient positive attitude toward sex as distinguished from a negative Christian assessment. Both traditions, he argued, contained prohibitions against incest, a preference for marital fidelity, a model of male superiority, caution regarding same-sex relations, respect for austerity, a positive regard for sexual abstinence, fears of male loss of strength through sexual activity, and hopes of access to special truths through sexual discipline. Nor were these basic prescriptions very different from what could be found in post-seventeenth-century Western society.

Yet there were clear discontinuities, even ruptures, between these historical periods. The reasons for moral solicitude regarding sexuality were different. In Foucault's reading, the ancients were concerned with health, beauty, and freedom, while Christians sought purity of heart before God, and bourgeois moderns aimed at their own self-idealization. The Greeks valued self-mastery; Christians struggled for self-understanding; and modern Western individuals scrutinized their feelings in order to secure compliance with standards of normality. Eroticism was channeled toward boys for the Greeks, women for the Christians, and a centrifugal movement in many directions for the Victorian and post-Victorian middle class. The Greeks feared the enslavement of the mind by the body; Christians dreaded the chaotic power of corrupted passion; post-nineteenth-century persons feared deviance and its consequent shame. Sexual morality was an aesthetic ideal, a personal choice, for an elite in antiquity; it became a universal ethical obligation under Christianity; and it was exacted as a social requirement under the power of the family and the management of the modern professional.

Foucault's study of the history of sexuality left open a question with which he had become preoccupied: How did contemporary Western culture come to believe that sexuality was the key to individual identity? How did sex become more important than love, and almost more important than life? He exposed the lack of freedom in past constructs of sexuality, and he critiqued past formulations of sexual prescriptions. But his presentation of current strategies for sexual liberation yielded no less skeptical a judgment. It suggested, rather, that however historically relative sexual ethics may be, moral solicitude regarding sexuality is not entirely a mistake.

**Catharine MacKinnon: A history of gendered violence.** Many Western feminists have shared Foucault's convictions that sexuality is socially constructed and the body is a site of power. Like Foucault, they have exposed continuing roles of medicine, education, and psychology in determining post-eighteenth-century sexual mores. With Foucault, they have emphasized discourse as a key to identifying underlying forces that link power, sexuality, and identity. But feminists fault Foucault for not extending his analytics of power to gender. Legal scholar Catharine MacKinnon, for example, opposes a Foucaultian history of desire on the grounds that the unacknowledged desiring subject is male. A history of sexuality that emphasizes sexual desire and change misses the enduring aspects of history—the unrelenting sexual abuse of women. History, then, remains silent regarding sexual exploitation, harassment, battery, and rape. Without attention to these unchanging experiences of women, MacKinnon argues, there can be no accurate analysis of sex and power.

A feminist theory of sexuality, according to MacKinnon, "locates sexuality within a theory of gender inequality" (1989, p. 127). It is a mistake, therefore, to adopt the stance that what sex needs is socially constructed freedom, that all sex can be good—healthy, appropriate, pleasurable, to be approved and expressed—if only it is liberated from ideologies of allowed/not allowed. Since sexuality is socially constructed not by a diffuse multiplicity of powers (in Foucault's sense) but by hegemonic male power, it is culturally determined as violent toward women. Pornography is a means through which this social construction is achieved.

Although not all feminists share MacKinnon's radical critique of historical and contemporary sexual understandings and practices, there is significant agreement that sexuality needs norms, and that past and present norms require gender analysis and critique. From this standpoint, a Foucaultian treatment of male discourse regarding sexuality perpetuates a view of sexuality as eroticized dominance and submission; it fails to expose this conflict as gendered.

**Evolutionary interpretations.** Foucault and MacKinnon represent interpretations of the history of sexuality and sexual ethics that deny any progress. They refuse to applaud advances in understandings of sexuality or to sanctify the present as enlightened and free. To some extent, they even reject notions of change in history—Foucault arguing for different, but not causally connected, historical perspectives; and MacKinnon focusing on similarities across time and cultures—indeed, a failure to change. Others, however, have charted an evolutionary process across the Western history of ideas about sex and the moral norms that should govern it. Those who believe that contemporary sexual revolutions have liberated persons and their sexual possibilities belong in this category. So do those who acknowledge the significance of advances in biology and psychology and call for appropriate adjustments in philosophical and theological ethics. Thoughtful commentators do not necessarily conclude that there has been real progress, though they identify evolutionary changes (Green, 1992; Shelp, 1987; Soble, 1991).

Richard Posner belongs to this latter group, offering what he calls an "economic theory of sexuality" (Posner, 1992). That is, he relies heavily on economic analysis both to describe the practice of sex and to evaluate legal and ethical norms in its regard. There are, he argues, three stages in the evolution of sexual morality. These stages correlate with the status of women in a given society (Posner, 1992). In the first stage, women's occupation is that of "simple breeder." When this is the case, companionate marriage is an unlikely possibility, and practices that are considered "immoral" are likely to flourish (e.g., prostitution, adultery, homosexual liaisons).

The second stage begins when women's occupations expand to include "child rearer and husband's companion." Here, companionate marriage is a possibility, and because of this, "immoral" practices that endanger it are vehemently condemned. When companionate marriage is idealized as the only possibility for everyone, societies become puritanical in their efforts to promote and protect it. In the third stage, women's roles are enlarged to include "market employment." Marriages will be fewer, but where they exist, they will be companionate. Other forms of sexual relationship, previously considered immoral, no longer appear to be either immoral or abnormal. This stage characterizes some Western societies more than others—notably, according to Posner, contemporary Sweden.

A very different kind of evolutionary theory can be found in the philosopher Paul Ricoeur's analysis of the symbolism of evil in Western history (Ricoeur, 1967). In this analysis, the Greco–Hebraic history of the consciousness of evil has three moments or stages: defilement, sin, and guilt. The sense of defilement is a pre-ethical, irrational, quasi-material sense of something that infects by contact. Sin is a sense of betrayal, of rupture in a relationship. And guilt is the subjective side of sin, a consciousness that the breakdown of a relationship is the result of an evil use of freedom. According to Ricoeur, sexual morality has appeared historically paradigmatic of the experience of defilement. This association has not been left behind; there remains in the implicit consciousness of the West an inarticulable but persistent connection between sexuality and evil. The result is that ethical wisdom regarding sexuality has remained far behind other developments in Western ethics, even though there has been a significant demythologizing of sex.

## Contemporary ethical reconstruction

The turn to history may have relativized much of traditional sexual ethics, but the motivation for the turn is more complicated. Given all the factors that have helped to weaken traditional sexual norms, ethical reflection has been left with very little anchorage. Science and medicine help, but they sometimes add to human suffering experienced in relation to sex. Philosophy and religion find their traditions struggling for relevance, for clarity, for reasonable guidance and more than reasoned inspiration. The turn to history has been an effort to find a truth that continues to be elusive. And history, like other disciplinary efforts, has probably both helped and heightened the need for the quest.

Contemporary efforts in sexual ethics recognize multiple meanings for human sexuality—pleasure, reproduction, communication, love, conflict, social stability, and so on. Most of those who labor at sexual ethics recognize the need to guide sexual behavior in ways that preserve its potential for good and restrict its potential for evil. Safety, nonviolence, equality, autonomy, mutuality, and truthfulness are generally acknowledged as required for minimal human justice in sexual relationships. Many think that care, responsibility, commitment, love, and fidelity are also required, or at least included as goals. With social construction no longer ignored, the politics of sex has become an ethical matter for persons and societies, institutions and professions. New questions press regarding the ways in which humanity is to reproduce itself and the responsibilities it has for its offspring. In all of this, sexual ethics asks,

How is it appropriate—helpful and not harmful, creative and not destructive—to live and to relate to one another as sexual beings?

MARGARET A. FARLEY

*Directly related to this entry are the entries* HUMAN NATURE; *and* MARRIAGE AND OTHER DOMESTIC PARTNERSHIPS. *For a further discussion of topics mentioned in this entry, see the entries* FEMINISM; HOMOSEXUALITY, *article on* ETHICAL ISSUES; PSYCHOANALYSIS AND DYNAMIC THERAPIES; *and* SEXUALITY IN SOCIETY. *This entry will find application in the entries* REPRODUCTIVE TECHNOLOGIES, *article on* ETHICAL ISSUES; SEX THERAPY AND SEX RESEARCH; *and* SEXUAL ETHICS AND PROFESSIONAL STANDARDS. *For a discussion of related ideas, see the entries* ABUSE, INTERPERSONAL, *article on* ABUSE BETWEEN DOMESTIC PARTNERS; FAMILY; GENDER IDENTITY AND GENDER-IDENTITY DISORDERS; MEDICAL ETHICS, HISTORY OF, *section on* EUROPE; SEXISM; SEXUAL DEVELOPMENT; SEXUAL IDENTITY; WOMEN, *article on* HISTORICAL AND CROSS-CULTURAL PERSPECTIVES. *Other relevant material may be found under the entries* ETHICS, *article on* SOCIAL AND POLITICAL THEORIES; FERTILITY CONTROL, *article on* ETHICAL ISSUES; INTERPRETATION; JUDAISM; PROSTITUTION; PROTESTANTISM; PUBLIC HEALTH AND THE LAW, *article on* LEGAL MORALISM AND PUBLIC HEALTH; ROMAN CATHOLICISM; *and* VALUE AND VALUATION. *See also the entry* NATURAL LAW.

## Bibliography

BAKER, ROBERT, and ELLISTON, FREDERICK, eds. 1975. *Philosophy & Sex.* Buffalo, N.Y.: Prometheus.

BIALE, DAVID. 1992. *Eros and the Jews: From Biblical Israel to Contemporary America.* New York: Basic Books.

BOROWITZ, EUGENE B. 1969. *Choosing a Sex Ethic: A Jewish Inquiry.* New York: Schocken.

BOSWELL, JOHN. 1980. *Christianity, Social Tolerance, and Homosexuality.* Chicago: University of Chicago Press.

BROWN, PETER. 1988. *The Body and Society: Men, Women, and Sexual Renunciation in Early Christianity.* New York: Columbia University Press.

CURRAN, CHARLES E., and McCORMICK, RICHARD A. 1993. *Dialogue About Catholic Sexual Teaching.* New York: Paulist Press.

D'EMILIO, JOHN, and FREEDMAN, ESTELLE B. 1988. *Intimate Matters: A History of Sexuality in America.* New York: Harper & Row.

EPSTEIN, LOUIS M. 1967. [1948]. *Sex Laws and Customs in Judaism.* New York: Block. Reprint. New York: KTAV.

FELDMAN, DAVID M. 1974. [1968]. *Marital Relations, Birth Control, and Abortion in Jewish Law.* New York: Schocken Books.

FOUCAULT, MICHEL. 1978. *The History of Sexuality.* Vol. 1, An Introduction. Translated by Robert Hurley. New York: Pantheon.

———. 1986. *The History of Sexuality.* Vol. 2, *The Use of Pleasure.* Translated by Robert Hurley. New York: Vintage.

———. 1988. *The History of Sexuality.* Vol. 3, *The Care of the Self.* Translated by Robert Hurley. New York: Vintage.

FOUT, JOHN C., ed. 1992. *Forbidden History: The State, Society, and the Regulation of Sexuality in Modern Europe.* Chicago: University of Chicago Press.

GREEN, RONALD M., ed. 1992. *Religion and Sexual Health: Ethical, Theological, and Clinical Perspectives.* Dordrecht, Netherlands: Kluwer.

GREENBERG, DAVID F. 1988. *The Construction of Homosexuality.* Chicago: University of Chicago Press.

LAMM, MAURICE. 1980. *The Jewish Way in Love and Marriage.* San Francisco: Harper & Row.

MACKINNON, CATHARINE A. 1989. *Toward A Feminist Theory of the State.* Cambridge, Mass.: Harvard University Press.

NELSON, JAMES B. 1978. *Embodiment: An Approach to Sexuality and Christian Theology.* Minneapolis, Minn.: Augsburg.

NOONAN, JOHN T., JR. 1986. *Contraception: A History of Its Treatment by the Catholic Theologians and Cannonists.* Enlarged ed. Cambridge, Mass.: Harvard University Press.

NOVAK, DAVID. 1992. "Some Aspects of Sex, Society, and God in Judaism." In *Jewish Social Ethics,* pp. 84–103. New York: Oxford University Press.

PEISS, KATHY, and SIMMONS, CHRISTINA, eds. (with ROBERT A. PADGUG). 1989. *Passion and Power: Sexuality in History.* Philadelphia: Temple University Press.

PLASKOW, JUDITH. 1990. *Standing Again at Sinai: Judaism from a Feminist Perspective.* San Francisco: Harper San Francisco.

POSNER, RICHARD A. 1992. *Sex and Reason.* Cambridge, Mass.: Harvard University Press.

RICOEUR, PAUL. 1967. *The Symbolism of Evil.* New York: Harper & Row.

SHELP, EARL E., ed. 1987. *Sexuality and Medicine.* 2 vols. Dordrecht, Netherlands: D. Reidel.

SOBLE, ALAN, ed. 1991. *The Philosophy of Sex: Contemporary Readings.* 2d ed. Savage, Md.: Rowman & Littlefield.

# SEXUAL ETHICS AND PROFESSIONAL STANDARDS

The Hippocratic oath gives early expression to a general prohibition against professionals taking advantage of the vulnerability of clients or patients and their families to enter into sexual relations: "Whatever house I may visit, I will come for the benefit of the sick, remaining free of all intentional injustice, of all mischief and in particular of sexual relations with both female and male persons, be they free or slaves" (Verhey, 1987, p. 72). The prohibition was reiterated for mental-health professionals by Sigmund Freud (Schoener et al., 1989). From these roots grows a general prohibition against professional–client sexual relations, including relations between teacher and student, supervisor and supervised, clergy and parishioner, therapist and client, and physician and patient. In some professions, the taboo has been so strong that sexuality is the problem professionals "don't talk about" (Rassieur, 1976) or "the problem with no name" (Davidson, 1977).

Yet some famous therapists (e.g., Carl Jung) have been notorious for having sexual relations with their clients (Schoener et al., 1989). Studies of various professions indicate a rate of sexual contact between professionals and clients or patients of between 5 and 11 percent (Schoener et al., 1989; Bonavoglia, 1992). The phenomenon has become sufficiently widespread to be called a "national disgrace" (Pope and Bouhoutsos, 1986) and an "epidemic" (Rutter, 1989).

In the ten years following the publication of *Betrayal* (Freeman and Roy, 1976), which described one woman's successful lawsuit over sexual misconduct by a psychiatrist, over $7 million was paid out in legal claims. In the face of revelations of misconduct, professional societies began to insert clear prohibitions into their codes: "sexual intimacies with clients are unethical" (American Psychological Association, 1981); "the social worker should under no circumstances engage in sexual activities with clients" (National Association of Social Workers, 1980); "sexual relations between analyst and patient are antithetic to treatment and unacceptable under any circumstance" (American Psychoanalytic Association, 1983). Even in the controversial field of sex therapy, direct sexual contact between therapist and client is discouraged; sexual surrogates are used instead (Masters et al., 1977).

Several jurisdictions have enacted laws making it a felony for a psychotherapist (including clergy) to have sexual contact with a client, and at least one holds the therapist's employer liable if the employer knew or should have known of a history of sexual abuse (Bonavoglia, 1992; for statutes, see Schoener et al., 1989). Sexual contact is variously defined, but generally includes not only sexual intercourse but also intimate touching and other sexualizing of the relationship.

The prohibition against professional–client sexual contact rests on three foundations: the likelihood of great harm from the sexual contact, the responsibility of the professional to work for the good of the client, and the vulnerability of the client and the power gap between client and professional, which raises questions even in the absence of demonstrable harm.

There is growing consensus that significant harm is done to patients or clients who enter sexual relations with professionals in whom they have vested trust: "[T]he balance of the empirical findings is heavily weighted in the direction of serious harm resulting to almost all patients sexually involved with their therapists" (Pope and Bouhoutsos, 1986, p. 63). A few therapists have argued for the beneficial effects of sexual relations between therapist and client (Shepard, 1971; Schoener et al., 1989), but their data have been challenged (Pope and Bouhoutsos, 1986; Schoener et al., 1989). Studies of women who have had sexual relations with their gynecologists, psychotherapists, and clergy all point to deleterious consequences including loss of trust, poor self-concept, loss of confidence in one's judgment, and difficulty establishing subsequent relationships (Pope and Bouhoutsos, 1986). Several commentators have noted the similarities to incest because of the power of the professional and have argued that the consequences are as deleterious as those of incest (e.g., Fortune, 1989). Others note that women who enter relations with therapists often have a history of sexual abuse, and thus are being revictimized (Rutter, 1989; Pope and Bouhoutsos, 1986).

Sexual contact between professional and client thus subverts the legitimate goal of the profession—the healing or making whole of one who is wounded and vulnerable (Verhey, 1987). There is both exploitation of the client for benefit of the professional and a failure to provide the services implied by the professional role.

However, harm and failure to help are not the only ethical issues at stake. Several commentators argue that the power of the professional is morally relevant (Lebacqz, 1985; Lebacqz and Barton, 1991). Professionals may hold several types of power: Asclepian power—the power of professional training; charismatic power—the power of personal magnetism and authority; social power—the power of the role and its authority (Brody, 1992). By contrast, the client lacks the power of the role and of its associated training. In addition, female clients facing male professionals generally lack the social power that men have in a sexist context (Lebacqz, 1985; Lebacqz and Barton, 1991). Clients are vulnerable.

The vulnerability of clients and the power of professionals mean that professionals can take advantage of clients. Sexual relations between professional and client are therefore an abuse of professional power—an illegitimate use of that power for the professional's own ends instead of for the ends of healing the client (Lebacqz and Barton, 1991; Schoener et al., 1989; Rutter, 1989; Fortune, 1989).

Moreover, the vulnerability of patients or clients and the power gap between client and professional may compromise the freedom needed to give truly informed consent for sexual intimacies (Pope and Bouhoutsos, 1986; Lebacqz and Barton, 1991). The psychotherapeutic notion of transference (redirecting childhood feelings toward a new object) suggests a special vulnerability that may literally paralyze patients, making them unable to resist a therapist's advances (Freeman and Roy, 1976). Noting special vulnerabilities in the sexual

arena, Karen Lebacqz and Ronald Barton (1991) propose that *sexual* intimacies differ from other acts to which patients, clients, and parishioners might continue to consent.

Some argue that vulnerability does not end when therapy ends and that there should be a prohibition on posttherapy sexual contact (Schoener et al., 1989; Rutter, 1989). John C. Gonsiorek and Laura S. Brown proposed that sexual relations posttherapy should never be permitted where there was significant transference or where the client was severely disturbed, but might be permitted after two years with former clients who were not disturbed and showed little transference (Gonsiorek and Brown, 1989). Such a proposal raises difficult issues regarding who would make this judgment, but it reflects a clear principle that the base for determining whether sexual relations are permissible is the relative power and vulnerability of professional and client. Sexual contact might not be wrong where the power gap is minimized. Although few codes of professional ethics address the posttherapy issue, in 1993, the American Psychiatric Association explicitly addressed it: "Sexual activity with a current or former patient is unethical" (APA, 1993).

In a similar vein, Lebacqz and Barton (1991) argue that romantic or sexual relations might be acceptable under circumstances where the power of professional and client is relatively equal and the relationship is under public scrutiny—for example, when clergy date parishioners with whom they are not involved in a pastoral counseling relationship and members of the church are informed.

All commentators agree, however, that "sexualizing . . . therapy is a betrayal of a trusting relationship" (Pope and Bouhoutsos, 1986, p. 54) and that no sexual relationship should be permitted where there is a counseling or therapeutic relationship involved (Pope and Bouhoutsos, 1986; Fortune, 1989; Rutter, 1989). The professional–client relationship that involves psychotherapy or particular vulnerability on the part of the client is a "forbidden zone" for sexuality (Rutter, 1989).

Professional–client sexual contact must be addressed on institutional, not just personal, levels. Professional societies and supporting organizations such as churches are complicit when they fail to punish offenders, try to cover up the problem, blame the victim, and otherwise minimize the issue (Fortune, 1989; Bonavoglia, 1992). Underreporting is a significant issue: 65 percent of therapists in one study had seen clients who were sexually abused by a previous therapist; they judged that abuse harmful in 87 percent of cases but reported it in only 8 percent (Schoener et al., 1989). Peter Rutter acknowledges the reluctance of men to blow the whistle on each other (Rutter, 1989). Gary Richard Schoener notes that the professional literature "documents more in the way of inaction than of active and creative study leading toward solutions" (Schoener et al., 1989). Professional misconduct damages the profession and institutions as well as individuals (Fortune, 1989). Lack of internal regulation within the professions has led some U.S. state legislatures (e.g., Minnesota) to pass laws that hold institutions as well as individuals responsible for sexual misconduct of professionals (Lebacqz and Barton, 1991).

Underlying social and cultural patterns—sexism, the eroticization of domination, and the maldistribution of power in society—are causal factors (Lebacqz and Barton, 1991; Rutter, 1989). Since Phyllis Chesler's early feminist exposé of therapy in *Women and Madness* (1972), feminists have paid attention to the ways in which traditional therapy often reinforces passive and self-destructive behaviors for women, including behaviors that would make women likely victims of sexual abuse. Dynamics of sexual contact cannot be understood without recognizing sex-role patterning and power imbalances in the general culture (Schoener et al., 1989; Lebacqz and Barton, 1991; Brown and Bohn, 1989). Evidence indicates, for example, that male clients may not experience the sexualizing of relationships to be as harmful as female clients do (Pope and Bouhoutsos, 1986). Such gender differences may reflect social patterning of male and female sexuality, in which men gain and women lose power when entering a sexual relationship. There is also evidence that women therapists do not engage in sexual contact with clients as frequently as male therapists do, and that they judge it more harmful (Schoener et al., 1989).

The traditional prohibition against sexual contact between professionals and their clients continues to be reaffirmed in spite of arguments and practices to the contrary. An adequate ethical framework requires attention not only to professional responsibility, harm, and power imbalances but also to institutional structures and to cultural dynamics of sexuality and power.

KAREN LEBACQZ

*For a further discussion of topics mentioned in this entry, see the entries* FEMINISM; GENDER IDENTITY AND GENDER-IDENTITY DISORDERS; SEXISM; SEX THERAPY AND SEX RESEARCH; SEXUAL ETHICS; SEXUAL IDENTITY; PROFESSIONAL–PATIENT RELATIONSHIP, *article on* ETHICAL ISSUES; PROFESSION AND PROFESSIONAL ETHICS; PSYCHOANALYSIS AND DYNAMIC THERAPIES; *and* WOMEN, *article on* HEALTH-CARE ISSUES. *For a discussion of related ideas, see the entries* AUTHORITY; FREEDOM AND COERCION; HARM; HEALING; *and* INFORMED CONSENT. *See also the* APPENDIX (CODES, OATHS, AND DIRECTIVES RELATED TO BIOETHICS), SECTION II: ETHICAL DIRECTIVES FOR THE PRACTICE OF MEDICINE, *especially* OATH OF HIPPOCRATES.

## Bibliography

AMERICAN PSYCHOLOGICAL ASSOCIATION. 1981. *Ethical Principles of Psychologists.* Washington, D.C.: Author.

BONAVOGLIA, ANGELA. 1992. "The Sacred Secret." *Ms.,* March–April, pp. 40–45.

BRODY, HOWARD. 1992. *The Healer's Power.* New Haven, Conn.: Yale University Press.

BROWN, JOANNE CARLSON, and BOHN, CAROLE R., eds. 1989. *Christianity, Patriarchy, and Abuse: A Feminist Critique.* New York: Pilgrim Press.

BURGESS, ANN W., and HARTMAN, CAROL R., eds. 1986. *Sexual Exploitation of Patients by Health Professionals.* New York: Praeger.

CHESLER, PHYLLIS. 1972. *Women and Madness.* New York: Avon Books.

DAVIDSON, VIRGINIA. 1977. "Psychiatry's Problem with No Name: Therapist–Patient Sex." *American Journal of Psychoanalysis* 37, no. 1:43–50.

FORTUNE, MARIE M. 1983. *Sexual Violence: The Unmentionable Sin.* New York: Pilgrim Press.

———. 1989. *Is Nothing Sacred? When Sex Invades the Pastoral Relationship.* San Francisco: Harper & Row.

FREEMAN, LUCY, and ROY, JULIE. 1976. *Betrayal: The True Story of the First Woman to Successfully Sue Her Psychiatrist for Using Sex in the Guise of Therapy.* New York: Stein and Day.

GABBARD, GLEN O., ed. 1989. *Sexual Exploitation in Professional Relationships.* Washington, D.C.: American Psychiatric Press.

GONSIOREK, JOHN C., and BROWN, LAURA S. 1989. "Post Therapy Sexual Relationships with Clients." In *Psychotherapists' Sexual Involvement with Clients: Intervention and Prevention,* pp. 289–301. Edited by Gary Richard Schoerer et al. Minneapolis, Minn.: Walk-in Counseling Center.

LEBACQZ, KAREN. 1985. *Professional Ethics: Power and Paradox.* Nashville, Tenn.: Abingdon.

LEBACQZ, KAREN, and BARTON, RONALD G. 1991. *Sex in the Parish.* Louisville, Ky.: Westminster/John Knox.

MASTERS, WILLIAM H.; JOHNSON, VIRGINIA E.; and KOLODNY, ROBERT C., eds. 1977. *Ethical Issues in Sex Therapy and Research.* Boston: Little, Brown.

NATIONAL ASSOCIATION OF SOCIAL WORKERS. 1980. *Compilation of Public Policy Statements.* Washington, D.C.: Author.

PLASIL, ELLEN. 1985. *Therapist: The Shocking Autobiography of a Woman Sexually Exploited by Her Analyst.* New York: St. Martin's/Marek.

POPE, KENNETH S., and BOUHOUTSOS, JACQUELINE C. 1986. *Sexual Intimacy Between Therapists and Patients.* New York: Praeger.

RASSIEUR, CHARLES L. 1976. *The Problem Clergymen Don't Talk About.* Philadelphia: Westminster.

RUTTER, PETER. 1989. *Sex in the Forbidden Zone.* Los Angeles: Jeremy P. Tarcher.

SANDERSON, BARBARA E., ed. 1989. *It's Never O.K.: A Handbook for Professionals on Sexual Exploitation by Counselors and Therapists.* St. Paul: Minnesota Department of Corrections.

SCHOENER, GARY RICHARD; MILGRAM, JEANETTE HOFSTEE; GONSIOREK, JOHN C.; LUEPKER, ELLEN T.; and CONROE, RAY M. 1989. *Psychotherapists' Sexual Involvement with Clients: Intervention and Prevention.* Minneapolis, Minn.: Walk-in Counseling Center.

SHEPARD, MARTIN. 1971. *The Love Treatment: Sexual Intimacy Between Patients and Psychotherapists.* New York: Peter H. Wyden.

VERHEY, ALLEN. 1987. "The Doctor's Oath—and a Christian Swearing It." In *On Moral Medicine: Theological Perspectives in Medical Ethics,* pp. 72–82. Edited by Stephen E. Lammers and Allen Verhey. Grand Rapids, Mich.: William B. Eerdmans.

# SEXUAL IDENTITY

Because some terms are deeply embroiled in controversial debates, the task of defining them itself becomes controversial. So it is with the term "sexual identity." Providing any definition immediately situates the definer within a particular perspective. One important perspective, which has served as the backdrop of much contemporary discussion, claims that the term refers to the distinct biological types of "male" and "female." This "traditionalist" definition of "sexual identity" has sometimes been associated with one or more of the following additional positions: that certain specific and "complementary" psychological attributes and social roles, specifically those of "masculinity" and "femininity," correspond to each of these distinct biological types; that a "natural" sexual attraction exists between these two biological types; that this attraction is most naturally satisfied through the act of intercourse; and that the act of intercourse, while naturally motivated by attraction, should also be motivated by other concerns, most importantly love and the desire to have children within the context of marriage.

One or all of these claims have been challenged over the last few decades by feminists; by those advocating various forms of sexual liberation; by gays and lesbians; and by scholars influenced (or not) by these movements. All of these challenges raise questions about what we mean by "sexual identity." Some of the positions developed in response to the above set of views have themselves been challenged. For the sake of clarity, we can group the challenges and counterchallenges around the following set of questions:

1. The sex question: Are there really two distinct biological types, "male" and "female"?
2. The gender question: How should we think about the relationship between biology and psychological attributes and forms of behavior?
3. The question of sexuality: What constitutes sexual desire? What are the various ways in which it can be characterized?
4. The question of sexual ethics: How ought we to think about sexual practices? Which, if any, should be condoned, which prohibited, and why?

## Sex

Over the past few decades, many have come to disbelieve the claim that there exist two sexes without gradations. Some feminists have argued that, biologically, it is more useful to think of many of the physical characteristics associated with sexual difference as manifested across the human species in a range of degrees, rather than as being associated exclusively with either sex. They claim that only a social desire to emphasize difference has caused us to think of such variations in stark, bipolar ways. Thus, for example, though we often think of men as "bigger" than women, many individual women are taller, heavier, longer limbed, and so forth, than many men. Similarly, while we tend to think of women and men as possessing very distinctive hormones, in actuality the situation is more complex. For example, the hormones estrogen and androgen are often thought of as the "female" and "male" hormones, respectively, suggesting that men have one and women the other. In reality, both hormones are found in both women and men, and after menopause, women often exhibit a lower ratio of estrogen to androgen than do men of a comparable age (Spanier, 1993). These feminists argue that many of the striking differences we see are at least partially the consequence of social pressures exerted on women and men to manifest such differences. Thus women are encouraged to remove body hair and to buy shoes that make their feet look as small as possible.

Some cultural historians claim that the view of men and women as possessing sharply differentiated bodies has developed only within the last few centuries. Thomas Laqueur (1990), for example, points out that prior to the eighteenth century, women's bodies were thought of as less developed versions of men's bodies. In this "one-sex" view, the vagina was not thought of as different from the male penis but, rather, as an inverted form of it. But during the eighteenth century, there emerged a view of "the two-sex body," that is, of female and male bodies being fundamentally different. With this new development, organs that had previously been referred to by the same name were given separate names. Thus, what had previously been "the testicles" now became differentiated into "the testicles" and "the ovaries." Others that previously had no name were given names, for example, the vagina. Even parts of the body remote from reproductive functions, such as the skeleton and the nervous system, began to be depicted as distinctive for women and men.

Recent research in biology suggests that differentiating the male from the female is no simple task. Various indicators of "maleness" and "femaleness" are individually sometimes ambiguous. Even when all of the indicators are clear, they do not necessarily cohere. For example, within contemporary science the standard distinguishing criterion has been taken to be the presence or absence of the Y chromosome. Most people possess two sets of chromosomes, one from each parent; females are understood to be those with two X chromosomes and males those with one X chromosome and one Y chromosome. However, there are problems with any neat application of this criterion. Some individuals inherit only one X chromosome but no Y chromosome. Or a piece of a Y chromosome may become attached to an X chromosome, producing an individual with an XXY pattern.

Even those individuals who possess a standard XX or XY pattern may exhibit characteristics that would incline many not to identify them by their chromosomal pattern. An XY individual may have testes that do not secrete the male hormone testosterone, or may have cells that are not sensitive to testosterone. That person will end up looking more like a female than a male (Lowenstein, 1987). There are also XY individuals who look female at birth and are raised as girls, but who develop masculine bodily features at adolescence. There are XX people whose adrenal glands secrete large amounts of male hormones. One consequence is clitoral enlargement, causing them to be taken for boys at birth. As adults they may also possess increased muscle mass and hairiness (Lowenstein, 1987). In short, recent scientific research has supported the point that even the biological distinction between male and female is not always clear-cut.

## Gender

Until the emergence of the second wave of feminism in the 1960s, the term "gender" was used primarily to indicate differences between female and male forms within language. Differences between women and men were commonly indicated by the term "sex," as in the phrase "the battle of the sexes." Feminists, however, began to use the term "gender" to refer to what they argued were socially constructed differences between women and men. It was felt that the term "sex," when applied to differences between women and men, suggested that such differences were biological in origin. A new term was needed to refer to differences that were a product of society.

Studies done within the social sciences pointed to the great differences among societies in expectations of what was appropriate behavior for men and women. For example, the anthropologist Michelle Zimbalist Rosaldo noted that there are some societies where women trade or garden, and others where men do; some where men are prudish and flirtatious, and others where women are (Rosaldo and Lamphere, 1974). Psychologists and other social scientists stressed the importance of socialization in structuring an individual's sense of self. Thus, John Money and Anke Ehrhardt (1972) reported that when children were assigned a gender at birth that did not match their chromosomal sex, it was most likely that their adult sense of self would conform to their assigned gender rather than to their chromosomal sex.

The term "gender" has been very useful in making possible a greater recognition of the social construction of differences between women and men. Recently, however, some scholars have been raising questions about how "gender" should be understood, and particularly how its relationship to "sex" should be interpreted. Using the term "sex" to describe biological differences, and "gender" to describe socially constructed ones, ignores the fact that biological distinctions are themselves social constructions. That modern biology, for example, interprets the penis as an organ distinct from the vagina is a social construction, more a consequence of changing cultural metaphors than of new scientific evidence (Laqueur, 1990).

Another problem is that the relationship between psychological traits and biological phenomena is still often understood to be that the former "follows" from the latter. While "gender" emphasizes that many psychological traits are social constructions, it does not necessarily undermine the view that such traits follow from biological differences. All it adds is that the path from biology to psychology proceeds by way of social construction.

Any model that claims that psychology follows from biology has problems accounting for those individuals whose socialization deviates from the norm. In other words, to the extent that "gender" is still viewed as tied to "sex," we have problems explaining the phenomena of girls who grow up exhibiting "masculine" psychological traits and boys who grow up with a "feminine" sense of self. The most striking examples of such cases are transsexuals, people who experience a dramatic misalignment between their physical features and their internalized sense of self. Such people frequently desire physical restructuring of their bodies to bring the physical and the psychic into alignment.

The term "gender" may still suggest, as did the term "sex," that people's psychic lives and behavior are necessarily unified, that it is appropriate to talk about a male or a female "identity." One suggestion has been that we talk about "gender" not as describing individual identity but as describing acts or performances we all play out (Butler, 1990). Such a model allows us to move the focus of "gender" from the individual to the activity. This type of shift is consistent with an overall tendency on the part of many contemporary scholars to think of "gender" as a type of social coding that is applied not only to behavior but also to psychic stances and to bodies. The recognition that bodies, like behavior, are socially coded in turn undermines the distinction between "sex" and "gender" insofar as the former had been understood as naturally "given" and the latter as the consequence of social construction (Scott, 1988).

## Sexuality

At least since the 1890s in industrialized Western countries, one paradigm of sexuality has been dominant: that which describes as "normal," genital–genital intercourse between one male and one female, and as "abnormal" or "perverse," sexual practices that fall outside that paradigm. "Perverse" practices include but are not limited to the following: voyeurism; exhibitionism; incest (sex between close relatives); oral sex; anal sex; sex with children (pedophilia); sex involving more than two persons; sex between humans and animals (zoophilia); sex with oneself (masturbation); sex involving the use of visual images (pornography); sex with a corpse (necrophilia); transvestism (an individual heightens his or her sexual pleasure by dressing in garments associated with the opposite sex); sex associated with the giving or experiencing of pain or humiliation (sadomasochism); sex strongly associated with a particular object or part of the body (fetishism); and sex between members of the same sex (homosexuality).

Homosexuality has, in particular, been the subject of much attention and debate over the last decades. The stigmatizing label "homosexuality" has been used to negatively characterize certain individuals since the late nineteenth century (Weeks, 1989); laws have been enacted against it and people have been jailed for practicing it (e.g., the English playwright Oscar Wilde). During the twentieth century, medical doctors and other scientific specialists have depicted it as a pathology and, as with other pathologies (but not accepted practices), have searched for causes (Bayer, 1987).

Much debate has centered on the question of whether homosexuality is a product of genetic inheritance or other biology, or is a consequence of socialization. During the 1960s and 1970s, homosexual men (who increasingly adopted the label "gay") and homosexual women (lesbians) began to form political organizations to resist the laws, practices, and beliefs that stigmatized them. They argued that homosexuality was not a perversion or a pathology, to be outlawed or cured, but a difference in preference that should be tolerated within a free and open society. The American psychiatric community has moved away from a description of homosexuality as pathology. In December 1973 the board of trustees of the American Psychiatric Association moved to delete the category "homosexuality" as necessarily a pathology from the second edition of the

*Diagnostic and Statistical Manual of Psychiatric Disorders,* retaining "ego dystonic homosexuality" to cover those not comfortable with their sexual orientation. In yet another revision, any specific reference to homosexuality was removed altogether, but the term "sexual orientation distress" was retained to permit treatment of those disturbed about their sexuality (Bayer, 1987).

Other questions have been added to the debate, among them whether homosexuality describes a particular kind of person or, more appropriate, a specific type of activity. Social historians have pointed out that the category "the homosexual" was constructed in the latter part of the nineteenth century to depict a specific type of person, followed shortly by the construction of "the heterosexual" (Katz, 1983; Halperin, 1990). Prior to the creation of "the homosexual," people who engaged in acts we would label as homosexual were not necessarily seen to require a special label. This is at least partially a consequence of the fact that the sex of one's partner has not always been viewed as an overriding feature of the sex act. For example, within many Native American societies, certain men, "the berdache," took on many of the tasks and characteristics associated with women. These men would have sex with other men. However, what was seen as distinguishing the sexual practices of the berdache was not that they had sex with other men but that they took the passive role in sex. Their male partners were not distinguished from men who had sex only with women (Williams, 1986). For such reasons, Eve Sedgwick has observed that given the many dimensions along which genital activity can be described, it is quite amazing that the sex of object choice has emerged as central during the twentieth century, and has come to define what we mean by "sexual orientation" (Sedgwick, 1990).

How we conceive of sexual practices defines much of our thinking about sexuality. The emphasis on the "normal" practice of heterosexual intercourse implies that sex between persons of the same gender and any sexual activity that does not lead to intercourse will be abnormal or "perverse" (or what Freud called "inverse"). These are not only clinical categories; they often function as strong moral terms of condemnation as well. Thus homosexuality is attacked both as pathology, and as voluntary wrongdoing, by those who see it not only as deviant but also as perverse behavior. The idea that homosexuality is normal sex, and neither pathology nor wrongdoing—an idea that has been widely accepted by many cultures throughout history—is discouraged by the heterosexual paradigm.

## Sexual paradigms

Just as matters of individual sexual identity have been oversimplified into a single male–female dichotomy, the many varieties of sexual behavior have often been reduced to a simple distinction between normality and perversion.

The condemnation of homosexuality and other deviant sexual activities and "perversions" brings us into the realm of sexual ethics and to the question of alternative sexual paradigms. A paradigm is an exemplary instance that serves as a standard. A sexual paradigm is an example of sexual activity that is taken as a standard for "normal" sexual behavior. The most obvious sexual paradigm is heterosexual genital–genital intercourse, but in order to employ this paradigm as a norm, we need to specify not only the overt activity but the aims and desires of the participants as well. Is the purpose of sexual intercourse, for example, to produce children? Or is it just "for fun"? Or an expression of love? Or a "conquest"? We can further distinguish between "minimalist" and "murky" paradigms of sexuality. Minimalist accounts tend to define sexuality as a simple, straightforward desire, while murky accounts dig deeper in order to find hidden or unconscious desires. Thomas Nagel (1969), for example, introduces the minimalist notion of "unadorned sexual intercourse," although he adds that such behavior, "unadorned," may well be perverse, and that a typical sexual encounter involves a complex of communicative gestures. Janice Moulton (1976) defines sexuality simply as the desire for physical contact, although she then provides a rich discussion of its many associated meanings. Alan Goldman (1977) isolates what he calls "plain sex," which he defines as "a desire for contact with another's body," and rejects accounts that try to define sexuality in terms of any further goal or purpose.

On the "murky" side, there is the lasting legacy of Plato's *Symposium* and its various discussions of eros. In particular, there is Aristophanes' famous tale about the divine fission of individual human beings out of complete wholes, according to which sexual desire is nothing less than the impossible desire to join together with "one's other half" and become "complete once again," and Socrates' much more effete conception of eros as the love of Beauty as such. Two thousand years of Christian theology have attempted both to chastise and to spiritualize sexuality, and the Tantric traditions of India and Tibet have refined sexuality into a spiritual road to enlightenment. More recently, Sigmund Freud and Carl Jung profoundly deepened our conceptions of sexuality, which is, in their accounts, no mere desire but a focus for the darkest and most explosive secrets of the psyche.

**The reproductive paradigm.** Biologically, sexuality can be defined in terms of a very specific genetic process, although even that has its ambiguities and confusions. This biological definition and its implied reproductive paradigm play an enormous role in our conceptions of sexuality. Whatever embellishments,

variations, and alternatives we and some of our fellow vertebrates have evolved or invented, heterosexual intercourse remains something of an "original text" in our sexual hermeneutics. It can be rejected, refuted, even reviled, but it must, first of all, be taken account of.

One might distinguish here, in line with a three-thousand-year-old moral tradition, between an individual's purpose and what we might call "nature's purpose." Until the end of the nineteenth century, when teleology or the purposiveness of nature was taken seriously, this phrase could be interpreted literally. Today, in the wake of increasingly antiteleological conceptions of evolution, the phrase "nature's purpose" must be taken as, at best, shorthand for a complex set of causal processes that are themselves the result of chance and natural selection. Even so, one might distinguish between the various drives and desires favored by natural selection because they increase the likelihood of a more adaptive genotype (what Richard Dawkins [1976] calls "the selfish gene"), and the more or less conscious and sometimes articulate desires of an adult human being. But we are not, like most creatures, mere sexual pawns of cunning nature. Some teenagers may not know of the various consequences and the significance of sexual activity, but for most adults this knowledge is profound, if not extensive, and sexuality may never be free of those associations. But whether or not this is the hidden purpose of *all* sexual desire and activity, it is clearly the conscious and conscientious choice of *some* sexual activity. Building a family is not, for most people, the only purpose of sexual activity; but by having sexual intercourse, it is possible to have children. Whatever creative alternatives may be dreamed up by medicine, one undeniable aspect of sexuality is, and will be, its traditional role in procreation.

The view that sexuality and sexual desire are really aimed at reproduction, even if the sexual participants desire only to perform a particular activity without thinking of the consequences, tends to move us from the minimalist view of sexuality to various murky views. The self-evident desires are no longer taken at face value, and a deeper biological (or theological) narrative, which may not be self-evident to the participants, comes into play. Thus the psychological consequences of thousands or millions of years of evolution manifest themselves in desires that may seem straightforward. Or, behind seemingly simple sexual desire lurks the secret of God's creation and the biblical injunction to be fruitful and multiply. But what links all the murky views is that sexuality does have a purpose or purposes, however they are to be explained, and these purposes are typically not self-evident. According to the minimalist views, sex is best understood as "plain" or "unembellished"; the murky views, on the other hand, insist that sex so understood is not understood at all.

**The pleasure paradigm.**    The target of many, if not most, of the minimalist accounts is the restricted reproduction of the "procreative" paradigm of sexual activity. For two thousand years, the harsher side of the Bible and the Christian theological tradition has insisted that sex is primarily, if not solely, procreative. The pleasures and desires associated with sexual activity not only are inessential but also are to be minimized. Emphasizing pleasure to the exclusion of the possibility of reproduction—for example, using contraception or engaging in activity that cannot result in impregnation—is forbidden. Essential to sexuality, in the reproductive paradigm, are male ejaculation, female receptivity, fertility, and conception.

In opposition to the reproductive model, with all of its strict prohibitions and limitations, and its suggestions of deep biological drives and purposes, the attractiveness of what we can call the pleasure paradigm is unmistakable. The availability of improved birth control methods since the 1960s has contributed greatly to its appeal. Sex is for pleasure, and what is desired is pleasure. There is nothing murky about this. Indeed, to many people it is self-evident. Accordingly, the restrictions on sexuality that limit and direct it toward heterosexual intercourse drop away, and in effect, anything that feels good is acceptable. Of course, one might well object that pleasure is not in itself sexual, and so one might want to circumscribe pleasures that are sexual from those that are not. But, for the defender of the pleasure paradigm, this requirement comes later. First comes the liberation from the restrictions of the reproductive model. Homosexuality, autosexuality, even bestiality seem to be normal on the pleasure paradigm. Heterosexual intercourse is but one of many activities serving the paradigm, and however many couples may continue to prefer it, it does not have any special claim to normality. According to this paradigm, good sex is that which provides maximum mutual pleasure; bad or mediocre sex is that which fails to satisfy either or both partners.

Once the reproduction model has been rejected, there are no longer the restrictions on either the objects or the obvious aims of sexual activity, but neither is it the case that "anything goes." Homosexuality is no longer a perversion of sex, but rape certainly will be. Almost any sexual activity between consenting adults is acceptable, but forcing sex on a person is not. Sexual activities that will not result in conception are no longer secondary, and sex that is conscientiously prevented from resulting in undesired conception becomes the norm. Masturbation becomes part of the paradigm of acceptable sexuality, even though its lacks the dimension of shared sexual enjoyment. The appeal of the paradigm and the cornerstone of most contemporary sexual ethics is the idea that sex ought to be pleasurable and, within moral but not particularly sexual bounds, unrestricted.

We might call the pleasure paradigm the "Freudian" model of sexuality, in order to pay homage to the person most responsible for its contemporary dominance. Sigmund Freud, in his *Three Contributions to the Theory of Sex* (1962), argued that sexuality should be conceived as enjoyable for its own sake, not as a means to further ends, whether natural or divine. But the centrality of Freud here also suggests that the pleasure paradigm may not be so simple and self-evident as we originally suggested. Freud is one of the great contemporary architects of "deep," if not labyrinthine, accounts of the psyche and of sexuality in particular. And so, for him and for us, pleasure and satisfaction are not to be construed so straightforwardly. Pleasure, as Aristotle noted more than two millennia ago, is not just a sensation. It is the "bloom" on successful activity. It accompanies but does not constitute satisfaction. But the difficult question is, Satisfaction of what? And here Freud's theory moves from an apparently minimalist physiological model to an extremely murky deep psychology.

In Freud's early theories, the pleasure paradigm rested on a male-dominated biological foundation, a "discharge" model in which sexual pleasure has its origins in the release of tension (catharsis). But the tensions released in sexual behavior are not merely physiological; they also arise from complexes of ego needs and identifications with various sexual "objects," usually (but not always) other people. Thus Freud distinguished, as we still distinguish, between mere physical gratification and "physical satisfaction."

The pleasure paradigm, for all of its seeming simplicity, invites murky interpretations. What is it that is enjoyed? What is it that is satisfied? A sensation is not pleasant in itself but in terms of its context, as a love bite on the shoulder by one's lover or a nasty passerby, respectively, makes evident. Indeed, even orgasm is not pleasant in itself, however often that might be fallaciously supposed; an orgasm in an inappropriate context is typically an extremely unpleasant experience. And so the pleasure Freud postulates is no simple release of tension but the satisfaction, often symbolic and indirect, of some of the murkiest of hidden and forbidden desires.

**The metaphysical paradigm.**    Some of these motives are so profound that they deserve to be called "metaphysical." Freud's discussion of the Oedipus complex sometimes takes on these ontological overtones, and Jung's various archetype theories surely do. But perhaps the most basic of all metaphysical paradigms of sexuality goes back (at least) to the fable told by Aristophanes in Plato's *Symposium,* and the idea that the gods split what we now call human beings out of complete wholes (with sexual desire being the desire to reunify the divided halves). One need not literally accept the more consciously absurd aspects of the story to appreciate the deep insight captured in the idea of "two out of one" or "merged selves" that Plato's Aristophanes is suggesting.

Sexual activity is an expression of a profound desire that has very little to do with merely physiological need or satisfaction, and the metaphysical paradigm is, accordingly, very much a part of the contemporary conceptions of romantic love and the idea that two people were "made for each other."

Indeed, despite the prevalence of the pleasure model in much of the current literature, there can be little doubt that much more is usually demanded of sexuality than mere pleasure, even mutual pleasure. People demand "meaningful" relationships. The metaphysical model provides this sense of "meaning." Pleasure, according to the metaphysical model, is no longer the purpose of sex, although it will surely appear as its accompaniment. But sex without love, no matter how enjoyable, is to be rejected on this paradigm. Even if it is not "perverse" or "immoral," "plain sex" will be meaningless, and the meaning of a relationship is primary for the metaphysical model.

**The communication paradigm.**    Sex is often "meaningful" without love, however, although sometimes those "meanings" are demeaning, as in a sadomasochistic relationship. What is one to say of the many varieties of sexual activity that are aimed neither at reproduction, nor at pure pleasure, nor at expressions of romantic love and togetherness? What of those relationships that seem to thrive on domination and pain? What does it say about our current paradigms of love that sadomasochistic relationships are now celebrated and preferred by some of our more avant-garde social visionaries? And what of those many tender encounters that, nonetheless, make no pretenses of love?

To explain such aspects of sexuality, a fourth paradigm is in order: sex as communication, as a physical form of expression of one's emotions and attitudes toward other people. It is a language, for the most part a body language, whose vocabulary consists of touches, gestures, and physical positions. It may be an expression of domination and submission; it may be an expression of respect, fear, tenderness, anger, admiration, worship, concern, or (of course) love. In the 1940s Jean-Paul Sartre defended a truncated version of this model in his classic *Being and Nothingness*. He interpreted all sexuality as the expression of conflict, a war for domination and freedom. But what is communicated in sex is rarely this alone, nor is sex plausibly always an expression of conflict. Nevertheless, Sartre forces us to see something that the defenders of the pleasure and metaphysical paradigms of sex prefer not to see: that sexual relationships, even normal, fully consensual sexual relationships, are not always innocent or loving. Sex is a medium for all sorts of emotions, some of them manipulative and even malicious.

The communication paradigm shifts the emphasis in sexuality from the more physical and sensual aspects of reproduction and pleasure to interpersonal roles and attitudes, and from expressions of love alone to expressions of all emotions and attitudes. Thus Sartre's model is clearly a communication model, but it is, like Sartre's view of emotions in general, too narrow, emphasizing only the more conflict-ridden and competitive interpersonal attitudes—one of which, he thinks, is love. In this view, certain sexual positions and activities are visibly more expressive of domination and submission, or equality and respect, or resentment and fear, or shyness and timidity. According to the communication model, these nonverbal expressions are essential to sexuality, its very purpose and content. This does not mean, however, that other sexual aspects need be excluded. The intention to impregnate a woman, for example, may be an expression of male domination and conquest, as in several of Normal Mailer's novels. Pleasure is quite obviously an important aspect of the communication model, but pleasure for its own sake is not. Pleasure—both the giving and the receiving of it, as well as the sharing of it—is vital to the communication of many emotions. But pain may be important as well, and inflicting small amounts of pain, as well as enduring moderate discomfort, is familiar as a means of expression in sex. What distinguishes the communication paradigm from the three more traditional ones is its emphasis on expression of interpersonal emotions and attitudes. These expressions are recognized by the other paradigms, but not as essential and primary.

Now it is evident that the answers to such questions as "What is normal sex?" and "What is perverse?" become immensely complicated. On a strict reproduction paradigm of sexuality, normal sex is whatever minimal genital activity is necessary to promote conception. All else is either irrelevant or immoral. In fact, of course, the reproduction paradigm is usually defended within the moral institution of marriage, and rarely defended without some reference to both love and mutual pleasure. On the pleasure paradigm, by contrast, whatever gives pleasure (to consenting adults) is normal and acceptable. Perversions of this paradigm provide pain instead of pleasure, ignore the pleasure of the other person, or produce pleasure in a manner that is, in the longer run, harmful. On the metaphysical paradigm, normality is sex as an expression of mutual meaningfulness such as mutual love. On the communication paradigm, what is normal becomes extremely complex, for one must view the emotions being expressed and the entire psyches of the people involved to make any intelligent judgment.

Human sexuality seems particularly appropriate for expressing the tender feelings of love and affection, but there are circumstances under which this is absolutely inappropriate (for example, with children); and all too often sexual activity that claims the expression of love as its aim may actually be an avoidance of intimacy. Indeed, the very context of sexual activity—two people alone, attending only to one another—is particularly conducive to intimate communication. What would be a perversion on this paradigm? Perhaps any form of deceit would be, just as lying is a "perversion" of verbal communication. And masturbation, while not exactly perverse, would surely be less than wholly sexual, just as talking to oneself is less than a whole conversation.

## Conclusion: The problem of normality

So long as biological specification and sexual intercourse alone define sexuality, "normality," as opposed to "perversion," seems to be easily defined. Males are equipped with certain obvious features, and females are differently equipped with equally obvious sexual features; and "normal" sex is intercourse between male and female. But as more is learned about the complexities of chromosome configuration and the biology of sex, the distinction between male and female—although usually still clear enough—becomes increasingly difficult. And as soon as one adds the essential concerns of psychology and the many worlds of cultural norms, practices, and paradigms to the unfolding medical complications, the traditional view of "normality" becomes a Pandora's box of problems.

This confusion extends to the task of defining a "normal" model of sexuality. Of the various cases and models we have considered, not a single one would be accepted as "normal" in every society and by everyone. Moreover, a pure instance of an ideal type or paradigm is probably nowhere to be found; not even the most pious proponent of a religiously oriented reproductive view would deny the desirability of love, pleasure, and emotional expression in sex, nor would the most enthusiastic hedonist deny the desirability of reproduction on at least some occasions, and perhaps of love and communication as well. And when these four models of sexuality are integrated with the matrix of possibilities that are to be found in the various combinations of gender identity and sexual orientation (and, in the most extreme cases, transsexual biological operations), the result is an enormous number of sexual lifestyles, desires, and activities, every one of which would be insisted upon as "normal," at least according to some people.

How does one decide what is normal and what is not? In one sense, "normal" simply means "statistically predominant," and there are still many people who would insist that this is a proper definition. But it is clear that, in ethical contexts, "normal" also means morally "correct." But in an area where most behavior is private, and involves only consenting adults and a great many individual differences, the relevance of statistics is easily challenged. Furthermore, what is statistically predominant in one portion of a population may be relatively rare and considered "perverted" in another. If sexual normality includes subjective preferences and psychological as well as biological considerations, then any definition of sexual normality will give priority to certain preferences and paradigms over others. But which ones? The traditional religious standards? The more modern "anything goes between consenting adults" attitude? The current "local standards" criterion of the courts, which assumes that it can be made clear how large or small a domain—a home, a town, or a state—is "local"?

The problem of normality thus becomes a dilemma. It begins with a built-in ambiguity between the statistically dominant and what ethically ought to be. The first is ascertained easily enough, assuming either truthful informants or extremely intrusive investigators; but the second, the quest for a sexual ethics, arises from within diverse psychological, cultural, and personal settings that presuppose many of the norms and attitudes that are to be investigated.

The result of these complexities should not be the abandonment of a search for ethical norms or the rejection of the concepts of normality and perversion. What emerges instead is an extremely complex matrix of considerations to be taken into account, in which tolerance is a wise approach and mutual understanding is the desirable outcome. In other words, what is needed in the examination of sexual identity is not just a good deal of medicine, biology, social psychology, and anthropology. It is also a good deal of appreciation for diversity and complexity. It is with this appreciation for diversity and complexity that the contemporary quest can proceed.

ROBERT C. SOLOMON
LINDA J. NICHOLSON

*Directly related to this entry are the entries* GENDER IDENTITY AND GENDER-IDENTITY DISORDERS; HOMOSEXUALITY; HUMAN NATURE; SEXUAL ETHICS; SEXUALITY IN SOCIETY; *and* BODY, *article on* SOCIAL THEORIES. *For a further discussion of topics mentioned in this entry, see the entries* FERTILITY CONTROL, *article on* SOCIAL ISSUES; GENETICS AND HUMAN SELF-UNDERSTANDING; LAW AND MORALITY; LOVE; *and* PSYCHOANALYSIS AND DYNAMIC THERAPIES. *For a discussion of related ideas, see the entries* FEMINISM; *and* SEX THERAPY AND SEX RESEARCH. *Other relevant material may be found under the entry* SEXUAL DEVELOPMENT.

## Bibliography

BAKER, ROBERT, and ELLISTON, FREDERICK, eds. 1975. *Philosophy and Sex.* Buffalo, N.Y.: Prometheus.
BAYER, RONALD. 1987. [1981]. *Homosexuality and American*

*Psychiatry: The Politics of Diagnosis.* Princeton, N.J.: Princeton University Press.

BENE, EVA. 1965a. "On the Genesis of Female Homosexuality." *British Journal of Psychiatry* 111:815–821.

———. 1965b. "On the Genesis of Male Homosexuality: An Attempt at Clarifying the Role of the Parents." *British Journal of Psychiatry* 111:803–813.

BIEBER, IRVING; DAIN, HARVEY J.; DINCE, PAUL R.; DRELLICH, MARVIN G.; GRAND, HENRY G.; GRUNDLACH, RALPH H.; KREMER, MALVINA W.; RIFKIN, ALFRED H.; WILBUR, CORNELIA B.; and BIEBER, TOBY B. 1962. *Homosexuality: A Psychoanalytic Study.* New York: Basic Books.

BUTLER, JUDITH. 1990. *Gender Trouble: Feminism and the Subversion of Identity.* New York: Routledge.

DAWKINS, RICHARD. 1976. *The Selfish Gene.* New York: Oxford University Press.

FREUD, SIGMUND. 1962. *Three Contributions to the Theory of Sex.* New York: Dutton.

GAGNON, JOHN H., and SIMON, WILLIAM. 1973. *Sexual Conduct: The Social Sources of Human Sexuality.* Chicago: Aldine.

GOLDMAN, ALAN. 1977. "Plain Sex." *Philosophy & Public Affairs* 6, no. 3:267–287.

GREENE, RICHARD. 1974. *Sexual Identity Conflict in Children and Adults.* New York: Basic Books.

HALPERIN, DAVID M. 1990. *One Hundred Years of Homosexuality.* New York: Routledge.

HUBBARD, RUTH. 1990. *The Politics of Women's Biology.* New Brunswick, N.J.: Rutgers University Press.

JAGGAR, ALISON. 1983. *Feminist Politics and Human Nature.* Totowa, N.J.: Rowman and Allanheld.

KATZ, JONATHAN. 1983. *Gay/Lesbian Almanac: A New Documentary.* New York: Harper and Row.

KETCHUM, SARA ANN. 1980. "The Good, the Bad and the Perverted: Sexual Paradigms Revisited." In *Philosophy of Sex: Contemporary Readings.* Edited by Alan Soble. Totowa, N.J.: Littlefield Adams.

KINSEY, ALFRED CHARLES; POMEROY, WARDELL; and MARTIN, CLYDE E. 1948. *Sexual Behavior in the Human Male.* Philadelphia: W. B. Saunders.

KOHLBERG, LAWRENCE. 1966. "A Cognitive-Developmental Analysis of Children's Sex-Role Concepts and Attitudes." In *The Development of Sex Differences,* pp. 82–173. Edited by Eleanor E. Maccoby. Stanford, Calif.: Stanford University Press.

KOLODNY, ROBERT C.; MASTERS, WILLIAM H.; HENDRYX, JULIE; and TORO, GELSON. 1971. "Plasma Testosterone and Semen Analysis in Male Homosexuals." *New England Journal of Medicine* 285:1170–1174.

LAQUEUR, THOMAS. 1990. *Making Sex: Body and Gender from the Greeks to Freud.* Cambridge, Mass.: Harvard University Press.

LOWENSTEIN, JEROLD M. 1987. "The Conundrum of Gender Identification: Two Sexes Are Not Enough." *Pacific Discovery* 40, no. 2:38–39.

MACCOBY, ELEANOR EMMONS, and JACKLIN, CAROL NAGY. 1974. *The Psychology of Sex Differences.* Stanford, Calif.: Stanford University Press.

MEAD, MARGARET. 1935. *Sex and Temperament in Three Primitive Societies.* New York: William Morrow.

MISCHEL, WALTER. 1970. "Sex-Typing and Socialization." In *Carmichael's Manual of Child Psychology,* vol. 2, pp. 3–72. 3d ed. Edited by Paul H. Mussen. New York: Wiley.

MONEY, JOHN, and EHRHARDT, ANKE A. 1972. *Man and Woman, Boy and Girl: The Differentiation and Dimorphism of Gender Identity from Conception to Maturity.* Baltimore: Johns Hopkins University Press.

MONEY, JOHN; HAMPSON, JOAN G.; and HAMPSON, JOHN L. 1955. "Hermaphroditism: Recommendations Concerning Assignment of Sex, Change of Sex, and Psychologic Management." *Bulletin of the Johns Hopkins Hospital* 97:284–300.

MONEY, JOHN, and TUCKER, PATRICIA. 1975. *Sexual Signatures: On Being a Man or a Woman.* Boston: Little, Brown.

MOULTON, JANICE. 1976. "Sexual Behavior: Another Position." *Journal of Philosophy* 73, no. 16:537–546.

NAGEL, THOMAS. 1969. "Sexual Perversion." *Journal of Philosophy* 66, no. 1:5–17.

NICHOLSON, LINDA. 1986. *Gender and History: The Limits of Social Theory in the Age of the Family.* New York: Columbia University Press.

OFFER, DANIEL, and SABSHIN, MELVIN, eds. 1984. *Normality and the Life Cycle: A Critical Integration.* New York: Basic Books.

———. 1966. *Normality: Theoretical and Clinical Concepts of Mental Health.* New York: Basic Books.

ROSALDO, MICHELLE ZIMBALIST; LAMPHERE, LOUISE; and BAMBERGER, JOAN, eds. 1974. *Woman, Culture, and Society.* Stanford, Calif.: Stanford University Press.

ROSE, ROBERT M.; BOURNE, PETER G.; POE, RICHARD O.; MOUGEY, EDWARD H.; COLLINS, DAVID R.; and MASON, JOHN W. 1969. "Androgen Responses to Stress: II. Excretion of Testosterone, Epitestosterone, Androsterone, and Etiocholanolone During Basic Combat Training and Under Threat of Attack." *Psychosomatic Medicine* 31, no. 5:418–436.

SANDERS, JUDITH ROSE. 1974. "Parental Sex Preference and Expectations of Gender-Appropriate Behavior in Offspring." M.A. thesis, Brooklyn College.

SARTRE, JEAN-PAUL. 1943. *L'Être et le néant: Essai d'ontologie phénoménologique.* Paris: Gallimard. Translated by Hazel Barnes as *Being and Nothingness: An Essay in Phenomenological Ontology.* New York: 1956.

SAYERS, JANET. 1982. *Biological Politics: Feminist and Anti-Feminist Perspectives.* New York: Tavistock.

SCOTT, JOAN. 1988. *Gender and the Politics of History.* New York: Columbia University Press.

SEARS, ROBERT RICHARDSON; MACCOBY, ELEANOR E.; and LEVIN, HARRY; in collaboration with LOWELL, EDGAR L.; SEARS, PAULINE S.; and WHITING, JOHN W. M. 1957. *Patterns of Child Rearing.* Evanston, Ill.: Row, Peterson.

SEDGWICK, EVE. 1990. *Epistemology of the Closet.* Berkeley: University of California Press.

SEIDMAN, STEVEN. 1992. *Embattled Eros: Sexual Politics and Ethics in Contemporary America.* New York: Routledge.

SOLOMON, ROBERT C. 1974. "Sexual Paradigms." *Journal of Philosophy* 71, no. 11:336–345.

———. 1975. "Sex and Perversion." In *Philosophy and Sex,* pp. 268–282. Edited by Robert Baker and Frederick Elliston. Buffalo, N.Y.: Prometheus. Reprinted in Solomon's *From Hegel to Existentialism,* pp. 122–136. Oxford: Oxford University Press, 1989.

SPANIER, BONNIE. 1993. *Gender Ideology in Science: Molecular Biology from a Feminist Perspective*. Bloomington: Indiana University Press.

VIDAL, GORE. 1991. "The Birds and the Bees." *Nation*, October 28, pp. 509–511.

WEEKS, JEFFREY. 1985. *Sexuality and Its Discontents: Meanings, Myths and Modern Sexualities*. London: Routledge & Kegan Paul.

————. 1989. "Inverts, Perverts, and Mary-Annes: Male Prostitution and the Regulation of Homosexuality in England in the Nineteenth and Early Twentieth Centuries." In *Hidden from History: Reclaiming the Gay and Lesbian Past*, pp. 195–212. Edited by Martin Duberman, Martha Vicinus, and George Chauncey, Jr. New York: Penguin.

WILDER, HUGH T. 1980. "The Language of Sex and the Sex of Language." In *Philosophy of Sex*. Edited by Alan Soble. Totowa, N.J.: Littlefield Adams.

WILLIAMS, WALTER L. 1986. *The Spirit and the Flesh: Sexual Diversity in American Indian Culture*. Boston: Beacon.

# SEXUALITY IN SOCIETY

I. Social Control of Sexual Behavior
   *Ernest Wallwork*
II. Legal Approaches to Sexuality
   *Clare Dalton*

## I. SOCIAL CONTROL OF SEXUAL BEHAVIOR

The twentieth century has witnessed an explosion of knowledge about the physiology, psychology, and sociology of human sexuality, thanks to the revolution in public acceptability of discourse about sexual conduct and the freeing of scholarly interest that followed the pathbreaking works published in the late Victorian era by Richard von Krafft-Ebing (1886), Havelock Ellis (1901), and Sigmund Freud (1955a, 1955b). However, controversy still rages over the basic issue of how sexual behavior is molded, encouraged, and discouraged by social customs and practices. Are males naturally more aggressive in seeking sexual contact than females, or is this a product of social patriarchy? Is homosexuality caused primarily by biological factors, or is it largely caused by social experiences during formative stages of the child's development? Is cultural permissiveness responsible for the dramatic increase in reports of sexual harassment and abuse, or are changing mores encouraging victims to name parents, doctors, and priests who were in the past able to hide their misconduct under a cloak of respectability?

The answers to these questions are not only empirical, they are also ethical and political. Our allegedly scientific beliefs about the "naturalness" of certain sexual acts often reflect unacknowledged cultural biases, and our thoughts and theories affect the behavior they label, characterize, and implicitly valorize or demean. As feminists, and historians such as Michel Foucault (1990), have pointed out, the neutral scientific language of medicine is no guarantor of the moral innocuousness of theories about gender and sexual behavior; to the contrary, claims of scientific objectivity about these topics are apt to be all the more dangerous morally for pretending to be value-free.

Theories of sexual behavior cannot avoid assumptions about power and domination that too frequently perpetuate injustices. Thus, Alfred Kinsey's claim that males are naturally more aggressive in initiating sex (Kinsey et al., 1948) is not merely the objective scientific statement it purports to be, but a statement that supports the power of men over women in society. Anyone who is concerned about power and justice needs continually to scrutinize and critique so-called scientific claims about human sexuality by attending to how they perpetuate social stereotypes that are not universal and, by assigning more value to the experiences of certain people (e.g., white heterosexual males), help to empower some and disempower others. One would expect social ethicists to be sensitized to these issues, but the most influential recent theorists of justice (e.g., John Rawls, Ronald Dworkin, Robert Nozick, Michael Walzer) scarcely even mention gender justice, much less consider sexual roles a central matter for ethical scrutiny (see Okin, 1989). One reason for this neglect is the traditional public/private dichotomy that assigns sexual behavior to a private arena outside the concerns of the social theorist. Employment of this dichotomy in the past to keep cases of domestic rape and child abuse out of American courts, on the grounds that they occur within a zone of privacy protected from public scrutiny, shows that it is scarcely an ethically neutral matter for a social scientist to point out how our sexual lives are influenced by a social ethos that makes such distinctions.

## Essentialism and constructionism

Theories about human sexual behavior in its social context range along a continuum stretching from essentialism (or naturalism), on the one hand, to social construction theory, on the other. Essentialism attributes certain sexual and gender behaviors to the unchanging nature of the human species. What is "natural" is "good"; what is social is "artificial" and tends to be "bad" insofar as it inhibits realization of the "proper" natural end of sexual conduct, be it erotic pleasure or procreation. Thomistic natural-law theory is explicitly essentialist in identifying procreation as the "natural" end of human sexuality, but modern sexologists assume essentialism in contending that a wide variety of pleasurable erotic acts are no less "natural" than heterosexual intercourse. Alfred Kinsey, for example, uses an essentialist argument when he draws on the sexual behavior of other mammals, "primitive" cultures, and human physiological capacities to contend that masturbation and homosexual acts are "natural" expressions of sexuality and, hence, irrationally condemned and punished by society. Kinsey also employs essentialist arguments, citing mammalian data, in support of such dubious contentions as that male extramartial coitus is more natural than female extramarital coitus (Kinsey et al., 1953; Irvine, 1990). William Masters and Virginia Johnson (1966) assume essentialism in viewing sex exclusively in terms of physiological responses, unencumbered by social and psychological factors. It is not an issue for Masters and Johnson that the socialization of Western women has discouraged female sexuality; rather the woman's naturally superior sexual responsiveness to the male, as evidenced by her capacity for multiple orgasms, is what counts for them (Irvine, 1990). What is missing in the sexologist's essentialist view of culture as an impediment is any acknowledgement of the multiple ways cultures give meaning to sexual behaviors and structure sexual and gender relationships beyond physiological responses.

According to social constructionists, sexual behavior and gender roles are products of a specific history, culture, and set of social institutions. Emile Durkheim succinctly expressed the constructionist emphasis on the primacy of culture over biology when he argued, at the end of the nineteenth century, that if an adolescent did not have cultural concepts to identify sexual desires, he or she might feel a vague urge but not know what it was, much less how to act on it (Durkheim, 1933; Wallwork, 1972, 1984). A second main feature of the social constructionist approach involves situating sexual role behavior within the prevailing economic and political system, with its male-dominated hierarchies of status and power. The constructionist perspective encourages exploration of the ways in which widespread cultural beliefs about sexual behavior (and the research projects they inspire) serve to perpetuate a patriarchal vision of human nature, social institutions, gender, and sex roles. Constructionists note with concern that the focus in research has more often than not been on the male sexual experience; Masters and Johnson's research, for example, limits sexuality to genitally oriented orgasm (Masters and Johnson, 1966). Feminist critics Alice Rossi (1973) and Leonore Tiefer (1978) complain that research focusing on genital physiology as the standard of sexual involvement evidences a "phallic fallacy" that implicitly devalues the pregenital or nongenital sexual experiences of women, such as the emotionally intense erotic feelings associated with looking at the beloved or anticipating a reunion with him or her.

The obvious strength of social constructionist theory is that it is able to account for the considerable diversity of sexual behavior and the meanings associated with such behavior cross-culturally, and to link these meanings to other role relationships. The power of society to mold human sexuality is evident in how nonerotic body parts—for example, crushed feet among the Chinese of a former era, the naked foot and even shoes in medieval Europe, and hair—have been eroticized by different peoples at different times (Stoller, 1991). The power of social custom is also obvious when one contrasts the negative conception of homosexuality in the Judaeo-Christian West with its positive evaluation among Melanesian societies and certain African tribes. Among the Sambia in the New Guinea highlands, boys from prepuberty to their mid-teens are expected to engage in oral-genital sexuality with the older teenage males with whom they live as a prerequisite to becoming heterosexual adult males (Herdt and Stoller, 1990). Because Sambians believe semen is essential for males to grow and mature physically, the ingestion of semen is deemed essential to becoming an adult heterosexual male and to fathering children.

Even within the same society, there are fads and fashions of sexual behavior. For instance, since the 1960s there has been a dramatic increase in oral-genital behavior in the United States (Janus and Janus, 1993; Walsh, 1989). Among contemporary males in the West, premature ejaculation is defined as a dysfunction for which medical treatment is often sought; but in many developing countries males are expected to reach orgasms quickly (in fifteen to twenty seconds in the East Bay society in Melanesia) and those who take a "long time" are ridiculed (Reiss, 1989).

But it would be a mistake to assume, from the considerable evidence for the importance of the elaborate cultural ideas, stimulants, and norms that surround the biologically limited range of sexual behaviors of which the human body is capable, that social constructionists are winning the battle with essentialists. In fact, the nature–nurture pendulum, which has swung back and forth several times already in the twentieth century, has been swinging back again toward the nature pole as the century ends. During the 1980s and 1990s, biological explanations have been on the ascendancy in many scientific circles. Sociobiologists challenge the constructionist assumption that most sexual behavior is determined by culture, arguing instead that certain basic mammalian and primate traits that lie beneath the social surface determine the configuration of human sexual behavior (Wilson, 1975). At the same time, the biologizing of psychology is well underway, as physiological models and research strategies are held to offer the best route to understanding traditional subjects of psychological inquiry such as mental illness and sexual preference.

## Interactionist model

The most plausible position on the essentialism–constructionism debate would appear to be that the biological factors in sexual desire, such as genes and hormones, do not act alone but instead interact with environmental factors, such as visual or auditory erotic stimuli, the significance of which depends in turn upon the individual's subjective erotic sensitivities, identities, fantasies, cognitive schemata, and behavioral patterns. These subjective factors, which lead some people to be excited by depictions of sadomasochistic acts and others not, are themselves influenced by the way a unique individual with certain inherited strengths and vulnerabilities interacts with significant others and specific sociocultural environments during the various psychosexual, ego-social, and cognitive stages of development. Biological factors certainly play a role; for example, testosterone appears to influence the intensity of sexual desire. But biological factors do not invariably cause sexual motives or behavior, for testosterone is itself highly responsive to environmental stimuli. Nurture, psychological development, subjective fantasies and beliefs, erotic stimuli, moral and aesthetic standards, social roles and expectations, and ego strengths and weaknesses all mold the range of the individual's sexual potentialities in certain directions rather than others. This molding is clear from the inability of biologists and sociobiologists, who study determinants that have operated within the species for thousands of years, to explain changes in sexual customs within a single generation or variations in sexual customs that occur in the same gender cross-culturally. Unfortunately, we do not yet possess a theoretical model sufficiently complex and nuanced to integrate and assign proper weight to all the multiple factors, including the individual's self-control, that influence human sexual behavior. The sociological point of view adopted here, which falls at the constructivist end of the essentialism–constructionism continuum, remains one among several plausible selective perspectives on social control of sexual behavior. Others are history, anthropology, ethnography, psychoanalysis, and social psychology.

## Social control requirements

Sexual behavior, defined broadly as any action or reaction involving erotic arousal or genital responses, is viewed by most sociologists as sufficiently problematic to require some degree of social control. One explanation often proffered for this social-control requirement, whether as controlled permission or regulated prohibition, is that at some point in the distant past human beings lost the preformed automatic sexual instincts of the lower animals—that is, the sexual control that is in nature—and came to depend upon culture and social institutions to guide the varied reproductive and nonreproductive behaviors that are considered sexual. The loss of preformed instinctual patterns of sexual behavior, by freeing human beings from the comparatively rigid behavior patterns of other animals, helped to create the great adaptability of the human species to its changing environment. It is also meant, with the human female's loss of the periodic estrus of other mammals, that the human female and male were potentially capable of sex at any time. Sexual motives came to pervade virtually all aspects of human life in a way that is uniquely characteristic of the species. At the same time, because the sexual drive differs from instinctual needs like respiration, thirst, and hunger, which must be gratified for the individual organism's survival, sexual desire was modified by subtle psychological and social influences.

Social control of sexual behavior has been necessitated in all social units—from the family to the clan, tribe, local community, and state—in part by the serious threats to social stability and maintenance of group life over time created by the potential for sex on demand all the year round. One such threat is incest, which is inimical to the group's evolutionary survival as well as to the psychological well-being and functioning of those who might be victimized by it. Another serious social consequence of sex on demand is the likelihood of children, which every society has a stake in limiting, assigning to families peacefully, and raising, educating, and training to be law-abiding, productive contributors. Still another consequence of sexual behavior that has required its social control is its potential for either reinforcing or disrupting existing roles and status hierarchies by creating strong new social bonds. Any rape or seduction of young girls or boys, or any adulterous relation, is liable to spark violence or some other disruption of the existing social order.

The transmission of family and communal property, prestige, and power is another crucial consequence of sexual liaisons that societies attempt to handle by means of legalized sexual union in marriage and the begetting of "legitimate children." Any dramatic increase in the number of illegitimate children and abandoned wives strains the system of distributing limited economic resources, shifting some of the burden from the family onto the rest of the community. The perpetuation of a society's religious ideals, moral norms, and laws is also intertwined with the monitoring of sexual conduct, since the way sexual conduct is controlled is often paradigmatic of the way the society expects individuals to pursue other moral and spiritual goals (Stone, 1985). The well-known sexual asceticism of the Puritan, for instance, was only one part of a lifestyle that affected every aspect of the Puritan's life, just as the idealization of female virginity affects every aspect of the life of the traditional Southern Italian villager (Parsons, 1969).

**Ideals and taboos.**    Social control of sexual behavior is exercised most obviously by widely shared, explicit ideals of sexual behavior that form the basis for taboos against inappropriate conduct. Taboos are backed by social punishments ranging from mild disapproval and loss of status to ostracism, imprisonment, and death. Within Judaism and Christianity, the standard-of-standards has been heterosexual intercourse in the context of marriage. Accordingly, masturbation, homosexuality, and extramarital sexuality have been condemned and often severely punished. Among the Greeks during the classical period, pederasty was idealized as the purest form of love, but it was also hedged about by rigid taboos. The relationship was limited to an older free man and a pubescent free boy. Oral and anal intercourse were unacceptable, and if a boy allowed himself to be penetrated anally, he lost his rights to citizenship. For the Greek male, what was important was not whether one's partner was male or female, but whether one was dominant or submissive.

**Social roles.** In addition to the values and norms shared throughout a culture, social control is also maintained by the basic institutions of society, especially the family, religion, schools, medicine, and law. An institution is defined sociologically as a stable cluster of values, norms, statuses, and roles that develop around a basic need of society. An important function of an institution is to socialize developing individuals through inculcation of social roles, which are social actions that take account of social expectations. A person's role is not simply what he or she habitually does (for this may not be socially significant), nor even what he or she is expected to do, if an expectation is only what one might predict from past actions. The role is what is expected of him or her, in the sense of what is approved or required, by, say, fashion, tradition, charismatic authority, or standards of rationality.

Gender roles, which indicate how males and females are expected to behave, significantly influence sexual behavior. In Western culture, the expectation has been that the woman is more passive and receptive, and more attuned to emotional connections, than the male, who is expected to be more aggressive, autonomous, and focused on power. Such gender roles have an effect on sexual conduct, independent of explicit sexual standards. For example, rape is strongly disapproved of in contemporary culture, yet date rape is disturbingly frequent, in part because males are socialized to dominate women in most social situations involving power. Hence, if a male's charm and powers of psychological persuasion fail in a sexual situation, coercion remains as a last resort. Here, as in most sexual acts, erotic desire is only one of several motivations that enter into the behavior. In addition, the need to maintain the male-dominant role identity and the propensity for males in Western societies to turn anger at frustration into aggression and violence are equally powerful motives.

Recently, sociologists have applied "script theory" to sexual behavior in order to account for the more spe-cific patterns that enable participants to make reasonably good guesses about the sequence of events probable in an otherwise loosely structured social situation (Gagnon and Simon, 1973; McKinney and Sprecher, 1989). Scripts are mental schemas that enable participants to jointly structure the interaction so that uncertainty is systematically reduced and cooperation enhanced. Sexual scripts enable participants to decode novel situations by reading the meaning of certain actions and to organize the situation into sequences of specifically sexual interactions (e.g., nonverbal courtship behaviors signaling availability like smiling, gazing, hair flipping, the "opening line," leaning close, and the proverbial invitation to see one's etchings). However, research on conflicts between the sexes in dating and marriage also shows that scripting is far from perfect, that the sexes often miscue each other or are dissatisfied in predictable ways—say, with the male's excessive sexual demands or emotional constriction, or the woman's unresponsiveness or moodiness.

Empirical beliefs—especially medically sanctioned ones—about the consequences for the individual's health of various sexual practices also play a significant role in the social control of sexual behavior. In classical Greece, for example, physicians recommended sexual moderation to prevent the excessive loss of life force in the too-frequent ejaculation of semen. In ancient China, somewhat similar beliefs about the consequences of excessive semen loss led to the cultivation of special techniques of intercourse without ejaculation in order to conserve the *yang* (the positive, light masculine principle whose interaction with *yin*—the negative, dark feminine principle—was believed to influence the destiny of creatures and things). And, of course, doctors within the Judaeo-Christian milieu have for millenia warned that masturbation would bring about some dreaded disease, disfigurement, or insanity. In our own time, fear of AIDS has dramatically changed sexual behavior, primarily by altering beliefs about the risks of unprotected sexual intercourse. It is one of Foucault's main contentions that medical beliefs, precisely because they are so important to patients, provide physicians with power that historically has often been used to dominate and control unjustly (Foucault, 1990).

It is easy to be impressed by the ideals, moral rules, and prudential teachings that are set forth so impressively in explicit doctrine by leading social authorities. But these action guides are not always reinforced by other cultures or even by other institutions in the same cultural context. Complex societies are not systematic cultural ensembles, despite the beliefs of sociological functionalists like Emile Durkheim and Talcott Parsons. Illicit sexual cultures—like red-light districts or the houses of prostitution that flourished in medieval Europe (Ariès and Bejin, 1985)—exist side by side with licit sexual cultures, counterbalancing and correcting excessive asceticism, and on some points canceling out the influence of the licit culture. A complex interrelationship often exists between these cultures, so there is often plenty of room for compromises and loopholes. Moreover, the different social-status groups and classes of the same society usually have different sexual cultures. For example, libertine elites, concentrated around courts (as in ancient Egypt, classical Greece and Rome, imperial China, India, and Japan) have surrounded themselves with a rich panoply of erotic art, pornographic literature, artificial physical stimuli, toys, and partners not encouraged among lower social ranks (Stone, 1985).

## Control and permissiveness

The so-called sexual revolution that occurred in the post–World War II epoch is sometimes viewed—erroneously—as releasing the individual from the constraining pressures of social control. But the new permissiveness is more accurately perceived as substituting new and, in some instances, somewhat different social standards, controls, and permissions for older ones. The most important contemporary cultural standards focus less on the legitimation of sex by marriage and more on the goods of sensual pleasure, intimacy, the autonomy of the parties (violated in the case of rape and harassment), and the basic equality of partners. Some salient features of the sexual revolution are the greater explicit public acknowledgment of sexuality (for example, in films, "soap operas," talk shows, and advice columns); the availability of cheap and reliable contraception, particularly birth control pills, which have for the first time in history released women from the fear of unwanted pregnancies; the increased availability of erotic stimulants (e.g., adult magazines, pornographic videos, computer networks); the rise of feminism and correlative decline in social inequality between the sexes; the increased acceptance or tolerance of sexual behaviors that were formerly disapproved, like masturbation, homosexuality, extramarital sexual affairs, and oral-genital sex; and the dramatic increase in teenage sexual conduct and at younger ages. There has also emerged in recent years a "recreational ideology," which holds that the purpose of sexual activity is not procreation or even mutual affection, but physical pleasure.

Although these changes reflect a certain permissiveness, there is evidence that men and women today have higher expectations, demands, and worries about their sexual performance (McKinney and Sprecher, 1989; Janus and Janus, 1993). The liberating views of sexologists have brought in their train new demands for mutual orgasm and standards of erotic performance that not all couples are capable of realizing at all times. Rising concern about date rape on university campuses in the United States is giving rise to explicit policies, sometimes accompanied by detailed lists of "do's" and "don'ts," designed to make sure there is willing and verbal consent to each individual sexual act, for example, kissing, fondling of breasts, touching of genitals, intercourse. New policies, grievance procedures, and punishments are proliferating to prevent and punish sexual harassment and rape (Gross, 1993).

The permissiveness associated with the sexual revolution also coexists with the continuation of strong cultural constraints on frank interpersonal communication about sexual behavior that has disturbing implications for preventing unwanted pregnancies and venereal diseases and for containment of the AIDS epidemic. Western society has a long history of prudishness about sexual topics that stretches back several millenia into the biblical period, when writers of the Hebrew Bible and Christian New Testament used euphemisms like "flesh," "loin," "thigh," "side," and "feet" (for penis), "lewdness" (for female genitals), and "one flesh" (for intercourse) in lieu of explicit sexual terms (Baab, 1962). Despite the new sexual permissiveness, and research showing that, for example, 20 percent of the American female population have had coitus by age 15 (Hayes, 1987) and that 59 percent of secondary school students have had sexual intercourse (Kann et al., 1991), parents continue to find it difficult to talk with their children in a knowledgeable way about sexual behavior. In a 1987 national survey, 69 percent of adult Americans viewed premarital coitus as "always wrong" for fourteen- to sixteen-year-olds (Davis and Smith, 1987). Research suggests that many adolescents perceive their parents as not very well informed about sex and as negative, rigid, and conservative in their attitudes toward sexuality (Metts and Cupach, 1989). Although adolescents tell researchers they would like to learn more about sex from their parents, their perceptions as well as the reported attitudes of many parents discourage open communication.

The difficulty parents have communicating information about sex is also found among many professionals charged with conveying information about sex to children, such as schoolteachers, clergy, and physicians. Research shows that adolescents learn most of their information about sexuality, such as petting and sexual intercourse, from same-sex peers, who are often ill-informed about contraception or the prevention of sexually transmitted diseases. However, some studies indicate that some sexuality education programs are able to convey factual information about anatomical and physiological aspects of sexuality, and to influence understanding of the risks of sexual behaviors (Orbuch, 1989; Metts and Cupach, 1989). Unfortunately, most teenagers remain unprepared for their first sexual encounters. Much remains to be done in communicating information about how to avoid unwanted pregnancies and infection by the human immunodeficiency virus (HIV) that causes AIDS.

Constraints on open discussion of sexual desires and practices is one factor in the high rape rates. Research shows that young men remain reluctant to declare their desire for sexual intercourse to a new date, while young women are less than open about their reluctance. Discussion of contraceptive measures is apparently still difficult for couples who have not had coitus, despite the threat of AIDS (Reiss, 1989). The culture of sexual permissiveness is thus riddled with constraints on forthright discussion of choosing among alternative sexual options. To help counter these constraints, health-care professions need improved educational programs on human sexuality, more training in public health, and opportunities to cultivate skills of communicating with patients as knowledgeable allies and responsible agents, not as passive recipients of authoritative information and advice.

A peculiar problem with many attempts to control sexual behavior is that the constraints and repressions designed to foster licit or safe sex often themselves contribute to the flourishing of illicit or unsafe sexual behavior, which becomes all the more alluring, exciting, and frequent precisely because it is prohibited. The firmest social controls of sexual behavior appear to be those that acknowledge the unique value of sexual desires, fantasies, and actions in human life in a spirit of tolerance toward nonharmful illicit wishes and behaviors, even as actual conduct is directed toward goals that are compatible with the best interests of the individuals involved and the groups of which they are a part.

ERNEST WALLWORK

*Directly related to this article is the companion article in this entry:* LEGAL APPROACHES TO SEXUALITY. *For a further discussion of topics mentioned in this article, see the entries* ABUSE, INTERPERSONAL; ADOLESCENTS; AIDS; AUTHORITY; CHILDREN; FAMILY; FEMINISM; FERTILITY CONTROL, *especially the article on* SOCIAL ISSUES; GENETICS AND HUMAN BEHAVIOR; HOMOSEXUALITY; HUMAN NATURE; JUSTICE; NATURAL LAW; PROSTITUTION; SEXISM; SEXUAL DEVELOPMENT; SEXUAL ETHICS; SEXUAL ETHICS AND PROFESSIONAL STANDARDS; SEXUAL IDENTITY; *and* VALUE AND VALUATION. *For a discussion of related ideas, see the entries* BODY; *and* LAW AND MORALITY.

## Bibliography

ARIÉS, PHILIPPE, and BEJIN, ANDRÉ, eds. 1985. *Western Sexuality: Practice and Precept in Past and Present Times.* Oxford: Basil Blackwell.

BAAB, OTTO J. 1962. "Sex, Sexual Behavior." In vol. 4 of *The Interpreter's Dictionary of the Bible,* pp. 296–301. Edited by George Arthur Buttrick. New York: Abingdon.

BEZEMER, WILLEKE; COHEN-KETTENIS, PEGGY; SLOB, KOOS; and VAN SON-SCHOONES, NEL, eds. 1992. *Sex Matters: Proceedings of the Xth World Congress of Sexology.* Amsterdam: Excerpta Medica.

BOSWELL, JOHN. 1980. *Christianity, Social Tolerance, and Homosexuality: Gay People in Western Europe from the Beginning of the Christian Era to the Fourteenth Century.* Chicago: University of Chicago Press.

DAVIS, JAMES A., and SMITH, TOM W. 1987. *General Social Surveys, 1972–1987: Cumulative Codebook.* Chicago: National Opinion Research Center.

DURKHEIM, EMILE. 1933. [1893]. *Emile Durkheim on the Division of Labor in Society.* Translated and edited by George Simpson. New York: Macmillan.

ELLIS, H. HAVELOCK. 1901. *Studies in the Psychology of Sex.* 7 vols. Philadelphia: F. A. Davis.

FOUCAULT, MICHEL. 1990. *The History of Sexuality.* Translated by Robert Hurley. New York: Vintage Books.

FREUD, SIGMUND. 1955a. *Studies on Hysteria.* Vol. 2 of *The Standard Edition of the Complete Psychological Works of Sigmund Freud.* Translated by James Strachey. London: Hogarth.

———. 1955b. [1905]. *Three Essays on the Theory of Sexuality.* In vol. 7 of *The Standard Edition of the Complete Psychological Works of Sigmund Freud,* pp. 130–243. Translated by James Strachey. London: Hogarth.

GAGNON, JOHN H., and SIMON, WILLIAM. 1973. *Sexual Conduct: The Social Sources of Human Sexuality.* Chicago: Aldine.

GROSS, JANE. 1993. "Combating Rape on Campus in a Class on Sexual Consent." *New York Times,* September 25, pp. A1, A9.

HAYES, CHERYL D., ed. 1987. *Risking the Future: Adolescent Sexuality, Pregnancy and Childbearing.* Washington, D.C.: National Academy Press.

HERDT, GILBERT H. 1981. *Guardians of the Flutes: Idioms of Masculinity.* New York: McGraw-Hill.

HERDT, GILBERT H., and STOLLER, ROBERT J. 1990. *Intimate Communications.* New York: Columbia University Press.

IRVINE, JANICE M. 1990. *Disorders of Desire: Sex and Gender in Modern American Sexology.* Philadelphia: Temple University Press.

JANUS, SAMUEL S., and JANUS, CYNTHIA L. 1993. *The Janus Report on Sexual Behavior.* New York: Wiley.

KANN, LAURA; ANDERSON, JOHN E.; HOLTZMAN, DEBORAH; ROSS, JIM; TRUMAN, BENEDICT I.; COLLINS, JANET L.; and KOLBE, LLOYD J. 1991. "HIV-Related Knowledge, Beliefs, and Behaviors Among High School Students in the United States: Results from a National Survey." *Journal of School Health* 61, no. 9:397–401.

KINSEY, ALFRED CHARLES; POMEROY, WARDELL B.; and MARTIN, CLYDE E. 1948. *Sexual Behavior in the Human Male.* Philadelphia: W. B. Saunders.

KINSEY, ALFRED CHARLES; POMEROY, WARDELL B.; MARTIN, CLYDE E.; and GEBHARD, PAUL H. 1953. *Sexual Behavior in the Human Female.* New York: Pocket Books.

KLASSEN, ALBERT D.; WILLIAMS, COLIN J.; and LEVITT, EUGENE E., eds. 1989. *Sex and Morality in the U.S.: An Empirical Enquiry Under the Auspices of the Kinsey Institute.* Middletown, Conn.: Wesleyan University Press.

KRAFFT-EBING, RICHARD VON. 1939. [1886]. *Psychopathia Sexualis: A Medico-Forensic Study.* New York: Pioneer.

MASTERS, WILLIAM H., and JOHNSON, VIRGINIA. 1966. *Human Sexual Response.* New York: Little, Brown.

MCKINNEY, KATHLEEN, and SPRECHER, SUSAN, eds. 1989. *Human Sexuality: The Societal and Interpersonal Context.* Norwood, N.J.: Ablex.

METTS, SANDRA, and CUPACH, WILLIAM R. 1989. "The Role of Communication in Human Sexuality." In *Human Sexuality: The Societal and Interpersonal Context,* pp. 139–161. Edited by Kathleen McKinney and Susan Sprecher. Norwood, N.J.: Ablex.

OKIN, SUSAN MOLLER. 1989. *Justice, Gender, and the Family.* New York: Basic Books.

ORBUCH, TEERI L. 1989. "Human Sexuality Education." In *Human Sexuality: The Societal and Interpersonal Context,* pp. 438–462. Edited by Kathleen McKinney and Susan Sprecher. Norwood, N.J.: Ablex.

PARSONS, ANNE. 1969. *Belief, Magic, and Anomie: Essays in Psychosocial Anthropology.* New York: Free Press.

REISS, IRA L. 1989. "Society and Sexuality: A Sociological Theory." In *Human Sexuality: The Societal and Interpersonal Context,* chap. 1, pp. 3–29. Edited by Kathleen McKinney and Susan Sprecher. Norwood, N.J.: Ablex.

ROSSI, ALICE S. 1973. "Maternalism, Sexuality, and the New Feminism." In *Contemporary Sexual Behavior: Critical Issues in the 1970s,* pp. 145–173. Edited by Joseph Zubin and John Money. Baltimore: Johns Hopkins University Press.

STOLLER, ROBERT J. 1991. *Porn: Myths for the Twentieth Century.* New Haven, Conn.: Yale University Press.

STONE, LAWRENCE. 1985. "The Strange History of Human Sexuality: Sex in the West." *New Republic,* July 8, pp. 25–37.

TIEFER, LEONORE. 1978. "The Context and Consequences of Contemporary Sex Research: A Feminist Perspective." In *Sex and Behavior: Status and Prospectus,* pp. 363–385. Edited by Thomas E. McGill, Donald A. Dewsbury, and Benjamin D. Sachs. New York: Plenum.

WALLWORK, ERNEST. 1972. *Durkheim: Morality and Milieu.* Cambridge, Mass.: Harvard University Press.

———. 1984. "Religion and Social Structure in *The Division of Labor.*" *American Anthropologist* 86, no. 1:43–64.

———. 1992. *Psychoanalysis and Ethics.* New Haven, Conn.: Yale University Press.

WALSH, ROBERT H. 1989. "Premarital Sex Among Teenagers and Young Adults." In *Human Sexuality: The Societal and Interpersonal Context,* pp. 162–186. Edited by Kathleen McKinney and Susan Sprecher. Norwood, N.J.: Ablex.

WILSON, EDWARD OSBORNE. 1975. *Sociobiology: The New Synthesis.* Cambridge, Mass.: Harvard University Press.

## II. LEGAL APPROACHES TO SEXUALITY

This article discusses law's relationship to sexuality from an explicitly American perspective, although the framework suggested here may lend itself to application in other cultural contexts.

### Sexual status and sexual conduct

From the point of view of American law, sexuality has two dimensions: status and conduct. Sexuality as status, in law as in the culture at large, contains two primary alternatives—heterosexuality and homosexuality—although recent efforts on the part of those claiming bisexual status to make political alliance with gay and lesbian activists may presage increased legal recognition of this third alternative. Law's affirmative involvement with issues of sexual status consists chiefly of the grant of the marriage license to heterosexual unions aspiring to some permanence, and the denial of that license to same-sex unions with the same aspiration. Less actively, but with greater impact on the lives of homosexual people, law has largely declined to recognize differential treatment on the basis of sexual orientation as a form of prohibited discrimination (Mohr, 1988).

Sexuality as conduct also has two principle aspects. The first encompasses explicitly sexual acts, of which intercourse is perhaps the paradigmatic example. Law prohibits intercourse, and sometimes other sexual activity, in a wide variety of situations, either where one of the parties has not consented or is deemed unable to consent, or where the intercourse or other activity, although consensual, is deemed to offend norms of public decency or order. Child sexual abuse, sexual assault and rape, statutory rape (intercourse with a woman, or in a few states with an individual, who is considered too young to provide meaningful assent), and incest are uniformly prohibited. Traditionally, a woman in the marriage relationship was, by law, sexually available at all times to her spouse. Since the 1970s, however, these laws have changed in many states and wives have legally charged husbands with rape. Prostitution—the buying and selling of sex—is authorized only in Nevada. Sodomy, both homosexual and heterosexual, is unlawful in a large minority of states. Sex before marriage and outside of marriage is still prohibited in some states, although enforcement of these prohibitions is virtually nonexistent because of the mismatch between the law and prevailing cultural practices and attitudes.

Another way in which law regulates sexual intercourse is by controlling or limiting the choices available to men and women before and after intercourse. The extent to which a state can limit access to abortion consistent with the mandates of federal and state constitutions has been a hotly contested issue, as the Supreme Court's decision in *Planned Parenthood of Southeastern Pennsylvania* v. *Casey* (1992) amply illustrates. The use of contraception by adults remains constitutionally protected, yet access to particular contraceptive techniques remains subject to regulation on health grounds, in a cultural context in which health concerns have frequently provided a pretext for political intervention.

President Bill Clinton's reversal in 1993 of the Bush administration's opposition to the introduction of RU-486, a "morning-after pill" and early abortifacient, provides a dramatic example of this interplay between policies and medicine. Unsuccessful battles to introduce contraceptives into the nation's high schools are reminders that contraceptive freedom does not generally extend to minors, despite everything known about their active sexuality and their exposure to sexually transmitted diseases (Miller et al., 1990).

In other contexts, law precludes procreation as a consequence of intercourse. The eugenics movement in the United States in the 1920s and 1930s produced laws compelling the sterilization of certain classes of criminals and those with mental disabilities or illness. These laws remain on the books in several states, and have never been deemed flatly unconstitutional, although they are no longer enforced. In the contemporary context, most if not all states provide a mechanism by which those legally responsible for sexually active people determined to be mentally incompetent can petition the state to authorize sterilization or contraception.

The second aspect of sexuality as conduct encompasses sexual displays the law views as expressing or arousing sexual receptivity or interest, and thereby offending norms of public decency or order. The sexual displays regulated by law are varied in character; they include solicitation, public nudity, and provocative dressing (toplessness for women) and cross-dressing (transvestism for men), as well as all forms of pornography. In this arena, too, enforcement is by no means uniform, and constitutional freedoms of speech and expression have created uncertainty even about the legitimacy of regulation.

## Law's multiple relationships to legal status and conduct

Law's relationship to sexuality is in part constituted by law's account of what in the sexual arena is permissible and what is prohibited, which behaviors are to be encouraged and which are to be discouraged. Statutes passed by legislatures establish guidelines for behavior and award privileges to those who comply or assess penalties against those who do not. Under the auspices of statutes, regulators promulgate implementing regulations. Judges determine the constitutionality of statutory law and the validity of regulation; they apply the language of statutes and regulations to particular individuals and circumstances, and they preside over the development and application of specific bodies of judge-made law. Thus, state criminal statutes have frequently made sodomy a crime, and the U.S. Supreme Court determined, in 1986, that these statutes violated no constitutional mandate (*Bowers* v. *Hardwick*, 1986).

States have traditionally controlled the provision of abortion through both statute and regulation, and the Supreme Court continues to decide, in a high-profile series of cases, which restrictions violate women's privacy or liberty interests (Dworkin, 1993). In the absence of statutes permitting the marriage of same-sex partners, the judge-made law of contract is occasionally invoked to regulate the distribution of assets upon dissolution of a gay or lesbian union. Judges may decline to make this body of law available to a nontraditional union in the same way that they routinely decline to enforce contracts of prostitution.

This relationship between law and sexuality is importantly shaped, however, by the fact that law's authority is actually invoked in sexual matters by public agencies or private parties in only a small fraction of the cases in which it might be. The gap between the law as announced and as invoked has a variety of origins.

Sometimes those who might initiate action against a violator do not know that the law offers them protection. For example, when Justice Clarence Thomas's nomination to the Supreme Court was threatened by the charge that he had harassed Professor Anita Hill while she was a young employee working under his supervision, the legal norms governing sexual conduct in the workplace received massive publicity. Sexual-harassment claims by female employees increased sharply in the months that followed.

Sometimes the enforcement of legal norms governing behavior that tends to be very private is simply impractical; sodomy, unlike public nudity, seldom comes to the attention of law-enforcement personnel. The norm serves, therefore, not as a general prohibition but as a tool in the arsenal of law-enforcement authorities wishing to target a particular individual or couple for enforcement action, a troublesome use of prosecutorial discretion. Sometimes police and prosecutors make conscious decisions not to investigate or prosecute certain offenses. This decision may be because investigation will be difficult or costly and the success of prosecution uncertain. It may be because the offenses in question constitute low priorities or particular victims belong to groups whose protection is a low priority. For example, prostitutes have not often been successful rape claimants, while "virtuous" white women raped by black strangers are the most favored rape complainants (Estrich, 1987). It may be because crimes have been left on the statute books long after public sentiment has changed. (Laws against adultery and premarital sexual contact have this character.) Or it may be because those charged with enforcement are dubious of the wisdom of the regulation or of its application to a particular situation. Many rape prosecutions, especially those involving parties who are not strangers, founder for one or more of these reasons. Those who have argued that specific victims of pornography should be allowed to bring civil actions against pornographers and distributors of pornography base their argument, in part, on the reluctance of public authorities to take appropriate action (MacKinnon, 1987).

Those who urge giving private parties greater responsibility for or authority to initiate legal action must also confront the reality that individuals are often unwilling or unable to invoke the law even when they understand that a legal norm has been violated. For example, the trauma of childhood sexual abuse often results in the repression of memory (Ernsdorff and Loftus, 1993). If the memory ever surfaces, it may be long after the time for bringing legal action has passed. Potential claimants may be fearful of retribution on the part of the one they accuse; this is often true for sexual-harassment claimants and battered women who charge their abusers with physical and sexual violence. They may be anxious about the costs, both financial and emotional, involved in being a complaining witness or a plaintiff. They may fear having their credibility challenged or their character impugned, and may see participation in the legal system as just another opportunity to be victimized; many sexual-harassment and rape victims articulate this concern. Finally, claimants in some circumstances may be able to resolve the situation without recourse to the formal mechanisms offered by the legal system.

If law's relationship to sexuality is influenced by the limited nature of actual legal interventions in sexual matters, it is just as crucially influenced by limited public understanding of the legal norms governing sexuality. How social actors perceive law's application to their own or others' sexual status or conduct may derive from actual individual or institutional knowledge of the law or of enforcement practices; but it may equally derive from impressions gleaned from a limited number of personal experiences or from stories emphasized by the media. Generalizations, often derived from limited information, then guide an individual's interaction with the legal system around sexual matters—setting standards for personal conduct, governing expectations about how the system will respond to legal violations, and providing the initiative for involvement in political efforts to change the law or replace its agents.

The national experience surrounding the charges that Clarence Thomas had sexually harassed Anita Hill illustrates this dynamic. The many interviews and polls conducted by the press demonstrated that public understanding of the law of sexual harassment was extremely limited prior to the publicity surrounding Thomas's confirmation hearings. In particular, many men expressed great surprise that behavior they had considered normal, playful, flattering, or flirtatious might be considered unlawful if addressed to a woman co-worker. In reaction, they interpreted the law as more draconian and restrictive than the history of its application warranted. This response led them to articulate a new code of conduct for themselves going well beyond any legal requirement, and at the same time to express the conviction that the law was unrealistic if not ridiculous.

Given this multilayered relationship between law and sexuality, it is as important to appreciate what law does not do as what it does, as important to know how laws are implemented as to know what they say, and as important to know what people think the law is as to know how it might be interpreted by some authoritative source.

## Victorian and modern visions of sexuality

In addressing issues of sexual status and performance, the contemporary legal system incorporates and reflects two very different visions of social and family life. Still influential is the vision we associate with the Victorian era. This vision incorporates an explicitly patriarchal family and social structure in which the interests of women and children are subordinated in culture and law to those of men, while women's value in the domestic sphere is emphasized and their opportunities outside that sphere are narrowly circumscribed. It also incorporates a sexually repressive culture in which sexual expression and practice is tightly controlled in law and in public while deviancy flourishes in private. The contrasting "modern" vision aspires to an egalitarian family and social structure that radically augments the rights of women and children both inside and outside the home, and to a culture of sexual tolerance and openness (Grossberg, 1985; Okin, 1989; Thorne and Yalom, 1992).

While there is no question that the law has gradually incorporated elements of the modern vision, an open struggle between the two visions continues within the legal system, as it does in the culture at large. For example, until the last quarter of the nineteenth century most states permitted a husband to use physical discipline to "chastise" his wife, and guaranteed him sexual access to her at all times. By the end of the century, wife abuse was no longer tolerated by the criminal law, and yet most states continued to grant husbands immunity from civil suit by their injured wives in the interests of domestic "harmony" and the privacy of family life. The right of sexual access, however, remained unimpaired, and the criminal justice system largely ignored wife abuse, refusing to arrest or prosecute batterers. Only in the 1970s, in the wake of the battered-women's movement, did the enforcement picture begin to change and marital rape immunities begin to erode. Many men and women, however, continue to believe that a marriage license takes away a woman's right to say no to sexual intercourse.

For many people the struggle between the two visions of social and family life is an attempt to find an appropriate balance. In the area of abortion, spousal and parental notification rules provide an example. In *Planned Parenthood* v. *Casey*, the one state regulation struck down as imposing an undue burden on women's exercise of their abortion rights was that requiring not spousal consent, but spousal notification (*Planned Parenthood*, 1992). The justices were explicit that the specter of an abusive and controlling husband doing violence to his pregnant wife drove this decision. On the other hand, parental notification and consent rules have been routinely upheld for minors, with only very narrow judicial bypass provisions for cases in which a young woman can justify to a judge both her capacity to make a mature decision and the need to withhold information from a parent. As a culture, we continue to support significant parental control over children, while we are much less tolerant of the idea that a husband should wield authority over his wife.

For some, particularly those conservatives influenced by religious fundamentalism, the struggle is largely to restore a Victorian vision of family and social life. Those who oppose abortion on this basis also frequently oppose contraception, believe that intercourse should be linked to procreation, and endorse a traditional division of family labor in which the woman attends to the home and the children, while the man is the principal breadwinner. While this constituency may be heartened by the erosion of women's freedom with respect to abortion since *Roe* v. *Wade* (1973), and by the Supreme Court's willingness to condemn consensual homosexual intercourse as a deviant social practice in *Bowers* v. *Hardwick* (1986), the legal system otherwise provides diminishing support for conservative family ideology.

### The tools of regulation

In situating itself with respect to sexuality, and in generating the specifics of regulation, the legal system draws on a variety of sources of cultural authority and deploys a variety of principles and policies. Sometimes the shift from the Victorian to the modern vision has involved reliance on new or different principles and policies, or the invocation of new sources of cultural authority and a frontal attack on the old. On other occasions, the very same principles and policies invoked to support the Victorian vision have proved adaptable enough to support the modern vision, when applied in new and different contexts. On many occasions, the same sources of cultural authority invoked by law in support of the Victorian vision have themselves abandoned or modified that support and now offer the law new support for the modern vision.

The two principal external sources of authority guiding legal regulation of sexuality have been morality and medical science. Morals derive either from secular ethical precepts or from religion, but the role of religion is complicated by the religious diversity within U.S. society and by the fact that its constitutional order insists on the separation of church and state. However, when moral precepts, even those rooted historically in specific religious traditions, are broadly accepted within society and thus secularized, they become a legitimate basis for legal intervention. When law steps in to regulate, it justifies its intervention by appeals to the secularized form of the moral mandate: to public decency or public order; to the value of life or the state's practical interest in heterosexual unions; to the "degeneracy" of certain sexual practices. When social consensus around a moral issue begins to erode, the link between particular moral notions and their specific religious underpinnings becomes exposed again, and law's endorsement of one side of the debate can be challenged as an improper conflation of church and state. In the United States of the 1980s and 1990s, this form of challenge to the moral basis of law can be seen most dramatically in the abortion debate and in the debate over the legitimacy of homosexual unions.

The issues involved in law's reliance on medical science have a different valence, since the concerns here are perceived to be those of knowledge rather than faith, of description rather than prescription. In areas involving sexuality, medical science has provided law with an understanding of what is necessary to protect public health and welfare and with guidelines about sexual status and conduct. In addressing the fundamental issue of sexual identity, medical science has drawn and redrawn the lines between aspects of sexuality that depend upon genetic programming, aspects that are the product of physical or mental disease or malfunction, and aspects that are the product of willed or chosen conduct. Changes in the medical understanding of homosexuality, for example, have in turn been central to legal debates about the appropriateness of regulating homosexual relationships and practices. In the abortion arena, law has turned to medicine in search of a scientific and secular ruling about when life begins, hoping to be able to adopt a definition free of religious bias.

The problems inherent in the relationship between law and medical science have two interrelated sources. First, medical science does not stand still, and law often lags behind the newest understanding. Compulsory sterilization laws provide a dramatic example; the genetic "science" on which these laws were based has been entirely discredited, and yet not all such laws have been repealed. Second, medical science is not as value-free as the deferential legal community often assumes; many shifts in the medical understanding of sexuality reflect shifts in values more than they do real advances in knowledge. Law's deference thus renders it susceptible to influence by medical science on matters about which medicine has no particular expertise or authority.

What of the legal principles governing the regulation of sexuality? Several of those legitimizing intervention have already been spelled out: maintaining public order, decency, health, and welfare. These laws fall within the traditional "police power" of the state. Another traditional basis for governmental intervention has been to encourage forms of association and sexuality that promote the state's conception of its interests. Matrimony and childbearing and rearing within matrimonial relationships are the clearest historical examples. However, the concepts of public order, decency, health, and welfare, and indeed of the state's interests, are malleable enough to serve the modern vision of social and family life.

The legal principles limiting regulation of sexuality have traditionally been those of privacy and autonomy, especially those forms of autonomy protected by First Amendment freedoms of thought and speech. Both these principles reflect a constitutional order that sees government as a threat to liberty; both are prepared to accord some cultural space to sexual activity and expression that deviate from widely held cultural norms, to guard against the erosion of liberty.

In the shift from the Victorian vision to the modern vision, the principles of privacy and autonomy have been pressed into service in new contexts while their hold over other arenas has been challenged. The privacy accorded family life was an important bulwark to the patriarchal authority of the male head of household, but it no longer serves to shield family members from charges of sexual abuse. Instead, privacy provides the foundation for the constitutional protection accorded both abortion and contraception, whose availability serves to bolster women's claims to sexual freedom and egalitarian participation in both private and public spheres. Efforts to have sodomy statutes declared unconstitutional, however, have demonstrated the limits of the privacy principle. In *Bowers* (1986), the Supreme Court declined to rule that private, consensual, homosexual conduct between adults was constitutionally protected.

Since the 1970s, the legal principle of equality has been invoked increasingly by champions of the modern vision of social and family life. Equality has provided a basis for the abolition of old intrafamilial immunities and has supported the exposure of family abuses. Equality has translated the private pain of sexual harassment in the workplace into a public claim of discrimination when the job itself or other workplace privileges are conditioned on consent to sexual activity, or when the harassment creates a hostile working environment (MacKinnon, 1979; *Meritor Savings Bank v. Vinson*, 1986).

Equality has also offered a new analysis of pornography. Where previous regulation of pornography depended on the "obscenity" that made it offensive to norms of public decency, the new analysis emphasizes the role pornography plays in endorsing and promoting the sexual objectification of women and thereby denying women equal status in society (MacKinnon, 1987, 1993). This characterization more properly represents what is at stake in the regulation of pornography. By the mid-1990s, however, none of the municipal ordinances based on it had survived constitutional scrutiny. The violation of women's right to be free of discrimination must still be weighed against the First Amendment freedoms of pornographers, distributors, and users; in this balance, the opponents of pornography have not prevailed. Importantly, women themselves are divided on this issue; many see the proliferation of pornography as enabling a liberating sexuality for women and support the First Amendment arguments made on pornography's behalf (Strossen, 1993).

Finally, equality is frequently offered by advocates as a basis for outlawing differential treatment on the basis of sexual identity and for providing a protected sphere in which gay and lesbian people can enjoy both privacy and autonomy in their experience of their sexuality (Mohr, 1988; "Sexual Orientation and the Law," 1993). As with pornography, this argument has made little headway within the legal system.

## Conclusion

In matters relating to sexuality, the balance law strikes between the impetus to regulate and the impetus to stay government's hand is an uncertain one, informed always by shifting cultural values. Issues resolved in the direction of regulation in one era may be revisited and resolved in the direction of abstention in the next. In the decades to come, it seems likely that the most contested territory is going to involve, first, the extent to which regulation of sexuality will be directed toward achieving the egalitarian vision of social and family life, freeing women and children from sexual exploitation and abuse, and second, the extent to which law will be persuaded to lift the burden of regulation currently imposed on homosexual conduct, and give protection in the name of equality to those who claim homosexual status.

CLARE DALTON

*Directly related to this article is the companion article in this entry:* SOCIAL CONTROL OF SEXUAL BEHAVIOR. *For a further discussion of topics mentioned in this article, see the entries* ABORTION; ABUSE, INTERPERSONAL; EUGENICS; FEMINISM; FERTILITY CONTROL; HOMOSEXUALITY;

Law and Bioethics; Law and Morality; Marriage and Other Domestic Partnerships; Prostitution; Rights; Sexism; Sexual Ethics; Sexual Ethics and Professional Standards; *and* Women, *article on* historical and cross-cultural perspectives. *For a discussion of related ideas, see the entry* Public Health and the Law.

## Bibliography

*Bowers* v. *Hardwick.* 1986. 485 U.S. 140.

Danielsen, Dan, and Engle, Karen, eds. 1994. *After Identity: A Reader in Law and Culture.* New York: Routledge.

Dworkin, Ronald. 1993. *Life's Dominion: An Argument About Abortion, Euthanasia, and Individual Freedom.* New York: Alfred A. Knopf.

Ernsdorff, Gary M., and Loftus, Elizabeth F. 1993. "Let Sleeping Memories Lie? Words of Caution About Tolling the Statute of Limitations in Cases of Memory Repression." *Journal of Criminal Law and Criminology* 84: 129–174.

Estrich, Susan. 1987. *Real Rape.* Cambridge, Mass.: Harvard University Press.

Frug, Mary Joe. 1992. "A Postmodern Feminist Legal Manifesto (An Unfinished Draft)." *Harvard Law Review* 105, no. 5:1045–1075.

Grossberg, Michael. 1985. *Governing the Hearth: Law and the Family in Nineteenth-Century America.* Chapel Hill: University of North Carolina Press.

Harvard Law Review. 1990. *Sexual Orientation and the Law.* Cambridge, Mass.: Harvard University Press.

Inness, Julie C. 1992. *Privacy, Intimacy, and Isolation.* New York: Oxford University Press.

Law, Sylvia A. 1988. "Homosexuality and the Social Meaning of Gender." *Wisconsin Law Review* 1988, no. 2: 187–235.

MacKinnon, Catharine A. 1979. *Sexual Harassment of Working Women: A Case of Sex Discrimination.* New Haven, Conn.: Yale University Press.

———. 1987. *Feminism Unmodified: Discourses on Life and Law.* Cambridge, Mass.: Harvard University Press.

———. 1993. *Only Words.* Cambridge, Mass.: Harvard University Press.

*Meritor Savings Bank* v. *Vinson.* 1986. 106 S.Ct. 2399.

Miller, H. G., et al., eds. 1990. *AIDS: The Second Decade.* Washington, D.C.: National Academy Press.

Mohr, Richard D. 1988. *Gays/Justice: A Study of Ethics, Society, and Law.* New York: Columbia University Press.

Okin, Susan Moller. 1989. *Justice, Gender, and the Family.* New York: Basic Books.

Olsen, Frances E. 1983. "The Family and the Market: A Study of Ideology and Legal Reform." *Harvard Law Review* 96, no. 7:1497–1578.

Petchesky, Rosalind P. 1984. *Abortion and Woman's Choice: The State, Sexuality, and Reproductive Freedom.* New York: Longman.

*Planned Parenthood of Southeastern Pennsylvania* v. *Casey.* 1992. 112 S.Ct. 2791.

Robson, Ruthann. 1992. *Lesbian (Out)law: Survival Under the Rule of Law.* Ithaca, N.Y.: Firebrand.

*Roe* v. *Wade.* 1973. 410 U.S. 113.

"Sexual Orientation and the Law." 1993. *Virginia Law Review* 79:1417–1902. Special issue.

Strossen, Nadine. 1993. "A Feminist Critique of 'The' Feminist Critique of Pornography." *Virginia Law Review* 79:1099–1190.

Thorne, Barrie, and Yalom, Marilyn, eds. 1992. *Rethinking the Family: Some Feminist Questions.* Rev. ed. Boston: Northeastern University Press.

Whisner, Mary. 1982. "Gender-Specific Clothing Regulation: A Study in Patriarchy." *Harvard Women's Law Journal* 5:73–119.

# SEXUAL ORIENTATION AND SEXUAL REORIENTATION

*See* Gender Identity and Gender-Identity Disorders; Homosexuality; *and* Sexual Identity.

# SIKHISM

## Origins and teachings

Sikhism began with Guru Nanak (1469–1539 C.E.), who was born a Hindu in the Punjab, which is still home for the vast majority of Sikhs. The word "Sikh" means "learner" or "disciple," and today the community numbers approximately 16 million. Nanak was the first of ten personal Gurus. Following the death in 1708 of the tenth Guru, Gobind Singh, the function of the Guru passed to the scripture and to the community. For this reason the Adi Granth (the Sikh scripture) is particularly venerated by the community.

In the North India of Nanak's day, a popular mode of religion among ordinary people was worship of a God of grace, immanent in all creation and never incarnated as a person or as an idol. This was the Sant Tradition and Nanak provided in his teachings its clearest statement. The presence of God is known through the *nam* (divine Name), mystically manifested in the beauty and order of the world around us, and one's duty is to meditate on the *nam*. This may be done by repeating a particular word or mantra, by singing hymns, or by silently meditating. In so doing one grows ever nearer to God, eventually achieving a condition of perfect union. In this union the cycle of transmigration (movement of the soul, at the death of the body, into a new body) is finally ended.

Those who accepted these teachings from Nanak were the first Sikhs. A line of successor Gurus followed him, the same divine spirit believed to inhabit each of them. The first four successors continued Nanak's teachings concerning the divine Name and, in 1603–1604 Arjan, the fifth Guru, collected their hymns and his own into a scripture, adding to it the works of other members of the Sant Tradition. During the time of the sixth Guru, Hargobind, the community attracted the attention of the Moghuls, at that time the rulers of northern India. By this time the community had grown noticeably large and the Moghuls were becoming suspicious of its increasing numbers. This danger receded, but it returned in the time of the ninth Guru, Tegh Behadur, who was executed by the Moghuls in 1675.

## The foundation of the Khalsa

In 1699 Tegh Bahadur's son and successor, Gobind Singh, inaugurated the Khalsa, a new order loyal Sikhs were summoned to join. Membership in the Khalsa was by an initiation ceremony and by a lifelong vow to maintain certain outward symbols, particularly uncut hair. Emphasis on the centrality of the divine Name was retained, but in place of the strictly inward faith taught by Guru Nanak, the tenth Guru created an organization that proclaimed the identify of his followers to all.

The inauguration of the Khalsa was crucial because it laid down for members an explicit code, or Rahit. Tradition records that the Guru promulgated all that the modern Khalsa observes today. In fact, many of the individual items of the Rahit can be traced to experiences that follow the actual foundation. The essential nature of the Khalsa, however, remains unaffected. Gobind Singh summoned loyal Sikhs to join his Khalsa; the Khalsa Sikh was to be known by certain outward features. These conspicuously included the obligation to bear arms and to retain uncut hair. Men were to add Singh ("Lion") to their name and women were to add Kaur ("Princess").

## Ranjit Singh, the Singh Sabha, and modern history

The eighteenth century, a time of much turbulence in the Punjab, was followed by a settled period during the early nineteenth century. Under Maharaja Ranjit Singh, who became ruler of the central Punjab in 1801, strong-government was introduced and during the next twenty-five years, the boundaries were enlarged in three directions. In the southeast, where the British advanced against Ranjit Singh, the border was drawn along the Satluj river, leaving many Sikhs in British territory or in the territory of their client states. Amritsar was not the capital city, but it was confirmed as the principal religious center. Ranjit Singh gilded the two upper storeys of its main temple, converting it into the famous Golden Temple.

His death in 1839 has been interpreted as marking the beginning of a steep decline in Sikh fortunes. In 1849, following two wars, the British annexed the Punjab. In 1873, however, the Singh Sabha (Singh Society) was founded and under its influence, the Sikh community was revived and reshaped. In 1920 the Singh Sabha was taken over by the more radical Akali movement, which was dedicated to the liberation of the gurdwaras (temples). With the partition of India in 1947, the Punjab was divided and the Sikhs in Pakistan moved across to the Indian area. Since then many Sikhs have claimed greater Punjab autonomy. The Indian army assault on the Golden Temple in 1984 led to decade-long demands by many Sikhs for Khalistan, a completely independent state. By 1993, however, these demands had subsided.

## The Singh Sabha and the Rahit

The dominant concern of the Singh Sabha reformers was to demonstrate that Sikhs formed an entirely distinct faith and that, in particular, they should not be confused with the Hindus. Special concern focused on the question of how a Sikh should behave. The intention was to show that the ways of the Sikh were emphatically not the ways of the other groups in India.

This required a restatement of the Rahit. According to tradition, Guru Gobind Singh had promulgated the Rahit in all its details, but by the late nineteenth century it had become impossible to determine his words with precision. The Rahit had been recorded for Sikhs in a number of Rahit-namas (Rahit manuals), none of which was entirely satisfactory. Those present at the founding of the Khalsa in 1699 would know what was required of them, and likewise those who associated with the Guru until his death in 1708. Most of the eighteenth century was, however, charged with warfare and persecution, and Sikhs had little time to record the Rahit that had been delivered to them. Ignorant or mischievous people might have corrupted the received Rahit, and the Rahit-namas could only be trusted after a scrupulous hand excised those portions that misled readers and restored those parts that had been lost.

The Singh Sabha leaders made unsuccessful attempts to produce an authentic Rahit-nama. Eventually, however, an acceptable version, Sikh Rahit Maryada, was issued in 1950, and appeals to this written authority are possible. The Sikhs have no clergy and so the publication of an authoritative text was truly significant. The question of orthodoxy, however, remains. Sikh Rahit Maryada represents the Khalsa version of orthodoxy, that is, the insistence on uncut hair; there is no doubt that since the days of the Singh Sabha, this has been the dominant style. There are, however, Sikhs who do not observe this version, preferring to venerate the

Gurus and scripture while cutting their hair. They do not observe the Rahit, yet still insist that they are Sikhs. It is here that Sikh identity becomes difficult to define and with it, the whole question of what constitutes Sikhism. The remainder of this article describes Khalsa Sikhism, but it is important to remember that many who call themselves Sikhs are not members of the Khalsa. This applies particularly to Sikhs living outside India.

## Khalsa regulations

Members of the Khalsa are identified by what are called the Five Ks (uncut hair, a comb, a steel wrist-band, a sword or dagger, and shorts). Smoking and intoxicants are firmly banned, the latter largely ignored but the former strictly maintained. Khalsa Sikhs are insistent on the right to carry a sword, a feature that enhances their reputation for violence. This reputation is greatly exaggerated. The Sikh should draw the sword (or use arms) only defensively, only when the cause is just, and only when all other methods have failed.

In Sikhism the key term when discussing ethical and moral issues is *seva* (service). Little guidance is given regarding health, disease, and the environment other than the most general principles. The objective is simply a life of personal righteousness, largely undefined. *Seva* is primarily considered a duty toward the gurdwara, and consists of obligations performed for the Guru on its holy ground. These include service in the *langar*, the free refectory that all gurdwaras are required to maintain, symbolizing the equality of all people. The concept is, however, further interpreted to mean genuine concern for the needs of others. According to Sikh Rahit Maryada, every Sikh is required to devote his or her entire life to the welfare of others.

In general, Sikhs are directed to see themselves as distinct from other faiths, particularly from all forms of Hindu tradition. This is the case with funerals, which involve a simple rite. Cremation follows death but all who assemble are required to restrict their lamenting. The corpse is dressed in clean garments, complete with the Five Ks, and the ceremony is conducted while hymns are sung. Such practices as laying the corpse on the floor or breaking the skull are sternly forbidden. Specific ethical injunctions are comparatively rare in Sikh Rahit Maryada, although those that are mentioned are clearly intended to be mandatory. The emphasis is, instead, placed on the duty of the individual Sikh to live a worthy life as circumstances of time and place dictate.

With two exceptions, matters of bioethical concern are not spelled out. Sikhs are left to determine them in the light of their religious faith. One exception is that female infanticide is strictly prohibited. This reflects an earlier period in Punjab history. The second exception is that, strictly speaking, initiated Khalsa members should not eat from the same dish as an uninitiated Sikh or one who has renounced the faith. All other issues, such as abortion, birth control, suicide, and euthanasia, are left to the individual or the family to decide.

W. H. McLeod

*For a further discussion of topics mentioned in this entry, see the entries* FAMILY; HINDUISM; *and* MEDICAL ETHICS, HISTORY OF, *section on* SOUTH AND EAST ASIA, *articles on* GENERAL SURVEY, *and* INDIA. *For a discussion of related ideas, see the entries* AFRICAN RELIGION; CONFUCIANISM; DEATH, ATTITUDES TOWARD; EASTERN ORTHODOX CHRISTIANITY; ISLAM; JAINISM; JUDAISM; LIFE; NATIVE AMERICAN RELIGIONS; PROTESTANTISM; ROMAN CATHOLICISM; *and* TAOISM. *Other relevant material may be found under the entries* DEATH, *article on* EASTERN THOUGHT; EUGENICS AND RELIGIOUS LAW; *and* HEALTH AND DISEASE, *article on* ANTHROPOLOGICAL PERSPECTIVES.

## Bibliography

AVTAR SINGH. 1970. *Ethics of the Sikhs.* Patiala, India: Punjabi University.
GREWAL, J. S. 1990. *The Sikhs of the Punjab.* Vol. II.3 of *The New Cambridge History of India.* Cambridge: At the University Press.
KOHLI, SURINDAR SINGH. 1975. *Sikh Ethics.* New Delhi: Munshiram Manoharlal.
McLEOD, W. H., ed. and trans. 1991. *Textual Sources for the Study of Sikhism.* Chicago: University of Chicago Press.
OBEROI, HARJOT. 1994. *The Construction of Religious Boundaries: Culture, Identity, and Diversity in the Sikh Tradition.* Delhi: Oxford University Press.
*Rehat Maryada: A Guide to the Sikh Way of Life.* 1978. English translation of the Sikh Rahit Maryada. Amritsar: Shiromani Gurdwara Parbandakh Committee.
*Sri Guru Granth Sahib in English Translation.* 1984–1991. 4 vols. Translated by Gurbachan Singh Talib. Patiala, India: Punjabi University.

# SMOKING

*See* SUBSTANCE ABUSE, *article on* SMOKING.

# SOCIAL MEDICINE

Throughout most of medical history the physician's role has been seen predominantly as a personal one in which, for the most part, the one-to-one patient–physician relationship is the one that is considered in medical ethical principles. Although the shocking evidence of physician participation in genocidal activities during World War II led to new ethical statements, such as the Declaration of Geneva, that place physicians' behavior in a social context, such statements nevertheless largely remain codifications of the ethical behavior of a physician toward a particular patient.

## Origin and meaning of social medicine

Enlargement of the role of the physician to include social and community aspects of disease prevention, diagnosis, and treatment is of relatively recent development, and is referred to as "social medicine." Many definitions of social medicine have been attempted, the more generally accepted ones reflecting the relationship of social factors to disease and death. Today there is a general consensus that social medicine represents the study of the medical needs of society and the interaction of medicine and society, along with the practice of inclusion of social factors in public health, preventive medicine, and the clinical examination and treatment of patients.

The concept grew from a variety of experiences over the centuries. In seventeenth-century London, weekly "Bills of Mortality" listing the previous week's deaths began to be published. Incomplete and inaccurate as they were, they inspired John Graunt (1620–1674) and, later, Edwin Chadwick (1800–1890) to relate social and economic circumstances to death rates.

Similarly, in Italy, Bernardino Ramazzini (1633–1714) documented the relationship of disease to a series of occupations. In the nineteenth century, these inchoate efforts came together into social-policy constructs. In Austria, Johann Peter Frank (1745–1821) published a monumental six-volume work on medical policy as a governmental endeavor—to ensure clean water and sewage disposal, for example, and to promote other regulatory efforts for the benefit of society. Chadwick, in Britain, urged government to take responsibility under the Poor Laws to protect the health of the growing population impoverished by increasing industrialization (Chadwick, 1965).

The industrial revolution fostered turmoil throughout Europe and increased the awareness of social causation of disease and death as it brought about far-reaching changes in the lives of working people. Friedrich Engels' study, *The Condition of the Working Class in England in 1844*, described the relationship of diseases such as tuberculosis, typhoid, and typhus to malnutrition, inadequate housing, contaminated water supplies, and overcrowding (Engels, 1968; Waitzkin, 1989).

The early nineteenth century therefore saw the beginning of a transformation of the physician's role (Rosen, 1974). As physicians increasingly recognized the impact of social factors on their patients' health, they saw that helping individual patients made it necessary to assess and respond to the social aspects of their lives along with everything else that might cause or prolong their patients' illnesses.

The term "social medicine" was first used in 1846 to mean "all those aspects of medicine that affect society" (Guérin, 1848, p. 203), but its popularization in Europe is usually attributed to Rudolf Virchow (1821–1902; see Ackerknecht, 1953, and Silver, 1987). Virchow, who later became a highly respected pathologist (known by his colleagues as the "Pope of Medicine"), was an early exponent of the importance of social factors as contributors to disease. In 1847, at the Prussian government's request, Virchow investigated a severe typhus epidemic in rural Upper Silesia. In his report he recommended a series of dramatic economic, political, and social changes that included increased employment, better wages, local autonomy in government, agricultural cooperatives, and a more progressive tax structure. He described disease causation as multifactorial, including the conditions of people's lives. To be effective, he argued, a health-care system must go beyond treating pathological problems in individual patients, and health professionals therefore must take responsibility for political action. In a radical medical-political newspaper he edited, the masthead read: "The physician is the natural attorney of (advocate for) the poor." Virchow insisted that "medicine is a social science, and politics nothing but medicine on a grand scale" (Silver, 1987, p. 85).

Early on, social medicine was basically an approach to medical practice; proponents recognized the effects of social conditions and took them into consideration in dealing with illness in patients. During the first half of the twentieth century, when Alfred Grotjahn published his *Soziale Pathologie* (1912) and René Sand his *Vers la Médecine Sociale* (1952), social medicine became more than an aspect of medical practice. These works, among others, established the importance and perhaps even the predominance of social factors in disease causation, maintenance, and remission. A whole new field of scholarly study emerged that understood health, disease, and the role of medicine in these terms. Beyond the traditional ethic of a physician's responsibility to a patient or to other physicians, social medicine, which was concerned with the relationship between health and the conditions of society, imposed an added discipline of responsibility to society (Grotjahn, 1912; Sand, 1952).

The discipline was further refined by John Ryle, professor of medicine at Cambridge University, who included social factors in the analysis of the varied responses of patients to illness. Since individual responses were influenced by the patient's family, work, and economic circumstances, he regarded the study and clinical application of these factors as part of the practice of social medicine (Galdston, 1949; Ryle, 1943). Ryle wrote that social medicine

> embodies the idea of medicine applied to the service of man as socius, as fellow or comrade, with a view to a better understanding and more durable assistance of all his main and contributory troubles which are inimical to active health. . . . It embodies also the idea of medicine applied in the service of societas, or the community of man with a view to lowering the incidence of all the preventable diseases and raising the general level of human fitness. (Ryle, 1943)

As it became clear that many of the causative agents were social in nature, social medicine embraced not only what is usually called "preventive medicine"—that is, advice on the prevention of illness provided to individuals and families within medical practice—but also what is usually called "public health"—efforts to prevent disease in whole communities. For health and disease, an interface was seen to exist between society and medicine, not just between the doctor and a patient. The family itself, the home, the workplace, the environment, and various other social conditions played a part in whether or not people became sick, how long they remained sick, whether they recovered, and even whether medical care and other health-care services were available.

Social medicine ranges from the doctor's use of social factors in making a better diagnosis or offering better treatment (that is, an approach to clinical problems) as well as providing preventive medicine, to helping the medical profession recognize social factors that are "pathological" or "therapeutic" in society (that is, an approach to public health). In its current interpretation, social medicine also means influencing the doctor's frame of mind as a professional, so he or she will recognize the need to modify social factors (in effect, an approach to social reform).

Social medicine therefore includes four components: (1) "medical care": treatment of the individual patient (or family) to provide comfort and hope, ease symptoms, and, when possible, prolong satisfying and productive life or even "cure" the disease; (2) "preventive medicine": guidance for the individual patient (or family) in promoting health and preventing disease; (3) "public health": advocacy and action for health promotion and disease prevention in the community; and (4) "social well-being" (as used in the definition of "health" in the Constitution of the World Health Organization), including amelioration of hunger, homelessness, unemployment, poverty, and hopelessness.

Social medicine in action attempts to (1) ensure equitable access to an effective and efficient medical-care system; (2) encourage preventive medicine by, for example, educating practitioners; (3) support extensive public-health activities; and (4) increase resources and services to improve social well-being.

## Social medicine as an ethical model

Physicians engaged in the field of social medicine must concern themselves with a wide variety of problems, disciplines, and factors that encompass what are conventionally understood to be outside the proper concerns of the medical profession. Once the physician recognizes a person as a social creature, the whole range of a patient's needs becomes relevant. Traditionally, physicians have rarely seen themselves as responsible for intervention to correct a social situation outside the family that might be contributing to the patient's illness or obstructing recovery. A socially oriented medical profession may need to take vigorous action in its patients' interest to promote improved housing, nutrition, and educational opportunities or to combat racism, discriminatory practices, or the inequities and inadequacies of the medical delivery system and its distribution or availability.

Social medicine holds that the physician has an ethical responsibility to take steps to change pathogenic situations to protect society, of which the particular patient for whom he or she bears responsibility is a part. In such circumstances, the practice of social medicine may place a physician in serious opposition to many powerful forces in society, not excluding the majority membership of his or her own profession. A physician may thereby incur social and professional opprobrium. This was the fate of Henrik Ibsen's Dr. Stockmann, described by his community as an "enemy of the people" because he questioned the safety of the town's springs, the source of its prosperity (Ibsen, 1935).

Even in milder efforts, physicians who undertake the practice of social medicine may face resistance in utilizing their professional role to ameliorate pathogenic social situations such as inadequate nutrition or malnutrition; accidents and disease that befall those who live in inadequate housing; unsafe working conditions; environmental hazards or decayed neighborhoods; and polluted air and water. Again, since many of these factors are the result of neglect commonly visited upon the poor, the physician who seeks to modify such situations may find it necessary to engage in social movements that attempt to mitigate or eliminate poverty and to encourage poor people to take action on their own. The physician may be forced to take a political position, even initiate political action, in pursuing this end, just as those who do not act or who oppose such actions are taking political positions.

The remainder of this article will cover specific aspects of social medicine. These aspects—environmental and occupational health, medical-care systems, responsibility of the profession, and medical education—illustrate the range of the field and its relevance to current issues.

## Environmental and occupational health

When a physician, as a responsible practitioner of social medicine, recognizes the potent and often baleful influence of industry on the health not only of its workers but of the community in which it is located, community education and further action may be indicated. There is increasing recognition of the environmental origins of cancer, for example, including the role of carcinogens in the workplace. Some workplaces are hazardous by the nature of the job; in others accidents, commonly the result of inadequate safety measures or careless disregard for safety standards, result in thousands of deaths and millions of injuries. Further, in an unfortunately large number of instances, the effluent of factories poisons rivers, lakes, and air, contributing to chronic morbidity and increased mortality among the workers and in the community.

The physician with social concern may find both political action and educational efforts unwelcome in a community torn between its need for the jobs provided by the industrial presence and fear of the industry's lethal qualities. In some communities, the answer has been to keep the lethal factory rather than accept unemployment, poverty, and starvation without it. Doctors and communities must begin to deal with a novel ethical conflict: How to modify the paradox of democratic capitalism—the need to restrain the profit motive in order to protect the community from destructive exploitation.

These actions include something more than professional response. The requirements for social change and political action (e.g., nutrition for the children of the poor or occupational safety measures) also demand that the physician act as citizen. In some situations the physician may very well be torn between social concern and his or her livelihood. The physician who works for an industry whose work processes are unsafe or pathogenic may jeopardize his or her job by taking a stand against the employer or the industry of which the employer is a part. Yet failing to take a stand makes him or her complicit and endangers the lives of countless others. A physician cannot be expected ethically to remain silent when the work situation is likely to produce trauma or disease.

Some employed physicians are expected to minimize reports of injury or disease in order to reduce the employer's financial commitment. That is the "job," as the employer sees it, for which the physician was hired. But is the physician's "job" to put first the interests of the employer who pays his or her salary, or the interests of the patient?

The dilemma of dual responsibility is most vividly apparent in wartime. In addition to the medical oath the physician may have taken at the completion of medical school, on entering military service the physician, like all military officers, must agree to obey military orders. These orders, for example, usually require the military physician to return wounded military personnel to action as quickly as possible. The decision as to which patient to treat first may therefore be determined by which one can be returned to duty most quickly rather than by the urgency of each patient's individual need for medical care. In an extreme case, the military physician would be expected to let a seriously wounded soldier die in order to save the life of one less seriously wounded who was able to return more quickly to battle. And if there were enemy wounded who were more urgently in need of care, when would their turn be?

## Medical-care systems

In its scholarly manifestation, social medicine initiates studies on a nation's economic and social systems' influence on the structure and function of its health-care system. Studies and procedures of health care in individual countries and cross-national comparisons are an important part of the analytic work of social medicine (Allende, 1939; Cochrane, 1972; Navarro, 1992; Roemer, 1991; Sidel and Sidel, 1982, 1983; Waitzkin, 1989).

The ethical imperative that arises from this work invites agitation for change and improvement in the structure of the medical-care system to improve its functioning. To that end the results of social medicine studies may generate promotion of the values and methods observed in other national systems, toward better access and improved quality in meeting the needs of the poor and the geographically isolated, and of marginally self-supporting workers. In today's situation, for example, the inflation of medical costs resulting from disorganization and inequities has bankrupted many families and barred adequate access to medical care for many others. What is the physician's role?

If access to medical care is dependent upon ability to pay, and many people are unable to obtain care for lack of funds, is the physician ethically obliged to oppose ability to pay as a condition for service? Of whom, if anyone, should the physician ethically demand payment? Should physicians demand that medical care be free to everyone at the time of service? When ability to pay interferes with access to medical care, does not the profit motive operate against the best interests of the patient and the ethical principles of the physician?

Newspaper reports and medical journal articles offer accounts of unequal medical treatment by race or gender. Blacks receive fewer advanced technological studies than whites for the same conditions (Kahn et al.,

1994; Kjellstrand, 1988; Wenneker and Epstein, 1989); women receive less intensive studies and procedures for heart disease than men (Ayaniah and Epstein, 1991; Kjellstrand, 1988). Ethical principles require reversal of such situations, and social medicine studies and principles guide physicians in taking action (Perkins, 1993; Hurowitz, 1993).

Evidence accumulates that with the increase of managed care as a method of cost control in medicine, physicians are urged to limit expenditures by reducing services or narrowing access to expensive studies, hospitalization, or medications. Physicians in medical groups under managed-care controls are offered incentives to conform with such regulations or may be punished financially for not complying.

Official reports as well as media accounts about the scandalous treatment of elderly people confined to nursing homes is another example in point. The profit motive too often leads not only to cutting corners on services and allowing short weights in food or supplies, but to making substitutions of less qualified staff, eliminating necessary services, and waiving safety and protective measures for the helpless inhabitants. Aside from the corrupt financial dealings it encourages in such cases, profit-making often prevents and obstructs both the best care and the provision of alternatives to institutional care. Physicians cannot insulate themselves morally from the mistreatment of elderly people in nursing homes nor from the exploitation of patients through the entrepreneurial mechanics of the pharmaceutical drug industry.

Is it part of the ethics of social medicine to condemn investment in drug industry stocks, in private proprietary hospitals, and in a variety of entrepreneurial enterprises such as laboratories, radiological centers, and other diagnostic and treatment modalities to which they refer their patients? The U.S. Congress and the American Medical Association have strongly condemned "self-dealing" of this nature.

## Responsibility of the profession

In addition to the question of the individual physician's ethics in financial dealings that may compromise patients' best interests, there is the associated question of the physician's responsibility for taking action when he or she observes any unethical or unprofessional behavior on the part of a colleague. If a physician knows first-hand about the poor quality of a particular nursing home, even if his or her particular patient is not affected by it, is the physician required to take steps to correct the situation? Legal steps? Professional steps? Or, more narrowly, if the physician knows of colleagues who do not or cannot adequately carry out their obligations as physicians because of incompetence or because of lack of training, illness, or addiction, what should be done about it? Social medicine holds that there is an ethical responsibility to call attention to these facts even if they do not cause risk to the physician's particular patients.

The physician as social medicine practitioner is asked to make a difficult choice, as a citizen and as a doctor. Social medicine as an ethical model imposes an obligation on the physician to serve his or her individual patient by serving all patients. And, as a member of a profession, the physician must act not only as an individual but as representative of that profession, adopting an advocacy role for the groups in society that require special attention and care. The profession is being asked to act toward society as the individual physician is asked in traditional ethical statements to act toward an individual patient.

Finally, the ethical physician has a responsibility to inform and educate the community on the social nature of health and illness. An educated and knowledgeable constituency is required to provide the necessary support for the political social action. Discussing the dangers of smoking, for example, is hardly enough. Physicians ought also to discuss the economics of the tobacco industry and suggest that steps need be taken to cushion workers from unemployment if the tobacco industry is diminished or eliminated. Moreover, if there is an industrial hazard that needs correction, physicians ought to advise not only on the danger but on means for correcting it.

It is clear, nonetheless, that for physicians to discharge social medical responsibilities in complex areas, they need to see themselves as part of a group larger than the medical profession alone. In 1956, Theodore Fox described the "Greater Medical Profession" and urged "converting the medical empire into a commonwealth" (Fox, 1956). To respond ethically to social needs is to recognize the contribution of all health workers and to act in concert with others in the health field and outside it. In doing this the physician may wish to join with others in professionally oriented groups—such as the American Public Health Association, the International Physicians for the Prevention of Nuclear War, Physicians for Human Rights, and Physicians for Social Responsibility.

## Social medicine in medical education

Medical education should include not only the technical, laboratory, and clinical models of what a physician can do, must know, and be able to deal with; it should also give the future physician the tools to recognize the social circumstances—industrial, neighborhood, legislative, administrative—that play a part in the production of disease or that influence medical care. Exposure to social medicine as an important component of medical education, along with the example of role models and the fact that faculty members have such interests, will influence students' and later practicing physicians' ideas as to what their responsibilities are and how these responsibilities can be discharged (Silver, 1973).

Although departments of social medicine had long existed in medical schools and hospitals in other countries, it was not until the 1950s that Ephraim Bluestone and Martin Cherkasky organized the first department of social medicine in a U.S. medical institution, Montefiore Medical Center in New York City (Levenson, 1984). Other institutions such as Harvard Medical School, the University of North Carolina College of Medicine, and the Albert Einstein College of Medicine later adopted the term in department names or titles of professorships, but the pace of this development in the United States has languished.

## Conclusion

Early medical ethics was largely restricted to the concept of a physician–patient dyad. Social relationships of pathogenic factors were unknown or ignored. In recent years it has become clearer that the social aspects of the prevention, causation, maintenance, or cure of disease cannot be adequately dealt with solely in the one-to-one relationship. Expanded notions of the physician's responsibility based on social factors ought to be included in modern medical ethics statements. The physician should learn to recognize and articulate social demands for change in situations that are harmful to patients and to the community, and not simply deal with problems as they arise in his or her patients.

To this end, physicians must know more about the social situations in which disease occurs or which contribute to disease; they must adopt an advocacy role in pursuing change, and join with other health workers in ensuring appropriate social action for correction. In addition to oaths and declarations in which physicians bind themselves to serve individual patients honorably and ethically, service to society must also be required of physicians. Social medicine deserves an integral place within a more traditional medical ethics. Unfortunately, issues of social medicine are often assigned low priority in medical education and in medical practice.

GEORGE A. SILVER
VICTOR W. SIDEL

*For a further discussion of topics mentioned in this entry, see the entries* AIDS, *article on* PUBLIC-HEALTH ISSUES; CONFLICT OF INTEREST; EPIDEMICS; EUGENICS, *article on* HISTORICAL ASPECTS; GENETICS AND ENVIRONMENT IN HUMAN HEALTH; HEALTH-CARE RESOURCES, ALLOCATION OF; HEALTH PROMOTION AND HEALTH EDUCATION; HEALTH SCREENING AND TESTING IN THE PUBLIC-HEALTH CONTEXT; MEDICAL EDUCATION; MEDICINE, ANTHROPOLOGY OF; MEDICINE, SOCIOLOGY OF; OCCUPATIONAL SAFETY AND HEALTH; POPULATION ETHICS, *section on* ELEMENTS OF POPULATION ETHICS; PUBLIC HEALTH; RACE AND RACISM; RESPONSIBILITY; SEXISM; WARFARE, *article on* MEDICINE AND WAR; *and* WHISTLEBLOWING. *For a discussion of related ideas, see the entries:* ABORTION; ABUSE, INTERPERSONAL; BIOETHICS EDUCATION; ECONOMIC CONCEPTS IN HEALTH CARE; FAMILY; FEMINISM; FOOD POLICY; HEALTH AND DISEASE, *article on* SOCIOLOGICAL PERSPECTIVES; PROFESSION AND PROFESSIONAL ETHICS; PUBLIC HEALTH AND THE LAW; SOCIAL WORK IN HEALTH CARE; STRIKES BY HEALTH PROFESSIONALS; *and* WOMEN, *article on* HISTORICAL AND CROSS-CULTURAL PERSPECTIVES.

## Bibliography

ACKERKNECHT, ERWIN HEINZ. 1953. *Rudolf Virchow: Doctor, Statesman, Anthropologist.* Madison: University of Wisconsin Press.

ALLENDE, GOSSENS SALVADOR. 1939. *La Realidad Medico-Social Chilena: Sintesis.* Santiago, Chile: Ministerio de Salubridad, Prevision y Asistencia Social.

AYANIAN, JOHN Z., AND EPSTEIN, ARNOLD M. 1991. "Differences in the Use of Procedures Between Women and Men for Coronary Heart Disease." *New England Journal of Medicine* 325:221–225.

CHADWICK, EDWIN. 1965. [1842]. *Report on the Sanitary Conditions of the Labouring Population of Great Britain.* Edited by M. W. Flinn. Edinburgh: Edinburgh University Press.

COCHRANE, ARCHIBALD LEMAN. 1972. *Effectiveness and Efficiency: Random Reflections on Health Services.* London: Neuffield Provincial Hospitals Trust.

ENGELS, FRIEDRICH. 1968. [1845]. *The Condition of the Working Class in England in 1844.* Stanford, Calif.: Stanford University Press.

FOX, THEODORE F. 1956. "The Greater Medical Profession." *Lancet* 2, no. 6946:779–780.

GALDSTON, IAGO, ed. 1949. *Social Medicine: Its Derivations and Objectives.* New York: Commonwealth Fund.

GROTJAHN, ALFRED. 1912. *Soziale Pathologie.* Berlin: A. Hirschwald.

GUÉRIN, JULES. 1848. "De l'intervention du corps médical dans le situation actuelle; programme de médecine sociale." *Gazette Médicale de Paris,* series 3, vol. 3, no. 12: 203.

HUROWITZ, JAMES C. 1993. "Toward a Social Policy for Health." *New England Journal of Medicine* 329, no. 2: 130–133.

IBSEN, HENRIK. 1935. [1882]. *An Enemy of the People.* In *Eleven Plays of Henrik Ibsen,* pp. 175–288. New York: Modern Library.

KAHN, KATHERINE L.; PEARSON, MARJORIE L.; HARRISON, ELLEN R.; DESMOND, KATHERINE A.; ROGERS, WILLIAM H.; RUBENSTEIN, LISA V.; BROOK, ROBERT H.; AND KEELER, EMMETT B. 1994. "Health Care for Black and Poor Hospitalized Medicare Patients." *Journal of the American Medical Association* 271:1169–1174.

KJELLSTRAND, C. M. 1988. "Age, Sex and Race Inequality in Renal Transplantation." *Archives of Internal Medicine* 148:1305–1309.

LEVENSON, DOROTHY. 1984. *Montefiore: The Hospital as Social Instrument: 1884–1984.* New York: Farrar Straus Giroux.

McKEOWN, THOMAS, and LOWE, CHARLES RONALD. 1974. *An Introduction to Social Medicine.* 2d ed. Oxford: Blackwell Scientific Publications.

NAVARRO, VICENTE. 1992. "Has Socialism Failed? An Analysis of Health Indicators Under Socialism." *International Journal of Health Services* 22, no. 4:563–601.

PERKINS, JANE. 1993. "Race Discrimination in the American Health Care System." *Clearinghouse Review* (special issue): 371–383.

ROEMER, MILTON. 1991. *National Health Systems: Comparative Strategies.* New York: Oxford University Press.

ROSEN, GEORGE. 1947. "What Is Social Medicine? A Genetic Analysis of the Concept." *Bulletin of the History of Medicine* 21, no. 5:674–733.

———. 1974. *From Medical Police to Social Medicine: Essays on the History of Health Care.* New York: Science History Publications.

RYLE, JOHN A. 1943. "Social Medicine: Its Meaning and Its Scope." *British Medical Journal 2*, no. 4324:633–636.

SAND, RENÉ. 1952. "The Advent of Social Medicine." In his *The Advance to Social Medicine,* pp. 507–589. London: Staples Press.

SIDEL, RUTH, and SIDEL, VICTOR W. 1982. *The Health of China.* Boston: Beacon Press.

SIDEL, VICTOR W., and SIDEL, RUTH. 1983. *A Healthy State: An International Perspective on the Crisis in U.S. Medical Care.* New York: Pantheon.

SILVER, GEORGE A. 1973. "The Teaching of Social Medicine." *Clinical Research* 21, no. 2:151–155.

———. 1987. "Virchow, the Heroic Model in Medicine: Health Policy by Accolade." *American Journal of Public Health* 77, no. 1:82–88.

WAITZKIN, HOWARD. 1989. "Marxist Perspective in Social Medicine." *Social Science and Medicine* 28, no. 11:1099–1101.

WENNEKER, MARK B., and EPSTEIN, ARNOLD M. 1989. "Racial Inequalities in the Use of Procedures for Patients with Ischemic Heart Disease in Massachusetts." *Journal of the American Medical Association* 261:253–257.

# SOCIAL WORK IN HEALTH CARE

Social workers have played a vital role in health care settings since the early twentieth century. Social work was introduced to medical settings in the United States by Dr. Richard C. Cabot in 1905. Cabot, a professor of both clinical medicine and social ethics at Harvard University, was instrumental in adding social workers to his clinic staff at Massachusetts General Hospital. Under the direction of their first department head, Ida Cannon, these social workers helped patients and their families cope with illness, disease, disability, and hospitalization by focusing particularly on their psychosocial needs, including their emotional reaction and adaptation (Rossen, 1987).

Over time, social work's function and influence in health-care settings have expanded significantly (Miller and Rehr, 1983). In addition to assisting hospitalized patients and their families, social workers provide genetic counseling, hospice services, psychotherapy and counseling in mental-health agencies, and treatment of people with eating disorders and substance abuse problems. These opportunities exist in hospitals, neighborhood health and family planning clinics, psychiatric institutions, community mental-health centers, nursing homes, rehabilitation centers, and other long-term care facilities. Social workers' specialized role is to help patients and their families cope with illness and disability.

Many social workers in health-care settings provide patients and their families with counseling, and information about and referral to needed resources (e.g., home health care, financial assistance, nursing home placement). Social workers are also skilled in organizing and facilitating support groups for various populations, such as cancer patients, rape victims, and parents of seriously impaired infants. They work to enhance the availability of community-based resources (e.g., health-care clinics in low-income neighborhoods or residential programs for children with AIDS), advocate on behalf of individual patients who are in need of services, and advocate to ensure that important public policy issues related to health care are addressed (e.g., funding for lead screening or guidelines concerning involuntary commitment of mentally ill individuals to psychiatric hospitals).

Social workers typically function as part of an interdisciplinary team, which may include physicians, nurses, nutritionists, rehabilitation staff, clergy, and health-care administrators. On occasion, they facilitate the process through which health-care professionals negotiate differences of opinion or conflict among themselves concerning specific ethical issues. Social workers' skilled use of mediation techniques can help to resolve disagreements that sometimes arise in health-care settings. Their sensitivity to ethnic and cultural diversity can be particularly helpful when there is a clash between patients' and families' ethnically or culturally based values and prevailing ethical norms, policies, and health-care practices (e.g., concerning the use of mood-altering medication, autopsy, or blood transfusion).

Bioethical issues in health-care settings present social workers with complex challenges (Reamer, 1985, 1987). Some of these ethical issues pertain to specific medical conditions. Examples include ethical dilemmas related to a family's decision about withdrawal of a patient's life support, abortion following a rape, organ transplantation, the use of restraints with a noncompliant psychiatric patient, or a patient's decision to refuse neuroleptic medication. When such issues arise, social workers often serve as important intermediaries in relationships among patients, their families, and health-care professionals. In these instances, social workers help patients and their families make difficult personal decisions, facilitate communication among members of the health-care team, advocate on a patient's or family's behalf, or raise policy issues that need to be addressed by a hospital, nursing home, or rehabilitation center.

Other bioethical issues concern the nature of relationships and transactions between social workers and patients or their families. For example, social workers in health-care settings must be familiar with privacy and confidentiality norms that govern relationships with patients and families. They must also be sensitive to complex ethical issues involving patients' right to self-determination, informed consent procedures, truth telling, professional paternalism, and whistleblowing (Loewenberg and Dolgoff, 1992; Reamer, 1990).

In particular, social workers can clarify differences among the ethical obligations that guide various professions. For example, social workers in a health-care setting can help clarify the ethical responsibilities of various professionals when staff suspect child abuse or that a patient with AIDS poses a threat to a third party.

Health-care social workers are also involved in discussion and formulation of the ethical aspects of health-care policy and administration. This may take several forms. Social workers may participate as members of institutional ethics committees (IECs) that discuss ethically complex cases and policies. They may have a particularly valuable perspective because of their extensive contact with patients and their families and can, therefore, contribute to discussions about, for example, resuscitation guidelines, patients' right to refuse treatment, advance directives, organ transplantation, treatment of severely impaired infants, and the privacy rights of AIDS patients. Similarly, social workers are active participants on institutional review boards (IRBs) that examine a variety of ethical issues in research on human subjects.

In addition, social workers may be involved in discussions about the ethical aspects of health-care financing mechanisms and cost-containment measures. They may also propose ways to advocate on patients' behalf or to advocate for policy reform that may provide a more just allocation of scarce health-care resources at the local, national, or international level. An example is social workers' participation on a hospital committee to assess the pressure to limit care provided to, and hasten discharge of, psychiatric patients covered under "managed care" programs operated by private insurers. In

these instances, social workers may help identify the psychosocial consequences of various strategies to allocate limited health-care resources.

As a profession, social work has its formal origins in nineteenth-century concern about the poor, and is an outgrowth of the pioneering work of charity organization societies and settlement houses, primarily in England and the United States (Brieland, 1987; Leiby, 1978). Thus, social workers are inclined to be attentive to the needs of low-income, culturally diverse, and oppressed patients and families.

Although contemporary social workers provide services to individuals and families at all points on the socioeconomic spectrum, the profession continues to have an abiding concern for the disadvantaged. As a result, social workers in health-care settings are alert to ethical issues that involve such populations as low-income patients, abused children and elders, women, refugees and immigrants, substance abusers, ethnic minorities, and gay or lesbian individuals. Concern about such vulnerable groups—for example, with respect to their access to health care, their privacy rights, or discrimination against them by health-care providers—is one of social work's principal hallmarks. Social workers may advocate for individual patients and families whose rights are threatened or who are victims of institutional abuse or discrimination. They also may advocate for public policy that will enhance protection of the rights of these populations.

Like all health-care professionals, in order to participate fully in discussions of bioethical issues and dilemmas, social workers need specialized knowledge and training. First, they need to be familiar with the history, language, concepts, and theories of bioethics, particularly as they have evolved since the early 1970s. Second, social workers should be knowledgeable about formal mechanisms that can help health-care professionals monitor and address bioethical issues. These include phenomena such as IECs, IRBs, utilization review and quality assurance committees, informed consent procedures, and advance directives. It is also useful for social workers to be acquainted with relevant codes of ethics and legal considerations (statutes and case law) related to patients' rights and health-care professionals' obligations.

Finally, social workers should be familiar with the various schools of thought that pertain to ethical decision making and ethical theory. This can be particularly useful when social workers are involved in discussion of cases with professional ethicists, for example, when a decision must be made about when and how to tell a fragile, terminally ill patient the truth about his or her diagnosis, or to disclose confidential information, against a patient's wishes, in order to protect a third party. This training may be offered as part of agency-based in-service education, professional conferences, or undergraduate and graduate social work education.

Especially since the early 1970s, social workers have been aware of the diverse and complex bioethical issues involved in health care, whether it involves acute or chronic, inpatient or outpatient, or medical, rehabilitative, nursing, or psychiatric care. Social workers' growing awareness of, and enhanced expertise in addressing, bioethical issues helps to ensure the protection of patients' and families' rights and the soundness of ethical decisions made in health-care settings.

FREDERIC G. REAMER

*Directly related to this entry are the entries* TEAMS, HEALTH-CARE; *and* ALLIED HEALTH PROFESSIONS. *For a further discussion of topics mentioned in this entry, see the entries* BIOETHICS EDUCATION, *article on* OTHER HEALTH PROFESSIONS; CLINICAL ETHICS, *article on* INSTITUTIONAL ETHICS COMMITTEES; CONFIDENTIALITY; FAMILY; INFORMED CONSENT, *articles on* MEANING AND ELEMENTS OF INFORMED CONSENT, *and* LEGAL AND ETHICAL ISSUES OF CONSENT IN HEALTH CARE (*with its* POSTSCRIPT); PATERNALISM; PRIVACY IN HEALTH CARE; PRIVILEGED COMMUNICATIONS; *and* WHISTLEBLOWING. *Other relevant material may be found under the entries* ETHICS; HEALTH POLICY, *article on* POLITICS AND HEALTH CARE; *and* LAW AND BIOETHICS.

## Bibliography

BRIELAND, DONALD. 1987. "History and Evolution of Social Work Practice." In *Encyclopedia of Social Work*, vol. 1, pp. 739–754. 18th ed. Edited by Anne Minahan. Silver Spring, Md.: National Association of Social Workers.

LEIBY, JAMES. 1978. *A History of Social Welfare and Social Work in the United States.* New York: Columbia University Press.

LOEWENBERG, FRANK, and DOLGOFF, RALPH. 1992. *Ethical Decisions for Social Work Practice.* 4th ed. Itasca, Ill.: F. E. Peacock.

MILLER, ROSALIND S., and REHR, HELEN, eds. 1983. *Social Work Issues in Health Care.* Englewood Cliffs, N.J.: Prentice-Hall.

NATIONAL ASSOCIATION OF SOCIAL WORKERS. 1979. *Code of Ethics of the National Association of Social Workers.* Silver Spring, Md.: Author.

REAMER, FREDERIC G. 1985. "The Emergence of Bioethics in Social Work." *Health and Social Work* 10, no. 4:271–281.

———. 1987. "Values and Ethics." In *Encyclopedia of Social Work*, vol. 2, pp. 801–809. 18th ed. Edited by Anne Minahan. Silver Spring, Md.: National Association of Social Workers.

———. 1990. *Ethical Dilemmas in Social Service.* 2d ed. New York: Columbia University Press.

ROSSEN, SALIE. 1987. "Hospital Social Work." In *Encyclopedia of Social Work*, vol. 1, pp. 816–821. 18th ed. Edited by Anne Minahan. Silver Spring, Md.: National Association of Social Workers.

## SOCIOBIOLOGY

*See* BIOLOGY, PHILOSOPHY OF; *and* GENETICS AND HUMAN SELF-UNDERSTANDING.

## SOCIOLOGY OF MEDICINE

*See* MEDICINE, SOCIOLOGY OF.

## SOUTH AFRICA

*See* MEDICAL ETHICS, HISTORY OF, *section on* AFRICA, *article on* SOUTH AFRICA.

## SOUTHEAST ASIA

*See* MEDICAL ETHICS, HISTORY OF, *section on* SOUTH AND EAST ASIA, GENERAL SURVEY, *and article on* SOUTHEAST ASIAN COUNTRIES.

## SOVIET UNION (FORMER)

*See* MEDICAL ETHICS, HISTORY OF, *section on* EUROPE, *subsection on* CONTEMPORARY PERIOD, *articles on* RUSSIA, *and* CENTRAL AND EASTERN EUROPE.

## SPAIN

*See* MEDICAL ETHICS, HISTORY OF, *section on* EUROPE, *subsection on* CONTEMPORARY PERIOD, *article on* SOUTHERN EUROPE.

## SPORTS

Sport and the ethics of sport do not receive the scholarly attention they deserve. Perhaps because scholars tend to dismiss sport as play, something not worth serious consideration, we overlook its enormous economic and political importance, as well as the ethical issues raised in it.

At least three issues in sport are pertinent to bioethics. First, the use of drugs and other performance aids raises questions about what is natural and what is fair.

Second, gender verification schemes in sport are motivated by concerns for fair competition but raise complex questions about gender identity. Third, health professionals in sport are confronted with occasionally vexing problems of divided loyalties.

### Performance enhancement

In competitions where the difference between winner and loser may be measured in fractions of seconds or inches, athletes are tempted to use anything that confers a competitive advantage. In addition to improvements in equipment and training, drugs and other biological manipulations have been used in an effort to gain an edge. For the most part, sports authorities have frowned on drugs and similar substances, calling the practice "doping" and imposing sanctions on athletes who use them. The International Olympic Committee, for example, bans a wide variety of stimulants, narcotics, anabolic steroids, diuretics, and other drugs. It also prohibits the practice of adding oxygen-carrying red blood cells, known as "blood doping," and taking the biosynthetic hormone erythropoietin, which accomplishes the same end, as well as drugs used to manipulate the urine in order to make detecting banned drugs difficult or impossible. The Council of Europe adopted a detailed *Anti-Doping Convention* in 1989 that pledged its signatories to redouble their efforts to discourage doping in sport.

The presence of apparent international consensus, however, does not mean that everyone behaves accordingly. Banned drugs have been used by athletes in many countries and in many different sports. Anabolic steroids, probably the most notorious performance-enhancing drugs, were used widely by athletes as early as the 1960s. The end of the Cold War revealed what many had suspected: that in some countries, the former East Germany in particular, using drugs to enhance the performance of athletes was systematic, organized, and sanctioned by the government (Hoberman, 1992). Drug use appears to have had broad appeal irrespective of political ideology, however. Athletes from western Europe, the United States, Canada, South America, and Asia have been suspected of, or caught using, banned drugs. The widespread adoption of performance-enhancing drugs by athletes is more a reflection of modern ideas about the body as an appropriate object of manipulation, and the inducement of huge financial rewards, than of political beliefs.

The discontinuity between official disapproval on the one hand, and widespread defiance on the other, has prompted debate about the ethical grounds for prohibiting performance-enhancing drugs in sport. Two reasons typically given in favor of such a ban are that the use of performance-enhancing drugs harms the athletes, and that using such drugs confers an unfair advantage and is a form of cheating. Some scholars are skeptical that either ethical justification for a ban can survive scrutiny (Fost, 1986).

The argument that drugs should be banned because they may be dangerous to the athletes who take them is a version of paternalism. As such, it is more plausible when applied to child and adolescent athletes than to adults. In sports such as swimming and gymnastics, athletes may reach their peak before the age of majority; in many other sports, intensive preparation, including drug use, may begin when an athlete is very young. Paternalism for children and adolescents can be justified when the risk of harm is significant.

Adult athletes who want to take drugs to improve their chances of success are unlikely to be persuaded by the argument that we ban drugs for their own good. They might point out that in certain sports the risks of the activity itself are probably far greater than the risks of taking performance-enhancing drugs. They might also argue—correctly—that any reasonable concept of freedom must accept the possibility that individuals may act unwisely. Further, they could claim that in their circumstances, the choice to use drugs is not irrational.

When athletes spend years seeking to be the best in their sport, only to discover that their competitors are using performance-enhancing drugs, their decision whether to use drugs often seems forced, almost to the point of coercion. They can abandon competition, compete at a disadvantage, or join in the doping (Murray, 1983). Athletes themselves lead the call for stringent penalties and strenuous enforcement, in part because they do not want to accept the risks of using drugs; but they are more likely to appeal to notions of fair play and, in their endeavor, the not-so-metaphorical "level playing field."

A second argument against banning drugs in sport is that no unambiguous distinction can be made between using a drug to restore someone to normal functioning and to boost function beyond the normal. Frustrating the effort to draw such a distinction is the ambiguity latent in the concept of disease, as well as the athlete's desire to push performance beyond the normal.

The pursuit of excellence leads athletes to condition themselves to perform well beyond any notion of "normal" as "average"; in actual competition, athletes such as marathon runners drive themselves to pathological states of exhaustion. Pointing to difficulties at the margin, however, can blind one to the obvious. Few people would doubt that diabetes is a disease, and insulin an appropriate treatment for it. Likewise, few would argue that a strong and healthy young man who takes massive doses of anabolic steroids to be able to lift heavier barbells is treating a disease. Distinctions useful, even crucial, in practice commonly contain gray areas where they are not helpful. But the existence of such regions of ambiguity is no proof that the distinction itself is useless or hopelessly flawed.

A third major argument against banning performance-enhancing drugs in sport is that they are not really unfair. Skeptics argue that there are many differences between victors and vanquished in sport: Some of these are the consequence of effort and can be said to have been earned; others are accidents of birth, or good fortune in having superior coaching, or equipment, or diet. Inequality is not equivalent to unfairness. Furthermore, skeptics claim, we allow athletes to eat special diets, take vitamin and nutritional supplements, and the like; therefore, it is inconsistent to object to their taking drugs. Perhaps, the skeptics argue, our real objection is that drug taking is unfair because not all athletes have access to the same drugs. That would be easily remedied by providing drugs to all who want them.

This argument, like the one before it, errs in presuming that a distinction is completely useless unless it is absolutely perfect. Defining the concept of "drug" is notoriously difficult, yet most people have no difficulty distinguishing between heroin and halibut, or steroids and spinach. A closer examination of the ethical significance of that distinction would probably reveal some deeply held notions about human nature, health, normality, and the purpose of sport. In any event, the distinction between drug and nondrug is not crucial. The critical distinction is between those substances and practices deemed to violate the spirit of sports competition, and those that pose no such threat.

It is likely that sports governing bodies reflect a widely held conviction that competitive sport is intended to display human excellences and that certain modifications in sport do not tarnish the meaning of the competition, but that performance-enhancing drugs clearly do. The public response to revelations of drug use, such as that by the Canadian sprinter Ben Johnson in the 1988 Olympics, suggests that the public shares a conception of sport that excludes performance-enhancing drugs. In particular, there has been no public clamor to allow an athlete found to have used such drugs to keep his or her medal.

At its core, the aversion to using performance-enhancing drugs in sport is as much aesthetic as ethical. Sport is an expression of human excellences such as strength, speed, grace, and cooperation. Any proposed change in rules, equipment, or technique should be evaluated according to whether it distorts the meaning of the sport by perverting the forms of human excellence the sport is believed to exhibit and reward. If a particular entity—for example, performance-enhancing drugs— violates the spirit of the competition, then it properly may be banned and the use of it deemed cheating.

## Gender verification

One way to gain a competitive advantage is to have a natural abundance of testosterone (by being a male) but to compete as a female. Testosterone is the hormone usually present in much higher concentrations in men than in women. It confers male secondary sex characteristics, including size and strength.

Reports appeared in the 1950s and 1960s that some men were competing as women. By the mid-1960s, tests were being carried out to confirm the sex of putatively female competitors. The initial tests were crude and sometimes humiliating. Contemporary alternatives include using techniques of molecular biology to detect the presence of a Y (male) chromosome, or simply requiring all athletes to undergo a standard physical examination (Ljungqvist and Simpson, 1992).

In gender testing, as in drug testing, it is essential to focus on why it is deemed important to exclude men from participating as women. The principal reason appears to be that in sports where size and strength are crucial, the advantage conferred by a male's higher testosterone level would be unfair. Here the simple equation between Y chromosomes and athletic performance collapses. There are syndromes in which a person has the normal male complement of chromosomes—an X and a Y—but the genitalia and secondary sexual characteristics of a woman. Such disorders may be caused by an abnormal form of testosterone or by insensitivity to testosterone. Persons with such syndromes are to all appearances women, despite their Y chromosome. They gain no performance advantage from it. Fairness would not be violated by allowing such XY females to compete as women.

## Divided loyalties in sports medicine

Divided loyalties occur when conflicting moral claims are made that cannot be honored simultaneously. They are frequent in certain kinds of medicine, including sports medicine. Two distinct forms of divided loyalties occur in sports medicine: conflicts between the athlete's welfare and the interests of others, and conflicts between the athlete's wishes and the athlete's good.

Team physicians are often agents of the team's ownership or management at the same time they are physicians to the individual athletes on the team. Management may want a key player to participate in an important competition, even at the risk of aggravating an injury. Numerous reports confirm this phenomenon. Team physicians may be coerced or seduced into deceiving an athlete about the severity of an injury. Or physicians may administer analgesics that disguise the extent of previous injuries. In such cases, the athlete's welfare is sacrificed for the interests of others, with the physician as agent.

Divided loyalties have recognizable features. They often appear when medicine is performing its social-control functions, such as declaring who is ill or injured. Expectations play a large role in determining their existence and severity. If someone is openly representing the interests of others, we do not expect him or her to look after ours. But when physicians minister to our medical needs, we typically assume that they are doing so for our benefit. The expectation that physicians will be loyal to patients serves as a regulative ideal for physician–patient interactions. It is an ideal in that it describes a desired form of behavior. It is regulative in that it both influences physician behavior and may be used as a standard against which to judge and—if necessary—impose sanctions against those who deviate significantly from the ideal. The ideal is frequently threatened and sometimes violated when divided loyalties arise.

Observers of sport note that the pressure to risk athletes' health at times comes from the athletes themselves. A marginal player may ask for an injection in an injured joint, hoping to compete and remain on the team. A star may do likewise for a key competition. Or athletes may ask physicians for help in obtaining or monitoring the effects of anabolic steroids or other performance-enhancing drugs. In such cases the conflict is between the athlete's wishes—to compete—and the athlete's good—at least that part of a person's good to which physicians typically minister, their physical well-being (Murray, 1986).

### Conclusion

Two factors suggest that current moral problems in sport may intensify in the near future. First, advances in biomedical research, such as the accelerated discovery of human genes controlling a host of physiological processes, provide the means for increased manipulation of human anatomy and physiology. Second, the already astounding financial importance of sport continues to grow, making the reward for successful manipulation ever greater. We will be challenged to articulate clearly and to preserve the value of sport in the face of these forces.

THOMAS H. MURRAY

*Directly related to this entry is the entry* CONFLICT OF INTEREST. *For a further discussion of topics mentioned in this entry, see the entries* FIDELITY AND LOYALTY; GENDER IDENTITY AND GENDER-IDENTITY DISORDERS; *and* GENETIC ENGINEERING, *article on* HUMAN GENETIC ENGINEERING. *For a discussion of related ideas, see the entries*

HEALTH PROMOTION AND HEALTH EDUCATION; MEDICINE AS A PROFESSION; PROFESSION AND PROFESSIONAL ETHICS; *and* TRUST. *Other relevant material may be found under the entries* AUTONOMY; *and* PATERNALISM.

### Bibliography

COUNCIL OF EUROPE. 1989. *Anti-Doping Convention.* Strasbourg: Author.

FOST, NORMAN. 1986. "Banning Drugs in Sports: A Skeptical View." *Hastings Center Report* 16, no 4:5–10.

HOBERMAN, JOHN M. 1992. *Mortal Engines: The Science of Performance and the Dehumanization of Sport.* New York: Free Press.

LJUNGQVIST, ARNE, and SIMPSON, JOE LEIGH. 1992. "Medical Examination for Health of All Athletes Replacing the Need for Gender Verification in International Sports: The International Amateur Athletic Federation Plan." *Journal of the American Medical Association* 267, no 6: 850–852.

MURRAY, THOMAS H. 1983. "The Coercive Power of Drugs in Sports." *Hastings Center Report* 13, no. 4:24–30.

———. 1986. "Divided Loyalties for Physicians: Social Context and Moral Problems." *Social Science and Medicine* 23, no. 8:827–832.

## SPOUSAL ABUSE

*See* ABUSE, INTERPERSONAL, *article on* ABUSE BETWEEN DOMESTIC PARTNERS.

## STERILIZATION

*See* FERTILITY CONTROL.

## STEWARDSHIP, PRINCIPLE OF

*See* ENVIRONMENT AND RELIGION; *and* ROMAN CATHOLICISM.

## STRIKES BY HEALTH PROFESSIONALS

Health professionals have engaged in collective protest labor actions at least since the physicians' strike in Cork, Ireland, in 1894. Between 1961 and 1966, physicians went on strike in ten countries: Austria, Belgium, Canada, Chile, France, Greece, Italy, Lebanon, Mexico, and the United States. Since then, labor conflicts and strikes have increased and continue to disrupt medical-care delivery throughout the world. Nurses have conducted scores of strikes in the United States following the 1968 repeal of their association's eighteen-year-old no-strike pledge. Notwithstanding, the American Association of Physician Assistants in 1990 adopted a policy position condemning "any action in the workplace that has an adverse effect on patient care," though it is not clear whether this prohibits strike actions.

These figures must be put into perspective. Since 1950, less than 1 percent of available work time has been lost to strikes in the United States in all fields of employment combined. Strikes are so uncommon, especially in health care, that virtually each one receives considerable news coverage.

## Unions and regulatory supervision

Until the National Labor Relations Act (NLRA) was passed in 1935, there was no significant government regulatory supervision of employment relations in health-care facilities in the United States. NLRA amendments in 1947 prohibited specific union activities, but exempted non-profit health-care institutions from having to recognize the bargaining rights of employees. That exemption ended with the 1974 amendments, which required mediation of labor disputes and specific notification procedures preceding any planned strike action, but only in health-care institutions. Government regulation continues to evolve through court rulings, legislation, and lobbying efforts by professional organizations.

A 1977 survey revealed that three-fourths of the contracts made between hospitals and their employees reached agreement on three key provisions. These include no-strike (employees agree not to strike), no-lockout (employers agree not to prohibit workers with grievances from working), and binding arbitration (settlement of the dispute by a person or persons chosen equally by the opposing sides). Most employers and employees further agreed to settle unresolved grievances in contract renewal negotiations. The group most noticeably missing from these contract agreements are physicians, with the exception of interns and residents, some of whom formed unions and organized strikes in several U.S. cities in the 1970s and 1980s. Because they are both employees and students, however, these physicians are unique in several regards.

As employed physicians, interns and residents are often responsible for teaching medical and other students, and except for psychiatry residents they can receive Medicare and Medicaid reimbursement for patient care delivered in hospitals and clinics. Their status as students is relatively short-term, student-body membership continually changes, and eligibility for collective bargaining is subject to challenge from administrators. These three features make union organization efforts for interns and residents especially difficult. In addition, physician solidarity in strike actions has been inconsis-

tent. In 1975 two physician strikes in New York City were publicly supported by the American Medical Association, while the twenty-three-day physician strike in Saskatchewan, Canada, in 1962, was hampered by the arrival of British and American physicians to provide medical care to local patients.

## Causes

Strike actions typically arise when continued conflict on contract issues becomes intolerable to the labor group and alternative methods of resolving the dispute have failed. They are designed to force management into contract concessions or resource reallocations through political pressure and public disapproval of the strike.

Health professionals who strike usually are those directly involved in patient care. Their concerns arise from either economic or management-based issues. Economic issues arise as a consequence of governmental or corporate policies that professionals believe will reduce their net income, including payment structures and rates for professional services, and malpractice premiums. Management issues focus on physical resource allocations, staffing, patient-care management, patient selection, admission and treatment requirements, and organizational decision making.

## Ethical issues

The moral permissibility of strikes based solely on economic self-interest issues is perceived as unprofessional and is more difficult to establish than those directly aimed at improving patient care. This difference reflects a felt moral tension between unionism and professionalism. Collective bargaining requries solidarity among employees and often is most effective against employers when it includes the threat of collective strike action. At the same time, strike action risks placing health professionals in conflict with their traditional ethical principle of patient advocacy. James Muyskens (1982) argues that nurses perhaps have been most troubled by this tension due to their lack of power relative to administrators and physicians. Allowing vulnerable patients to suffer as a means to a political end—even one that will ultimately benefit all patients—requires very strong justification, reasonable assurance of success, and careful precautions to minimize harm to patients. Comprehensive ethical analysis is complex, but the following points can be applied to most strike situations:

1. Most goods and services provided to patients by health-care professionals are absolutely necessary, with very limited possibility of adequate substitution. Whether patients can be treated at other facilities depends on community resources, the jurisdiction of the strikers, and the willingness by nonstriking professionals to perform out-of-contract work.

2. The interdependence of the various groups of health-care professionals renders effective patient care a necessarily collective enterprise. A strike by one group creates a conflict of duties for the other groups, who have professional allegiances to their patients as well as to their colleagues. It strains the fibers of professional solidarity.

3. According to Norman Daniels (1978), health care is an unequally distributed good of great strategic importance for securing an equality of opportunity in society. This conception limits the medical services that may be withheld justifiably and provides the basis for a moral obligation to announce in advance the intent to strike. For critically ill and emergency-care patients, for example, care deferred is care denied. These patients may therefore have special entitlement claims for care that supersede any particular labor dispute arising from economic or management concerns. In virtually all strikes, emergency facilities and care of critically ill patients have been continued.

4. Health-care professionals have duties to both present and future patients. The second duty entails a significant professional share in the larger community obligation to secure adequate health resources in the future. Muyskens (1982) and others have argued that when future resources are threatened by current labor conflict and alternative negotiating strategies have failed, collective strike action by professionals may be necessary to secure such resources, including those needed for attracting and retaining qualified professionals.

5. Two ethical theories can serve as bases for the justification of a strike aimed at improved patient care. Utilitarians would compute the aggregate health-care harms and benefits to current versus future patients and compare the relative overall goods of continued care under current conditions with the likely improved care following a strike action. This argument's persuasiveness depends in part on how certain the strikers are about retaining improved patient benefits despite future economic and administrative changes in the institution(s). The other basis is deontological, or based on moral obligation, and arises from the health-care professionals' collective judgment that current conditions are so substandard as to be unacceptable in good conscience, and they must not be associated with them, lest they fail in their duty to their own professional integrity and standards of care.

## Future directions

Three conceptual advances in developing ethical frameworks appropriate to health-care issues may prove useful in finding new ways to resolve conflicts in employment relations. The first involves moving from autonomy-based conceptions of individual rights and obligations toward communitarian models involving social solidarity. This is especially relevant in light of two emerging trends in health care: direct employment of professionals by corporations, and the need explicitly to ration access to medical services. To the extent that the economics of health care shapes the relationships among professionals, patients, and management, unionization and the threat of strike actions among professionals may increase as a result of these evolving arrangements. On the other hand, making physicians employees may improve the working conditions of nurses and other professionals, thereby reducing the risk of strikes overall.

The second advance examines power in the professional–patient relationship. Strikes by professionals are essentially power struggles to force management into employment concessions with workers. As such, power deserves careful analysis as a moral value in this context. Brody (1992) argues that the morally responsible use of power requires the more powerful party to recognize openly its relative advantage, to use that advantage in a directed way, and to share selflessly with the other party the benefits of mutual cooperation. Finally, to pursue improved patient care and to reduce strikes, the creative labor conflict resolution mechanisms, including fact-finding, mediation-arbitration, and final arbitration, warrant study and experimentation.

PAUL J. REITEMEIER

*Directly related to this entry is the entry* CIVIL DISOBEDIENCE AND HEALTH CARE. *For a further discussion of topics mentioned in this entry, see the entries* CONFLICT OF INTEREST; PROFESSIONAL–PATIENT RELATIONSHIP, *article on* ETHICAL ISSUES; *and* PROFESSION AND PROFESSIONAL ETHICS. *This entry will find application in the entries* ALLIED HEALTH PROFESSIONS; MEDICINE AS A PROFESSION; NURSING AS A PROFESSION; *and* TEAMS, HEALTH-CARE. *For a discussion of related ideas, see the entries* FIDELITY AND LOYALTY; HARM; RESPONSIBILITY; *and* UTILITY. *Other relevant material may be found under the entry* MEDICAL EDUCATION.

## Bibliography

BADGLEY, ROBIN F., and WOLFE, SAMUEL. 1967. *Doctors' Strike: Medical Care and Conflict in Saskatchewan.* Toronto: Macmillan of Canada.

BRODY, HOWARD. 1992. *The Healer's Power.* New Haven, Conn.: Yale University Press.

DANIELS, NORMAN. 1978. "On the Picket Line: Are Doctors' Strikes Ethical?" *Hastings Center Report* 8, no. 1 (February): 24–29.

———. 1985. *Just Health Care.* Cambridge: At the University Press.

HOFFMAN, LILY M. 1989. *The Politics of Knowledge: Activist Movements in Medicine and Planning.* Albany: State University of New York Press.

MESLIN, ERIC M. 1987. "The Moral Costs of the Ontario Physicians' Strike." *Hastings Center Report* 17, no. 4:11–14.

METZGER, NORMAN; FERENTINO, JOSEPH M.; and KRUGER, KENNETH F. 1984. *When Health-Care Employees Strike: A Guide for Planning and Action.* Rockville, Md.: Aspen.

MILLER, RICHARD U.; BECKER, BRIAN E.; and KRINSKY, EDWARD B. 1979. *The Impact of Collective Bargaining on Hospitals.* New York: Praeger.

MUYSKENS, JAMES L. 1982. "Nurses' Collective Responsibility and the Strike Weapon." *Journal of Medicine and Philosophy* 7, no. 1:101–112.

PETERSEN, DONALD J.; REZLER, JULIUS S.; and REED, KEITH A. 1981. *Arbitration in Health Care.* Rockville, Md.: Aspen.

THOMASMA, DAVID C., and HURLEY, R. MORRISON. 1988. "The Ethics of Health Professional Strikes." In *Medical Ethics: A Guide for Health Professionals,* pp. 358–374. Edited by John F. Monagle and David C. Thomasma. Rockville, Md.: Aspen.

WERTHER, WILLIAM B., JR., and LOCKHART, CAROL ANN. 1976. *Labor Relations in the Health Professions: The Basis of Power—the Means of Change.* Boston: Little, Brown.

WOLFE, SAMUEL, ed. *Organization of Health Workers and Labor Conflict.* 1978. Farmingdale, N.Y.: Baywood.

# STUDENTS AS RESEARCH SUBJECTS

Using students as research subjects is a special issue when the researcher, or the institution sponsoring the research, is in a position of power or authority over the students' educational progress. Though persons of college age may or may not be the age of majority, depending on the law of their state, they are mature enough to make competent decisions about whether to participate in research. However, faculty have great power over students: Students are dependent on teachers for good grades, favorable recommendations, opportunities for rewards such as teaching or research assistantships, and the less tangible benefit of being known and respected by someone who may be a role model. This dependency, coupled with the ready availability of students as a subject pool, raises questions about the validity of students' participation as subjects in research conducted by their teachers or educational institutions. Students may not be able to resist the pressure to consent.

The Department of Health and Human Services regulations on research reflect ethical concern for dependent subjects. Specific provisions require informed consent to be obtained under conditions that "minimize the possibility of coercion or undue influence," and that "Where some or all of the subjects are likely to be vulnerable to coercion or undue influence, such as persons with acute or severe physical or mental illness, or persons who are economically or educationally disadvantaged, appropriate additional safeguards have been included in the study to protect the rights and welfare of these subjects" (DHHS, 1983, secs. 46.116, 46.111). While students are not as vulnerable as the categories of persons mentioned above, the circumstances of the student–teacher relationship and the methods of recruiting subjects may combine to constitute undue influence.

Students recruited from introductory courses in psychology and other behavioral sciences are commonly used as subjects in behavioral research. Participation in research may be a course requirement for all students, it may be a requirement for which there are alternatives such as writing a research paper, or it may be a fully voluntary activity in response to an invitation.

An argument in favor of a strict requirement to be a research subject is the educational benefit of participation. The experience of being a subject adds meaning to the study of behavioral science that cannot be gained through reading, lecture, and discussion (Gamble, 1982). But it is doubtful that educational benefit is the primary motivation for the strict requirement; more likely, it is the need for subjects for faculty and graduate student research. Yet if all participation in research constitutes a unique educational benefit, then the strict requirement would be justified. Whether participation is educationally beneficial will depend on the features of the protocol and on whether and how the protocol is explained to the students, either before or after their participation. Simply completing a survey instrument or a standard psychological test will offer little educational benefit to the vast majority of students who have prior experience with such activities. But if, in addition, methods, objectives, and results of the research are explained to the students, the total experience may be educationally significant. That may not be practical for all research: The research may involve deception, and an explanation to one group of students may be communicated to other students, who then will not be naive subjects; also, the collection and analysis of data may not be complete before the end of the course. Therefore, unless the research projects presented for required student participation are screened to eliminate those with minimal opportunity for educational benefit, a strict requirement for all students to be research subjects is not justifiable on educational grounds.

The argument against the strict requirement, even if all projects are screened for educational benefit, is that it conflicts with the provision found in every code of ethics, set of principles, and other regulations regarding research that subjects must give their informed consent—which clearly entails that prospective subjects may refuse to participate and may withdraw at any time. The American Psychological Association does not condone a strict requirement for students to participate in research. Its *Ethical Principles in the Conduct of Research with Human Participants* (1973) stated that an investigator's respect for an individual's freedom to decline to participate in research requires careful thought and consideration when the investigator is in a position of authority over the participant, as when the participant is his or her student. In a revision, "Ethical Principles of Psychologists and Code of Conduct" (1992), the association explicitly rejects a strict requirement: "When research participation is a course requirement or opportunity for extra credit, the prospective participant is given the choice of equitable alternative activities" (p. 1608).

Several conditions must be met to avoid undue influence on students to participate in research. For any research in which students are the primary subjects, solicitations must be presented in a general way to all students and not be made individually. Individual solicitations could be perceived by students as a request the refusal of which could jeopardize their grades or their relationship with the teacher. A solicitation from an instructor to the students in his or her course to participate in the instructor's own research project will be more likely to exert or seem to exert undue influence than a solicitation by the instructor to participate in one of several projects being carried out by faculty. Where participation is part of a course, there must be an alternative educational activity. The reward, or course credit, for participating in research or the alternative activity should be a minor portion of students' grades for the course. If a student's grade can be raised from a B to an A by putting in time as a subject, that would be undue influence on the decision whether to participate. Finally, the alternatives should be comparable with participation in terms of the time and effort required. It will be difficult to set up alternatives, such as research assignments, that will be comparable in all respects. In order that particular protocols not be seen by prospective subjects as much easier tasks, the alternatives should be comparable to the kind of research participation that would take the least time and effort. Given the reluctance of many students to do research projects and write reports, the pressure to be a subject may be great. Hence, voluntary consent will be obtained only if participation in research is completely optional.

Behavioral research with undergraduate students is more common than medical research using medical students as subjects. The general problems of undue influence and voluntariness of consent are equally significant, though it is arguable that pressure to participate is greater in the medical context because of a closer relationship between faculty and students, greater power over students for recommendations to residency programs, and greater relevance of participation in research to students' careers in medicine. Additional pressure to participate may come from payment to subjects, which is more common in medical research. In some cases the amounts are considerable, given the finances of most medical students.

Some medical schools have policies on student participation that are more restrictive than those that apply to other subjects (Shannon, 1979; Christakis, 1985). Students may not participate in research that poses more than minimal risk or in research that would interfere with their studies. The basis of this policy may be that students' primary objective is medical education, or that medical students are especially susceptible to the influence of faculty researchers, or that the power of faculty over medical students is greater than that over nonstudent subjects. Any one of these may cause students to consent to research that is not in their interest.

This restrictive approach has been criticized as elitist or paternalistic (Christakis, 1985; Nolan, 1979). It is elitist if the motivation is that medical students are a special class of citizens, distinct from other subjects, and therefore should have greater protection from the risks and inconveniences of research to pursue their higher calling. It is paternalistic if the motivation is to protect medical students from mistaken judgments about their own interests when they are deciding whether to consent to participation in research. Since the federal regulations aim to protect all potential subjects from giving uninformed or involuntary consent, the more stringent protections for medical students seem to imply that the standard ones are not sufficient and that all potential subjects should have greater protection. Alternatively, the greater paternalism may have an elitist basis.

The restrictive policy for medical students has been rejected by the argument that medical students are surely not any "less free" than the general population, and very likely are more capable of autonomous decision making because they have cleared hurdles to get to medical school. Further, the greater willingness and knowledge of medical students make their consent more voluntary and informed than that of the general population (Angoff, 1985). However, there is evidence that medical students consider themselves under pressure to consent, and believe that the consent process used by their professors is inadequate (Kopelman, 1983).

The Institutional Review Board at one medical school approved a research protocol only if the subjects were restricted to third- and fourth-year medical students and medical professionals. These medically educated and experienced persons could be expected to understand and assess the risks and discomforts of several invasive procedures that would be employed, whereas "ordinary" subjects could not (Angoff, 1985). This preference is consistent with the view of Hans Jonas that healthy volunteers should be recruited on a "descending order of permissibility": Those who are poorest in knowledge, motivation, and freedom should be the last to be used; those on the other end of this scale have the capacity to identify with research and should be the first to be subjects (Jonas, 1970). This view supports a policy of encouraging medical students to participate in research because of their greater knowledge and their commitment to medicine. However, it does not respond to the problem of greater pressure to participate, which is the central concern for students as research subjects.

BRUCE L. MILLER

Directly related to this entry are the entries AUTHORITY; FREEDOM AND COERCION; INFORMED CONSENT, article on CONSENT ISSUES IN HUMAN RESEARCH; and RESEARCH POLICY, article on SUBJECT SELECTION. For a further discussion of topics mentioned in this entry, see the entries MEDICAL EDUCATION; and PATERNALISM. See also the APPENDIX (CODES, OATHS, AND DIRECTIVES RELATED TO BIOETHICS), SECTION IV: ETHICAL DIRECTIVES FOR HUMAN RESEARCH.

## Bibliography

AMERICAN PSYCHOLOGICAL ASSOCIATION. 1973. Ethical Principles in the Conduct of Research with Human Participants. Washington, D.C.: Author.
———. 1992. "Ethical Principles of Psychologists and Code of Conduct." American Psychologist 47, no. 12:1597–1611.
ANGOFF, NANCY R. 1985. "Against Special Protections for Medical Students." IRB 7, no. 5:9–10.
CHRISTAKIS, NICHOLAS. 1985. "Do Medical Student Research Subjects Need Special Protection?" IRB 7, no. 3:1–4.
DEPARTMENT OF HEALTH AND HUMAN SERVICES (DHHS). 1983. "Protection of Human Subjects." 45 CFR 46.
GAMBLE, HAROLD F. 1982. "Case Study: Students, Grades and Informed Consent." IRB 4, no. 5:7–10.
JONAS, HANS. 1970. "Philosophical Reflections on Experimenting with Human Subjects." In Experimentation with Human Subjects, pp. 1–31. Edited by Paul A. Freund. New York: George Braziller.
KOPELMAN, LORETTA. 1983. "Cynicism Among Medical Students." Journal of the American Medical Association 250, no. 15:2006–2010.
LEVINE, ROBERT L. 1988. Ethics and Regulation of Clinical Research. 2d ed. New Haven, Conn.: Yale University Press.
NOLAN, KATHLEEN A. 1979. "Protecting Medical Students from the Risks of Research." IRB 1, no. 5:9.
SHANNON, THOMAS A. 1979. "Case Study: Should Medical Students Be Research Subjects?" IRB 1, no. 2:4.

# SUB-SAHARAN AFRICA

See MEDICAL ETHICS, HISTORY OF, section on AFRICA, article on SUB-SAHARAN COUNTRIES.

# SUBSTANCE ABUSE

## I. ADDICTION AND DEPENDENCE

Addiction has been called a "victimless crime." Nothing could be further from the truth. Every day we read about, hear about, or know someone who is a victim of a crime caused by those who use or seek drugs. On a different level we are frequently exposed to the environmental effects of addiction—secondary cigarette smoke, for example, or accidents on the road or in the workplace caused by excessive alcohol use.

Few people disagree that addiction and dependence are destructive health behaviors, yet there seems to be a vast sea of confusion surrounding addictive behavior. The facts are clear: Addiction to and dependence on tobacco, alcohol, illicit and legal drugs, and possibly biologically driven behaviors such as sex and eating, and social activities such as gambling, are widespread and very destructive.

Addiction has wide-ranging consequences: According to U.S. Surgeon General Antonia Novello, 52 percent of college students report using alcohol before committing crimes, and 70 percent of attempted suicides were linked to alcohol. Novello also reports that alcohol use is associated with over 27 percent of all murders, 30 percent of rapes, 33 percent of property offenses, and 37 percent of robberies perpetrated by young people (Novello, 1993).

In addition, the cost of treating infants exposed to cocaine is estimated to be $500 million a year, and hospital emergency room mentions of cocaine increased in the first two quarters of 1991 to 47,652, from 41,306 in 1990.

Drug and alcohol dependence and addiction cut across all geographic, ethnic, and social boundaries. According to the Drug Enforcement Agency, the total sales of illicit drugs in the United States in 1993 amounted to $100 billion (Alden, 1993). This makes drug abuse as large as a top ten company on the Fortune 500 list.

The business community is so concerned about the problem that preemployment drug screening of prospective employees has become commonplace. The majority of Fortune 500 companies have some sort of drug-testing program. Drug testing is the norm in the U.S. armed forces, and many current court cases are examining if and when the government has the right to test its employees.

The death toll from health problems caused by smoking is staggering. In 1990, 418,690 Americans died prematurely due to the effects of cigarettes. Yet, there are 46 million smokers in the United States who shorten their lives and increase their health risk for lung disease, cancer, and heart disease with each puff (*Substance Abuse*, 1993). According to the Centers for Disease Control and Prevention, every time they light up, they lose seven minutes of life (Centers for Disease Control, 1993).

Smoking affects both smokers and those who are exposed to smoke through passive inhalation, employers whose smoking workers are sick more often, and the health-care system, which must treat disorders caused by smoking. Smoking, according to the U.S. Surgeon General's Office, costs the United States over $65 billion per year. Tobacco, it points out, "is the only product that when used as directed, results in death and disability" (Novello, 1993, p. 806).

Beyond the health consequences for adults, smoking is a serious threat to young people on several levels. Despite widespread antismoking programs, 3 million teenagers smoke on a regular basis, a number that has remained constant since 1980 (Elders et al., 1994). Every year a million new teenage smokers light up—every day 3,000 teens begin to use a drug that will cause lifelong damage. Most of these smokers will have been smoking for several years by the time they graduate from high school. It is, of course, illegal to sell cigarettes to minors.

Smoking is not the only potential threat from addictive substances to young people. National surveys show that 41 percent of teenagers indulge in "binge drinking" and 5 percent of teenagers drink daily (Johnston et al., 1993). The 1991 Household Survey on Drug Abuse found that 33 percent of the household population, age twelve or older, had used marijuana in their lifetime (National Household Survey, 1991). In 1989, 5.1 percent of college students had used a hallucinogen during the past year; by 1992 the number had risen to 6.8 percent (Johnston et al., 1993). Data from the 1992 National High School Senior Survey indicate that drug use among eighth graders—specifically LSD, marijuana, and inhalants—is increasing (Johnston et al., 1993).

Why would anyone engage in such behavior in the face of such obvious and dire consequences? What are the root causes of such behavior? Why is there any debate about drug use when the frightening consequences are known? Part of the answer comes from exploring the question of what addiction really means.

## What is addiction?

The concept of addiction—whether to alcohol, cigarettes, heroin, or sexual behavior—is widely misunderstood. Although there is room for debate about the "levels" of addiction caused by different substances, and perhaps about the "rights" of people to use addictive substances, there is no debate about what constitutes addiction. Addictive disease is defined by compulsion, loss of control, and continued, repeated use despite adverse consequences. Even though a person knows what will happen, he or she will use the addictive substance again. It is impossible to stop. Thus, addiction is a disease characterized by repetitive and destructive use of one or more substances, and stems from a biological vulnerability exposed or induced by environmental factors such as drug taking.

Until scientists learned how popular "recreational" drugs such as cocaine affected the brain, it was thought that addiction required a physical withdrawal syndrome. That is not necessarily true. While a mild withdrawal has been described, compulsive use of cocaine is driven by positive effects. This information has contributed to research that clearly indicates there is no valid distinction between physical and psychological addiction.

Anyone who uses any chemical in the way described above is suffering from addictive disease. Users are distinguished by the type of drug, genetic vulnerabilities, individual predisposition to addiction, and the setting in which the drug is used.

Addiction includes preoccupation with the acquisition of a drug. In general, when obtaining a drug plays a central role in a person's life, addiction is present or near. Many studies have shown that addicts rank finding and using their drug above work, family, religion, hunger, sex, and survival. Even when the high is no longer achieved, the drug and its use are paramount. Drug taking fools the brain, giving the user a false sense of accomplishment that is at odds with reality, to the point that denial is common.

Since drugs cause a chronic disease in an otherwise healthy person, staying clean or straight becomes a daily problem. Relapse, therefore, is another significant and expected part of addictive disease. It is common for addicts to have relatively long periods of abstinence intermingled with drug-use binges. Chemical addiction does not happen overnight. Addicts are not moral failures but victims of a disease.

If addiction is understood as defined above, it is easy to see why it can be called a process: Use leads to tolerance . . . leads to abuse . . . leads to chemical dependence and addiction.

## Who becomes addicted?

Anyone can become addicted. After all, most Americans use drugs—whether caffeine, nicotine, or more powerful substances. And anyone who takes cocaine or other narcotics frequently for a long enough time becomes addicted to the drug regardless of any genetic predisposition. However, rarely do cancer patients become addicts. It is more than a simple drug–dose–duration equation. It is motivation and intent. It may turn out that some people—perhaps 10 percent of the population—have a preexisting biological, or genetic, predisposition to drug and alcohol dependency.

Establishing the genetic basis of addiction may be the most important part of proving beyond a doubt that addiction is a disease. For example, studies of identical twins (who share the same genetic information) have shown that if one twin is an alcoholic, there is a 74 percent chance that the other twin will also be an alcoholic. Fraternal twins, who do not share the same genetic makeup, have only a 32 percent chance of each being an alcoholic. Studies of children born to alcoholic parents, but adopted during infancy by nonalcoholic parents, were more likely to become alcoholics than children born to nonalcoholic parents (Miller and Gold, 1991).

A 1991 review of studies in which offspring of alcoholic parents were compared with offspring of nonalcoholic parents concluded that those with a family history of alcoholism found alcohol to be more rewarding than those without such a family history. The adult children of alcoholic parents found greater pleasure and excitement, and less anxiety and depression, associated with drinking than did the offspring of nonalcoholic parents (Helzer and Burnam, 1991).

In animal studies, researchers have been able to breed rats with a genetic preference for alcohol and rats with no desire to consume alcohol. The rats bred to like alcohol act like alcoholics, choosing to drink to the point of getting drunk even in the presence of food and water. Studies of these two breeds show biological differences among neurotransmitters (the chemical messengers between nerve cells) that may account for the alcohol-consuming rats' strong desire to drink.

In April 1990, the genetic basis of human addiction was supported by a report suggesting that alcoholics have a genetic variation that results in a more frequent occurrence of a receptor for a particular neurotransmitter, dopamine. In December 1990, a government study was unable to verify this report's findings. However, in July 1991, two studies not only supported the initial study but also linked the genetic variation to other disorders, such as hyperactivity. While much work remains to identify the specific genetic link for addiction, the preliminary results are encouraging.

It is also possible to develop addictive disease with no biological predisposition. One reason may be the particular action of the drug itself. Researchers are now demonstrating that drug exposure can, for a time, alter genetic expression so that the brain redefines "normal." Another may be emotional triggers that set off addiction, or the availability of a drug. One study showed that an estimated 20 percent of GIs in Vietnam developed heroin addiction. Interestingly, 90 percent were able to give up heroin once they returned from Vietnam. Finally, as Ivan Pavlov proved, whether it is food and a bell or a drug and a bell, salivation is salivation. Drugs are powerful conditioners shaping behavior and responses.

Traditionally, psychiatry in particular and medicine in general have been slow to respond to the medical and societal challenges posed by addiction. Even the *DSM-III-R* (American Psychiatric Association, 1987), the "bible" of psychiatric diagnosis, does not mention addiction per se but instead discusses dependence.

## What is dependence?

What is meant by "dependence"? Is there a distinction between dependence and addiction? Is addiction dependence and dependence addiction? If addiction is defined as a disease characterized by repetitive and destructive use of one or more mood-altering substances and stems from a biological vulnerability exposed or induced by environmental forces, is the difference between them only semantic?

Traditionally, those who have seen addiction as a consequence of choice have made a distinction. They suggest that dependence is a stage below addiction, where the choice to continue taking drugs or alcohol or continuing certain behaviors can be stopped "if the person really wants to stop." One drug policy expert, Mark A. R. Kleiman, refers to this as a "failure of self command." Drug taking, he says, inherently "affects decisions. It is commonplace that people behave differently under the influence than they do sober." Making decisions such as "having another round," Kleiman points out, may lead to further bad choices. The nature of the drug—to reduce inhibition when intoxicated—brings about "drugged choices" (Kleiman, 1992).

However, Kleiman says, "For most drug takers the decision to start any given drug use session is made while sober. Intoxication can account for excess once use has started, but it cannot explain starting too often or why the (sober) decision to start does not correctly allow for the possibility of an intoxicated decision to continue too long" (Kleiman, 1992, p. 31).

The answer to that question is in the "medical" definition of dependence and the understanding and acceptance of addiction of any kind as a biological process that—for genetic reasons—affects some people more intensely than others.

### Is addiction a "real" disease?

There is another major factor, beyond genetics, that supports the disease model of addiction: neuroanatomy or the vulnerable brain chemistries that affect all sorts of emotions, from elation, joy, and pleasure to unhappiness and dysphoria.

Since addiction has become so widespread among so many diverse groups, scientists, physicians, psychologists, and others have searched for biological explanations. One well-known and accepted biological basis for addiction is the fact that the brain has been around far longer than addictive substances. So if the brain lacks a special section called "the addiction center," why do humans become physiologically hooked?

Two decades of research have produced dramatic breakthroughs in the understanding of the neuroanatomical aspects of addiction. For example, most researchers first viewed addiction as resulting primarily from attempts to avoid the pain and discomfort associated with withdrawal. However, in the 1950s researchers began to explore the role of abuse-prone substances in activating specific neurochemicals in the brain that are basic to the "reward/reinforcement" system. This area of the brain is where the "action" takes place when humans conduct any activity that makes them feel good: the good feelings that come from doing a good job at work, hitting a home run in a softball game, making love, or seeing a beautiful sunset.

All drugs that are addictive in humans are now considered to be "reinforcing" in that their use stimulates further use. Animals will press a lever for a drug injection or a puff of cocaine. Once they learn that pressing the lever gives them cocaine, they press and press and press, frequently at the expense of eating—and their lives. This reinforcing property is one of the key elements of the drugs' addictive nature. While this may seem obvious, until recently many people believed that drugs were not addictive unless they caused withdrawal effects. As a result, some drugs with overt withdrawal symptoms, such as heroin, were considered addictive, while drugs such as cocaine, with less obvious with-

drawal symptoms, were considered to be nonaddictive. It is now known that all drugs are reinforcing.

Two types of reinforcement occur in the reward system. Positive reinforcement results from a stimulus that brings pleasure to a subject who is in a normal mood state. The identification of positive reinforcers is complicated by the highly subjective nature of pleasure and by the difficulties of defining normal mood states. Negative reinforcement is produced by discontinuing unpleasant feelings and the subsequent return to a normal state. Popular analgesics such as aspirin and acetaminophen can be viewed as negative reinforcers.

Survival drives, such as eating, drinking, copulating, and seeking shelter, are positive reinforcers. But—and this is one of the most important reasons why drug addiction is so powerful—drugs of abuse, including cocaine, amphetamines, opiates, barbiturates, benzodiazepines, alcohol, nicotine, caffeine, cannabis, and phencyclidine, are positive reinforcers. They reinforce drug-taking through the immediate pleasure that results—the high. Then they create a biological desire for more—as is true of any pleasurable experience—by releasing neurochemicals such as dopamine, which is directly involved in mood regulation.

Addictive substances also contribute to "priming" in the brain, which is similar to the feeling a person gets upon seeing a bowl of salted pretzels. The person may not miss the pretzels when he or she is full or not around them, but seeing them on the table sets off an immediate desire because the brain remembers what it feels like to eat pretzels.

Other factors besides the pharmacological effects of drugs may lead to positive reinforcement. For example, drug use may enhance a person's social standing, encourage approval by drug-using friends, and convey a special status to the user.

Researchers have discovered that an addict's body responds differently to various chemicals and environmental factors, and that this different response may increase the risk of addiction (Gawin, 1991; Killam and Olds, 1957). Many of these varying responses occur in the area of the brain called the limbic system. The limbic system contains nerve cells that help to regulate moods. It is also involved in the perception of reward. In this case, "reward" refers to the pleasure felt after doing something good. (Eating, for example, is essential for survival. The limbic system rewards eating and makes it a pleasurable activity that humans are likely to look forward to repeating.)

Drugs like cocaine trick the limbic system by triggering the reward response through the release of neurotransmitters. Neurotransmitters are chemical messengers between nerve cells that are intricately involved in regulating moods. Cocaine, for example, leads to the increased availability of the neurotransmitter dopamine.

Dopamine causes specific nerve cells to fire, and the result is endogenous brain reward or euphoria. Since cocaine uses brain systems normally reserved for species survival reward, the user feels as if he or she has just accomplished something important. The euphoria and brain reward produced by cocaine make the brain view it as a substance necessary for survival. Hence the brain asks for more cocaine and excessive amounts of dopamine are released. Normally, any surplus dopamine released by the nerve cells is reabsorbed by them; however, cocaine interferes with this reabsorption. Finally, the brain's store of dopamine is depleted. With their supply of neurotransmitters depleted, cocaine users experience intense depression and cravings for more cocaine. In addition, the limbic system remembers cocaine's pleasurable response, a memory that can be triggered by talking about the drug, or smelling it, or even a visual stimulus such as talcum powder. It is believed that the action of drugs in a section of the brain called the nucleus accumbens is primarily responsible for the feelings of positive reinforcement that result from use of virtually all the addictive drugs.

Given enough repetitions, drug and alcohol use become as entrenched as the desire for food, water, or sex. Furthermore, the dopamine pathways have many other influences, from the hypothalamus and hormones to the frontal lobe of the brain—the area responsible for judgment and insight. Not only do drugs cause the addict's brain to demand more drugs; the addict's ability to handle this demand rationally in the context of other everyday demands (such as work, family responsibilities, health and safety concerns) is distorted. Tormented by the acquired drive for the drug, memory of euphoria, and denial of obvious consequences, the addict becomes out of control.

Obviously, the complexity of the body and the brain means that no simple answer for the cause of addiction will be found. However, researchers are using sophisticated diagnostic examinations to uncover more information in an attempt to understand better the effects of drugs upon the brain. While it is doubtful that these procedures will provide a definitive, simple answer to the cause of addiction, the information gleaned from them may result in more effective treatment and prevention strategies.

## What is tolerance?

Tolerance may occur when the brain environment redefines "normal" and resets that level of feeling due to continued drug abuse. If drugs are taken to seek pleasure, they develop a life of their own as the brain redefines normal to require their presence in expected quantities. In other words, it takes more and more just to feel normal.

Interestingly, the emphasis on drug reward in the addiction process paves the way for other conditions, such as eating disorders and even sexual or gambling disorders, to be considered addictions. Eating disorders, in particular, share common behavioral symptoms, biological reward pathways, high relapse rates, and treatment strategies with other forms of substance abuse. More research is necessary to establish the legitimate inclusion of sexual and gambling behaviors with other expressions of addiction.

## Drug triggers: The brain learns

Drug use provides a quick and powerful means of changing one's moods and sensations. In a cost–benefit analysis, the user seeks the immediately gratifying effects as a "benefit" that outweighs the long-term cost of drug use. Other users may be influenced by physical or psychological states such as depression, pain, or stress that may be temporarily relieved by drug consumption. Drug use is such a powerful reinforcer and shaper of behavior that drug paraphernalia and virtually all of the events associated with finding and using drugs become reinforcers.

A variety of nondrug factors, including psychological states such as depression or anxiety, and/or environmental factors (drug paraphernalia, drug-using locations or friends, etc.) can become so associated with drug taking that merely being depressed or seeing drug paraphernalia may trigger the urge to use drugs.

**Withdrawal.** While significant evidence supports the role of dopamine in the reward process, the neuroanatomy of withdrawal is not as clearly defined. However, a wide variety of abused drugs, with apparently little in common pharmacologically, have common withdrawal effects in certain areas of the brain. Opiates, benzodiazepines, nicotine, and alcohol have all had their withdrawal symptoms treated effectively with clonidine, a medication that works in an area of the brain called the locus coeruleus.

Unlike opiate and alcohol withdrawal, symptoms of cocaine withdrawal are relatively mild and disappear relatively quickly. This dearth of withdrawal symptoms helps to explain the episodic pattern of use reported by many cocaine addicts: periods of intense bingeing alternate with intervals of abstinence. The intense craving and high relapse rate associated with cocaine use appear to derive more from a desire to repeat a pleasurable experience than to avoid the discomfort of withdrawal.

In fact, for all drugs, reward may be more important than withdrawal in the persistence of addiction and relapse, in that successful treatment of withdrawal has not generally improved recovery.

**Treatment implications.** The disease model of addiction is supported by the high degree of addiction that various substances of abuse cause and the likelihood that a drug addict will be using more than one drug. This multiple addiction is a major factor and plays a significant role in the treatment of addiction. Treatment strategies aimed at eliminating one specific form of addiction, such as cocaine abuse, without addressing other mood-altering substances, have usually failed. The addict who abuses only one drug is very rare. The Epidemiologic Catchment Area study of over 20,000 respondents found that 16 percent of the general population experienced alcoholism at some point during their lifetime—with 30 percent of these alcoholics also abusing other drugs. Alcoholics were 3.9 times more likely than nonalcoholics to have comorbid drug abuse. Similarly, the rates of alcohol abuse among other drug addicts were high: 36 percent of cannabis addicts, 62 percent of amphetamine addicts, 67 percent of opiate addicts, and 84 percent of cocaine addicts were also alcoholics. These studies, combined with clinical observations regarding the concurrent use of multiple substances, suggest common biological determinants for all addiction (Miller and Gold, 1991).

The success of Alcoholics Anonymous, with its broad ban of all mood-altering substances, lends further support to the unified disease concept of addiction. Similarly, naltrexone, a medication known previously for its efficacy in helping opiate addicts to recover, has been used successfully to treat alcoholism, cocaine addiction, and eating disorders. Although naltrexone can block the effects only of opiates, it appears to be effective against other drugs of abuse primarily because of the involvement of the opiate system in reward. According to this theory, naltrexone's opiate inhibition makes other drug use less reinforcing and ultimately prevents full-blown relapse to drug use as the addict's body learns not to associate drug use with reward. However, even with the use of Alcoholics Anonymous and viable pharmacological therapies like naltrexone, addiction remains difficult to treat primarily because drug use is so intertwined with the biological reward system.

For an addict, drug use becomes an acquired drive state that permeates all aspects of life. Withdrawal from drug use activates separate neural pathways that cause withdrawal events to be perceived as life-threatening, and the subsequent physiological and psychological reactions often lead to renewed drug consumption. The treatment research consensus that time in treatment and/or abstinence is the greatest predictor of treatment success may reflect the time required to reinstate predrug neural homeostasis, fading of memory of euphoria and conditioned cues, and the reemergence of endogenous reinforcement for work, friends, shelter, food, water, and copulation.

Drug reinforcement is so powerful that even when it is eliminated by pharmacological blockade (e.g., nal-trexone), humans quickly identify themselves as opiate available or unavailable and change their behavior without changing their attachment to the drug and its effects. Once pharmacological intervention is discontinued, the addict resumes self-administration.

Moods and other mental states, such as drug-craving and anxiety, can become conditioned stimuli that may lead to drug use. Clinicians have used relaxation training, in which patients are taught relaxation and breathing techniques, to use in the presence of drug-related stimuli or the mental states they would normally associate with the need to use drugs.

Clearly, relapse prevention and successful treatment of addiction require much more than the alleviation of withdrawal symptoms. It is well known that patients with higher pretreatment levels of social support, employment, and productivity have a better prognosis for successful response to initial treatment and long-term abstinence. Treatment outcomes for these patients may improve because they perceive the long-term cost of drug use (loss of family or job) as outweighing the short-term "benefit" of drug use. Educational efforts that stress the risks associated with drug abuse help individuals to avoid drug use. No pharmacological or nonpharmacological treatment strategy can match the success of prevention.

The disease model of addiction should not be used to excuse the addict's responsibility; abuse has to begin somewhere. The addict remains culpable for the initial decision to use the drug and for continuing to use it despite adverse consequences. Nevertheless, an understanding of addiction and the addiction process allows us to comprehend the existence of addiction as well as why abstinence in treatment is difficult to achieve.

## Summary

All abuse-prone drugs are used, at least initially, for their positive effects and because the user believes the short-term benefits of this experience surpass the long-term costs. Once initiated, drug use permits access to the reinforcement reward system, which is believed to be anatomically distinct from the negative/withdrawal system in the brain. This positive reward system provides the user with an experience that the brain equates with profoundly important events like eating, drinking, and sex.

While studies have confirmed an encouraging decline in the number of illicit drug users, substance abuse continues to be a national problem. National Household Surveys have found that over 13 percent of Americans had tried at least one illegal drug during a given year, with an estimated 6–7 million cocaine users and at least 700,000 people having used heroin (National Household Survey, 1991). Estimates of LSD use among high school seniors have increased, according to 1993 reports from the National Institute on Drug Abuse (Johnston et al., 1993). In addition, seizures of LSD were the third highest among illegal drugs. Ecstasy (another hallucinogen) use among adolescents is on the rise.

Better news is increased understanding of the role that genetics and inheritance play in possible predisposition to addiction. And the best news of all is the widespread acceptance of the biological nature of drug addiction and the disease model, which brings hope to millions of people who now think they are at fault because they cannot overcome their body's desires. The future will being greater understanding of the biological pathways and, with that, cures for addiction and dependence.

MARK S. GOLD

*Directly related to this article are the other articles in this entry:* SMOKING, ALCOHOLISM, ALCOHOL AND OTHER DRUGS IN A PUBLIC-HEALTH CONTEXT, *and* LEGAL CONTROL OF HARMFUL SUBSTANCES. *For a further discussion of topics mentioned in this article, see the entries* GENETICS AND HUMAN BEHAVIOR, *article on* SCIENTIFIC AND RESEARCH ISSUES; LIFESTYLES AND PUBLIC HEALTH; OCCUPATIONAL SAFETY AND HEALTH; RACE AND RACISM; *and* SEXUALITY IN SOCIETY, *article on* SOCIAL CONTROL OF SEXUAL BEHAVIOR. *For a discussion of related ideas, see the entries* AUTONOMY; BEHAVIOR MODIFICATION THERAPIES; FREEDOM AND COERCION; HEALTH PROMOTION AND HEALTH EDUCATION; *and* SEXISM. *Other relevant material may be found under the entries* ABUSE, INTERPERSONAL; AIDS, *article on* PUBLIC-HEALTH ISSUES; HARM; HEALTH SCREENING AND TESTING IN THE PUBLIC-HEALTH CONTEXT; PROSTITUTION; RIGHTS; *and* SOCIAL MEDICINE.

## Bibliography

ALDEN, WILLIAM. 1991. Personal communication with Alden (director of the U.S. Drug Enforcement Administration Congressional Liaison Office).

AMERICAN PSYCHIATRIC ASSOCIATION. 1987. *Diagnostic and Statistical Manual of Mental Disorders (DSM-III-R).* 3d ed., rev. Chicago: Author.

CENTERS FOR DISEASE CONTROL AND PREVENTION. 1993. Statement on health effects of smoking, August 26. Discussed in "Smoking's Annual Cost Is Put at 5 Million Years of Life," *New York Times,* August 27, p. A19.

DACKIS, CHARLES A., and GOLD, MARK S. 1988. "Psychopharmacology of Cocaine." *Psychiatric Annals* 19, no. 9:528–530.

ELDERS, M. JOYCELYN; PERRY, CHERYL L.; ERIKSEN, MICHALE P.; and BIOVINO, GARY A. 1994. "Report of the Surgeon General: Preventing Tobacco Use Among Young People." *American Journal of Public Health* 84, no. 4:543–547.

GAWIN, FRANK H. 1991. "Cocaine Addiction: Psychology and Neurophysiology." *Science* 251, no. 5001:1580–1586.

GOLD, MARK S. 1991. *The Good News About Drugs and Alcohol: Curing, Treating, and Preventing Substance Abuse in the New Age of Biopsychiatry.* New York: Villard.

———. 1994. *The Facts About Drugs and Alcohol.* 4th ed. New York: Bantam.

GRIFFITHS, ROLAND R.; BIGELOW, GEORGE E.; and HENNINGFIELD, JACK E. 1980. "Similarities in Animal and Human Drug Taking Behavior." *Advances in Substance Abuse: Behavioral and Biological Research* 1:1–90.

HELZER, JOHN E., and BURNAM, M. AUDREY. 1991. "Epidemiology of Alcohol Addiction: United States." In *Comprehensive Handbook of Drug and Alcohol Addiction,* pp. 9–38. Edited by Norman S. Miller. New York: Marcel Dekker.

JOHNSTON, LLOYD; O'MALLEY, PATRICK M.; and BACHMAN, JERALD G. 1993. *National Survey Results on Drug Use from the Monitoring the Future Study, 1975–1992.* 2 vols. Washington, D.C.: National Institute on Drug Abuse.

KILLAM, K. F., and OLDS, J. SINCLAIR. 1957. "Further Studies on the Effects of Centrally Acting Drugs on Self-Stimulation." *Journal of Pharmacology and Experimental Therapy* 119:157. Abstract of a paper given at the Fall Meeting of the American Society for Pharmacology and Experimental Ethics, November 8–10, 1956.

KLEIMAN, MARK A. R. 1992. *Against Excess: Drug Policy for Results.* New York: Basic Books.

McLELLAN, A. THOMAS; LUBORSKY, LESTER; WOODY, GEORGE E.; O'BRIEN, CHARLES P.; and DRULEY, KEITH A. 1983. "Predicting Response to Alcohol and Drug Abuse Treatments." *Archives of General Psychiatry* 40, no. 6:620–625.

MILLER, NORMAN S., and GOLD, MARK S. 1991. *Alcohol.* New York: Plenum Medical.

*National Household Survey on Drug Abuse.* 1991. Rockville, Md.: U.S. Department of Health and Human Services, Public Health Administration.

NOVELLO, ANTONIA C. 1993. "From the Surgeon General, U.S. Public Health Service." *Journal of the American Medical Association* 270, no. 7:806.

PROCHASKA, JAMES O.; DiCLEMENTE, CARLO C.; and NORCROSS, JOHN C. 1992. "In Search of How People Change: Applications to Addictive Behaviors." *American Psychologist* 47, no. 9:1102–1114.

ROBINS, LEE N.; HELZER, JOHN E.; PRZYBECK, THOMAS R.; and REGIER, DARREL A. 1988. "Alcohol Disorders in the Community: A Report from the Epidemiologic Catchment Area." In *Alcoholism: Origins and Outcome,* pp. 15–29. Edited by Robert M. Bose and James E. Barrett. New York: Raven.

*Substance Abuse: The Nation's Number One Health Problem: Key Indicators for Policy.* 1993. Princeton, N.J.: Robert Wood Johnson Foundation.

WIKLER, ABRAHAM. 1973. "Dynamics of Drug Dependence: Implications of a Conditioning Theory for Research and Treatment." *Archives of General Psychiatry* 28, no. 5:611–619.

*Youth and Alcohol: Selected Reports to the Surgeon General.* 1993. Washington, D.C.: U.S. Department of Education.

## II. SMOKING

From the time native peoples of the Americas introduced Europeans to tobacco until the second decade of the twentieth century, smoking and other forms of tobacco use posed questions of etiquette and morality rather than of medicine. The first public-policy issues concerning tobacco centered on its role as an important cash crop and a potential source of tax revenue. Medical questions about tobacco use failed to materialize because, until the 1920s, there were no scientific grounds for supposing that smoking endangered the health of smokers. Half a century more passed before epidemiologists began making a case for the dangers of environmental tobacco smoke (ETS) to nonsmokers.

Scientists began building the case for the dangerousness of smoking when A. C. Broders (1920) published an article correlating tobacco use with lip cancer. Subsequent studies repeatedly linked tobacco use, and in particular smoking, with a variety of diseases, with the correlation of lung cancer and smoking being salient. Evidence was derived from epidemiologic studies, typically retrospective; laboratory studies; and findings at autopsy. By 1957, the federally sponsored Study Group on Smoking and Health had concluded that a *causal* link existed between smoking and lung cancer. The U.S. Public Health Service (U.S. PHS) affirmed a causal link between smoking and numerous cancers, as well as other diseases, in 1964 when Surgeon General Luther Terry issued an advisory report titled *Smoking and Health* (U.S. Surgeon General's Advisory Committee, 1964). Since 1964 the U.S. PHS has continued to publish reports to or from the surgeon general detailing the deleterious effects of smoking (U.S. Department of Health, Education and Welfare [U.S. DHEW], 1971, 1972, 1974, 1975, 1978, 1979; U.S. Department of Health and Human Services [U.S. DHHS], 1980, 1981, 1982, 1983, 1984, 1985, 1986, 1989, 1990, 1992; U.S. PHS, 1968; National Clearinghouse for Smoking and Health, 1969) and the addictive properties of smoking (U.S. DHHS, 1988, 1990).

The United States was not alone in noting the causal role smoking plays in the generation of various cancers and other diseases. In the United Kingdom, for example, the Royal College of Physicians (1962) had already published findings similar to those in *Smoking and Health*. Undoubtedly part of the reason for the relatively slower acceptance of the health risks of smoking in the United States arose, and continues to arise, from a politically powerful tobacco industry. The British Medical Association (1986) also describes vigorous tobacco industry opposition to its antismoking campaign. As Peter Taylor (1984) has made clear, the public has every reason to doubt all tobacco industry claims to plain dealing and honest brokering.

Reflection on just a few facts gives a sense of the ethical and policy problems posed by smoking. Males who smoke twenty cigarettes a day have a seven- to ninefold increase in their likelihood of developing lung cancer. The U.S. Environmental Protection Agency (U.S. EPA) in 1992 estimated nonsmoking wives of smokers are about 1.3 times more likely to develop diseases that regular smokers are likely to get. Michael Siegal (1993), after reviewing studies of the effects of ETS on nonsmoking restaurant workers, concluded that they were 1.5 times more likely to develop lung cancer than nonsmokers exposed to ETS at home, and nonsmoking bartenders were 4.4 times more likely to develop lung cancer. A review by J. Michael McGinnis and William H. Foege (1993) of U.S. mortality studies for 1990 says much. In 1990, smoking accounted for 30 percent of lung cancer deaths and 21 percent of deaths from cardiovascular disease. In the same year, smoking ranked as the leading cause of death in the United States, with 400,000 deaths (19% of all deaths). Alcohol, by comparison, killed 100,000 Americans, and illicit drugs 20,000. Only poor diet and activity patterns—killers of 300,000 Americans (or 14% of deaths) in 1990—came anywhere near smoking as a cause of death. Smoking is *the* leading cause of preventable death in industrialized countries.

### Restrictive policies

Given the risks that smoking poses for smokers and nonsmokers, two obvious considerations shape public policy on smoking. First, the risks to smokers themselves suggest that at least some restrictive policies designed to protect smokers from themselves may be in order. Second, the risks that smokers impose on nonsmokers support policies designed to keep smokers from exposing nonsmokers to ETS or from forcing nonsmokers to carry the social costs of smoking. In addition to these two obvious considerations, the promotion of health ideals has served as a third consideration for restrictive policy. For example, in 1992 the Joint Commission on the Accreditation of Health Care Organizations (JCAHO), the chief hospital accreditation agency in the United States, began requiring hospitals to forbid smoking within their premises, in the absence of a physician's order to the contrary, as a condition of accreditation. Robert Goodin (1989) uses these kinds of considerations to develop a vigorous case for a public policy aimed at a total ban on smoking.

Despite the risks smokers cause themselves, policies designed to stop smokers from smoking are difficult to justify within the Anglo-American moral tradition. The more restrictive a policy is, the more difficult it is to justify. Difficulties for justification arise from a repugnance for paternalistic interferences in the lives of others. At least since John Stuart Mill's *On Liberty* (1859), antipaternalistic sentiment has been widespread in the English-speaking philosophical community, with Joel Feinberg (1986) being one of its best contemporary voices. Feinberg has emphatically rejected legal paternalism, the doctrine that "[i]t is always a good reason in support of a prohibition that it is necessary to prevent harm (physical, psychological, or economic) to the actor himself" (p. xvii). Most people probably share Feinberg's reluctance to prohibit a person's acting on a self-regarding choice made in a cool moment with full knowledge of the facts. Hence philosophers distinguish strong and weak paternalism (Sartorius, 1983). Strong paternalists permit interference with competent choices that fail to promote the chooser's best interests. Weak paternalists allow interference with risky, incompetent choices. Despite an absence of consensus on what constitutes a competent choice, factors such as coercion, ignorance, mental impairment, addiction, and the like serve as grounds for challenging the competence of a choice.

If smoking is a competent choice, then public policies that would overrule competent choices face mighty objections. It requires breathtaking confidence to assume that overruling a competent choice is more likely to promote a person's well-being than respecting it. In the case of smoking, the probable ground for forbidding competent choices to smoke is almost certain to center on the health benefits of not smoking. But not all people value health. Moreover, they may suffer from diseases that make health risks of smoking beside the point. What overwhelmingly good reason does a twenty-year-old woman with ovarian cancer have for not smoking? And why select smoking for special attention? Many other activities and habits also negatively affect a person's health. Working as a collier, wolfing down cheeseburgers, and a preference for sitting instead of walking all have baleful effects on a person's health. But nobody seriously suggests making a low cholesterol count a condition for buying potato chips. So long as one accepts value pluralism, the connection of not smoking with a person's best interests is going to depend on that person's values and circumstances. What citizens in a free society value varies. That is a fact with which policymakers in a free society must live.

## Arguments for paternalistic policies

Smoking may be significantly different from many other risky behaviors for a variety of reasons. Four will be considered. All undermine the suggestion that smokers choose to smoke on the basis of a full understanding of the relevant facts in a cool moment, providing weakly paternalistic grounds for restrictive smoking policies.

First, many smokers have a meager comprehension of the risks of smoking. Although education and warnings have improved the public's knowledge of the dangers, a stunning number of people still fail to appreciate them. In the United States, the surgeon general (U.S. DHHS, 1989) has reported that 8 million smokers (15%) do not believe smoking causes lung cancer; 15 million (29%) do not believe it causes heart disease. Female smokers of childbearing age often do not understand the risks of smoking during pregnancy: 32 percent are ignorant of the increased risk of stillbirth; 24 percent do not know that smoking can cause premature birth; and 15 percent do not know that smoking increases the likelihood of a low-birth-weight baby. Smokers also underestimate their personal risk. In 1986, only 18 percent of smokers claimed to be very concerned about their smoking, 24 percent were not at all concerned, and almost 50 percent believed they had to smoke more than ten cigarettes per day to affect their health adversely.

Many high school students labor under misapprehensions about the risks of smoking, with 34 percent not believing smoking a pack or more of cigarettes per day puts one at great risk of serious harm. These figures do represent substantial progress over beliefs that had existed during the 1950s, 1960s, and 1970s, and will undoubtedly continue to change in the direction of knowledge, but substantial numbers of adults and adolescents still lack accurate knowledge of the risks of smoking. This kind of ignorance might be thought to cast doubt on the competence of the decision to start smoking.

Second, a consensus has emerged that nicotine is an addictive substance. Although the surgeon general's 1964 report (U.S. PHS, 1964) classified smoking as a habit, not an addiction, thinking has changed. In 1964, much emphasis was placed on the role of physiological dependency. The 1964 report made a special effort to determine if smoking satisfied the World Health Organization's requirements for addiction, and concluded that it did not. As research on addiction developed over the ensuing years, however, the concept of addiction expanded to accommodate psychosocial, in addition to pharmacologic, factors. To reflect this shift, "dependency" has come to be a preferred term. In any case, the relevance of classifying smoking as a dependency or an addiction serves to buttress a case for weak paternalism. Dependency or addiction casts doubt on either the competence or voluntariness of the choice to smoke. If smokers cannot help themselves, perhaps others should help them.

Third, the age at which smoking is begun has steadily declined. The surgeon general's report (U.S. DHHS, 1989) cited 17.2 as the average age of initiation for male smokers and 19.1 for female smokers. These ages have declined steadily over the years. Among smokers born since 1935, the same report noted that almost half began smoking before age eighteen. Such early commencement of smoking erodes the presumption that smoking is a competent, informed decision. Adolescents are often thought to underestimate future risks. Moreover, social pressures, including advertising, might be hypothesized as the true causes of the decision to smoke. Hence choosing to smoke might not be a voluntary choice but a child's incompetent decision. Thus, a weak paternalist has the option of arguing that smoking is born of incompetent choice, often made by a minor, and sustained by addiction (Levanthal et al., 1987).

Fourth, the tobacco industry has labored shamelessly to mislead the public about the risks of smoking. Advertisements, for example, brim with images of handsome, hard-muscled men and women playing sports or cavorting joyously together. The industry has made countless lying representations about the safety of its products, the knowledge it had of smoking's dangers, and the target audience of its advertisements. The young and women are frequent targets. Children five years and older identify Joe Camel as readily as Mickey Mouse. In 1983, children in the United Kingdom bought £60 (about $100) worth of cigarettes apiece (British Medical Association, 1986). Virginia Slims' advertisements exploit feminist ideals. The tobacco industry refuses to accept responsibility for its actions. Straightforward arguments reach an easy conclusion. Tobacco companies have striven to prevent people from making informed, rational choices about whether to smoke.

## Replies and concessions to paternalistic policies

Despite the force of these four considerations, they fail to justify such extreme antismoking measures as total bans, bans on the sale of high-tar cigarettes, or requiring a medical prescription to buy cigarettes, but they do make a strong case for education. First, if smokers have inadequate knowledge of the risks of smoking, the nonpaternalistic response of improved education is available. As the surgeon general's 1989 report (U.S. DHHS, 1989) made clear, the public is vastly better informed about the risks of smoking than in 1964. Also, the warnings on the sides of cigarette packs sold in the United States and Canada make it likely that those who are "unaware" of the risks of smoking either cannot read or are refusing to believe the evidence. The fact that 90 percent of smokers express a desire to quit suggests a better grasp of the risks than denials of risks suggest.

Nor do the addictive qualities of tobacco justify prohibition or medicalization. First, it strains the evidence to claim, as does Robert Goodin (1989), that smoking is as addictive as heroin, citing the similarity in the quit rates of heroin addicts and smokers. Cigarettes are cheap, well advertised, publicly consumable, and legal. Heroin is not. It would be rash to conclude that the quit rates would be the same if smoking and heroin had the same level of social acceptability. Second, even though smoking is addictive, many people have quit smoking. From 1965 to 1987, smoking prevalence for males fell from 50.2 percent to 31.7 percent. In 1987, 44.8 percent of adults who had ever smoked had quit. Figures available in 1992 estimate that 28 percent of the adult population in the United States smokes. Evidently, many smokers have proven to be far from slaves to their habit. To force smokers who have not quit into treatment for their addiction would require, within the prevailing antipaternalistic, liberal tradition, a demonstration that smoking has made them incapable of competently refusing care. There is no evidence that smokers have so clouded their minds that they cannot make competent decisions about whether to enter smoking-cessation programs.

The deplorably young age at which many smokers begin smoking does justify some restriction, but not bans. First, laws prohibiting the sale of cigarettes to minors should be enforced. Second, cigarettes should no more be dispensed from vending machines than alcohol is. Third, minors are extremely sensitive to the price of cigarettes (Warner, 1986). Price increases should be instituted to discourage the purchase of cigarettes and tobacco products by minors. All of these measures are weakly paternalistic: They do not target competent adults.

Finally, the issues raised by the lying advertisements of tobacco companies must be addressed. Given the demonstrable dangers of cigarettes, advertisements designed to produce false beliefs about the safety of smoking should be suppressed. At a minimum, a policy similar to that in the United Kingdom, which limits advertisements to "tombstones" advertisements, like those found on financial pages for underwriting a stock sale, accompanied by a warning of the product's dangers, should be legislated. Further, to the extent a person is harmed as a result of false beliefs created by deceptive tobacco advertising, a strong case exists for allowing that he or she has suffered a tort. The law on this will undoubtedly evolve in the future. To date, courts in the United States have found against plaintiffs, but that could well change as the duplicity of tobacco companies becomes established in court. None of these considerations, however, would justify prohibitions on the sale of tobacco products to save smokers from self-inflicted harm.

For those who have no native distaste for paternalistic intervention, as do some utilitarians, the arguments against paternalistic intervention have limited force.

For utilitarians, the case for intervention turns on whether particular policies enhance the well-being of smokers after subtracting any disutilities that arise from restricting their liberty to smoke. In fact, the utilitarian case is general. For those who accept the utilitarian perspective, the case for restrictive policies to protect smokers from themselves is a powerful one, as would be the case even more assuredly for policies meant to protect nonsmokers.

## Protecting nonsmokers: Pros and cons

In the absence of good nonutilitarian rationales for highly restrictive smoking policies for adult smokers, powerful rationales do exist for restricting smoking to protect nonsmokers. The rationales are in two general forms: social costs and health risks.

Smoking imposes an array of social costs. Smokers get sick more often than nonsmokers. Robert Goodin (1989) cites studies that estimate the economic costs to the U.S. economy at between $52 and $62 billion. In 1993 the American Heart Association and the American Lung Association put the cost at over $112 billion per annum. Although federal tax revenues from the sale of tobacco products amounted to over $4 billion in 1990, Goodin concedes that the economic costs of smoking probably are covered by producers and users of tobacco products. He cites a study by Christine Goodfrey and Alan Maynard (1988) and statistics from Ontario, Canada, revealing that in the province of Ontario, a mere 8 percent of total tobacco revenues covers all health costs connected with smoking-related diseases. Though Canadian tax rates are higher than the U.S. tax rates, federal excise taxes on cigarettes in the United States more or less match the health costs of smoking to smokers. The studies do underestimate the costs of ETS. And, like Daniel Wikler (1983), one must wonder why the economic costs of smoking excite so much more public attention than the economic costs of obesity, daily omelets, or living in a house suffused with radon. On the darker side, smokers' premature deaths reduce pension costs. From the liberal perspective, a chief concern must center on the *harm* smokers may be doing to nonsmokers. This harm, if construed in terms of economics, could be handled by increasing taxes on tobacco products to allow damaged nonsmokers to recover for injuries suffered. But harms to nonsmokers might also be used as grounds for substantial limitations on smoking.

All defensible theories of just laws recognize a conduct's harmfulness to others as a good reason for regulating it (Feinberg, 1986). Over the past several decades evidence has continued to mount that exposure to ETS causes the same kind of harms to nonsmokers that directly inhaling smoke causes to smokers (U.S. DHHS,

1986; Wald et al., 1986; National Institute for Occupational Safety and Health [NIOSH] 1991). And though the evidence for the harmfulness of ETS to nonsmokers has yet to prove as overwhelming as the evidence for the harmfulness of smoking to smokers, the evidence *is* impressive. Some argue for the safety of ETS (Ecobichon and Wu, 1990; Tollison, 1988), but the U.S. EPA's report (1992) puts the health risks of ETS beyond serious doubt. James Repace (1985) had estimated the risk at about the same level as drowning. The 1992 U.S. EPA report agrees with him. Moreover, many nonsmokers incur the risks attendant to ETS exposure involuntarily.

Justifying policies to save nonsmokers from the risks of ETS raises two kinds of questions. How risky must an activity be to nonparticipants to justify restricting the liberty interests of participants? Second, in instances where the case for regulation is strong, how restrictive can regulations be? Granted, smoking poses enough risk to nonsmokers to justify its restriction. But what restrictions are justified? Again, it depends on how great the risks of ETS are. If policy considerations concern health-care facilities, it seems unlikely that the desire to save nonsmokers from ETS would justify such policies as the JCAHO's decision to impose what amounts to a ban on smoking within accredited hospitals or the U.S. PHS's ban on the sale or use of tobacco products in its facilities. Protecting nonsmokers could be achieved by confining smoking to designated, well-ventilated areas. Moreover, smokers could be charged a premium that allowed hospitals to reduce risks from other sources. In any case, no studies have shown that patients are at increased risk from ETS in hospitals that provide designated smoking areas. Consideration for the safety of nonsmokers, whether patients or employees, fails to justify the increasingly popular total bans on smoking and/or the sale of tobacco in hospitals. If grounds for extremely restrictive policies on tobacco use, such as prohibition of sales or consumption, exist, they depend on rationales other than the dangers tobacco poses to smokers or nonsmokers. Tobacco prohibitionists might enlist health ideals to justify restrictive policies.

## Health ideals

Medical and nursing organizations have long played a role in advocating better public health. Advocacy can run from leading by example (e.g., few doctors smoke) to pushing for measures designed to make unhealthy lifestyles less attractive. As temples of health values, hospitals have a special role. Patients entering hospitals often forgo their insalubrious pleasures, as those with a taste for martinis and sirloin quickly learn. Since tobacco use is the preeminent cause of preventable deaths, institutions created for the delivery of health care have good reason for actively enforcing good health practices on their premises or through their offices and officers. Tobacco use stands at odds with the avowed mission of medical and nursing institutions. At a minimum, these institutions should not promote unhealthy living.

Historically, particularly in mental hospitals, medical institutions have failed to do enough to discourage the use of tobacco. Patients in mental hospitals often received cigarettes as rewards for good behavior, making beds, complying with ward rules, and other measures meant to facilitate a smoothly running institution. Perhaps in consequence, psychiatric patients with histories of major mental illnesses smoke at shockingly high rates. Estimates typically are 70 percent or higher (Hughes et al., 1986). Moreover, nursing homes and regular hospitals routinely accommodated smokers without regard to the safety of nonsmoking patients and staff.

In addition, the policies of various governmental agencies stand at odds. In the United States, the DHHS develops programs to discourage smoking while the Departments of Agriculture (USDA) and State develop and defend programs to encourage the growth of tobacco for consumption in the United States and abroad, most notoriously in Third World markets, where sales of cigarettes and cigarette tobacco have offset declines in U.S. consumption (USDA, various). Nobody contends that tobacco policies in the United States form a coherent whole.

Despite the attractiveness of policies aimed at the prevention of tobacco use via the imposition of health ideals, the moral defensibility of policies that go beyond education and the protection of nonsmokers is suspect (Brock, 1983; Lavin, 1990). It is difficult to discern what moral grounds could support such policies, if the grounds are neither weakly paternalistic nor rooted in the harm principle. The remaining grounds for compelling compliance with health values that many people do not share are likely to center on the objective good of health ideals. Dan Brock (1983) has offered powerful arguments for caution when organizations propose to force allegedly objective goods on people.

Policies on the sale of tobacco to foreign countries also raise a number of difficult issues. Perhaps the chief problem comes from the collusion of federal agencies with tobacco companies to sell cigarettes to people who lack adequate information about the risks of smoking. After all, the federal government forbids the sale of cigarettes on those terms in the United States. Ubiquitous, vigorous opposition by tobacco companies to all efforts to inform Third World consumers of the risks of smoking exacerbates the problem. The moral terrain is familiar. First, since many Third World governments have neither the money nor the inclination to educate their citizens about the health risks of smoking, a strong case

exists for policies discouraging tobacco sales to countries whose citizens lack the chance to make informed choices about smoking. Second, a case also exists for policies discouraging sales to countries where many nonsmoking citizens are likely to be harmed by an increase in smoking prevalence. Such policies stay within the traditional, albeit liberal, grounds for restrictive policies. The restrictions should protect inadequately informed, incompetent, and involuntarily exposed individuals from uncompensated harms.

MICHAEL LAVIN

*Directly related to this article are the other articles in this entry:* ADDICTION AND DEPENDENCE, ALCOHOLISM, ALCOHOL AND OTHER DRUGS IN A PUBLIC-HEALTH CONTEXT, *and* LEGAL CONTROL OF HARMFUL SUBSTANCES. *For a further discussion of topics mentioned in this article, see the entries* ADOLESCENTS; ADVERTISING; AUTONOMY; FREEDOM AND COERCION; HARM; HEALTH PROMOTION AND HEALTH EDUCATION; LIFESTYLES AND PUBLIC HEALTH; PATERNALISM; PATIENTS' RESPONSIBILITIES, *article on* DUTIES OF PATIENTS; PATIENTS' RIGHTS, *article on* ORIGIN AND NATURE OF PATIENTS' RIGHTS; PUBLIC HEALTH, *articles on* HISTORY OF PUBLIC HEALTH, *and* PHILOSOPHY OF PUBLIC HEALTH; PUBLIC HEALTH AND THE LAW; *and* UTILITY. *For a discussion of related ideas, see the entries* BEHAVIOR CONTROL; BENEFICENCE; FEMINISM; INFORMED CONSENT, *article on* MEANING AND ELEMENTS OF INFORMED CONSENT; RACE AND RACISM; RESPONSIBILITY; SEXISM; SOCIAL MEDICINE; WOMEN, *articles on* HISTORICAL AND CROSS-CULTURAL PERSPECTIVES, *and* HEALTH-CARE ISSUES. *Other relevant material may be found under the entries* BEHAVIOR MODIFICATION THERAPIES; FETUS, *article on* PHILOSOPHICAL AND ETHICAL ISSUES; HEALTH-CARE FINANCING, *article on* HEALTH-CARE INSURANCE; HOSPITAL, *article on* MODERN HISTORY; INTERNATIONAL HEALTH; OCCUPATIONAL SAFETY AND HEALTH, *article on* ETHICAL ISSUES; *and* RIGHTS.

## Bibliography

BRITISH MEDICAL ASSOCIATION. 1986. *Smoking Out the Barons: The Campaign Against the Tobacco Industry.* Chichester, U.K.: Wiley.

BROCK, DAN. 1983. "Paternalism and Promoting the Good." In *Paternalism,* pp. 237–260. Edited by Rolf E. Sartorius. Minneapolis: University of Minnesota Press.

BRODERS, A. C. 1920. "Squamous-Cell Epithelioma of the Lip: A Study of Five Hundred and Thirty-seven Cases." *Journal of the American Medical Association* 74, no. 10: 656–664.

ECOBICHON, DONALD J., and WU, JOSEPH W., eds. 1990. *En-*

*vironmental Tobacco Smoke: Proceedings of the International Symposium at McGill University, 1989.* Lexington, Mass.: Lexington Books.

FEINBERG, JOEL. 1986. *Harm to Self: Moral Limits of the Criminal Law.* Vol. 3. Oxford: Oxford University Press.

GIBSON, MARY, ed. 1985. *To Breathe Freely: Risk, Consent, and Air.* Totowa, N.J.: Rowman and Allanheld.

GODFREY, CHRISTINE, and MAYNARD, ALAN. 1988. "Economic Aspects of Tobacco Use and Taxation Policy." *British Medical Journal* 297, no. 6644:339–343.

GOODIN, ROBERT E. 1989. *No Smoking: The Ethical Issues.* Chicago: University of Chicago Press.

HUGHES, JOHN R.; HATSUKAMI, DOROTHY K.; MITCHELL, JAMES E.; and DAHLGREN, LISA A. 1986. "Prevalence of Smoking Among Psychiatric Outpatients." *American Journal of Psychiatry* 143, no. 8:993–997.

LAVIN, MICHAEL. 1990. "Let the Patients Smoke: A Defence of a Patient Privilege." *Journal of Medical Ethics* 16, no. 3:136–140.

LEVENTHAL, HOWARD; GLYNN, KATHLEEN; and FLEMING, RAYMOND. 1987. "Is the Smoking Decision an 'Informed Choice'? Effect of Smoking Risk Factors on Smoking Beliefs." *Journal of the American Medical Association* 257, no. 24:3373–3376.

MCGINNIS, J. MICHAEL, and FOEGE, WILLIAM H. 1993. "Actual Causes of Death in the United States." *Journal of the American Medical Association* 270, no. 18:2207–2212.

MILL, JOHN STUART. 1975. [1859]. *On Liberty.* New York: Norton.

NATIONAL CLEARINGHOUSE FOR SMOKING AND HEALTH. 1969. *The Health Consequences of Smoking: 1969 Supplement to the 1967 Public Health Service Review.* Washington, D.C.: U.S. Government Printing Office.

NATIONAL INSTITUTE FOR OCCUPATIONAL SAFETY AND HEALTH (NIOSH). 1991. *Environmental Tobacco Smoke in the Workplace: Lung Cancer and Other Health Effects.* Cincinnati: Author.

REPACE, JAMES L. 1985. "Risks of Passive Smoking." In *To Breathe Freely,* pp. 3–30. Edited by Mary Gibson. Totowa, N.J.: Rowman and Allanheld.

ROYAL COLLEGE OF PHYSICIANS. 1962. *Smoking and Health: Summary and Report of the Royal College of Physicians of London on Smoking in Relation to Cancer of the Lung and Other Diseases.* New York: Pitman.

SARTORIUS, ROLF E., ed. 1983. *Paternalism.* Minneapolis: University of Minnesota Press.

SIEGEL, MICHAEL. 1993. "Involuntary Smoking in the Restaurant Workplace: A Review of Employee Exposure and Health Effects." *Journal of the American Medical Association* 270, no. 4:490–493.

STUDY GROUP ON SMOKING AND HEALTH. 1957. "Smoking and Health: Joint Report of the Study Group on Smoking and Health." *Science* 125, no. 3258:1129–1133.

TAYLOR, PETER. 1984. *The Smoke Ring: Tobacco, Money, and Multinational Politics.* New York: Pantheon.

TOLLISON, ROBERT D., ed. 1988. *Cleaning the Air: Perspectives on Environmental Tobacco Smoke.* Lexington, Mass.: Lexington Books.

U.S. DEPARTMENT OF AGRICULTURE (USDA). Various. *Tobacco situation outlook reports.*

U.S. DEPARTMENT OF HEALTH, EDUCATION AND WELFARE (U.S. DHEW). 1971. *The Health Consequences of Smoking: A Report of the Surgeon General, 1971.* Washington, D.C.: U.S. Government Printing Office.

———. 1972. *The Health Consequences of Smoking: A Report of the Surgeon General.* Washington, D.C.: U.S. Government Printing Office.

———. 1973. *The Health Consequences of Smoking.* Washington, D.C.: U.S. Government Printing Office.

———. 1974. *The Health Consequences of Smoking.* Washington, D.C.: U.S. Government Printing Office.

———. 1975. *The Health Consequences of Smoking.* Washington, D.C.: U.S. Government Printing Office.

———. 1978. *The Health Consequences of Smoking, 1977–1978.* Washington, D.C.: U.S. Government Printing Office.

———. 1979. *Smoking and Health: A Report of the Surgeon General.* Washington, D.C.: U.S. Government Printing Office.

U.S. DEPARTMENT OF HEALTH AND HUMAN SERVICES (U.S. DHHS). 1980. *The Health Consequences of Smoking for Women: A Report of the Surgeon General.* Washington, D.C.: U.S. Government Printing Office.

———. 1981. *The Health Consequences of Smoking: The Changing Cigarette: A Report of the Surgeon General.* Washington, D.C.: U.S. Government Printing Office.

———. 1982. *The Health Consequences of Smoking: Cancer: A Report of the Surgeon General.* Washington, D.C.: U.S. Government Printing Office.

———. 1983. *The Health Consequences of Smoking: Cardiovascular Disease: A Report of the Surgeon General.* Washington, D.C.: U.S. Government Printing Office.

———. 1984. *The Health Consequences of Smoking: Chronic Obstructive Lung Disease: A Report of the Surgeon General.* Washington, D.C.: U.S. Government Printing Office.

———. 1985. *The Health Consequences of Smoking: Cancer and Chronic Lung Disease in the Workplace: A Report of the Surgeon General.* Washington, D.C.: U.S. Government Printing Office.

———. 1986. *The Health Consequences of Involuntary Smoking: A Report of the Surgeon General.* Washington, D.C.: U.S. Government Printing Office.

———. 1988. *The Health Consequences of Smoking: Nicotine Addiction: A Report of the Surgeon General.* Washington, D.C.: U.S. Government Printing Office.

———. 1989. *Reducing the Health Consequences of Smoking: 25 Years of Progress: A Report of the Surgeon General.* Washington, D.C.: U.S. Government Printing Office.

———. 1990. *The Health Benefits of Smoking Cessation: A Report of the Surgeon General.* Washington, D.C.: U.S. Government Printing Office.

———. 1992. *Smoking and Health in the Americas: A Report of the Surgeon General.* Washington, D.C.: U.S. Government Printing Office.

U.S. ENVIRONMENTAL PROTECTION AGENCY (U.S. EPA). 1992. *Respiratory Health Effects of Passive Smoking: Lung Cancer and Other Disorders.* Washington, D.C.: U.S. Government Printing Office.

U.S. PUBLIC HEALTH SERVICE (U.S. PHS). 1963. *Smoking and Health: Report of the Advisory Committee to the Surgeon*

*General of the Public Health Service.* Washington, D.C.: U.S. Government Printing Office.

―――. 1968. *The Health Consequences of Smoking: A Public Health Service Review, 1967.* Washington, D.C.: U.S. Government Printing Office.

WALD, NICHOLAS J.; NANCHAHAL, KIRAN; THOMPSON, SIMON G.; and CUCKLE, HOWARD S. 1986. "Does Breathing Other People's Tobacco Smoke Cause Lung Cancer?" *British Medical Journal* 293, no. 6556:1217–1222.

WARNER, KENNETH E. 1986. "Smoking and Health Implications of a Change in the Federal Cigarette Excise Tax." *Journal of the American Medical Association* 255, no. 8:1028–1023.

WIKLER, DANIEL. 1983. "Persuasion and Coercion for Health." In *Paternalism,* pp. 35–59. Edited by Rolf E. Sartorius. Minneapolis: University of Minnesota Press.

## III. ALCOHOLISM

What are the benefits and problems that attend the use of alcoholic beverages? In what ways may drinking cause harm? Is the use of alcohol hazardous for all individuals or only for some? Who is at risk? Should an intoxicated person be held accountable for his or her actions while "under the influence"? How is excessive drinking like or unlike other self-injurious appetitive behaviors such as overeating, smoking, or other substance abuse? Should society limit or control the use of alcohol, and should it warn consumers of potential risks associated with drinking? Is alcoholism a disease, primarily a medical rather than a moral problem?

Opinion remains divided on many of these issues, reflecting the diversity of beliefs, practices, and emotions surrounding the use of beverage alcohol in various cultures. Historical and cross-cultural investigations indicate that prevailing cultural beliefs about alcohol and alcohol problems play an important role in determining moral attitudes. Research continues to generate new data about the biomedical and behavioral aspects of drinking. An informed consideration of the use of alcohol must attend simultaneously to the implications of new information and the influence of shifting values.

### Alcohol: Blessing or curse?

A product of natural fermentation, beverage alcohol, or ethanol, is perhaps the oldest known and most universally consumed psychoactive substance. Ancient peoples drank copious amounts of wine, beer, and other naturally fermented alcoholic beverages, praising their ability to lift the spirits, relieve fatigue, and enhance health. In many societies, alcohol was regarded as a divine gift and was incorporated into religious rituals. Early historical records indicate, however, that alcohol also brought problems. The Hebrew Bible, for example, tells how Noah embarrassed his sons by getting drunk (Gen.

9:20–24) and warns of calamity for "those who tarry long over wine" (Prov. 23:29–35).

Ambivalence toward alcohol use has persisted into modern times and is expressed cross-culturally in a wide diversity of attitudes, beliefs, and practices. The French, for example, regard wine as essential to their diet and lifestyle, and tend to view abstainers as deviant. Millions of Muslims, by contrast, forswear all alcohol as evil. Even within a particular society, attitudes may be heterogeneous and historically variable. Seventeenth-century colonial settlers in North America, for example, viewed drink as the Good Creature of God; three centuries later, the United States banned Demon Rum (Rorabaugh, 1979).

Empirical evidence suggests that the use of alcohol offers both modest benefits and significant hazards. In moderate amounts, alcohol is a mild relaxant that stimulates appetite and facilitates social interaction. Sociocultural norms play an important role in determining specific contexts in which drinking may normally occur and influence the experience and behavior of the drinker as well. Aside from alcohol's subjective benefits, there is evidence that moderate drinking may reduce the risk of coronary artery disease in some individuals (Klatsky, 1990).

### Hazards of alcohol use

The potential social and economic costs of alcohol use to society can be staggering. In the United States alone, it is estimated that abuse of alcohol cost $136.3 billion in 1990 for alcohol-related diseases, accidents, lost productivity, and rehabilitation (Harwood et al., 1985). Three aspects of alcohol use may present problems: drinking itself, acute intoxication, and chronic heavy drinking, commonly referred to as alcoholism.

Ethanol is a simple yet highly toxic molecule that is rapidly absorbed throughout the body and brain. While moderate consumption of alcohol (no more than two drinks per day) does not appear to pose significant health risks for most individuals, there are some populations for whom even moderate drinking may be ill-advised. Specifically, there is now evidence that drinking by pregnant women may expose the fetus to serious risk of a number of permanent morphological and cognitive defects collectively known as fetal alcohol syndrome (FAS) (U.S. Department of Health and Human Services, 1990). The relatively recent discovery of FAS (and its milder form, fetal alcohol effects [FAE]) has raised vexing ethical questions concerning the moral and legal culpability of women who drink during pregnancy. Acknowledging society's duty to warn consumers about this previously unrecognized hazard, the U.S. government passed legislation in 1988 that requires manufacturers, bottlers, and importers of alcoholic beverages to include a surgeon general's health warning on all containers.

Acute intoxication and chronic heavy use of alcohol pose the greatest hazards and raise the most pressing ethical concerns. Acute intoxication directly impairs a range of perceptual and motor functions, thereby increasing the risk of accidental injury and death by motor vehicle accidents, falls, slips, drownings, and other mishaps. The risk of serious accidental injury is greatly increased in modern technological societies, where alertness is required to safely operate heavy machinery and high-powered vehicles. In recent years, there has been a growing movement in many countries to reduce alcohol-related automobile injuries and fatalities through tougher laws and preventive education aimed at deterring drunk driving. The current legal consensus appears to be that while intoxication undoubtedly affects judgment and competence, the drunk driver should be held accountable for the decision to drive while impaired. Doubts about the ability of some individuals to make this choice when drinking is reflected in the enactment of new laws that hold bartenders, party hosts, and other servers of alcoholic beverages responsible for monitoring consumption and refusing drinks to inebriated individuals.

Intoxication may also lead to harm through its apparent ability to break down inhibitions on sexual and aggressive impulses in some individuals. In the United States, for example, alcohol intoxication has been strongly associated with assault, murder, rape, spousal violence, and other types of violence. It has not been established that intoxication itself is the direct cause of these outcomes, since in some societies drinking and intoxication are not commonly associated with such violence. Personality variables and culturally influenced expectations regarding intoxication may be important in mediating the relationship between alcohol and violence (Anglin, 1982).

In addition to the problems directly related to episodes of acute alcohol intoxication, there is widespread recognition of the harm caused by chronic excessive drinking, commonly referred to as alcoholism. At sufficient doses, the daily or frequent drinker may experience increased tolerance and, eventually, physiological dependence and withdrawal symptoms. Prolonged heavy drinking is implicated in a number of serious and potentially fatal health problems, including cirrhosis, pancreatitis, peptic ulcer, hypertension and cardiovascular disease, and various cancers. Moreover, both the central and the peripheral nervous systems are damaged by chronic alcohol abuse. In addition to well-known complications such as peripheral neuropathy, ataxia, and alcohol-related dementias, researchers have discovered more subtle cognitive deficits resulting from chronic alcoholism (Tarter et al., 1989).

Epidemiological studies indicate that about one person in ten in the United States is a problem drinker. The persistence of excessive drinking in the face of adverse consequences is the primary criterion in the diagnosis of alcohol abuse; alcohol dependence is diagnosed if tolerance and withdrawal symptoms have developed. Sex, age, and ethnicity are significant variables in the distribution of problem drinking. Men are at least four times as likely to be diagnosed with alcohol dependence as women. D.W.I.-related accidents and fatalities are most frequent among the young. In some ethnic groups, such as Chinese-Americans and Orthodox Jews, alcohol problems are rare, while in certain Native American tribes alcoholism is a leading cause of death.

Alcoholism is associated with an increased prevalence of psychiatric disorders, although symptoms of anxiety and depression may often abate following detoxification and a period of abstinence. Whether alcoholism is a cause or a consequence of other mental disorders continues to be debated. An important longitudinal study challenges the view that alcoholism is but a symptom of preexisting emotional problems with the finding that the mental health of nonalcoholics and future alcoholics does not differ significantly in childhood (Vaillant, 1983).

## Is alcoholism a disease?

Beliefs about the cause or causes of alcoholism and the nature of drinking problems exert an important influence on public perceptions, institutional responses, and treatment and prevention, and shape the framework that guides ethical inquiry and response.

The disease concept of alcoholism, first articulated by Elvin M. Jellinek in the 1940s, was actively promoted by a loose coalition of reformers, service providers, and recovering alcoholics (Jellinek, 1960). Since then, it has become the official view of the American medical profession and the World Health Organization, and has gained wide acceptance among the public at large in the United States and many other Western countries. Proponents of the disease concept argue that alcoholism, like diabetes, essential hypertension, and coronary artery disease, is a biologically based disease precipitated by environmental factors and manifested in an irreversible pattern of compulsive, pathological drinking behavior in individuals who are constitutionally vulnerable. Central to the disease model is the belief that the alcoholic effectively loses control over his or her consumption of alcohol and can never safely drink again. The disease model also holds that alcoholism is a progressive disease that may be arrested by abstinence but never cured.

Although subsequent research has provided evidence of a genetic predisposition for some types of alcoholism (Goodwin, 1985), attempts to demonstrate empirically a biological basis for alcoholism have yielded inconclusive results. Whatever influence genetics and biology have in the pathogenesis of alcoholism, many authorities agree that psychosocial variables are of equal importance to the onset and course of drinking problems. The current consensus among researchers and scholars is that alcoholism is a complex biopsychosocial disorder in which multiple factors play a role.

Critics of the disease concept argue that empirical research has failed to support its basic tenets. Herbert Fingarette refers to the disease concept as a myth, asserting that "almost everything that the American public believes to be the scientific truth about alcoholism is false" (Fingarette, 1988, p. 1). Reviewing research, Fingarette challenges the following tenets of the disease concept of alcoholism: (1) irresistible craving and loss of control after the first drink; (2) inevitable progression; and (3) the impossibility of a return to controlled drinking. More specifically, he cites studies that show alcoholics do not always experience craving and retain a considerable degree of volition in their actual drinking behavior (Mello and Mendelson, 1972); epidemiological studies that suggest patterns of alcohol abuse are highly variable and may spontaneously remit without intervention (Cahalan and Room, 1974); and, finally, evidence that at least some alcoholics have successfully returned to more moderate drinking (Davies, 1962; Polich et al., 1980).

Arguing that the disease concept is pseudoscientific, Fingarette and other critics (Peele, 1989) imply that by lending the legitimizing mantle of medical science to the disease concept—at least as it is currently formulated—proponents deprive the public of accurate information that forms the necessary basis for informed consent regarding treatment. Others (Vaillant, 1983), while conceding that alcoholism is not a disease in the strict medical sense, continue to defend the disease model; they argue that its value in destigmatizing alcoholism and legitimizing treatment outweighs issues of epistemological rigor.

The modern disease concept emerged and gained acceptance primarily in response to humanitarian concerns rather than on the basis of scientific evidence. Eager to undo the religious underpinnings and moralistic legacy of the American temperance movement and prohibition, advocates of the disease concept correctly perceived its ability to recast the alcoholic as sick rather than as morally deviant. If the alcoholic is unable to control self-destructive drinking because of an incurable illness, then he or she deserves compassion and treatment rather than blame. Paradoxically, the attempt to reconceive alcoholism in medical rather than moral terms can be seen as fulfilling a moral agenda, that is, a desire to help rather than condemn the problem drinker.

This ethical stance can be seen, in turn, as part of a broader movement in modern society to destigmatize deviant behavior of all types by promoting understanding and compassionate intervention. Thus, much of the controversy surrounding the disease model arises out of a tacit conflict between scientific and moral agendas, a confounding of facts and values in society's response to alcohol.

Anthropology offers a possible semantic solution to the disease controversy by distinguishing between *illness* and *disease* (Chrisman, 1985). Whereas diseases are defined by objective scientific criteria, social anthropologists view illnesses as cultural constructions defined by subjective distress, loss of normal social functioning, and adoption of the sick role. Within these terms, alcoholism can be seen as a culturally defined illness or *folk disease* for which society has sanctioned the sick role and compassionate intervention.

## The role of Alcoholics Anonymous

Despite the widespread acceptance of the disease concept, the leading approach to overcoming alcoholism in the United States is, ironically, not a medical treatment but a self-help program based on principles of moral and spiritual renewal. Founded in 1935 by Bill Wilson, an alcoholic stockbroker, Alcoholics Anonymous (AA) borrowed many of its ideas from an evangelical Christian movement known as the Oxford Group. Though it embraces the disease concept as part of its holistic view of alcoholism as a threefold illness (physical, mental, and spiritual), AA's primary emphasis is on achieving sobriety through a process of moral-spiritual renewal as set forth in the Twelve Steps. Central to AA's approach is the alcoholic's decision to abstain from alcohol "one day at a time." Believing alcoholism to be a disease that may be arrested but never cured, AA views "recovery" as a lifelong process requiring constant vigilance and regular attendance at meetings where members "share their experience, strength, and hope." The Twelve Steps encourage AA's members to admit their faults, make amends to those they have hurt, and help other alcoholics achieve sobriety. Members are also encouraged to select sponsors, experienced AA members who are available for advice and support.

How effective is AA? AA's membership, estimated at 1.5 million worldwide (General Service Office, 1987), provides impressive evidence of its success in reaching problem drinkers. However, the overwhelming majority of alcoholics remain untreated. Of those who are exposed to AA, many drop out; those who remain may constitute a self-selected group receptive to its message and style. Moreover, because of the methodological difficulties of conducting research on a self-help group of anonymous individuals, few controlled studies exist on AA's effectiveness compared with other treatment approaches (Ogborne and Glaser, 1985). Nonetheless, AA has come to exercise a pervasive influence over both inpatient and outpatient treatment programs in the United States, where the primary goal is often to motivate the alcoholic to participate in AA.

Advocates of AA's approach to treatment have been accused of intolerance toward alternative approaches, especially behavior modification therapies that pursue the goal of controlled drinking rather than total abstinence. Despite evidence that not all problem drinking follows a progressive, deteriorating course and that some problem drinkers are able to return to more moderate patterns of consumption, controlled drinking advocates have been criticized as irresponsible for even suggesting an alternative to abstinence (Pendery et al., 1982). AA's success presents a curious dilemma for researchers and clinicians: The very elements that may contribute to its effectiveness as a self-help group—simple beliefs, group loyalty and cohesiveness, and an emphasis on personal experience and testimony—leave it resistant to outside influence and to new information that appears to contradict its core assumptions (Galanter, 1990). The employment of large numbers of recovering alcoholics as counselors and administrators in alcohol treatment programs has further complicated the situation as personal loyalty to AA's "one disease, one treatment" approach has come into conflict with the more empirically based, eclectic approach of researchers and of clinicians trained in the mental-health professions. The difficulty of reconciling these two orientations finds expression in a growing trend toward "dual diagnosis" in which alcoholics are assigned an additional psychiatric diagnosis and treated with medication. Wary of all drugs as potentially addictive, many AA-based paraprofessionals have been uneasy with psychiatric diagnosis and medication; in turn, mental-health professionals have viewed alcoholism counselors as insufficiently aware of psychiatric disorders and treatments. Such tensions point to fundamental differences in the assumptive frameworks that each group brings to diagnosis and treatment.

The first of AA's Twelve Steps declares that the alcoholic is powerless over alcohol and must therefore surrender to a "higher power." Believing this to be a self-defeating prescription for helplessness and relapse in the face of a needlessly mystified "disease," Stanton Peele has argued for restoring an explicitly moral model of alcoholism and other addictions that emphasizes the alcoholic's ability rationally to choose sobriety and commit to new values (Peele, 1988). Advocates of AA's approach argue, however, that this is precisely what AA accomplishes: a daily commitment to abstinence and "a new way of life." That alcoholics may regain a sense of control by admitting powerlessness, they say, may simply reflect a spiritual paradox rather than a contradiction.

Medicalization of alcohol problems has yet to resolve the question of what causes alcoholism or to provide satisfactory solutions to the moral problems posed by the use and misuse of alcohol. Motivated by the desire to destigmatize alcoholism in order to promote compassionate treatment, the disease model still has not adequately disposed of the issue of personal responsibility. The drinker makes choices, but these choices are significantly influenced by biological, psychological, and sociocultural forces beyond conscious control. An important element of AA's success may be that it embraces both aspects of this duality: It holds that alcoholics do not choose their condition—they are subject to multiple systemic forces beyond their awareness—yet, with support, they can effectively assume responsibility for their problem and choose to abstain. Meaningful ethical inquiry must embrace both poles of this duality by recognizing the complex interplay of personal choice with the many factors that may influence or limit it.

RICHARD W. OSBORNE

*Directly related to this article are the other articles in this entry:* ADDICTION AND DEPENDENCE, SMOKING, ALCOHOL AND OTHER DRUGS IN A PUBLIC-HEALTH CONTEXT, *and* LEGAL CONTROL OF HARMFUL SUBSTANCES. *For a further discussion of topics mentioned in this article, see the entries* ABUSE, INTERPERSONAL; FETUS, *articles on* HUMAN DEVELOPMENT FROM FERTILIZATION TO BIRTH, *and* PHILOSOPHICAL AND ETHICAL ISSUES; GENETICS AND HUMAN SELF-UNDERSTANDING; HARM; HEALTH AND DISEASE, *article on* ANTHROPOLOGICAL PERSPECTIVES; HOMICIDE; INJURY AND INJURY CONTROL; OCCUPATIONAL SAFETY AND HEALTH, *article on* ETHICAL ISSUES; RESPONSIBILITY; *and* SELF-HELP. *For a discussion of related ideas, see the entries* AUTONOMY; BEHAVIOR MODIFICATION THERAPIES; FREEDOM AND COERCION; GENETICS AND ENVIRONMENT IN HUMAN HEALTH; GENETICS AND HUMAN BEHAVIOR, *article on* SCIENTIFIC AND RESEARCH ISSUES; HEALTH PROMOTION AND HEALTH EDUCATION; MEDICINE, ANTHROPOLOGY OF; PATERNALISM; RACE AND RACISM; REHABILITATION; SEXISM; SEXUALITY IN SOCIETY, *article on* SOCIAL CONTROL OF SEXUAL BEHAVIOR; *and* SOCIAL MEDICINE. *Other relevant material may be found under the entries* ADVERTISING; ALTERNATIVE THERAPIES, *article on* SOCIAL HISTORY; FAMILY; IMPAIRED PROFESSIONALS; MATERNAL–FETAL RELATIONSHIP; *and* PROSTITUTION.

## Bibliography

ALCOHOLICS ANONYMOUS WORLD SERVICES. 1976. *Alcoholics Anonymous.* 3d ed. New York: Author.

AMES, GENEVIEVE M. 1985. "American Beliefs About Alcoholism: Historical Perspectives on the Medical–Moral

Controversy." In *The American Experience with Alcohol: Contrasting Cultural Perspectives*, pp. 23–39. Edited by Linda A. Bennett and Genevieve M. Ames. New York: Plenum.

ANGLIN, DOUGLAS M. 1982. "Alcohol and Criminality." In *Encyclopedic Handbook of Alcoholism*, pp. 383–394. Edited by E. Mansell Pattison and Edward Kaufman. New York: Gardner.

CAHALAN, DON, and ROOM, ROBIN. 1974. *Problem Drinking Among American Men*. New Brunswick, N.J.: Rutgers Center of Alcohol Studies.

CHRISMAN, NOEL J. 1985. "Alcoholism: Illness or Disease?" In *The American Experience with Alcohol: Contrasting Cultural Perspectives*, pp. 7–21. Edited by Linda A. Bennett and Genevieve M. Ames. New York: Plenum.

DAVIES, D. L. 1962. "Normal Drinking in Recovered Alcohol Addicts." *Quarterly Journal of Studies on Alcohol* 23: 94–104.

FINGARETTE, HERBERT. 1988. *Heavy Drinking: The Myth of Alcoholism as a Disease*. Berkeley: University of California Press.

GALANTER, MARC. 1990. "Cults and Zealous Self-Help Movements: A Psychiatric Perspective." *American Journal of Psychiatry* 147, no. 3:543–551.

GENERAL SERVICE OFFICE OF ALCOHOLICS ANONYMOUS. 1987. *World AA Directory*. New York: Alcoholics Anonymous World Services.

GOODWIN, DONALD W. 1985. "Genetic Determinants of Alcoholism." In *The Diagnosis and Treatment of Alcoholism*, 2d ed., pp. 65–87. Edited by Jack H. Mendelson and Nancy K. Mello. New York: McGraw-Hill.

HARWOOD, HENRICK J.; KRISTIANSEN, P.; and RACHEL, J. V. 1985. *Social and Economic Costs of Alcohol Abuse and Alcoholism*. Issue Report no. 2. Research Triangle Park, N.C.: Research Triangle Press.

HEATH, DWIGHT B. 1982. "In Other Cultures They Also Drink." In *Alcohol, Science, and Society Revisited*, pp. 63–80. Edited by Edith L. Gomberg, Helene R. White, and John A. Carpenter. Ann Arbor: University of Michigan Press.

HELZER, JOHN E., and PRYZBECK, THOMAS R. 1988. "The Co-Occurrence of Alcoholism with Other Psychiatric Disorders in the General Population and Its Impact on Treatment." *Journal of Studies on Alcohol* 49, no. 3:219–224.

HESTER, REID K., and MILLER, WILLIAM R. 1989. *Handbook of Alcoholism Treatment Approaches: Effective Alternatives*. New York: Pergamon.

JELLINEK, ELVIN M. 1960. *The Disease Concept of Alcoholism*. New Haven, Conn.: Hillhouse.

KLATSKY, ARTHUR L. 1990. "Alcohol and Coronary Artery Disease." *Alcohol, Health & Research World* 14, no. 4: 289–300.

KURTZ, ERNEST. 1979. *Not-God: A History of Alcoholics Anonymous*. Center City, Minn.: Hazelden, Educational Services.

MARLATT, G. ALAN. 1983. "The Controlled Drinking Controversy." *American Psychologist* 38, no. 10:1097–1110.

MARLATT, G. ALAN, and ROHSENOW, DAMARIS J. 1980. "Cognitive Processes in Alcohol Use: Expectancy and the Bal-

anced Placebo Design." *Advances in Substance Abuse: Behavioral and Biological Research* 1:159–199.

MELLO, NANCY K., and MENDELSON, JACK H. 1972. "Drinking Patterns During Work-Contingent and Noncontingent Alcohol Acquisition." *Psychosomatic Medicine* 34, no. 2: 139–164.

OGBORNE, ALAN C., and GLASER, FREDERICK B. 1985. "Evaluating Alcoholics Anonymous." In *Alcoholism and Substance Abuse: Strategies for Clinical Intervention*, pp. 176–192. Edited by Thomas E. Bratter and Gary G. Forrest. New York: Free Press.

PATTISON, E. MANSELL, and KAUFMAN, EDWARD. 1982. *Encyclopedic Handbook of Alcoholism*. New York: Gardner Press.

PEELE, STANTON. 1988. "A Moral Vision of Addiction: How People's Values Determine Whether They Become and Remain Addicts." In *Visions of Addiction: Major Contemporary Perspectives on Addiction and Alcoholism*, pp. 201–233. Edited by Stanton Peele. Lexington, Mass.: Lexington Books.

———. 1989. *The Diseasing of America: Addiction Treatment out of Control*. Lexington, Mass.: Lexington Books.

PENDERY, MARY L.; MALTZMAN, IRVING M.; and WEST, L. JOYLON. 1982. "Controlled Drinking by Alcoholics? New Findings and a Re-Evaluation of a Major Affirmative Study." *Science* 217, no. 4555:169–175.

POLICH, J. MICHAEL; ARMOR, DAVID J.; and BRAIKER, HARRIET B. 1980. *The Course of Alcoholism: Four Years After Treatment*. Santa Monica, Calif.: Rand.

RORABAUGH, W. J. 1979. *The Alcoholic Republic: An American Tradition*. Oxford: Oxford University Press.

TARTER, RALPH E.; ARRIA, AMEILIA M.; and VAN THIEL, DAVID H. 1989. "Neurobehavioral Disorders Associated with Chronic Alcohol Abuse." In *Alcoholism: Biomedical and Genetic Aspects*, pp. 113–129. Edited by H. Werner Goedde and Dharam P. Agarwal. New York: Pergamon.

U.S. DEPARTMENT OF HEALTH AND HUMAN SERVICES. ALCOHOL, DRUG ABUSE, AND MENTAL HEALTH ADMINISTRATION. NATIONAL INSTITUTE ON ALCOHOL ABUSE AND ALCOHOLISM. 1990. *Seventh Special Report to the U.S. Congress on Alcohol and Health*. Rockville, Md.: Author.

VAILLANT, GEORGE E. 1983. *The Natural History of Alcoholism*. Cambridge, Mass.: Harvard University Press.

WANCK, BICK. 1990. "Mentally Ill Substance Abusers." In *Handbook of Outpatient Treatment of Adults: Nonpsychotic Mental Disorders*, pp. 577–603. Edited by Michael E. Thase, Barry A. Edelstein, and Michel Hersen. New York: Plenum.

WORLD HEALTH ORGANIZATION. 1978. *Mental Disorders: Glossary and Guide to Their Classification in Accordance with the Ninth Revision of the International Classification of Diseases*. Geneva: Author.

## IV. ALCOHOL AND OTHER DRUGS IN A PUBLIC-HEALTH CONTEXT

Psychoactive drugs are substances that alter the mental state of humans when ingested. There are a wide variety of such substances, naturally occurring and synthesized, including tobacco, alcoholic beverages, coffee, tea, chocolate, and some spices, as well as substances legally available only through medical channels, such as benzodiazepines, cannabinoids, opiates, and cocaine. Such substances often have other use-values along with their psychoactive properties. Users may like the taste or the image of themselves that the use conveys. Use may be a medium of sociability (Partanen, 1991) or part of a religious ritual. Some substances have other useful properties; alcohol, for example, is a source of calories and is also the solvent in many tinctures.

Psychoactive drugs differ in their metabolic pathways and mechanisms of action in the human body, in the strength of their effects, and in the states of mind and feelings they induce. But the effects of drug use are also powerfully dependent on the pattern of use and on set and setting, that is, the expectations of the user and of others present and the context of use (Zinberg, 1984). Although the psychoactive effect of tobacco may not even register in the consciousness of a habituated cigarette smoker, in other circumstances the effect of tobacco use may be so strong that the user is rendered unconscious, as early Spanish observers reported concerning native South Americans (Robicsek, 1978).

Psychoactive substances are frequently valued by potential consumers well above the cost of production. On the one hand, this means that taxes on alcohol, tobacco, and other drugs have long been an important fiscal resource for the state. On the other hand, it means that there are substantial incentives for an illicit market to emerge where sale of drugs is forbidden or stringently restricted.

A consideration of drugs in a public-health context may appropriately start from a consideration of general cultural patternings and understandings of drug use. This is followed by a discussion of the major approaches to limiting harms from drug use. The article concludes with a characterization of the major directions in the development of drug policies in the United States and other industrialized countries.

## General cultural framings of drug use

Three social patternings of psychoactive drug use can be distinguished as prototypical: medicinal use, customary regular use, and intermittent use. In many traditional societies, particular drugs or formulations have been confined to medicinal use, that is, use under the supervision of a healer to alleviate mental or physical illness or distress. For several centuries after the technique for distilling alcoholic spirits had diffused from China through the Arab world to Europe, for instance, spirits-based drinks were regarded primarily as medicines (Wasson, 1984). This way of framing drug use has been routinized in the modern state through a prescription system,

with physicians writing the prescriptions and pharmacists filling them. Drugs included in the prescription system are usually forbidden for nonmedicinal use.

Where a drug becomes a regular accompaniment of everyday life, its psychoactivity is often muted and even unnoticed, as is often the case for a habitual cigarette smoker. Likewise, in southern European wine cultures, wine is differentiated from intoxicating "alcohol"; wine drinkers are expected to maintain the same comportment after drinking as before. We may call this a pattern of "banalized use": A potentially powerful psychoactive agent is domesticated into a mundane article of daily life, available relatively freely on the consumer market.

Intermittent use—for instance, on sacred occasions, at festivals, or only on weekends—minimizes the buildup of tolerance to the drug. It is in the context of such patterns that the greatest attention is likely to be paid to the drug's psychoactive properties. The drug may be understood by both the user and others as having taken over control of the user's behavior, thus explaining otherwise unexpected behavior, whether bad or good (see the "disinhibition hypothesis" in Pernanen, 1976; see also Room and Collins, 1983). As in Robert Louis Stevenson's fable of Dr. Jekyll and Mr. Hyde, normal self-control is expected to return when the effects of the drug have worn off. Given the power attributed to the substance, access to it may be limited—in traditional societies, by sumptuary rules keyed to social differentiations; in industrial societies, by other forms of market restriction.

In industrial societies, a fourth pattern of use is commonly recognized for certain drugs: addicted or dependent use, marked by regular use, often of large doses. Since the pattern of use of the drug in question is not banalized in the society, addiction to it is defined as an individual failing rather than as a social pattern. Although attention is paid to physical factors sustaining regular use, such as use to relieve withdrawal symptoms, most formulations of addiction focus on psychological aspects, including an apparent commitment to drug use to the exclusion of other activities and despite default of major social roles. An addiction concept thus also focuses on loss of normal self-control, but the emphasis is not so much on the immediate effects of the drug as on a repeated or continuing pattern of an apparent inability to control or refrain from use, despite adverse consequences.

## Addiction as a modern governing image

The concept of addiction as an affliction of the habituated drug user first arose in its modern form for alcohol, as heavy drinking lost its banalized status in the United States and some other countries under the influence of the temperance movement of the nineteenth century

(Levine, 1978, 1992). Habitual drunkenness had been viewed since the Middle Ages as a subclass of gluttony; now, abstinence from alcohol was singled out as a separate virtue and as an important sign of the key virtue in a democracy of autonomous citizens: self-control. Along with other mental disorders, "chronic inebriety," as alcohol addiction was usually termed, was reinterpreted as a disease appropriate for medical intervention (although without losing all of its negative moral loading).

In nineteenth-century formulations, addictiveness was seen as an inherent property of alcohol, no matter who used it, and this perception justified efforts to prohibit its sale. By the late nineteenth century, such addiction concepts were being applied also to opiates and other drugs, and this formulation has remained the governing image for these drugs to the present day (Room, 1974). But as temperance thinking became unpopular with the repeal of national alcohol prohibition in the United States (1933), for alcohol the concept was reformulated to be a property of the individual "alcoholic," who is mysteriously unable to drink like a normal drinker. This "disease concept of alcoholism" received its classic scholarly formulation by Elwyn M. Jellinek (1952), who later (1960) retreated to a broader formulation of alcohol problems.

In popular thinking and often in official definitions, addiction has remained a property of the *drug* for illicit drugs but of the *person* for alcohol (Christie and Bruun, 1968). The inherent addictiveness attributed to illicit drugs is the primary rationale for their prohibition. The extent of the anathema imposed in U.S. cultural politics by labeling a substance as "addictive" can be gauged from the unanimous testimony of cigarette company executives to the U.S. Congress in 1994 that they do not believe that cigarettes are addictive, despite the evidence of their own corporate research (Hilts, 1994a, 1994b, 1994c).

American philosophers have begun to question and rethink the meaning of addiction concepts (Szasz, 1985; Fingarette, 1988; Seeburger, 1993) and to consider the implications for drug policy (Husak, 1992). In a related initiative, economists have begun propounding and testing theories of "rational addiction," which is how they define a behavior that one engages in repeatedly while fully taking into account its future effects (Grossman, 1993). By the mid-1990s, this critical thinking had had no discernible influence on the American political consensus around an addiction-based policy for illicit drugs.

## Approaches to limiting the problems resulting from drug use

Most human societies have known of and used psychoactive drugs, and most have also made efforts to limit the use of one or more drugs, customarily if not legisla-

tively. Historically, the main aim of restrictions was to diminish threats to the social order or to maximize the labor supply. Public-health concerns were sometimes expressed in justifying restrictions—for instance, in the efforts of James I of England to stem tobacco smoking (Austin, 1979)—but such concerns were rarely decisive. The restrictions on the spirits market adopted in Britain as a response to the extreme alcoholization of eighteenth-century London (depicted in Hogarth's famous print of "Gin Lane") are an early example of limits substantially motivated by public-health concerns (Coffey, 1966). Only in recent decades have public-health concerns become a major element in discussions of drug policies, although the concerns are often subordinated for legal drugs to fiscal and economic considerations, and for illicit drugs to moral and lifestyle issues.

The health hazards from psychoactive drugs occur in two main ways: in connection with particular occasions of use or in connection with the patterning of use over time. Thus an overdose from barbiturates, a traffic casualty from drunk driving, or an HIV infection from sharing a needle to inject heroin are all consequences associated with a particular occasion of use; while lung cancer from tobacco smoking, liver cirrhosis from alcohol use, and (by definition) addiction all reflect a history of heavy use (Room, 1985). As we shall note, measures to prevent event-related problems often differ from and may even conflict with measures to prevent cumulative, condition-related problems. For alcohol, the ethical situation with regard to public-health measures is now complicated by the possibility of a protective effect against heart disease to be balanced against the undoubted negative health effects (Schmidt, 1985; Edwards et al., 1994).

Efforts to limit problems from drug use can be seen as oriented to controlling whether the drug is used at all; to influencing the amount, context, and pattern of use; or to preventing harmful consequences of use (Bruun, 1970; Moore and Gerstein, 1981).

**Prohibiting use to all or some.**    Efforts to impose a general prohibition on the use of a drug for all members of a society have a lengthy history, although the efforts have frequently ended in failure (Austin, 1979). Perhaps the most sustained such effort has been the prohibition on alcoholic beverages in Islamic societies. In general, religious taboos on drug use tend to have had more lasting effect than state prohibitions. Prohibiting the sale or use of a drug that some might choose to use and enjoy involves a degree of intervention in the marketplace and in private behavior unusual for modern democratic states. If there are those who use the drug without problems, the prohibition on their use must be justified as for the benefit of others who would have or would cause problems if they used the drug. In societies with a strong tradition of individual liberties and consumer sovereignty, the discomfort with this line of argument in support of prohibition is commonly resolved by presumptions that users will sooner or later become addicted and that users without problems do not really exist.

A common form of prohibition on use in village and tribal societies has been sumptuary rules restricting use to particular status groups, most commonly to the most powerful segments of the society. Depending on the culture, a variety of arguments are offered for the inability of lower-status groups to handle drug use appropriately. Since psychoactive drugs offer visions of an alternative reality (Stauffer, 1971) and may be associated with disinhibition, dominant groups may fear challenges to their power if subordinates have access to drugs (Morgan, 1983). The universalist ethic of modern states has made such explicit sumptuary restrictions untenable, with the substantial exception of prohibitions on use by children. Even the provisions, still common in U.S. state laws, that the names of habitual drunkards should be posted and that those listed should be refused service of alcoholic drinks are unenforced because of their perceived interference with individual liberties.

A third form of modified prohibition of use, common in modern societies, is the limitation to medicinal use. The individual's supply of such medications is controlled by state-licensed professionals, backed up by a state system of market controls. National controls on psychopharmaceuticals are backed up by an unusual and elaborate international control structure (Bruun et al., 1975; Nadelmann, 1990). In principle, prescription and use of the drugs are limited to therapeutic purposes. For psychoactive drugs, commonly prescribed to relieve negative affective states or mental distress, the leeway for what constitutes therapeutic use is often quite wide, and a substantial part of the resources of the health system in industrial societies is absorbed in superintending the provision of psychoactive drugs. Except for methadone as a remedy for heroin addiction and nicotine as a remedy for tobacco smoking, it is generally considered illegitimate to prescribe a drug in order to maintain a habitual pattern of use without withdrawal or other distress. Use for pleasure or for the sake of the psychoactive experience is considered nontherapeutic, so the functions of drugs considered as psychopharmaceuticals are always described in terms of the relief of distress rather than of the provision of pleasure. To some extent, the medical prescription system in a modern state serves as a covert form of control by status differentiation according to the prejudices of the prescriber; for instance, older and more "respectable" adults will find it easier than the younger and more "disreputable" to obtain prescriptions for a psychopharmaceutical.

**Influencing the pattern of use.** An enormous variety of strategies, formal and informal, have been used to influence the amount, pattern, and context of drug use. Among the potential aims of such strategies is the public-health aim of reducing the prevalence of hazardous use.

*Controlling availability.* One class of such strategies attempts to reduce drug-related problems by controlling the market in drugs, whether by taxes, by general restrictions on availability, or by user-specific restrictions (Room, 1984; Edwards et al., 1994). Public-health considerations are one reason among several that governments tax legally available drugs such as alcohol and tobacco. Such taxes often constitute a substantial portion of the price to the consumer. Raising taxes does diminish levels of use among heavier as well as lighter users, although demand usually diminishes proportionately less than the proportional increase in price (i.e., it is relatively inelastic). Thus, short of levels that create an opening for a substantial illicit market, raising taxes on drugs tends both to have positive public-health effects and to increase government revenues.

Governments also often control the conditions of availability, particularly for alcohol. Through a system of retail licenses or by a government monopoly of sales, limits are placed on the hours and conditions of sale. Changes in these limits have sometimes been found to affect patterns of consumption and of alcohol-related problems (Smith, 1988). However, with the strengthening of the ideology of consumer sovereignty—that legal goods should be readily available, with purchases limited only by the consumer's means—controls on availability tend to have been loosened in recent decades (Mäkelä et al., 1981).

A generally stronger and more direct effect on hazardous alcohol consumption has been found from measures that ration or restrict the availability of alcohol for specific purchasers (Edwards et al., 1994). A general ration limit for all purchases particularly restricts heavy consumption, or at least raises its effective price, but such measures strongly conflict with the ideology of consumer sovereignty and are thus now politically impracticable nearly everywhere. As noted above, proscriptions or limits on sales to named heavy users have also fallen out of favor as infringements on individual liberty.

*Controlling the circumstances of use.* Another class of strategies aims to deter drinking or drug use in particularly hazardous circumstances, usually with criminal sanctions. The prototype situation here is driving after drinking. Given that alcohol consumption impairs vehicle-driving ability, most countries now treat driving with a blood-alcohol level above a set limit as a criminal offense, and enforcement of these laws often absorbs a substantial part of the criminal justice system's resources. Popular movements as well as policymakers have expended much energy, particularly in the United

States and other Anglophone and Scandinavian countries, in seeking a redefinition of drunk driving as a serious rather than a "folk" crime (Gusfield, 1981). This type of situational limit or prohibition has been extended to other skill-related tasks and has also been applied to driving after using other psychoactive drugs, particularly illicit drugs. A related development has sought to eliminate illicit drug use in working populations and alcohol use in the workplace through random urine testing, with job loss as the sanction (Zimmer and Jacobs, 1992). The ethics of this measure, strongly pushed by the U.S. government in the 1980s, are controversial, particularly since the tests detect illicit drug use that has not necessarily affected work performance (Macdonald and Roman, 1994). Random blood-alcohol tests of drivers to deter drinking while driving have also proved controversial; they are well accepted and widely applied in Australia (Homel et al., 1988), legally permissible but not intensively applied in the United States, but viewed as an impermissible infringement on individual liberty and privacy in many countries.

*Education and persuasion about use.* A third class of strategies seeks to educate or persuade against hazardous drug use. Since such strategies are seen as the least coercive, at least for those beyond school age, they are used very widely and commonly, despite the frequent lack of clear evidence on their effectiveness (Moskowitz, 1989). Some education of schoolchildren about the hazards of drug use is very widespread, indeed nearly ubiquitous, in the United States. Most countries in the world have also made at least a token effort at public information campaigns about the hazards of tobacco smoking; poster and slogan campaigns against drinking while driving and against illicit drug use are also widespread. Other public information campaigns on alcohol have promoted limits on drinking (e.g., suggestions of safe levels in Britain and Australia) or campaigned against drinking in various hazardous circumstances. Often these public information campaigns compete for attention in a media environment saturated with advertising on behalf of various tobacco and alcohol brands. Since the 1970s, some governments have imposed substantial restrictions on tobacco and (to a lesser extent) alcohol advertising, for example, banning advertisements on electronic media and requiring warning labels in advertisements or on product packages. These restrictions have often precipitated court fights over the constitutional permissibility of restrictions on the freedom of "commercial speech."

**Reducing the harm from use.** The strategies considered so far are primarily directed at influencing the fact or pattern of use. They thus fall into the categories either of supply reduction or demand reduction, to use terminology commonly applied concerning addictive drugs. Since the late 1980s, substantial attention has been directed to a third option—harm reduction;

that is, strategies that reduce the problems associated with drug use without necessarily reducing the drug use itself (O'Hare et al., 1992; Heather et al., 1993). Attention to this class of strategies has a somewhat longer history for alcohol (Room, 1975). Such strategies usually focus on the physical or social environment of drug or alcohol use, seeking physical, temporal, or cultural insulation from the harm it may engender. Thus, needle exchanges aim to remove the risk of HIV infection from injection drug use, and seat belts and air bags help to insulate drinking drivers—and those around them—from potential casualties.

The debate over harm-reduction strategies for illicit drugs has raised classic ethical issues for public health. Some argue that insulating the behavior from harm will encourage and thus increase the prevalence of the behavior. A further consideration is the actual effectiveness of the insulation provided. Thus, efforts to provide a safer tobacco cigarette have been largely undercut by compensatory changes in puffing and inhaling by smokers. At an empirical level, it seems that insulating drug use from harm does not necessarily increase the prevalence of drug use. Even if it did, an old public-health tradition, epitomized by the operation of venereal disease clinics, would argue that reducing the immediate risk of harm takes a higher ethical priority than affecting the prevalence of disapproved behaviors.

## The political reality in the mid-1990s: Lopsided policies

The United States and many other countries have experienced recurring "moral panics" in recent decades concerning illicit drug use and have invested substantial resources in efforts to prevent such use. These resources have been largely invested in two directions: a particular preventive strategy—interdicting the illicit market—and the provision of treatment. The first of these directions has received the greatest investment of government resources. There was indeed a substantial decrease in illicit drug use in North America in the late 1980s and early 1990s (possibly due primarily to the normal ebb and flow of youth fashions), though data from 1993 and 1994 suggested the decline might have been ending. But the illicit market remains strong, while drug-related imprisonments have helped propel the United States to the highest rate of incarceration among industrial societies. Meanwhile, preventing the very substantial health harm from legal drugs such as alcohol and tobacco has received a much lower priority. In government policymaking, public-health considerations have often been subordinated to economic concerns. In recent years, for example, the United States has successfully attacked control structures and forced a greater availability of both alcohol and tobacco in other countries with suits under the General Agreement on Tariffs and Trade (Ferris et al., 1993).

A substantial emphasis on the treatment of addiction has accompanied the attention to prevention. But in this mixed policy environment, the role of treatment has been highly differentiated by type of drug. To a large extent, tobacco smoking has remained defined as a health rather than as a social problem, with the emphasis on the health consequences of smoking rather than on the physical dependence of smokers on tobacco. Thus there has been very little public provision of treatment for smoking addiction; most of those who have quit have done it by themselves or in mutual-help groups. At the other extreme, the goals for an illicit-drug treatment system have been highly ambitious: In the mid-1970s and again in the late 1980s, the United States aspired in theory to provide treatment to every unincarcerated addict. Quite explicitly, treatment for illicit drug use has been seen as a form of social control, and a high degree of coercion to treatment has been taken for granted (Gerstein and Harwood, 1990). On occasion, U.S. drug strategies have argued for the provision of treatment as a means to encourage courts to be tougher on those who will then have chosen not to accept it (Strategy Council on Drug Abuse, 1973, p. 38).

In the case of alcohol, there has also been a large growth in treatment provision, not only in the United States (Klingemann et al., 1992). But alcohol treatment in the United States was until recently less an adjunct of the criminal justice system, and it remains quite separate in other countries. The growth of alcohol treatment provision, it has been argued, accompanied and served as a "cultural alibi" for the dismantling of the alcohol control structure left behind by the temperance era (Mäkelä et al., 1981). Although there is an increasing contradiction between the demands for sobriety in a technological environment and the increased market availability of alcohol, managing this contradiction is seen as a character test for the individual consumer, with treatment for alcoholism provided for those deemed to have failed the test.

These policy trends for alcohol and tobacco apply in broad terms also to other industrial countries, although high-tax strategies have been more commonly applied outside the United States, particularly for tobacco. For illicit drugs, the U.S. "drug war" ideology has been strongly exerted internationally as well as at home (Traver and Gaylord, 1992). Through such mechanisms as the international narcotic-control conventions and through active multilateral and bilateral diplomacy, the United States has been relatively successful in maintaining and indeed strengthening legal prohibitions. Nevertheless, the international illicit market continues to grow. In debates about drug policies in the mid-1990s, the practical relevance as well as the ethics of current U.S. policies were increasingly questioned by scholars (e.g., Graubard, 1992).

ROBIN ROOM

*Directly related to this article are the other articles in this entry:* ADDICTION AND DEPENDENCE, SMOKING, ALCOHOLISM, *and* LEGAL CONTROL OF HARMFUL SUBSTANCES. *For a further discussion of topics mentioned in this article, see the entries* ADVERTISING; BEHAVIOR CONTROL; ECONOMIC CONCEPTS IN HEALTH CARE; FREEDOM AND COERCION; HARM; HEALTH PROMOTION AND HEALTH EDUCATION; LIFESTYLES AND PUBLIC HEALTH; OCCUPATIONAL SAFETY AND HEALTH, *especially the article on* TESTING OF EMPLOYEES; PHARMACEUTICS, *especially the article on* ISSUES IN PRESCRIBING; PHARMACY; PUBLIC HEALTH AND THE LAW; RIGHTS; RISK; *and* SELF-HELP. *For a discussion of related ideas, see the entries* HEALTH OFFICIALS AND THEIR RESPONSIBILITIES; MENTAL HEALTH; *and* MENTAL ILLNESS.

## Bibliography

AUSTIN, GREGORY A. 1979. *Perspectives on the History of Psychoactive Substance Use.* DHEW publication no. (ADM) 79–810. Washington, D.C.: U.S. Government Printing Office.

BRUUN, KETTIL. 1970. "Finland: The Non-Medical Approach." In *Proceedings of the 29th International Congress on Alcoholism and Drug Dependence: Sydney, Australia, February 1970,* pp. 545–558. Edited by L. G. Kiloh and David S. Bell. Chatswood, Australia: Butterworths.

BRUUN, KETTIL; PAN, LYNN; and REXED, INGEMAR. 1975. *The Gentlemen's Club: International Control of Drug and Alcohol.* Chicago: University of Chicago Press.

CHRISTIE, NILS, and BRUUN, KETTIL. 1968. "Alcohol Problems: The Conceptual Framework." In vol. 2 of *International Congress on Alcohol and Alcoholism (Washington, D.C.),* pp. 65–73. Edited by Mark Keller, Maria Majchrowicz, and Timothy G. Coffey. Washington, D.C.: Program Publications Committee, 28th International Congress on Alcohol and Alcoholism.

COFFEY, TIMOTHY C. 1966. "Beer Street, Gin Lane: Some Views of 18th-Century Drinking." *Quarterly Journal of Studies on Alcohol* 27, no. 4:669–692.

EDWARDS, GRIFFITH; ANDERSON, PETER; BABOR, THOMAS F.; CASSWELL, SALLY; FERRENCE, ROBERTA; GIESBRECHT, NORMAN; GODFREY, CHRISTINE; HOLDER, HAROLD D.; LEMMENS, PAUL; MÄKELÄ, KLAUS; MIDANIK, LORRAINE T.; NORSTRÖM, THOR; ÖSTERBERG, ESA; ROMELSJÖ, ANDERS; ROOM, ROBIN; SIMPURA, JUSSI; and SKOG, OLE-JØRGEN. 1994. *Alcohol Policy and the Public Good.* Oxford: Oxford University Press.

FERRIS, JACQUELINE; ROOM, ROBIN; and GIESBRECHT, NORMAN. 1993. "Public Health Interests in Trade Agreements on Alcoholic Beverages in North America." *Alcohol Health and Research World* 17:235–241.

FINGARETTE, HERBERT. 1988. *Heavy Drinking: The Myth of Alcoholism as a Disease.* Berkeley: University of California Press.

GERSTEIN, DEAN R., and HARWOOD, HENRICK J., eds. 1990. *A Study of the Evolution, Effectiveness, and Financing of Public and Private Drug Treatment Systems.* Vol. 1 of *Treating Drug Problems.* Washington, D.C.: National Academy Press.

GRAUBARD, STEPHEN R., ed. 1992. "Political Pharmacology: Thinking About Drugs." *Daedalus* 121, no. 3. Special issue.

GROSSMAN, MICHAEL. 1993. "The Economic Analysis of Addictive Behavior." In *Economics and the Prevention of Alcohol-Related Problems,* pp. 91–123. Edited by Michael E. Hilton and Gregory Bloss. NIAAA research monograph no. 25, NIH publication no. 93–3513. Washington, D.C.: National Institute on Alcohol Abuse and Alcoholism.

GUSFIELD, JOSEPH R. 1981. *The Culture of Public Problems: Drinking-Driving and the Symbolic Order.* Chicago: University of Chicago Press.

HEATHER, NICK; WODAK, ALEX; NADELMANN, ETHAN; and O'HARE, PAT, eds. 1993. *Psychoactive Drugs and Harm Reduction: From Faith to Science.* London: Whurr.

HILTS, PHILIP J. 1994a. "Embattled Tobacco: Cigarette Makers Debated the Risk They Denied." *New York Times,* June 16, p. A1.

———. 1994b. "Embattled Tobacco: Tobacco Maker Studied Risk but Did Little About Results." *New York Times,* June 17, p. A1.

———. 1994c. "Embattled Tobacco: Grim Findings Scuttled Hope for 'Safer' Cigarette." *New York Times,* June 18, p. A1.

HOMEL, ROSS; CARSELDINE, DON; and KEARNS, IAN. 1988. "Drunk-Driving Countermeasures in Australia." *Alcohol, Drugs and Driving* 4, no. 2:113–144.

HUSAK, DOUGLAS N. 1992. *Drugs and Rights.* Cambridge: At the University Press.

JELLINEK, ELWYN M. 1952. "Phases of Alcohol Addiction." *Quarterly Journal of Studies on Alcohol* 13, no. 4:673–684.

———. 1960. *The Disease Concept of Alcoholism.* New Haven, Conn.: Hillhouse Press.

KLINGEMANN, HARALD; TAKALA, JUKKA-PEKKA; and HUNT, GEOFFREY, eds. 1992. *Cure, Care or Control: Alcoholism Treatment in Sixteen Countries.* Albany: State University of New York Press.

LEVINE, HARRY GENE. 1978. "The Discovery of Addiction: Changing Concepts of Habitual Drunkenness in American History." *Journal of Studies on Alcohol* 39, no. 1:143–174.

———. 1992. "Temperance Cultures: Concerns About Alcohol Problems in Nordic and English-Speaking Cultures." In *The Nature of Alcohol and Drug Related Problems,* pp. 15–36. Edited by Griffith Edwards, Malcolm Lader, and D. Cohn Drummond. Oxford: Oxford University Press.

MACDONALD, SCOTT, and ROMAN, PAUL M., eds. 1994. *Drug Testing in the Workplace.* Vol. 11 of *Research Advances in Alcohol and Drug Problems.* New York: Plenum.

MÄKELÄ, KLAUS; ROOM, ROBIN; SINGLE, ERIC; SULKUNEN, PEKKA; and WALSH, BRENDAN. 1981. *A Comparative Study of Alcohol Control.* Vol. 1 of *Alcohol, Society, and the State.* Toronto: Addiction Research Foundation.

MOORE, MARK HARRISON, and GERSTEIN, DEAN R., eds. 1981. *Alcohol and Public Policy: Beyond the Shadow of Prohibition.* Washington, D.C.: National Academy Press.

MORGAN, PATRICIA. 1983. "Alcohol, Disinhibition, and Domination: A Conceptual Analysis." In *Alcohol and Disinhibition: Nature and Meaning of the Link,* pp. 405–420. Edited by Robin Room and Gary Collins. NIAAA research monograph no. 12, DHHS publication no. (ADM) 83–1246. Washington, D.C.: U.S. Government Printing Office.

MOSKOWITZ, JOEL M. 1989. "The Primary Prevention of Alcohol Problems: A Critical Review of the Research Literature." *Journal of Studies on Alcohol* 50, no. 1:54–88.

NADELMANN, ETHAN A. 1990. "Global Prohibition Regimes: The Evolution of Norms in International Society." *International Organization* 44, no. 4:479–526.

O'HARE, PATRICK A.; NEWCOMBE, RUSSELL; MATTHEWS, A.; BUNING, ERNST C.; and DRUCKER, ERNEST, eds. 1992. *The Reduction of Drug-Related Harm.* London: Routledge.

PARTANEN, JUKA. 1991. *Sociability and Intoxication: Alcohol and Drinking in Kenya, Africa, and the Modern World.* Helsinki: Finnish Foundation for Alcohol Studies.

PERNANEN, KAI. 1976. "Alcohol and Crimes of Violence." In *Social Aspects of Alcoholism,* pp. 351–444. Edited by Benjamin Kissin and Henri Begleiter. Vol. 4 of *The Biology of Alcoholism.* New York: Plenum.

ROBICSEK, FRANCIS. 1978. *The Smoking Gods: Tobacco in Maya Art, History and Religion.* Norman: University of Oklahoma Press.

ROOM, ROBIN. 1974. "Governing Images and the Prevention of Alcohol Problems." *Preventive Medicine* 3, no. 1:11–23.

———. 1975. "Minimizing Alcohol Problems." In *Proceedings of the Fourth Annual Alcoholism Conference of the National Institute on Alcohol Abuse and Alcoholism: Research, Treatment and Prevention,* pp. 379–393. Edited by Morris Chafetz. DHEW publication no. (ADM) 76–284. Washington, D.C.: National Institute on Alcohol Abuse and Alcoholism.

———. 1984. "Alcohol Control and Public Health." *Annual Review of Public Health* 5:293–317.

———. 1985. "Alcohol as a Cause: Empirical Links and Social Definitions." In *Currents in Alcohol Research and the Prevention of Alcohol Problems,* pp. 11–19. Edited by Jean-Pierre von Wartburg, Pierre Magnenat, Richard Müller, and Sonja Wyss. Berne, Switzerland: Hans Huber.

ROOM, ROBIN, and COLLINS, GARY, eds. 1983. *Alcohol and Disinhibition: Nature and Meaning of the Link.* NIAAA research monograph no. 12, DHHS publication no. (ADM) 83–1246. Washington, D.C.: U.S. Government Printing Office.

SCHMIDT, WOLFGANG. 1985. "Regulating the Supply of Alcoholic Beverages—A New Concept for an Old Ideology?" In *Currents in Alcohol Research and the Prevention of Alcohol Problems,* pp. 107–117. Edited by Jean-Pierre von Wartburg, Pierre Magnenat, Richard Müller, and Sonja Wyss. Berne, Switzerland: Hans Huber.

SEEBURGER, FRANCIS F. 1993. *Addiction and Responsibility: An Inquiry into the Addictive Mind.* New York: Crossroad.

Smith, David Ian. 1988. "Effectiveness of Restrictions on Availability as a Means of Preventing Alcohol-Related Problems." *Contemporary Drug Problems* 15, no. 4:627–684.

Stauffer, Robert B. 1971. *The Role of Drugs in Political Change.* New York: General Learning Press.

Strategy Council on Drug Abuse. 1973. *Federal Strategy for Drug Abuse and Drug Traffic Prevention, 1973.* Washington, D.C.: U.S. Government Printing Office.

Szasz, Thomas. 1985. *Ceremonial Chemistry: The Ritual Persecution of Drugs, Addicts, and Pushers.* Rev. ed. Holmes Beach, Fla.: Learning Publications.

Traver, Harold, and Gaylord, Mark S., eds. 1992. *Drugs, Law and the State.* New Brunswick, N.J.: Transaction.

Wasson, R. Gordon. 1984. "Distilled Alcohol Dissemination." *Drinking and Drug Practices Surveyor* 19:6.

Zimmer, Lynn, and Jacobs, James B. 1992. "The Business of Drug Testing: Technological Innovation and Social Control." *Contemporary Drug Problems* 19, no. 1:1–26.

Zinberg, Norman E. 1984. *Drug, Set and Setting: The Basis for Controlled Intoxicant Use.* New Haven, Conn.: Yale University Press.

## V. LEGAL CONTROL OF HARMFUL SUBSTANCES

At the close of the twentieth century, opium, its constituent morphine, and the derivative heroin are viewed with fear and suspicion. As both popular and professional attitudes turned against drug use in the United States around 1980, physicians began to fear prescribing potentially addictive analgesics, and likewise patients began to fear taking them. This attitude contrasts sharply with that of one of America's leading physicians in the mid-nineteenth century, George Wood, of the University of Pennsylvania, who wrote in 1868 that opium produces "an exaltation of our better mental qualities, a warmer glow of benevolence, a disposition to do great things, but nobly and beneficently, a higher devotional spirit, and withal a stronger self-reliance, and consciousness of power" (Wood, 1868, vol. 1, p. 712).

Clearly, the ethical position one takes regarding the availability of a drug is profoundly affected by whether one believes that the drug is risky in any amount or that reasonable doses of the drug are a boon to humankind. These two positions have alternately influenced experts and the public since at least the eighteenth century in English-speaking countries. While one of these attitudes has held sway, the opposite ethical position has been dismissed as wrongheaded and refuted both morally and scientifically.

### Attitudes toward alcohol

Alcohol, a drug with a long history of easy availability and widespread consumption in the West, provides instructive examples of these dramatic shifts of opinion and their impact on ethical positions. The history of fermented beverages like beer and wine goes back millennia, and distilled spirits began to be produced by about 1300 in Europe. For centuries thereafter, nearly pure alcohol was produced in small amounts, and extraordinary characteristics were attributed to it. *Aqua vitae*, as certain distilled alcohol products were termed, was said to prolong life. In its qualities it approached the quintessence, or fifth element (along with earth, air, fire and water). The "spirit" derived from distillation, according to John French, a seventeenth-century English physician, has wonderful "vertues . . . for there is no disease, whether inward or outward, that can withstand it" (French, 1667, p. 132).

Faith in the life-sustaining and tonic qualities of distilled spirits became embedded in European culture and aided the spiraling rise in consumption of spirits in parts of Europe during the sixteenth and seventeenth centuries. By the late seventeenth century, when civil authorities and religious leaders were becoming alarmed by the effects of increased consumption, widespread assumptions about the beneficial effects of alcohol frustrated their attempts to control it. It was the effects of consumption—drunkenness, poverty, violence, and neglect—that bothered community leaders. Yet most medical authorities continued to praise distilled spirits for their mysteriously restorative qualities.

In England, new scientific data challenged the old beliefs during the "gin epidemic" of the eighteenth century. For the first half of the century a battle raged between the populace—especially in London, where gin was cheaper than an equal volume of beer—and some religious and secular leaders who were appalled by the spiraling number of public drunks, "weak, feeble, and distempered children," (Plant, 1985, p. 9) and deaths attributed to the massive and cheap consumption of distilled spirits. Hogarth's prints, *Gin Lane* and *Beer Street* of 1751, capture the social destruction resulting from a substance once thought an unadulterated good.

Rebutting prior claims for the beneficial effects of alcohol was a new series of medical studies, spurred by alarm generated by the "epidemic" and aimed specifically at distilled spirits. These studies distinguished between distilled spirits, an artificially concentrated form of alcohol, and the naturally fermented beer and wine. Distilled spirits now appeared in two opposing guises: a good substance that promoted life and health, and an evil substance that destroyed the body and mind.

This new view of distilled spirits was incorporated into voluntaristic plans for self-improvement, most notably the religious movement led by John Wesley. In his attempt to revitalize the Church of England and establish a strict morality of behavior, Wesley argued a distinction between fermented and distilled spirits. He described the latter as "a certain, tho' a slow poison," although he conceded that it might have medicinal uses (Wesley, 1747, p. xix). Eventually Wesley's Methodism moved, especially in the United States under the guidance of Wesley's chosen missionary Francis Asbury, to a rejection of alcohol in any form.

Opposition to alcohol also drew on the Christian ascetic tradition, which had a long history before the eighteenth century but was being revived by religious movements in the later part of that century. Along with Methodism, Quaker antagonism toward alcohol gradually spread in America, and by the early decades of the nineteenth century, similar sentiments were strong in many Congregationalist and Presbyterian congregations.

In addition to moral objections, in the United States criticism of alcohol was based upon social and medical observations. Benjamin Rush, perhaps the most distinguished American physician of his time, launched an attack on alcohol based on his experiences as a physician in the War for Independence. Rush countered the popular notion that distilled spirits were a healthy means of invigorating soldiers and field workers, or a stimulant to intellectual activity. However, like Wesley, he focused on spirits, not all forms of alcohol. His pamphlet *An Enquiry into the Effects of Spirituous Liquors upon the Human Body*, written in the 1780s, was distributed by the thousands throughout the nation and was still being reprinted and distributed four decades later.

**Temperance movements.**    Later reformers, most notably Lyman Beecher in his monumental *Six Sermons on Intemperance*, which first appeared in 1826, moved to more extreme attitudes, condemning not only distilled spirits but all alcoholic beverages. Moderation was no longer recommended as an ideal; rather, it was presented as a dangerous delusion that would draw many into alcohol abuse. Alcohol itself, Beecher argued, not the amount or type consumed, was an evil.

The first American temperance movement, imbued with Beecher's condemnation of a naturally produced substance, was broadly successful, at least for a brief period; a dozen states enacted prohibition during the 1850s. For the purposes of understanding the great shifts in attitude toward alcohol and other drugs, it is important to note the total denigration of alcohol that accompanied the American temperance movement. The effort to make alcohol an outlaw substance was not blocked by favorable references to wine in the Bible. Some Protestants postulated that there were "two wines" mentioned in the New Testament—a dangerous, intoxicating wine and another wine that was nonintoxicating—and that the variable references to wine were only to the second, safe variety.

The use of alcohol as a medicine by many physicians was viewed with great suspicion and irritation by the temperance movement because any useful characteristic of alcohol contradicted the position that alcohol had no redeeming qualities. Temperance hospitals—where alcohol was not used even medicinally—sprang up along with temperance hotels and restaurants.

The impact of the Civil War weakened the temperance movement. Per capita consumption of alcohol, which had reached a low point in the 1850s, began to rise again until a second peak was reached shortly before World War I. The image of alcohol during this second temperance movement also was heatedly contested. Alcohol maintained its medical image as a body restorative and strengthener, but at the same time it was denounced by the Woman's Christian Temperance Union and other religious temperance leaders as Demon Rum, the destroyer of families and productivity. An attack on the system of distributing alcohol through saloons, led by the Anti-Saloon League, grew again into an attack on alcohol in any form. In 1920, a year after ratification of the Eighteenth Amendment to the Constitution, which prohibited "manufacture, sale or transportation" of intoxicating liquors for "beverage purposes," the entire nation went dry.

Thus, the United States experienced a positive attitude toward alcohol consumption in the eighteenth century, followed by a reversal dominated by the image of alcohol as a fundamentally evil substance that led to widespread prohibition in the 1850s. This first peak of prohibition faded under the resentment of the public, the difficulty of enforcement, and the monumental distraction of the Civil War. Later in the nineteenth century, opposition to alcohol revived, centering on the burgeoning urban saloon, a center of political and moral corruption, and a symbol of the rising fear of recent immigrants crowding into the cities. This anti-alcohol campaign proved even more successful than the previous crusade, achieving a total legal prohibition except for sacramental and medicinal uses.

**Post-Prohibition.**    After 1933, the year of the Eighteenth Amendment's repeal, the backlash against Prohibition made advocacy of alcohol control an object of ridicule until about 1980; then another change in attitude toward alcohol—perhaps the beginning of a third temperance movement—once again put the issue of alcohol's damaging social consequences in the forefront of public concern. In 1984 the federal government established a national drinking age of twenty-one, and since 1989, all containers for beverage alcohol manufactured for sale in the United States have been required by federal law to bear a government label warning against the dangers of alcohol. Meanwhile, since the 1980s state drunk-driving laws have been made much more punitive. Per capita consumption of alcohol, which hit a third historical peak in 1980, has since then been gradually in decline.

## Attitudes toward other drugs

Alcohol's image did not wax and wane in isolation from drugs like morphine, heroin, and cocaine, although the peaks of their favorable and unfavorable public images did not coincide precisely with those of alcohol. Cocaine use rose rapidly following its introduction into the United States in the mid-1880s. Not until the Harrison Act (1914) did the federal government prohibit sale of cocaine without a prescription. A similar restriction on alcohol, National Prohibition, was enacted five years later, and by the mid-1920s the federal government moved to eliminate heroin completely as a legally obtainable substance.

When we review the history of drugs and alcohol in the United States, it is apparent that the ethical debate and extent of control have been related to the healthy or poisonous image of these powerful substances. Interestingly, one extreme or the other was not buried by the victory of its contrary position. The ascendancy of one point of view seems to have created the conditions for the gradual emergence of the opposite attitude. A further point worth noting is that in the campaign against drugs and alcohol, the American practice has been to condemn them as being without any but the most limited value as medicine, and to hedge that exemption with tight restrictions. The periods of favorable and unfavorable attitudes are rather lengthy compared with the human life span, so each tends to be seen as the settled opinion of science and society, and the presence or absence of controls seems based on what appear to be established premises.

## The control of drugs and alcohol

**Effect of licensing and taxation.** The control of these substances involves both practical and philosophical considerations. Practically, a nation or locality has a limited array of controls, and these usually rest on the compliance of the public. During the English gin epidemic, Parliament was limited to using a variety of license fees and taxes, which were not always easily enforced, to curb the production of gin. Success in the campaign did not begin to be acknowledged by observers until after 1750, when, presumably, the baleful effects of gin and the prolonged campaign against it by reformers had changed public attitudes toward this form of alcohol. Beer consumption, it should be noted, was not targeted by the campaign in London, which was against distilled spirits, not alcohol itself.

In the United States the campaign initiated by Rush and perfected by Beecher rested on changing the attitude of the public and then employing law to confirm the rejection of alcohol. Beecher worked through national voluntary organizations, established a printing house, and encouraged traveling organizers. In 1851, Maine enacted the first comprehensive prohibition of alcohol. State laws prohibiting alcohol relied on local enforcement, which in the mid-nineteenth century was quite modest compared with the battery of tax laws and federal enforcement agencies that would be brought to bear on the problem a century later.

Control of opiates and cocaine initially took a different turn because, by the late nineteenth century, the licensing of physicians and pharmacists had become widespread in the United States. As a result, the first control over these drugs, after a period of free access, was to make them available by prescription only, although commonly a small amount would be permitted in an over-the-counter remedy. To alert the public, the Pure Food and Drug Act (1906) required that the amount of drugs in a remedy be included on the label. Due to the peculiarities of the U.S. Constitution, the federal government had little power to interfere with drug distribution within the nation. The appropriate police powers were relegated to the individual states.

During the Progressive Era (approximately 1890–1920), reformers worked to give the central government more power so that the benefit of uniform national laws could be applied to problems like tainted meat, adulterated medicines, destruction of forests, and drug abuse. With regard to drug abuse, the knotty constitutional problem was addressed by basing the Harrison Act of 1914, meant to regulate the distribution of opiates and cocaine, on the federal power to tax. Each transaction, from importation to retail purchase, had to be recorded and a small tax paid. Evasion of this law would be punished as a violation of the tax statutes. The restriction on maintenance doses of opiates to addicts was effected through Treasury Department regulations promulgated to carry out the Harrison Act. This part of the regulation was overturned by the U.S. Supreme Court in 1916 as a violation of states' rights, but it was effectively reinstated on another basis by the Court in 1919 during a peak of concern over drug addiction and in the face of the impending prohibition of alcohol.

The impact of impending alcohol prohibition on the severity of other drug laws illustrates a common factor in the control of drugs, what one might call the "hydraulic model," which implies that repression of one drug shifts use to another substance. This analysis encourages a blanket control of drugs and is especially popular when it is believed that abuse of a particular drug is a sign of an "addictive personality" (late twentieth century) or the affliction of "inebriety" (late nineteenth century). These diagnoses suggest that the afflicted individual is pressured to use alcohol and drugs, and that if one substance is not available, he or she will switch to another.

**Effectiveness of drug control measures.** The question of "availability" raises the controversial issue of the effectiveness of control measures. Do laws against drugs accomplish much more than raising the price of drugs? Can prescription controls or international interdiction reduce the supply of drugs? Can prohibition reduce the supply of alcohol? Here the answers are difficult, but one can say that in general the reduction in drug and alcohol use that accompanied the restrictions in the United States beginning with World War I (and ending with the start of a second drug epidemic in the 1960s) occurred during a period of extraordinary antagonism toward drugs. Laws against them grew progressively more severe, with the exception of alcohol, whose prohibition was repealed in 1933. Confidence in legal control was reinforced by the obvious decline in drug use (and alcohol consumption fell from 1.7 U.S. gallons per capita in 1910, to about .6 gallons between 1920 and 1930, and did not return to the 1910 level until the mid-1960s [Rorabaugh, 1979, p. 232]). Antidrug legislation became increasingly severe, even after Prohibition was repealed in 1933, including mandatory minimum sentences and, in 1956, federal enactment of the death penalty as an option for some cases of drug trafficking.

In order to understand the doubts concerning legal sanctions in the late-twentieth-century "epidemic," we must compare the two drug epidemics. During the first wave of drug use, laws did not exist until the public's fear demanded them. The more recent wave of drug use found the most severe drug laws in effect when a favorable attitude toward drug use was spreading across many sectors of American life. The apparent weakness in the enforcement of these laws, their clash with a new attitude among experts and the public, and the failure to recall the earlier experience with drugs led to ridicule and comfortable evasion of the law. A renewed harmony between anti-drug attitudes and anti-drug laws followed.

In the 1930s, at the end of the epidemic that peaked about the time of World War I, the United States, after having had general anti-drug and anti-alcohol education required by state laws, adopted a policy of silence regarding drugs. When silence was not possible, exaggeration was instituted to complement the increasing severity of the drug laws. This policy may account for the loss of public memory of that early "epidemic"; the style of making any drug use fraught with extreme danger (with the purpose of discouraging experimentation) contributed to the lack of balanced knowledge about drugs that characterized both adults and youth in the 1960s. The ultimate effect of the policy was to undercut the credibility of official statements on drug use.

In addition to the questions of changes in attitudes toward drugs and the practical problem of what control mechanisms exist, there is the broader question of control philosophy. Should drugs be controlled at all?

Should the state try to protect citizens from their own desire to use drugs? Is drug control a law-enforcement problem, a public-health task, or a moral or religious issue? For Beecher, alcohol had to be controlled because, while drunkenness ruined health and family life, it also impaired the individual's ability to hear and respond to God's message of salvation. Alcohol produced temporal death and eternal damnation.

Beecher's British contemporary, John Stuart Mill, rejected American prohibition laws and similar restrictions on the buyer of alcohol as an unjustified interference with liberty. Mill was particularly harsh on actions designed to protect individuals from themselves. To questions of policy he applied this prime principal: "Over himself, over his own body and mind, the individual is sovereign" (Mill, 1975, p. 11).

The debate between law-enforcement and public-health approaches to drug and alcohol abuse is particularly sensitive to public attitudes toward the nature of the drugs themselves. In an era of drug toleration, public-health methods and medical treatment in general are advocated and practiced. The concern is not so much with the drug as with the bad effects the drug may have on an unwise or excessive user. As the attitude turns against drugs in any amount, frustration and anger support police action, arrests, and punishments for violations of a strict rejection of drug use that leaves no area for "recreational" drug use.

**Decriminalization.** In the era of increased drug use beginning about 1965, an attack on prohibitory laws began with criticism of extraordinarily long sentences meted out to persons who possessed small amounts of marijuana. By 1970 the federal law had been softened and advocates of legalizing marijuana were organized. With the rise in cocaine and heroin use, many called for legalizing or "decriminalizing" these drugs on grounds that their dangers had been exaggerated. In 1972 the term "decriminalization" was proposed in the first report of the U.S. Commission on Marihuana and Drug Abuse as a compromise between arresting persons with small amounts of marijuana for personal use, and a free market in marijuana. Decriminalization would allow use while still permitting a national policy warning against the drug and maintaining legal sanctions against those producing and distributing large amounts of the plant.

Libertarians, such as the economist Milton Friedman, added a philosophy of freedom from state interference in private acts, such as drug use, to the debate over controls. Although the public has been increasingly opposed to drug use (reflected also in reduced consumption of tobacco and alcohol) and in favor of strict anti-drug laws since about 1980, analyses questioning the campaign against drugs have continued (Friedman, 1991).

Opposition to the "war against drugs" has centered on two themes: interdiction of drugs from foreign nations and domestic enforcement of stricter anti-drug laws. Critics have argued that interdiction has not affected the availability of drugs, especially cocaine, the chief target of the U.S. Coast Guard and the other services as well as the U.S. Drug Enforcement Administration. With regard to domestic policy, application of harsh criminal penalties to drug offenders is condemned as a source of prison crowding that does little or nothing to reduce crime or hard-core drug use.

A recent suggestion offered by those opposed to overreliance on the criminal justice approach is "harm reduction," a phrase that attempts to describe Dutch drug policy. The Netherlands is noted for allowing personal use of drugs, providing sterile needles to drug injectors, and generally tolerating drug availability. The expectation is that in the long run this policy will allow more users to survive into a life less dominated by, or free from, drug use.

Criticism of any policy that would appear to encourage or facilitate drug use has been severe. Arguments against legalization include the observation that laws pressure users into treatment, the symbolic importance of an anti-drug policy, and the fear that drug use would increase if drugs were easily available and inexpensive.

In conclusion, the history of drug and alcohol control illustrates the slowly shifting assumptions societies make regarding these powerful substances. At the extreme of each attitude their good or evil nature seems so obvious that contrary notions are rejected with dispatch. Consequently, the ethical debate is deeply influenced by these alterations in attitude. These contrary positions also make an indefinitely sustainable drug policy difficult to frame.

DAVID F. MUSTO

*Directly related to this article are the other articles in this entry:* ADDICTION AND DEPENDENCE, SMOKING, ALCOHOLISM, *and* ALCOHOL AND OTHER DRUGS IN A PUBLIC-HEALTH CONTEXT. *Also directly related is the entry* LIFESTYLES AND PUBLIC HEALTH. *For a further discussion of topics mentioned in this article, see the entries* LAW AND BIOETHICS; LAW AND MORALITY; PATERNALISM; *and* PRIVACY IN HEALTH CARE. *Other relevant material may be found under the entries* BEHAVIOR CONTROL; FREEDOM AND COERCION; HEALTH AND DISEASE, *article on* HISTORY OF THE CONCEPTS; *and* HEALTH POLICY, *article on* POLITICS AND HEALTH CARE.

### Bibliography

AARON, PAUL, and MUSTO, DAVID F. 1981. "Temperance and Prohibition in America: A Historical Overview." In *Alcohol and Public Policy: Beyond the Shadow of Prohibition*, pp. 127–181. Edited by Mark H. Moore and Dean R. Gerstein. Washington, D.C.: National Academy Press.

BEECHER, LYMAN. 1828. *Six Sermons on Intemperance*. 4th ed. Boston: T. R. Marvin.

FRENCH, JOHN. 1667. *The Art of Distillation; or, A Treatise of the Choicest Spagyrical Preparations, Experiments, and Curiosities Performed by Way of Distillation*. London: E. Coles for T. Williams.

FRIEDMAN, MILTON. 1991. "The War We Are Losing." In *Searching for Alternatives: Drug-Control Policy in the United States*, pp. 53–67. Edited by Melvyn B. Krauss and Edward P. Lazear. Stanford, Calif.: Hoover Institution.

KLEIMAN, MARK. 1992. *Against Excess: Drug Policy for Results*. New York: Basic Books.

LENDER, MARK E., and MARTIN, JAMES K. 1982. *Drinking in America: A History*. New York: Free Press.

MILL, JOHN STUART. 1975. [1859]. *On Liberty*. Edited by David Spitz. New York: W. W. Norton.

MUSTO, DAVID F. 1987. *The American Disease: Origins of Narcotic Control*. Enl. ed. New York: Oxford University Press.

NADELMANN, ETHAN A. 1991. "Thinking Seriously About Alternatives to Drug Prohibition." *Daedalus* 121, no. 3:85–132.

PLANT, MOIRA. 1985. *Women, Drinking, and Pregnancy*. New York: Tavistock Methuen.

RORABAUGH, WILLIAM J. 1979. *The Alcoholic Republic*. New York: Oxford University Press.

RUSH, BENJAMIN. n.d. *An Enquiry into the Effects of Spirituous Liquors upon the Human Body, and Their Influence upon the Happiness of Society*. Philadelphia: Thomas Bradford.

U.S. NATIONAL COMMISSION ON MARIHUANA AND DRUG ABUSE. 1972. *Marihuana: A Signal of Misunderstanding*. Washington, D.C.: U.S. Government Printing Office.

U.S. OFFICE OF NATIONAL DRUG CONTROL POLICY. 1989. *National Drug Control Strategy*. Washington, D.C.: U.S. Government Printing Office.

WESLEY, JOHN. 1747. *Primitive Physick; or, An Easy and Natural Method of Curing Most Diseases*. London: Thomas Trye.

WILSON, JAMES Q. 1990. "Against the Legalization of Drugs." *Commentary* 88, no. 2:21–28.

WOOD, GEORGE B. 1868. *A Treatise on Therapeutics, and Pharmacology, or Materia Medica*. 3d ed. 2 vols. Philadelphia: J. B. Lippincott.

# SUBSTITUTED JUDGMENT

*See* DEATH AND DYING: EUTHANASIA AND SUSTAINING LIFE, *articles on* ETHICAL ISSUES, *and* PROFESSIONAL AND PUBLIC POLICIES. *See also* CHILDREN, *articles on* HEALTH-CARE AND RESEARCH ISSUES.

# SUFFERING

*See* PAIN AND SUFFERING.

# SUICIDE

Philosophical issues concerning suicide arise in a wide range of contemporary end-of-life dilemmas: the withdrawal or withholding of medical treatment; involuntary treatment; high-risk, experimental, and unconventional treatment; euthanasia, assistance, and physician assistance in suicide; requests for maximal treatment; and many others. Although suicide is often popularly understood in a narrower sense of active, pathological self-killing, traditionally abhorred, the underlying issue most broadly conceived concerns the role the individual may play in bringing about his or her own death.

Two focal issues concerning suicide are evident in these broader dilemmas. First, should suicide be recognized as a right, and if so, under what conditions? On this first question rest the foundations for various applications of the "right to die," as well as a variety of other issues in high-risk and self-sacrificial behavior.

Second, what should the role of other persons be toward those intending suicide? On this second question rest practical, legal, and public-policy issues in suicide prevention and suicide assistance. Both focal issues concerning suicide raise larger questions about the nature of choices to die and the relevance of mental illness, about the role of the state, about conceptual issues in determining what actions are to be counted as suicide, about the role of religious belief concerning suicide, about the possibility of an autonomous choice of suicide, and about the moral status of suicide.

## The incidence of suicide

The United States exhibits a rate of reported suicide—12.2/100,000 per year (1991 figures)—that falls approximately midrange between societies in which reported suicide rates are extremely low, such as the Islamic countries, and those in which reported rates are extremely high, for example, Hungary. In the United States, there are over 30,000 reported suicides per year and about eight to twenty times that many reported attempts; the worldwide suicide rate can be estimated at about 13/100,000 or about 728,000 deaths per year in a world population of 5.6 billion. In the United States, suicide is the third leading cause of death for those in the fifteen- to twenty-four-year age group; it is the eighth highest cause of death for the population as a whole. Suicide rates are approximately equivalent across socioeconomic groups. Suicide rates are four times higher for males, but attempted suicide rates are three or four times higher for females. Attempt rates for whites and blacks are equivalent; rates of death by suicide are twice as high for whites. For white males, suicide rates increase with age, rising to a peak of 72.6/100,000 in the age range eighty to eighty-four; for women, suicide rates peak in midlife, declining thereafter; and black women in the age range eighty to eighty-four have the lowest rate of all adult groups, 1.2/100,000. There are no reliable estimates of the number of unreported suicides, particularly in medical situations involving terminal illness. Suicide statistics reflect primarily suicides in the narrower sense of active, pathological self-killings, while deaths brought about by refusal of treatment, by self-sacrifice or voluntary martyrdom, by high-risk behavior, or by self-deliverance in terminal illness are rarely described or reported as suicides.

## Scientific models of suicide

Contemporary scientific understandings of the nature of suicide, primarily in the narrower sense, tend to fall into three groups: the "medical" model; the "cry-for-help," "suicidal career," or "strategic" model; and the "sociogenic" model.

**The medical model.** This model, heavily influential throughout most of the twentieth century, has understood suicide in terms of *disease*: If suicide is not itself a disease, then it is the product of disease, usually mental illness. Suicide is understood as involuntary and nondeliberative, the outcome of factors over which the individual has no control; it is something that "happens" to the victim. Studies of the incidence of mental illness in suicide often tactily appeal to this model by attempting to show that mental illness—usually depression, less frequently other mental disorders—is always or almost always present in suicide. This invites the inference that the mental illness or depression "caused" the suicide.

**The cry-for-help model.** A second model, developed in the pioneering work of Edwin Schneidman and Norman Farberow in the 1950s, understands suicide as a communicative strategy: It is a cry for help, an attempt to seek aid in altering one's social environment. Thus it is primarily "dyadic," making reference to some second person (or less frequently, an institution or other entity) central in the suicidal person's life. In this view, it is the suicidal gesture that is clinically central; the completed suicide is an attempt that is (often unintentionally) fatal. While the cry for help is manipulative in character, it is also often quite effective in mobilizing family, community, or medical resources to assist in helping change the circumstances of the attempter's life, at least temporarily. Later theorists have developed related models that also interpret suicide attempts as strategic: The concept of "suicidal careers" interprets an individual's repeated suicide threats and attempts as a method of negotiating the world, though—as for Sylvia Plath—such an attempt may prove fatal.

**The sociogenic model.** Originally developed by sociologist Emile Durkheim (1858–1917) in his landmark work *Suicide*, the sociogenic model sees suicide as the product of social forces varying with the type of social organization within which the individual lives. "It is not mere metaphor," Durkheim wrote in 1897, "to say of each human society that it has a greater or lesser aptitude for suicide . . . a collective inclination for the act, quite its own, and the source of all individual inclination, rather than their result" (Durkheim, 1951, p. 299). In societies in which individuals are very highly integrated into the society and their behavior is rigorously governed by social codes and customs, suicide tends to occur only when it is institutionalized and required by the society (as, for example, in the Hindu practice of *sati*, or voluntary widow-burning); this is termed "altruistic" suicide. In societies in which individuals are very loosely integrated into the society, suicide is "egoistic," almost entirely self-referential. In still other societies, Durkheim claims, individuals are neither over- nor underintegrated, but the society itself fails to provide adequate regulation of its members; this situation results in "anomic" suicide, typical of modern industrial society. In Western societies of this sort, institutionalized suicide has been extremely rare but not unknown, confining itself to highly structured situations: The sea captain was expected to "go down with his ship," and the Prussian army officer was expected to kill himself if he was unable to pay his gambling debts.

Like the medical model, the sociogenic model understands suicide as "caused," but it identifies the causes as social forces rather than individual psychopathology. Like the cry for help model, the sociogenic model sees suicide as a responsive strategy, but the responses are not so much matters of individual communication as conformity to social structures and reaction to the social roles a society creates.

## Prediction and prevention

Two principal strategies are employed for recognition of the prospective suicide *before* the attempt: the identification of verbal and behavioral clues; and the description of social, psychological, and other variables associated with suicide. Suicide prevention includes alerting families, professionals (especially those likely to have contact with suicidal individuals, such as schoolteachers), and the public generally to the symptoms of an approaching suicide attempt. They are trained to recognize and take seriously both direct warnings (e.g., "I feel like killing myself") and indirect warnings (e.g., "I probably won't be seeing you anymore") and behavior (e.g., giving away one's favorite possessions). They are also encouraged to be especially sensitive to these symptoms in those at highest risk: those who are older, live alone, are alcoholic, have negative interactions with important others or are isolated, and especially those

with a history of previous suicide attempts. Prevention strategies take a vast range of forms, from the "befriending" techniques developed by the Samaritans in England and the crisis "hotlines" widely used in the United States to involuntary commitment to a mental institution. Prevention strategies also include "postvention," or postoccurrence intervention, for the survivors—spouse, parent, child, or important other—of a person whose suicide attempt was fatal, since such survivors are themselves at much higher risk of suicide, especially during the first year.

These models of suicide and the associated forms of prediction and prevention are ubiquitous in contemporary medical and psychiatric practice. Yet although suicide has been treated largely as a medical or psychiatric matter, the conceptual, epistemological, and ethical problems it raises have reemerged as right-to-die issues in bioethics and redirected attention to the individual's role in his or her own death. It is no longer clear that these views of suicide, which reinforce a narrower conception of suicide, are appropriate in situations of terminal illness and other serious medical conditions, or that they can illuminate a broader range of individual roles in one's own death.

## Conceptual issues

The term "suicide" carries extremely negative connotations. However, there is little agreement on a formal definition. Some authors count all cases of voluntary, intentional self-killing as suicide; others include only cases in which the individual's primary intention is to end his or her life. Still others recognize that much of what is usually termed suicide neither is wholly voluntary nor involves a genuine intention to die, such as suicides associated with depression or other mental illness. Many writers exclude cases of self-inflicted death that, while voluntary and intentional, appear aimed to benefit others or to serve some purpose or principle—for instance, Socrates' drinking the hemlock, Captain Oates's walking out into the Arctic blizzard to allow his fellow explorers to continue without him, or the self-immolation of war protesters. These cases are usually not called suicide, but "self-sacrifice" or "martyrdom," terms with strongly positive connotations. However, attempts to differentiate these positive cases from negative ones often seem to reflect moral judgments, not genuine conceptual differences.

Cases of death from self-caused accident, self-neglect, chronic self-destructive behavior, victim-precipitated homicide, high-risk adventure, and self-administered euthanasia—all of which share many features with suicide but are not usually termed such—cause still further conceptual difficulty. Consequently, some authors claim that is is not possible to reach a rigorous formal definition of suicide, and prefer a "criterial" or operational approach to characterizing the term, noting its varied, shifting, and often inconsistent range of uses. Nevertheless, conceptual issues surrounding the definition of suicide are of considerable practical importance in policy formation, affecting, for instance, coroners' practices in identifying causes of death, insurance disclaimers, psychiatric protocols, religious prohibitions, codes of medical ethics, and laws prohibiting or permitting assistance in suicide.

## Suicide in the Western tradition

Much of the extremely diverse discussion of suicide in the history of Western thought has been directed to ethical issues. Plato (ca. 430–347 B.C.E.) acknowledges Athenian burial restrictions—the suicide was to be buried apart from other citizens, with the hand severed and buried separately—and in the *Phaedo,* he also reports the Pythagorean view that suicide is categorically wrong. But Plato also accepts suicide under various conditions, including shame, extreme distress, poverty, unavoidable misfortune, and "external compulsions" of the sort imposed on Socrates by the Athenian court. In *Republic* and *Laws,* respectively, Plato obliquely insists that the person suffering from chronic, incapacitating illness or uncontrollable criminal impulses ought to allow his life to end or cause it to do so. Aristotle (384–322 B.C.E.) held more generally that suicide is wrong, claiming that it is "cowardly" and "treats the state unjustly." The Greek and Roman Stoics, in contrast, recommended suicide as the responsible, appropriate act of the wise man, not to be undertaken in emotional distress, but as an expression of principle, duty, or responsible control of the end of one's own life, as exemplified by Cato the Younger (95–46 B.C.E.), Lucretia (sixth century B.C.E.), and Seneca (ca. 4 B.C.E.–65 C.E.).

Although Old Testament texts describe individual cases of suicide (Abimilech, Samson, Saul and his armor-bearer, Ahithophel, and Zimri), nowhere do they express general disapproval of suicide. However, the Greek-influenced Jewish general Josephus (37–100 C.E.) rejects it as an option for his defeated army, and clear prohibitions of suicide appear in Judaism by the time of the Talmud during the first several centuries C.E., often appealing to Gen. 9:5, "For your lifeblood I will demand satisfaction." The New Testament does not specifically condemn suicide, and mentions only one case: the self-hanging of Judas Iscariot after the betrayal of Jesus. There is evident disagreement among the early Church Fathers about the permissibility of suicide, especially in one specific circumstance: Although some disapproved, Eusebius (ca. 264–340), Ambrose (d. 397), and Jerome (ca. 342–420) all held that a virgin may kill herself in order to avoid violation.

While Christian values clearly include patience, endurance, hope, and submission to the sovereignty of God, values that militate against suicide, they also stress willingness to sacrifice one's life, especially in martyrdom, and absence of the fear of death. Some early Christians (e.g., the Circumcellions, a subsect of the rigorist Donatists) apparently practiced suicide as an act of religious zeal. Suicide committed immediately after confession and absolution, they believed, permitted earlier entrance to heaven. Augustine (354–430) asserted that suicide violates the commandment "Thou shalt not kill," and is a greater sin than any that could be avoided by suicide. Whether he was simply clarifying earlier elements of Christian faith or articulating a new position remains a matter of contemporary dispute. In any case, it is clear that with this assertion the Christian opposition to suicide became unanimous and absolute.

This view of suicide as morally and religiously wrong intensified during the Christian Middle Ages. Thomas Aquinas (ca. 1225–1274) argued that suicide is contrary to the natural law of self-preservation, injures the community, and usurps God's judgment "over the passage from this life to a more blessed one" (*Summa theologia* 2a 2ae q64 a5). By the High Middle Ages the suicide of Judas, often viewed earlier as appropriate atonement for the betrayal of Jesus, was seen as a sin worse than the betrayal itself. Enlightenment writers began to question these views. Thomas More (1478–1535) incorporated euthanatic suicide in his *Utopia* (1516); John Donne (ca. 1572–1631) treated suicide as morally praiseworthy when done for the glory of God (as, he claimed in *Biathanatos* [1608, published posthumously in 1647], was the case for Christ); David Hume (1711–1776) mocked the medieval arguments, justifying suicide on both autonomist and beneficent grounds.

Later thinkers such as Mme. de Staël (Anne Louise Germaine, née Necker, the baroness Staël-Holstein, 1766–1817)—although she subsequently reversed her position—and Arthur Schopenhauer (1788–1860) construed suicide as a matter of human right. Throughout this period, other thinkers insisted that suicide was morally, legally, and religiously wrong, for instance, John Wesley (1703–1791), who said that suicide attempters should be hanged, and Sir William Blackstone (1723–1780), who described suicide as an offense against both God and the King. Immanuel Kant (1724–1804) used the wrongness of suicide as a specimen of the moral conclusions the categorical imperative could demonstrate. In contrast, the Romantics tended to glorify suicide, and Friedrich Nietzsche (1844–1900) insisted that "suicide is man's right and privilege."

In Western thought, the volatile discussion of the moral issues in suicide ended fairly abruptly at the close of the nineteenth century. This was due in part to Emile Durkheim's insistence (1897) that suicide is a function of social organization, and also to the views of psychological and psychiatric theorists, developing from Jean Esquirol (1772–1840) to Sigmund Freud (1856–1939), that suicide is a product of mental illness. These new "scientific" views reinterpreted suicide as the product of involuntary conditions for which the individual could not be held morally responsible. The ethical issues, which presuppose choice, have reemerged only in the later part of the twentieth century, stimulated primarily by discussions in bioethics of dilemmas at the end of life.

## Non-Western religious and cultural views of suicide

Among religious moralists, Christian thinkers variously assert that divine commandment categorically prohibits suicide, that suicide repudiates God's gift of life, that suicide ruptures covenantal relationships with other persons, or that suicide defeats the believer's obligation to endure suffering in the image of Christ. But the prohibition of suicide is apparently absolute only in Christianity and Islam. Many other world religions hold the view that suicide is prima facie wrong, but that there are certain exceptions. Judaism, for example, prohibits suicide, but venerates the suicides at Masada and accepts *kiddush hashem,* self-destruction to avoid spiritual defilement. (Martyrdom to avoid apostasy, accepted and venerated by Christianity, may seem very closely to resemble this practice, but since the time of Augustine, Christianity has uniformly rejected self-caused death, as distinct from allowing oneself to be killed.)

Many traditional societies have exhibited institutionalized suicide practices: the *sati* of a Hindu widow, who was expected to immolate herself on her husband's funeral pyre; the *seppuku* or *hara-kiri* of traditional Japanese nobility out of loyalty to a leader or because of infractions of honor; and, in cultures as diverse as Sumer and China, the apparently voluntary submission to sacrifice by a king's retainers at the time of his funeral in order to accompany him into the next world. Eskimo, Native American, and some traditional Japanese cultures have practiced voluntary abandonment of the elderly, a practice closely related to suicide, in which the elderly are left to die, with their consent, on icefloes, on mountaintops, or beside trails.

In addition, some religious cultures have held comparatively positive views of suicide, at least in certain circumstances. The Vikings recognized suicide, as a form of violent death, as guaranteeing entrance to Valhalla. The Jains, and perhaps other groups within traditional Hinduism, honored deliberate self-starvation as the ultimate asceticism, and also recognized religiously motivated suicide by throwing oneself off a cliff. The Maya held that a special place in heaven was reserved for those who killed themselves by hanging (though other methods of suicide were considered disgraceful), and recognized a goddess of suicide, Ixtab. Many other pre-Columbian peoples in the Western hemisphere engaged in apparently voluntary ritual self-sacrifice, notably the Aztec practice of heart sacrifice, which was generally characterized at least at some historical periods by enhanced status and social approval. The view that suicide is intrinsically and without exception wrong is associated most strongly with post-Augustinian Christianity of the medieval period, surviving into the present; this absolutist view is not by and large characteristic of other cultures.

## Contemporary ethical issues

Is suicide *morally* wrong? Both historical and contemporary discussions in the Western tradition exhibit certain central features. Consequentialist arguments tend to focus on the damaging effects a person's suicide can have on family, friends, coworkers, or society as a whole. But, as a few earlier thinkers saw, such consequentialist views would also recommend or require suicide when the interests of the individual or others would be served by suicide. Deontological theorists have tended to treat suicide as intrinsically wrong, but, except for Kant, are typically unable to produce support for such claims that is independent of religious assumptions. Contemporary ethical argument has focused on such issues as whether hedonic calculus of self-interest, where others are not affected, provides an adequate basis for an individual's choice about suicide; whether life has intrinsic value sufficient to preclude choices of suicide; and whether any ethical theory can show that it would be wrong, rather than merely imprudent, for the ordinary, nonsuicidal person, not driven by circumstances or acting on principle, to end his or her life.

## Epistemological issues

Closely tied to conceptual issues, the central epistemological issues raised by suicide involve the kinds of knowledge available to those who contemplate killing themselves. The issue of what, if anything, can be known to occur after death has, in the West, generally been regarded as a religious issue, answerable only as a matter of faith; few philosophical writers have discussed it directly, despite its clear relation to theory of mind. Some writers have argued that since we cannot have antecedent knowledge of what death involves, we cannot knowingly and voluntarily choose our own deaths; suicide is therefore always irrational. Others reject this and instead attempt to establish conditions for the rationality of suicide. Others consider whether death is always an evil for the person involved, and whether death is appropriately conceptualized as the cessation of life. Still other writers examine psychological and situational constraints on decision making concerning suicide. For instance, the depressed, suicidal individual is described as seeing only a narrowed range of possible future outcomes in the current dilemma, the victim of a kind of "tunnel vision" constricted by depression. Also, the possibility of preemptive suicide in the face of deteriorative mental conditions like Alzheimer's disease is characterized as a problem of having to use that very mind which may already be deteriorating to decide whether to bear deterioration or die to avoid it.

### Public-policy issues

It is often, though uncritically, assumed that if a person's suicide is "rational," it ought not to be interfered with or prohibited. However, this raises policy issues about the role of the state and other institutions in the prevention of suicide.

**Rights and the prevention of suicide.**  In the West, both church and state have historically assumed roles in the control of suicide. In most European countries, ecclesiastical and civil law imposed burial restrictions on the suicide as well as additional penalties, including forfeiture of property, on the suicide's family. In England, suicide remained a felony until 1961. Suicide has been decriminalized in most of the United States and in England, primarily to facilitate psychiatric treatment of suicide attempters and to mitigate the impact on surviving family members, although in many U.S. states, assisting another person's suicide is a violation of statutory law, case law, or recognized common law. In Germany, assisting a suicide is not illegal, provided the person is competent and acting voluntarily; in the Netherlands, physician-assisted suicide is tolerated under the same guidelines as voluntary active euthanasia.

In recent years, suicide-prevention strategies have been enhanced by considerable advances in the epidemiological study of suicide, in the identification of risk factors, and in forms of clinical treatment. Suicide-prevention professionals welcome increased funding for education and prevention measures targeted at youth and other populations at high risk of suicide. Nevertheless, philosophers are increasingly alert to the more general theoretical issues these strategies raise, for example, the effect of high false-positive rates on the right to avoid unjustified coercion. Restrictions to prevent suicide—such as involuntary incarceration in a mental hospital or suicide precautions in an institutional setting—typically limit liberty, but because the predictive measures of suicide risk that are available are neither perfectly reliable nor perfectly sensitive, they will identify some fraction of persons as potential suicides who would not, in fact, kill themselves and fail to identify others who will. There are two distinct issues here: first, how great

an infringement of the liberty of those erroneously identified is to be permitted in the interests of preventing suicide by those correctly identified; and, second and more generally, whether restrictive measures for preventing suicide can even be justified at all, even for those who will actually go on to commit suicide. Civil rights theorists are generally disturbed by the first of these problems; libertarians by the second.

Although U.S. law does not prohibit suicide, it is not usually interpreted to recognize suicide as a right. There is considerable pressure from right-to-die groups in favor of recognizing a broad right to self-determination or "self-deliverance" in terminal illness not only by refusal of life-prolonging treatment but by bringing about one's own death. Other right issues are also raised by suicide, for example, freedom of expression. When Hemlock Society president Derek Humphry's *Final Exit*—a book addressed to the terminally ill that provided explicit instructions on how to commit suicide, including lethal drug dosages—was published in the United States in 1991 and sold over half a million copies, its publication was protected on the grounds of freedom of expression; yet in several other countries, including France and Australia, *Final Exit* was banned.

**Physician-assisted suicide.**  Although issues of the permissibility of suicide generally have been the focus of sustained historical discussion, contemporary public-policy debate tends to focus on a narrower, specific issue: that of physician-assisted suicide, usually coupled with the question of voluntary active euthanasia. There are two principal arguments advanced for the legalization of these practices. First, claims about autonomy appeal to a conception of the individual as entitled to control as much as possible the course of his or her own dying. To restrict the right to die to the mere right to refuse unwanted medical treatment and so be "allowed" to die, this argument holds, is an indefensible truncation of the more basic right to choose one's death in accordance with one's own values. Thus, advance directives, such as living wills and durable powers-of-attorney, do-not-resuscitate orders, and other mechanisms for withholding or withdrawing treatment, are inadequate to protect fundamental rights. Second, arguments for the legalization of physician-assisted suicide, usually together with euthanasia, involve an appeal to what is variously understood as mercy or nonmaleficence. Since not all terminal pain can be controlled and since suffering encompasses an even broader, less controllable range than pain, it is argued, it is defensible for a person who is in irremediable pain or suffering to choose death if there is no other way to avoid it.

Two principal arguments form the basis of the opposition to legalization of these practices: First, it is claimed that killing (in both suicide and euthanasia) is simply morally wrong, and hence wrong for doctors to facilitate or perform; and second, that legalization would invite a "slippery slope" leading to involuntary killing. The slippery slope argument contends, among other things, that permitting assistance in suicide or the performance of euthanasia would make killing "too easy," so that doctors would turn to it for reasons of bias, greed, impatience, or frustration with a patient who was not doing well; that it would set a dangerous model for disturbed younger persons who were not terminally ill; and that, in a society marked by prejudice against the elderly, the disabled, racial minorities, and many others, and motivated by cost considerations in a system that does not guarantee equitable care, "choices" of death that were not really voluntary would be imposed on vulnerable persons. Suicide in these circumstances would become a matter of social expectation or imperative. The counterargument for legalization replies that more open attitudes toward suicide would reduce psychopathology by allowing more effective counseling, and that, by bringing out into the open—and hence under adequate control—practices that have always gone on in secrecy, legalization would provide the most substantial protection for genuine patient choice.

Particularly relevant to public-policy discussions is the contention of some contemporary writers that suicide will become "the preferred way of death," since it allows control over the time, place, and circumstances of dying. Others claim that as pain control in terminal illness improves, all interest in physician-assisted, euthanatic suicide will disappear. These may seem to be mere predictive claims. But in the technologically developed nations, where the epidemiologic transition in causes of death now means that the majority of the population will die not of parasitic and infectious disease, as was the case in all societies until the middle of the nineteenth century and is still the case in many less developed nations, but of late-life degenerative diseases with prolonged downhill courses, these claims may seem to harbor quite different normative visions of the role a person may—and should—play in his or her own death.

MARGARET PABST BATTIN

*Directly related to this entry is the entry* DEATH, ATTITUDES TOWARD. *For a further discussion of topics mentioned in this article, see the entries* DEATH; DEATH AND DYING: EUTHANASIA AND SUSTAINING LIFE; ETHICS; MEDICAL ETHICS, HISTORY OF, *section on* EUROPE; MENTAL ILLNESS; *and* RIGHTS, *article on* RIGHTS IN BIOETHICS. *For a discussion of related ideas, see the entries* AUTONOMY; COMPETENCE; FREEDOM AND COERCION; LIFE; NATURAL LAW; PAIN AND SUFFERING; *and* UTILITY. *Other relevant material may be found under the entry* COMMITMENT TO MENTAL INSTITUTIONS.

## Bibliography

ALVAREZ, ALBERT. 1971. *The Savage God: A Study of Suicide.* London: Weidenfeld and Nicolson. Includes historical essay and study of Sylvia Plath.

ANDERBERG, THOMAS. 1989. *Suicide: Definitions, Causes, and Values.* Lund, Sweden: Lund University Press.

AUGUSTINE. 1972. *Concerning the City of God Against the Pagans.* Translated by Henry S. Bettenson. London: Penguin.

BAECHLER, JEAN. 1979. *Suicides.* Translated by Barry Cooper. Oxford: Basil Blackwell.

BARRACLOUGH, BRIAN M. 1992. "The Bible Suicides." *Acta Psychiatrica Scandinavia* 86, no. 1:64–69.

BATTIN, MARGARET PABST. 1982. *Ethical Issues in Suicide.* Englewood Cliffs, N.J.: Prentice-Hall.

———. 1994. *The Least Worst Death: Essays in Bioethics on the End of Life.* New York: Oxford University Press.

BATTIN, MARGARET PABST, and MARIS, RONALD W., eds. 1983. "Suicide and Ethics." *Suicide and Life-Threatening Behavior* 13, no. 4. Special issue.

BATTIN, MARGARET PABST, and MAYO, DAVID J., eds. 1980. *Suicide: The Philosophical Issues.* New York: St. Martin's Press. Collection of classic essays on conceptual, moral, and epistemological issues, psychiatry, and law.

BRODY, BARUCH A., ed. 1989. *Suicide and Euthanasia: Historical and Contemporary Themes.* Dordrecht, Netherlands: Kluwer. Collection of scholarly essays on classical philosophy, Jewish casuistry, early Christianity, and Renaissance, Reformation, and Enlightenment thought, plus contemporary essays.

DAUBE, DAVID. 1972. "The Linguistics of Suicide." *Philosophy and Public Affairs* 1, no. 4:387–437.

DONNE, JOHN. 1982. *Biathanatos.* Edited by Michael Rudick and Margaret Pabst Battin. New York: Garland.

DONNELLY, JOHN, ed. 1990. *Suicide: Right or Wrong?* Buffalo, N.Y.: Prometheus Books. Includes selections from Seneca, Aquinas, Hume, Kant, and contemporary authors.

DURKHEIM, EMILE. 1951. *Suicide: A Study in Sociology.* Translated by John A. Spaulding. Edited by George Simpson. New York: Free Press.

FEDDEN, HENRY ROMILLY. 1938. *Suicide: A Social and Historical Study.* London: Peter Davies.

HORAN, DENNIS J., and MALL, DAVID, eds. 1980. *Death, Dying and Euthanasia.* Lanham, Md.: University Publications of America.

HUME, DAVID. 1963. [1777]. "Of Suicide." In *Essays: Moral, Political and Literary,* pp. 586–596. London: Oxford University Press.

HUMPHRY, DEREK. 1991. *Final Exit: The Practicalities of Self-Deliverance and Assisted Suicide for the Dying.* Eugene, Oreg.: National Hemlock Society.

HUMPHRY, DEREK, with WICKETT, ANN. 1978. *Jean's Way.* London: Quartet Books. Personal account of assistance in terminal-illness suicide by founders of the Hemlock Society, a right-to-die organization.

JOHNSON, GRETCHEN L. 1987. *Voluntary Euthanasia: A Comprehensive Bibliography.* Los Angeles, Calif.: National Hemlock Society. Includes section on suicide and assisted suicide.

KANT, IMMANUEL. 1980. *Lectures on Ethics*. Translated by Louis Infield. Indianapolis, Ind.: Hackett.

——. 1983. *Ethical Philosophy: The Complete Texts of the Grounding for the Metaphysics of Morals, and Metaphysical Principles of Virtue, Part II of the Metaphysics of Morals*. Translated by James W. Ellington. Indianapolis, Ind.: Hackett.

——. 1993. *The Critique of Practical Reason*. Translated by Lewis White Beck. 3d ed. New York: Macmillan.

LANDSBERG, PAUL-LOUIS. 1953. *The Experience of Death; The Moral Problem of Suicide*. Translated by Cynthia Rowland. New York: Philosophical Library.

MARIS, RONALD W.; BERMAN, ALAN L.; MALTSBERGER, JOHN T.; and YUFIT, ROBERT I., eds. 1992. *Assessment and Prediction of Suicide*. New York: Guilford.

MARIS, RONALD W., and LAZERWITZ, BERNARD M. 1981. *Pathways to Suicide: A Survey of Self-Destructive Behaviors*. Baltimore: Johns Hopkins University Press.

NOVAK, DAVID. 1975. *Suicide and Morality: The Theories of Plato, Aquinas and Kant and Their Relevance for Suicidology*. New York: Scholars Studies Press.

PERLIN, SEYMOUR, ed. 1975. *A Handbook for the Study of Suicide*. Oxford: Oxford University Press.

PRADO, CARLOS G. 1990. *The Last Choice: Preemptive Suicide in Advanced Age*. Westport, Conn.: Greenwood.

SCHNEIDMAN, EDWIN S., ed. 1976. *Suicidology: Contemporary Developments*. New York: Grune and Stratton.

SCHNEIDMAN, EDWIN S., and FARBEROW, NORMAN I., eds. 1957. *Clues to Suicide*. New York: McGraw-Hill. An anthology assembled by the founders of contemporary suicidology.

SENECA, LUCIUS ANNAEUS. 1920. "Letter on Suicide" and "On the Proper Time to Slip the Cable." In *Ad Lucilium Epistulae Morales*. Translated by Richard M. Gummere. London: W. Heinemann.

SPROTT, SAMUEL E. 1961. *The English Debate on Suicide: From Donne to Hume*. La Salle, Ill.: Open Court.

# SUPEREROGATION

*See* OBLIGATION AND SUPEREROGATION.

# SURGERY

*The following is a revision and update of the first-edition entry "Surgery" by Judith P. Swazey and Paul S. Russell.*

Surgery is the branch of medicine using manual skills (from the Greek *cheirourgos*, working with the hand) to accomplish the goals of medicine: to relieve suffering, provide cures, prevent disease, and improve function. Surgeons therefore must master the essential motor skills enabling them to perform operations successfully. Although manual skills are a necessary feature of surgical competence, modern surgery values a host of other skills as well. Surgeons are expected to take histories, examine patients, order tests, and make accurate diagnoses. They are also supposed to know the pathophysiology of many diseases, some of which are never treated with an operation. Patients with chronic lung disease, for instance, have varying degrees of incapacity that influence their recovery from surgery. Surgeons are expected to know how such diseases affect decisions for and against an operation as well as how to manage them after an operation.

Even more relevant to bioethics, surgeons are expected to possess the skills and attitudes that promote good doctor–patient relationships, to interact with families, and to know the community's resources for assisting in patient care (Peterson, 1992). Surgeons play a role in persuading hospitals, HMOs, insurance companies, and government agencies to provide the resources to prevent illness or disability (such as alcoholism and traumatic injuries) and to ensure optimal recovery and rehabilitation. Thus, in addition to the essential manual skills, medical knowledge, and clinical judgment, surgeons are expected to possess the ethical attitudes and skills expected of all physicians (Parmer, 1982). This union of hand and mind, technical skills and intellectual ability, forms an important basis for understanding the ethical issues facing surgeons.

The importance of the surgeon's nontechnical skills becomes apparent in an assessment of the outcome of surgical care. The platitude "The operation was a success but the patient died" ironically reflects the serious truth that a technically excellent operation may still represent a bad surgical outcome. A heart attack following technically perfect gallbladder surgery, for example, represents a surgical failure. Surgical success ultimately depends on contributing to overall patient welfare, and the evaluation of surgical outcomes depends on results that matter most to patients: relief of suffering, optimizing function, and so on.

Acquiring and maintaining manual skills requires surgeons to spend more time than other doctors in training and hands-on practice—five to ten years, compared to nonsurgeons' usual three to five (Pories and Askalson, 1990). Surgical practitioners also spend more time directly involved in patient care than do nonsurgeons. The extra time and effort influence those who go into surgery, and their behavior as practitioners. Students often select a surgical career because of a background belief in a work ethic. Surgical training and practice, by virtue of the long hours and physical challenges, further reinforce such a belief.

Another basic feature of surgery is the requisite injuring of the (patient's) body in order to provide benefit. The craft of surgery can be traced back to one of the earliest documents in ancient civilization, the Smith Papyrus (Majno, 1975). The earliest surgeons in both

Western and non-Western cultures repaired wounds, stopped hemorrhages, and set fractures. Although in the Middle Ages surgery was often performed by barbers rather than the university-educated physicians, by the eighteenth century surgery had reached equal educational status with medicine (Zimmerman and Veith, 1967). The earliest medical schools in America, for instance, all had professors of surgery (Moore, 1976). Elective or planned operations, however, were extremely rare until the development of anesthesia and antisepsis in the mid-nineteenth century. Following those developments, the number of elective operations increased dramatically.

Because surgery usually involves an injury or intervention, there is often a more obvious connection between surgical care and outcome. This means that surgeons are held more liable than other physicians, a situation instilling in them a strong sense of individual responsibility. This sense of responsibility is associated with traits like decisiveness, certitude, self-discipline, compulsiveness, and tenacity (Cassell, 1991). Such traits, in turn, translate into a greater sense of professional autonomy that sometimes reaches arrogance (Bosk, 1979). Patients often seek out confident, paternalistic surgeons with positive attitudes, and there are reasons to believe that the reassurance and comfort such patients derive may improve the objective outcomes of surgical care. It is ethically challenging for the surgeon to be a decisive, paternalistic practitioner while at the same time ensuring patient autonomy.

The invasive nature of surgical treatment, as opposed to treatment by diet, drugs, or rest, creates a strong need for patient consent. The practice of consent to surgery can be found in eighteenth-century records, but the modern notion of informed consent does not appear until the twentieth century. Historically, informed consent became attached to surgical operations via assault and battery law and hence has failed to be recognized as necessary for other medical treatments (or nontreatment). Although surgery has become safer and more generally accepted, it continues to require special consent forms in the United States even though some riskier and more innovative nonsurgical treatments still do not. This anachronism needs revision to promote a better and more general practice of informed consent in medicine.

In the United States, surgical organizations took the lead in establishing safety standards for hospitals and operating rooms, organizing blood banks, and beginning the systematic assessment of outcomes (Moore, 1976). These important areas are now critical for improving the quality of medical care and the capacity to benefit patients.

As of 1987, 8.6 percent (11,421) of U.S. surgeons were women. This proportion had increased dramatically from 1970, when only 2.5 percent were women (Peebles, 1989). The 3.5-fold increase roughly parallels the 3.5-fold increase in female medical school graduates over the same seventeen-year period. Thus, the same proportion (28 percent) of female medical school graduates were in surgery in 1987 as in 1970. However, for the purpose of these calculations, obstetricians/gynecologists are counted as surgeons. The approximately 20 percent of practicing OB/GYN physicians who are women constitute more than half of the female surgeons in the United States. If the female OB/GYN practitioners are subtracted, the percentage of female surgeons drops to 5.5 percent. Thus, as of 1987, only 1 in 20 practicing surgeons in the United States was a woman. This small representation might reflect different lifestyles that encourage alternative choices, combined with a paucity of female role models in surgery.

The number of minority physicians (blacks, Hispanics, and American Indians) in American medicine remains extremely low relative to the proportion in the population overall—21 percent of the U.S. population are in a minority group but only 6.5 percent of practicing physicians are. There are no readily available figures for the distribution among surgeons, but the proportion is likely to be relatively lower.

The seven topics discussed below represent important ethical issues in modern surgery. None is unique to surgery, but they are more prominent and controversial in surgery. These issues exist at an intermediate level between the microethics of individual virtue and the macroethics of social policy. Surgeons and their organizations play an important role in shaping surgical practice and health-care delivery by their actions at this level. The American College of Surgeons has an ethical pledge for its members to take and a set of ethical bylaws; there are otherwise no official ethical guidelines for surgeons beyond those mandated for physicians in general. In each case an ethical practice or policy needs to be consistent with broader social values and norms so that surgical practices can truly serve the welfare of patients. Many other topics could be discussed—such as fetal surgery, the surgeon's role in transplant allocation, do-not-resuscitate orders, and interprofessional rivalries—but these issues are less specific to surgery and will be found covered in more detail elsewhere in the Encyclopedia.

## Ghost and itinerant surgeons

Ghost surgery occurs when a surgeon takes credit for an operation he or she does not perform. General anesthesia makes it impossible for patients to know who was actually present in the operating room, and some surgeons who have assigned surgical assistants to perform operations then take the credit and collect the fees.

Professional surgical organizations condemn ghost surgery across the board, not only because it is fraudulent but also because it undermines the trust between patient and doctor that forms the basis for all good medical care. However, there are some practices resembling ghost surgery that deserve closer scrutiny. In teaching hospitals, senior surgeons frequently share operative responsibility with surgical trainees. Surgeons may become unavailable because of other professional obligations, illness, or vacations, thus requiring a colleague to step in. In small community hospitals, surgeons may follow an older standard of care no longer used in larger centers. For example, in large hospitals vascular surgeons perform arterial bypass surgery, whereas in a community hospital the same operation might be done by a general surgeon. These practices share with ghost surgery the substitution of one surgeon or practice for another, and the possibility of misleading patients. As long as the quality of care is competent, the ethical problem can be resolved by informing patients ahead of time about the need for surgical residents and shared responsibilities, the potential exigencies requiring a substitute, and the existence of alternative practices. This gives patients an opportunity to ask questions and even to choose a different setting for their care, if they so wish.

Itinerant surgery, a relative of ghost surgery, occurs when surgeons travel from hospital to hospital because small hospitals lack the caseload for regular, on-site surgeons. These surgeons visit hospitals, perform operations, and leave, delegating preoperative and postoperative care to a community-based physician. When performed on a limited scale, with a competent surgeon and an adequate facility, this practice seems justified. However, some surgeons conclude from this practice that the responsibility for pre- and postoperative care can always be assumed by other physicians or assistants. Most surgical organizations disapprove of this practice and assert that, whenever possible, the surgeon performing the operation should also be responsible for preoperative and postoperative care.

### Innovative technology

New operations and instruments are less regulated than new drugs. This is partly because the art of surgery already has substantial individual variability. Different surgeons frequently do the same operations differently and use different instruments; what works for one surgeon may not work for another. In addition, surgeons have traditionally honored inventive colleagues by naming new operations or instruments for them. This intrinsic variability and the tradition of honoring innovative methods make it very difficult to draw a sharp line between acceptable and unacceptable innovation.

In addition, the American public becomes fascinated by new procedures even before they can be proved safe or effective. If the media portray a new method favorably, patients often demand it before it can be subjected to critical review. Manufacturers and hospitals also promote new methods because it is in their best interest to do so. Indeed, publicizing and selling new technology are appropriate ways to ensure prompt technology transfer. Problems occur, however, when safety and efficacy are compromised.

Controlled trials, the gold standard for evaluating new drugs, are ethically more problematic for innovative surgical procedures. It is difficult, if not impossible, to ethically ask a patient to undergo a simulated operation for the sake of control. But for new treatments promising only marginal benefits, the absence of controls creates major problems.

Despite the necessary "art" (Selzer, 1976) or variability in surgical treatment, and despite the need for innovation, surgical organizations need to be involved in efforts to assess new treatments. There has been some limited involvement; however, gastric freezing, intestinal bypass for obesity, and mammary artery ligation are only a few examples of surgical methods that were applied in good faith to large numbers of patients without prior assessment and were later found to be ineffective and harmful.

### AIDS and other blood-borne infections

The AIDS epidemic has forced surgeons to consider more carefully the duty to care, the right to refuse to provide care, the degree of danger they must accept, and the right to test patients for the surgeon's sake rather than for the patient's benefit. The incidence of workplace-acquired hepatitis is much higher among surgeons than other physicians, but this has not been true for AIDS (Sim and Jeffries, 1990). As of 1994, there have been no reports of a surgeon acquiring AIDS during an operation. Thus the danger to surgeons seems remote.

Maintaining a minimal level of danger, however, requires surgeons and operating rooms to observe high standards of safety. Eliminating unnecessary sharp instruments, using trays to pass knives, and using special forceps to handle needles are technical refinements that reduce the chance of injury. Wearing gloves, masks, eye protection, and impermeable gowns are all standard, universal practices. Screening all patients preoperatively for HIV is not warranted because of the low incidence of the virus, problems with false positives and negatives, and the protection achieved with universal precautions (Peterson, 1990). If a needle-stick injury occurs, testing both parties makes sense from an epidemiological point of view. But laws in some states require a special consent for HIV testing, and patients sometimes refuse to be tested. Committees or courts in some jurisdictions can override the patient's refusal, but in others the legal course of action is unclear. On ethical grounds the surgeon has some right to know a patient's HIV status when a positive test result will affect a potentially infected surgeon's own decisions concerning sexual relations, blood donation, and family planning.

Reports of an infected dentist transmitting HIV to four patients in 1990 created an uproar over the potential danger of infected surgeons (Centers for Disease Control, 1991). As a result, the CDC issued a policy telling surgeons to voluntarily undergo mandatory testing, ordering lists of seriously invasive procedures, and declaring that infected surgeons should stop doing procedures and be monitored. Since then retrospective studies of thousands of patients operated on by infected surgeons have not found a single patient infected in this manner. Surgical organizations therefore refused to develop the lists and disagreed openly with the CDC policy. While the potential danger exists it does seem extremely remote, and screening surgeons or limiting their activities does not seem justified.

Finally, HIV-positive patients should receive the same surgical care as anyone for surgery that prolongs life, relieves suffering, or restores function (Diettrich et al., 1991). However some surgical care is discretionary and would not ordinarily be undertaken by people with serious coexisting conditions or limited life expectancies. Patients with metastatic cancer who have asymptomatic hernias, for instance, would not ordinarily have the hernia repaired. Thus, for asymptomatic and non-health-threatening conditions, elective surgery would ordinarily not be performed on HIV-positive people.

## Malpractice

Because surgery invades or injures the body in order to heal it, and because the connection between an operation and an injury is relatively easy to establish, surgeons face more lawsuits than other physicians (Harvard Medical Practice Study, 1990). This means that they pay more for malpractice insurance, face more angry patients, and experience the trauma of a lawsuit more often. Tort law (litigation) plays an ethical role by preventing injury and by compensating injured persons. It prevents injury by sending a deterrent signal to be careful to all surgeons, not just the defendant surgeon. If the signal produces excessive caution, then surgical practice becomes too defensive and expensive. In addition to producing fear in all surgeons, litigation makes defendant surgeons feel guilty even without a trial. Some become seriously depressed and stop practicing. In addition, the costs and the time spent on legal defense produce enormous strain. Even if a jury finds in favor of a surgeon, the ordeal of a trial takes a heavy toll.

The other ethical role of litigation concerns compensating injured patients. While many studies find that tort law deters injury, most find the compensation aspect insufficient; too few victims receive funds, and the

system's costs are excessive (Harvard Medical Practice Study, 1990). Furthermore, there are other possible ways to compensate for injuries. An insurance mechanism in the U.S. compensates workplace injuries. In New Zealand and Sweden medical injuries are handled by an administrative board that decides whether an injury was caused by medical care and, if it was, sets a level of compensation based on the patient's loss. Such systems compensate more victims promptly than does tort litigation, since they do not require proving a deviation from a standard of care. In the New Zealand and Swedish systems, if medical care caused the injury, patients are compensated promptly. Although a compensation system has its own administrative costs and involves more patient payments, it saves the hefty legal expenses of a malpractice trial. It also avoids the emotional costs and distress that would be experienced by patients and surgeons. Overall the financial costs of the two systems are about the same.

Many surgical organizations and individual surgeons work with lawyers, government agencies, and elected officials to address problems with the malpractice system. Replacing the tort system with an injury compensation system makes sense on the grounds of justice. But this would mean finding a replacement for litigation's deterrent effect. This in turn would require more regulation of surgical practice, which runs contrary to the surgeon's individualistic character. Nevertheless, it makes sense to consider accepting restraints on independence in order to compensate injured patients and alleviate some of the burden of lawsuits.

## Specialization

Specialization is an important ethical issue because of its mix of potential benefits along with social and professional costs (Colwell, 1992). Specialists benefit individual patients, especially those with rare diseases, by making available greater knowledge and experience. They also benefit society when they report new knowledge and try new methods. It is impossible to imagine the emergence of modern surgery without the benefit of extensive specialization.

At the same time, specialist care costs more, and the number of specialists plays a role in determining the amount of care available in a given area; the supply plays an important role in determining the demand. The mounting costs of specialist care arise because a "need" for care tends to generate a right to that care, thereby creating a social or insurance mechanism to pay for it. In the case of surgery as compared to other forms of medical care, specialization greatly increases costs.

There are social costs in addition to the financial ones (Jordan, 1991). Creation of a specialty removes an area of expertise from the generalist. This is especially true as new specialists and generalists are trained. For instance, general surgeons used to deal with major trauma; creation of a trauma specialty means that general surgeons no longer have as much training and experience in trauma care. As a result, community-based general surgeons may no longer be familiar enough with major trauma to expertly manage such patients. This becomes problematic in rural areas with small numbers of cases; such patients may have to be transported long distances, with added hazards and extra expense. Is this worthwhile, or should all surgeons learn how to handle these cases?

Fragmentation of care and specialty rivalries are other costs of specialization (Silen, 1992). When care is fragmented, patients may suffer from one condition while being treated for another, less significant condition. For instance, a patient with major heart disease may suffer a heart attack while having a prostate problem treated. Complications like these can sometimes be avoided by the more holistic, less fragmented care offered by a generalist rather than a specialist.

Since surgical organizations have some control over (responsibility for) the rate of specialization, they need to consider more than technical proficiency (Organ, 1990). Justifying a new specialty depends on a cost/benefit calculation that includes the costs of limiting generalists as well as how a new specialty will affect the entire fabric of health care (Council on Long Range Planning, 1989).

## Remuneration

American surgeons have been better compensated than other physicians because of their scarcity, the greater costs of training, and the increased effort required for surgical care. This custom has recently been challenged by nonsurgeons who contend that cognitive work (the intellectual activity of history taking, test ordering, diagnosing, and nonsurgical treatment) is just as valuable and receives relatively too little compensation. Surgeons, they argue, should be paid less and cognitive physicians more. Now that the supply of surgeons has increased, the gap between demand and supply has narrowed and, at present, there is an even greater need for primary-care physicians (Colwell, 1992). Need or scarcity as a basis for extra compensation, therefore, no longer exists. The increased costs of training and effort, however, persist.

Recently, the U.S. government began setting fees for Medicare patients based on a formula determined by resource costs (the resource-based relative value scale) (Hsiao et al., 1988). This limits the surgeon's freedom to set fees and the money thus spent on surgical care. Surgical organizations oppose fee setting on the grounds that it fails to recognize fully the value of surgical care (Maloney, 1991). They suppose that, given the freedom to choose and adequate resources, patients would be willing to pay more for surgical than for cognitive care. This argument rests on the idea that regulating fees interferes with market demand, and that ultimately this would produce inferior surgical care.

On the other hand, there are enormous discrepancies between the incomes of surgical and some nonsurgical physicians as well as numerous examples of excessive rates of surgery in some localities. Furthermore, insurance companies, not individual consumers, generally pay for medical care, thereby reducing the ability of a market-oriented approach to establish appropriate fees. These factors favor some readjustment to recognize the value of cognitive care and reduce excessive surgery.

## Supply of surgeons

By regulating the number of trainees, surgical organizations determine the number of surgeons available to meet societal needs. Since the number of applicants usually exceeds the number of training positions, these calculations sometimes deny qualified physicians completely free career choices.

Shortly after World War II there was a great influx of surgeons. Large numbers of military surgeons returned to civilian life, and many foreign physicians came to the United States for surgical training (Moore, 1976). As a result, some surgeons found that after investing years in training, there were few job opportunities (Nickerson et al., 1976). Even more important were the findings that the supply of surgeons tended to determine the amount of surgical care and that this contributed to escalating health-care costs.

As a result of a number of studies demonstrating a relative oversupply, surgical organizations began measuring current needs for surgical care and predicting future needs. These estimates were used to determine the number of trainees and of training programs approved in the United States. Although the regulation of surgical personnel seems justified in order to reduce the volume of excessive surgery and improve professional work satisfaction, two important assumptions in the calculation of needs raise important questions. The first concerns assumptions about the number of surgical operations required to maintain competence. Some studies have suggested that a larger volume correlates with better results (Luft et al., 1979; Hannan et al., 1989). But other data suggest that larger volumes of operations correlate more closely with less stringent criteria and with patients receiving surgery with less justification. Undue emphasis on the volume requirement could drive these rates even higher. There is, however, a distribution problem in that while certain regions do have an oversupply of surgeons, others have an undersupply. Overcoming this problem may lead to exorbitant costs.

Second, little attention has been paid to the amount of time spent by surgeons outside operating rooms, making hospital rounds and seeing patients in offices and clinics (Wheeler, 1992). Little is known about the impact of this aspect of surgical work on factors like patient function, the degree of suffering, efficiency, and patient satisfaction. As these factors become more measurable, they need to be fed back into calculations of the numbers of surgeons and the kind of training needed.

LYNN M. PETERSON

*For a further discussion of topics mentioned in this entry, see the entries* AIDS; HEALTH-CARE FINANCING, *article on* PROFIT AND COMMERCIALISM; INFORMED CONSENT; MEDICAL MALPRACTICE; PROFESSIONAL–PATIENT RELATIONSHIP; TECHNOLOGY; *and* WOMEN, *section on* WOMEN AS HEALTH-CARE PROFESSIONALS. *This entry will find application in the entries* MEDICINE AS A PROFESSION; ORGAN AND TISSUE TRANSPLANTS; *and* TEAMS, HEALTH-CARE. *For a discussion of related ideas, see the entries* AUTONOMY; HARM; *and* PATERNALISM.

## Bibliography

BOSK, CHARLES L. 1979. *Forgive and Remember: Managing Medical Failure.* Chicago: University of Chicago.

CASSELL, JOAN. 1991. *Expected Miracles: Surgeons at Work.* Philadelphia: Temple University Press.

CENTERS FOR DISEASE CONTROL. 1991. "Update: Transmission of HIV Infection During an Invasive Dental Procedure—Florida." *Journal of the American Medical Association* 265, no. 5:563–568.

COLWELL, JACK M. 1992. "Where Have All the Primary Care Applicants Gone?" *New England Journal of Medicine* 326, no. 6:387–393.

COUNCIL ON LONG RANGE PLANNING AND DEVELOPMENT (AMA). 1989. "The Future of General Surgery." *Journal of the American Medical Association* 262, no. 22:3178–3183.

DIETTRICH, NANCY A.; CACIOPPO, JOHN; KAPLAN, GERALD; and COHEN, STEVEN M. 1991. "A Growing Spectrum of Surgical Disease in Patients with Human Immunodeficiency Virus/Acquired Immunodeficiency Syndrome: Experience with 120 Major Cases." *Archives of Surgery* 126, no. 7:865–866.

HANNAN, EDWARD L.; O'DONNELL, JOSEPH F.; KILBURN, HAROLD, JR.; BERNAND, HARVEY R.; and YAZICI, ALTAN. 1989. "Investigation of the Relationship Between Volume and Mortality for Surgical Procedures Performed in New York State Hospitals." *Journal of the American Medical Association* 262, no. 4:503–510.

HARVARD MEDICAL PRACTICE STUDY. 1990. *Patients, Doctors, and Lawyers: Medical Injury, Malpractice Litigation, and Patient Compensation in New York.* Boston: Author.

HSIAO, WILLIAM C.; BRAUN, PETER; DUNN, DANIEL; and BECKER, EDMUND R. 1988. "Resource-Based Relative Values: An Overview." *Journal of the American Medical Association* 260, no. 16:2347–2353.

JORDAN, GEORGE L. 1991. "The Future of General Surgery." *American Journal of Surgery* 161, no. 2:194–202.

LUFT, HAROLD S.; BUNKER, JOHN P.; and ENTHOVEN, ALAIN C. 1979. "Should Operations Be Regionalized? The Empirical Relation Between Surgical Volume and Mortality." *New England Journal of Medicine* 301, no. 25:1364–1369.

MAJNO, GUIDO. 1975. *The Healing Hand: Man and Wound in the Ancient World.* Cambridge, Mass.: Harvard University Press.

MALONEY, JAMES V., JR. 1991. "A Critical Analysis of the Resource-Based Relative Value Scale." *Journal of the American Medical Association* 266, no. 24:3453–3458.

MOORE, FRANCIS D. 1976. "American Surgery." In vol. 2 of *Advances in American Medicine: Essays at the Bicentennial,* pp. 614–684. Edited by John Z. Bowers and Elizabeth Purcell. New York: Josiah Macy, Jr., Foundation.

NICKERSON, RITA J.; COLTON, THEODORE; PETERSON, OSLER; BLOOM, BERNARD; and HAUCK, WALTER W., JR. 1976. "Doctors Who Perform Operations." *New England Journal of Medicine* 295, no. 17:921–925; no. 18:982–989.

ORGAN, CLAUDE H., JR. 1990. "The Future of General Surgery." *Archives of Surgery* 125, no. 2:145–146.

PARMER, MICHAEL A. 1982. "Ethics of a Professional Surgeon." *Bulletin of the American College of Surgeons* 67, no. 7:2–5.

PEEBLES, RHONDA. 1989. "Female Surgeons in the U.S.: An Eighteen-Year Review." *Bulletin of the American College of Surgeons* 74:18–23.

PETERSON, LYNN M. 1990. "AIDS and Surgical Care: A Challenge for the 90s." *Bulletin of the American College of Surgeons* 75:20–24.

———. 1992. "Advance Directives, Proxies, and the Practice of Surgery." *American Journal of Surgery* 163:277–282.

PORIES, WALTER J., and ASKALSON, HAZEL M. 1990. "The Surgical Residency: The Job Description Does Not Fit the Job." *Archives of Surgery* 125:147–150.

SELZER, RICHARD. 1976. *Mortal Lessons: Notes on the Art of Surgery.* New York: Simon and Schuster.

SILEN, WILLIAM. 1992. "Where Have the Surgeons (Doctors) Gone?" *American Journal of Surgery* 163, no. 1:2–4.

SIM, ANDREW J. W., and JEFFRIES, DONALD J., eds. 1990. *AIDS and Surgery.* Oxford: Blackwell Scientific.

WHEELER, H. BROWNELL. 1992. "The View of Surgery from Space." *Archives of Surgery* 127, no. 5:511–515.

ZIMMERMAN, LEO M., and VEITH, ILZA. 1967. *Great Ideas in the History of Surgery.* 2d rev. ed. New York: Dover.

# SURROGACY

*See* REPRODUCTIVE TECHNOLOGIES, *articles on* SURROGACY, ETHICAL ISSUES, *and* LEGAL AND REGULATORY ISSUES.

# SURROGATE DECISION MAKING

*See* DEATH AND DYING: EUTHANASIA AND SUSTAINING LIFE, *articles on* ETHICAL ISSUES, *and* PROFESSIONAL AND PUBLIC POLICIES. *See also* CHILDREN, *article on* HEALTH-CARE AND RESEARCH ISSUES.

# SUSTAINABLE DEVELOPMENT

The idea of sustainable development dominates late-twentieth-century discussions of environment and development policy. It is a key term in international treaties, covenants, and programs and is being written into the constitutions of nation-states. An immense literature has gathered around it (Marien, 1992). Even those who reject the term must define their views in reference to it. In spite of this influence, serious empirical, conceptual, and normative problems must be addressed if the term is to serve as a comprehensive framework for efforts to sustain the biosphere and advance human fulfillment, economic security, and social justice throughout the world.

## The appeal of sustainable development

If the peoples of the world are to cooperate in solving their economic, social, and environmental problems, they must share a common understanding of the relationships among these problems and a common vision of a sustainable and just future. The economic expansion that began in the West several centuries ago has spread to embrace the world, transforming all societies in its wake and creating a global economic system and attendant monoculture with powerful human and environmental impacts. Given the dominance of this system, there needs to be a comprehensive policy framework to guide it—even if the framework adopted is critical of the system itself and seeks to redirect or even dismantle it.

Sustainable development is an appealing candidate for this office. "The key element of sustainable development is the recognition that economic and environmental goals are inextricably linked" (National Commission on the Environment, 1993, p. 2). This premise, bolstered by empirical claims that poverty and environmental degradation feed one another and that conservation need not constrain development nor development result in environmental degradation, has obvious political advantages. It allows persons with conflicting positions in the environment–development debate to search for common ground without appearing to compromise their positions. New coalitions of nongovernmental organizations (NGOs) concerned for justice, population, environment, and development issues have formed under the flag of sustainable development. Business leaders have come forward to propose new business-to-business and business-to-government partnerships in the name of sustainable development (International Chamber of Commerce, 1991; Schmidheiny, 1992). In addition, sustainable development has broad moral appeal among those motivated by concern for present as well as future generations, since it purports to be the

name for a process and a future state in which everyone and the environment as a whole will benefit.

"Sustainable" qualifies the idea of development. After World War II it was widely assumed that economic development would lead to greater freedom, justice, and security for the world's peoples. When environmental issues first appeared on the international agenda at the Stockholm Conference on the Human Environment in 1972, the debate was whether—and how—concerns for environment and equity could be reconciled with economic development. In succeeding years, as economic development strategies failed to close the gap between rich and poor, within or between nations, and studies showed growth in world population and consumption approaching Earth's biophysical limits, questions were raised about whether the theory of development could serve either human or environmental needs and whether it did not need to be modified to include ecological, political, social, cultural, and spiritual considerations.

By 1992, for most participants at the World Conference on Environment and Development (UNCED) held at Rio de Janeiro, these issues appeared settled. The principal agreement of the conference, *Agenda 21*, affirms that "integration of environment and development . . . will lead to the fulfillment of basic needs, improved living standards for all, better protected and managed ecosystems and a safer, more prosperous future. No nation can achieve this on its own; but together we can—in a global partnership for sustainable development" (United Nations, 1993, p. 15).

This entry analyzes why the concept of sustainable development occupies the center of thought on development and environment policy, how it is being defined, what criticisms are being raised about it, and what kind of work is needed if the concept truly is to meet the needs of the planet.

Sustainable development nicely expresses the progressive evolutionary worldview that emerged in the West in the late nineteenth century, with all the presumed objective support of the natural sciences, and the positive attitude toward social change often associated with it (Esteva, 1992). This progressivist ideology recognizes the problems posed by the interactions of population growth, resource use, and environmental degradation but is guardedly optimistic about the capacities of modern societies to solve those problems, given public understanding, technological and structural improvements in keeping with sound scientific research, and strong political leadership. As the Stockholm Declaration affirmed: "[T]he capability of man to improve the environment increases with each passing day" (Weston et al., 1980, p. 344).

The discourse of sustainable development thus occupies a middle-of-the-road position between those perspectives that take an uncritically optimistic attitude toward growth and technological change and those that predict the inevitability of global collapse. It also confirms the liberal insistence that the meaning of the goal of human development, fulfillment, or quality of life be stated in purely formal terms so that individuals and groups have the opportunity to define it for themselves (Kidd, 1992).

## The meaning of sustainable development

Mainstream thinking on sustainable development views it as a form of societal change that adds the objective or constraint of resource sustainability to the traditional development objective of meeting basic human needs (Lélé, 1991). "Mainstream thinking" refers to those ideological frameworks typical of international environmental agencies such as the United Nations Environment Programme (UNEP); international development agencies, including the World Bank; research organizations such as the International Institute for Environment and Development; and NGOs such as the Washington-based Global Tomorrow Coalition.

The concept of resource sustainability originated in the late nineteenth century in the context of renewable resources such as forests or fisheries, where it informed such ideas as "maximum sustainable yield." When the language of "sustainable development" came into international usage with the publication by the International Union for the Conservation of Nature and Natural Resources (IUCN), UNEP, and the World Wildlife Fund (WWF) of the *World Conservation Strategy* in 1980, this original meaning was retained but broadened to include the maintenance of ecosystem "carrying capacity" and the management and conservation of all living resources as a necessary prerequisite to development. Thus a clear line of intellectual (and often institutional and professional) descent runs from Gifford Pinchot, the first director of the U.S. Forest Service, and other turn-of-the-century advocates of the "resource conservation ethic" in Europe and the United States, to contemporary mainstream thought on sustainable development. Pinchot's utilitarian notion that "conservation . . . stands for development . . . the use of natural resources . . . for the greatest number for the longest time" remains at the root of contemporary thinking on sustainable development (Pinchot, 1910, pp. 42–48).

It is possible to interpret "sustainable development" literally to mean sustaining indefinitely the process of economic growth, change, or development. But this viewpoint is not representative of the U.N. World Commission on Environment and Development, chaired by Gro Harlem Brundtland, prime minister of Norway, the group most responsible for marshaling the data, argument, and political influence necessary to put the term on the agenda of international debate. In the commis-

sion's view, although a new era of more efficient technological and economic growth is needed in order to break the link of poverty and environmental degradation, "ultimate limits [to usable resources] exist" and indefinite economic expansion is therefore impossible (World Commission on Environment and Development, 1987, pp. 8–9).

Nonetheless, like the goal of equity, the prerequisite of ecological sustainability is often either downplayed or presumed, as in the classic definition offered by the World Commission on Environment and Development: "Sustainable development is development that meets the needs of the present without compromising the ability of future generations to meet their own needs" (World Commission on Environment and Development, 1987, p. 43). Ecological sustainability is more likely to be mentioned in a list of "requirements" of sustainable development, such as those composed by the organizers of the Ottawa Conference on Conservation and Development in 1986 (Jacobs and Munro, 1987):

- integration of conservation and development
- satisfaction of basic human needs
- achievement of equity and social justice
- provision for social self-determination and cultural diversity
- maintenance of ecological integrity

## Issues of sustainable development

For many critics, sustainable development lacks clarity of definition, including criteria for and examples of successful achievement (Yanarella and Levine, 1992). As early as 1984, UNEP Executive Director Mostafa K. Tolba lamented that sustainable development had become "an article of faith, a shibboleth; often used, but little explained" (Lélé, 1991, p. 607). A recent survey of the literature on sustainable development found that "case studies are surprisingly few and often hard to come by" (Slocombe et al., 1993). It is notable that the second version of the World Conservation Strategy, *Caring for the Earth*, acknowledges the ambiguity of the term, and places its emphasis on "building a sustainable society" (ICUN, UNEP, WWF, 1991).

For other critics, the concept of sustainable development is all too clear and fundamentally mistaken. Negative critiques of sustainable development cluster around its (1) empirical accuracy; (2) idea of justice; (3) idea of sustainability; (4) economic assumptions; (5) view of science; and (6) metaphorical and spiritual assumptions.

**Empirical accuracy.**    The empirical basis of sustainable development thinking is criticized both for its analysis of the problems of poverty and environmental degradation and for its proposed solutions to them. Thijs de la Court (1990) and Richard B. Norgaard (1988a), among others, argue that mainstream thinking typically ignores the two major factors responsible for both of these problems—the shift of local economies to production of exports for the world market and the adoption by traditional societies of the values of Western urban and capitalist society. Thus global free trade, the solution often offered by sustainable development proponents as the way to greater integration of the local community into the world economic system, will only intensify the problems, lending support to massive, hierarchically managed, capital-intensive industrial projects—dams, plantations, factories, urban settlements—that destroy the diversity and integrity of human communities and environments alike (Sachs, 1993). Nor will most of the other policies typically promoted in the name of sustainable development be of much help: more scientific data, more efficient technology, improved managerial capabilities, and more effective environmental education. Much more fundamental and difficult actions are necessary, such as community control of the economy, land reform, changes in cultural values, and reductions in the consumption of industrial commodities and in birthrates (Lélé, 1991).

**Social justice.**    Most pronouncements on sustainable development hold that social justice, especially in the form of equity between wealthy and poor nations, is essential to the process. Critics contend that these ideas are seldom explicated in any detail, however. The issue of population stabilization is generally avoided, conflicting claims of intragenerational versus intergenerational equity are not addressed, and fundamental civil and political rights are seldom mentioned. In keeping with traditional development theory, there is abstract emphasis on meeting "basic human needs" and, in recent years, "participation of all stakeholders," but it is seldom clear what these needs are, which ones should have priority, what kind of participation is required, or how sustainable development will result in greater justice or environmental protection.

These questions have become especially acute in the sphere of gender. One of the primary challenges to mainstream thinking on sustainable development has come from the international women's movement through organizations such as INSTRAW (United Nations International Research and Training Institute for the Advancement of Women) and ecofeminist theoretical perspectives, such as those of Vandana Shiva and Maria Mies (Braidotti et al., 1994). Within the women's movement there is widespread recognition of the deep-seated patriarchal assumptions in development discourse and the connections between the destruction of nature and the exploitation of women and other marginal groups in the development process. Mainstream sustainable development theory does little to change this. *Agenda 21*, the blueprint for sustainable development

adopted by the United Nations Conference on Environment and Development in 1992, retains a patriarchal orientation, evident in its failure to recognize the special role of "subdominants"—women, people of color, children, native and indigenous people—in each of its seven major themes (Warren, 1994). In order to address this problem, the Women's Environmental and Development Organization (WEDO) and other organizations have argued for the need for women to gain control over natural resources and the benefits that are derived from them and for recognition of women's special knowledge and skills in environmental care.

**Idea of sustainability.**    Environmental ethicists and scientific ecologists are critical of the idea of sustainable development because of its reductionist approach to environmental values. Discussions of sustainable development typically assume that what needs to be sustained is human use, especially human agricultural use and industrial production. Yet instrumental value is only one of the many environmental values that need to be sustained in the complex interplay of human enjoyment, respect, use, and care of nature, and there is empirical evidence that single-minded pursuit of instrumental value through such policies, for example, as "maximum sustainable yield" seldom succeeds (Ludwig et al., 1993). *Agenda 21* is criticized for its exclusive concentration on the need to sustain the environment for human use. Chapter 15, for example, argues that the primary reason for preserving biodiversity is that it provides a potential source of genetic materials for biotechnological development (Sagoff, 1994). This emphasis reflects a strong anthropocentric value orientation, explicit in Principle 1 of the Rio Declaration on Environment and Development: "Human beings are at the centre of concerns for sustainable development" (United Nations, 1993, p. 9).

In an unprecedented policy decision in 1991, the Ecological Society of America challenged the widely held assumption that what ought to be sustained is human use of the biosphere. It set the goal of a "sustainable biosphere" as its priority for research in ecology in the closing decade of the twentieth century, thus implying that the biosphere has value in and for itself and that above all else this is the value that must be sustained (Risser et al., 1991).

Failure to recognize that nature has value of its own (as well as for the sake of humans) has serious practical consequences. Not only does it inhibit acceptance of the idea of sustainable development by many environmental and religious groups whose traditions embrace a more generous understanding of nature's values, but it eliminates consideration of those meanings of sustainability having to do with the way life nourishes life—with sustenance. Certain methods of subsistence agriculture, for example, built up over many generations, especially by women, simultaneously nourish human communities and the soil, yet fail to receive public recognition and support (Shiva, 1988).

**Economic assumptions.**    Criticisms of the economic analysis and prescriptions of sustainable development thinking have been suggested above and may be summarized under two primary headings. First, and most generally, are those criticisms that find in the idea of sustainable development only another example of the triumph of *homo economicus* in modern society. There is a prevalent assumption that sustainable development is equivalent to sustainable *economic* development. Thus economists at the International Institute for Environment and Development argue in circular fashion that their "sustainability paradigm," a version of the "conventional economic paradigm, illustrated by utilitarian benefit–cost analysis," if modified to allow for the concept of intergenerational equity, is preferable to the "bioethics paradigm" that recognizes intrinsic values in nature, because, among other things, the latter "inhibits [economic] development" (Turner and Pearce, 1990, p. 2).

The second sort of criticism concentrates on the failure of sustainable development thinking to challenge the assumption that economic growth can break the link between poverty and environmental degradation. Although the Brundtland commission recognized "ultimate limits," it nonetheless recommended a five- to tenfold increase in global economic productivity to reduce poverty and provide the resources for environmental protection (World Commission on Environment and Development, 1987). Ecological economists such as Herman Daly point out the biophysical impossibility of such growth and the need to arrest, or even reduce, the total "throughput" or flow of matter-energy, from natural sources, through the human economy, and back to nature's sinks. They believe that a strict distinction should be made between "growth," defined as "quantitative expansion in the scale of the physical dimensions of the economic system," which cannot be sustained indefinitely, and "development," defined as the "qualitative change of a physically nongrowing economic system in dynamic equilibrium with the environment," which can be so sustained (Daly and Cobb, 1989, p. 71). In their view, limited progress can be made in arresting economic growth by enforcing accepted maxims of sound economics, for example, increased resource efficiency and environmental accounting to show how income is actually a drawdown of natural capital or stock resources. Such measures alone, however, will be insufficient without redistribution of wealth and income between nations and classes, as well as population stabilization.

**View of science.**    Mainstream sustainable development thinking is dominated by the policy languages of science, economics, and law. Typical of such discourse is the view that science can provide a value-neutral definition of sustainability acceptable to persons with widely differing value perspectives (Brooks, 1992). But critics point to hidden norms in scientific methodology that support the status quo and are inconsistent with the personal and political transformations needed for justice and care of Earth. Moreover, only a very narrow range of considerations can be scientifically determined, thereby effectively eliminating challenges to established value judgments. In addition, the use of "risk analysis" focuses on involuntary costs that ecological changes may impose on society rather than on what should be the most important concern: the altering of ecosystems that risk-free business-as-usual will effectuate (Sagoff, 1994). Donald Ludwig, Ray Hilborn, and Carl Walters (1993) argue that the history of resource exploitation teaches the necessity of action before scientific consensus is achieved and that while science can help recognize problems, it cannot provide solutions. They caution that spending money on more scientific research is often a way to avoid addressing problems of population growth and excessive use of resources.

**Metaphorical and spiritual assumptions.** Some critics consider the concept of "development" a dangerous mystification of history and do not believe adding the adjective "sustainable" appreciably alters the difficulty. Biologically speaking, "development" means progress from earlier to later, or from simpler to more complex, stages in the growth of an organism. In post–World War II development discourse, it was used as a metaphor for the transition of traditional societies into modern industrial societies (leading to distinctions between "underdeveloped," "developing," and "developed" societies). Used in this way, the metaphor implies a step forward in a linear progression, a natural, organic flowering, rather than a deliberate, culturally specific invention. It also implies that the most modern nations, such as the United States, are the most civilized and therefore models to imitate. Adding "sustainable" to "development" only confirms these biological connotations and hence strengthens its potential to obscure differences among cultures and the drawbacks of modernization.

But more than a misplaced analogy is at issue. "Development" is a powerful secular religion, in the words of Peter Berger, "the focus of redemptive hopes and expectations" (Berger, 1976, p. 17). Viewed in these terms, "development" means more than an improvement in material living standards. Development as religion means that human fulfillment is to be found in activities that improve material living conditions, for oneself and for others. Development as religion is a messianic mission to bring the fruits of material progress to the world, and it is questionable whether the idea of "sustainable development" substantially changes this. To depart from the religion of development would require defining the ends of development in terms of qualitative, as well as quantitative, goods—goods such as truth, beauty, freedom, friendship, humility, simplicity. Not only are such moral and spiritual goods the most worthy ends of human life; they may be the only way to empower persons to reduce their consumption, limit their procreation, and live sustainable lives (Goulet, 1990).

## The future of sustainable development

Given the value placed upon unthrottled economic growth in industrial and nonindustrial societies alike, acceptance of the goal of sustainable development, even in a weak sense, is a remarkable and positive step (Marien, 1992). Moreover, acceptance of the idea of sustainable development in international circles and by the government, business, and NGO leadership of many nations, north and south, means that there now exists an opportunity for dialogue and new social compacts between diverse political constituencies. It is possible to argue, therefore, that the idea of sustainable development offers a realistic way of effecting a potentially radical transformation in global environment and development policy. The question is whether (1) these diverse constituencies can be engaged in a process of mutual inquiry, criticism, and discussion that will lead, step by step, toward improvements in the empirical, conceptual, and normative adequacy of the idea and in meaningful attempts to embody it in practice; and (2) an international political constituency, uniting mainstream and marginal groups and actors, can be mobilized to challenge the entrenched powers that will inevitably be threatened by changes in policy. There is also the question of whether these things can happen quickly enough, before disillusionment sets in and a fragile consensus is shattered. There are several ways of advancing this kind of agenda over the next decade.

Empirical understanding of sustainable development will improve with a more issue-driven and democratically structured scientific approach that recognizes the uncertainty of facts, conflicts in values, and the urgency of decisions. Such an approach needs to be transdisciplinary and practically focused on the dynamics responsible for poverty, injustice, and environmental degradation and on how these dynamics may be changed without economic growth through resource depletion. It requires analyses of factors such as human motivation and ownership patterns, neglected in most studies to date. Studies of alternative development policies in the Indian state of Kerala present good examples (Franke and Chasin, 1992).

Empirical adequacy also will improve through initiatives such as those now underway to design quantitative "indicators" of sustainability (Trzyna, 1994),

especially those indexes that can challenge, and eventually replace, the Gross National Product (GNP) as the measure of economic and social well-being. For example, Daly and Cobb (1989) propose an Index of Sustainable Economic Welfare that measures not only levels of consumption but also income distribution, natural resource depletion, and environmental damage. Macroeconomic criteria and indicators of sustainability have been proposed in areas such as population stability, greenhouse gases, soil degradation, and preservation of natural ecosystems (Ayres, 1991). Specific moral and material incentives to meet these criteria are also being developed (Goulet, 1989).

The conceptual and normative adequacy of the idea of sustainable development will improve as it is expanded to include the full range of moral and public-policy criteria necessary to sustain the biosphere and advance human fulfillment, economic security, and social justice throughout the world (Corson, 1994). Such a redefinition of the goals of sustainable development will need to include (1) development conceived primarily as improvement in the quality of human life; (2) sustainability conceived as the sustainability of Earth's biosphere, with protection and restoration of ecosystems and biodiversity and sustainable use of renewable resources contributing to that end; (3) the transition to a steady-state global economy by reducing consumption among affluent classes while at the same time promoting economic growth in poor communities to meet basic human needs and provide the resources necessary for environmental protection; (4) redistribution of wealth and income between rich and poor nations; (5) population stabilization and eventual reduction to more optimal levels; (6) guarantees of basic human rights, including environmental rights, to all persons, with special attention to the empowerment of women and children; (7) new nondominating and nonreductionsitic ways of producing and transmitting knowledge of the environment and sustainable livelihood; and (8) freedom for local cultures, Western and non-Western, to pursue a variety of alternative visions and strategies of sustainable development.

The philosophy of sustainable development will also improve as discussion moves beyond the confines of economics and resource management into larger multidisciplinary and public arenas. Most mainstream thought on sustainable development has taken place without the benefit of philosophy, theology, the arts, or humanities and with only limited benefit from scientific ecology. Yet intellectual leaders in these fields, from diverse cultures and faiths throughout the world, have been trying to understand the meaning of just, participatory, and sustainable ways of life for several decades (Engel and Engel, 1990). Citizens also have substantial contributions to make to an enlarged understanding of sustainable development, as the peoples' alternative treaties signed at the NGO-led Global Forum at Rio de Janiero demonstrate (Rome et al., 1992).

Nowhere is the challenge to mainstream sustainable development thinking more difficult—or more fateful—than in the area of comprehensive spiritual values and morals. In 1987 the U.N. Commission on Environment and Development concluded that "human survival and well-being could depend on success in elevating sustainable development to a global ethic" (World Commission on Environment and Development, 1987, p. 308). Faced with the prospect that the mainstream interpretation of sustainable development might well become a global ethic, critics argue for what they believe to be more adequate understandings of human nature and destiny, calling instead for "authentic development," "just, participatory ecodevelopment," or simply "good life." Sustainable development need not be anthropocentric or androcentric; it may be theocentric or coevolutionary (Norgaard, 1988b), a human activity that nourishes and perpetuates the historical fulfillment of the whole community of life on Earth.

J. RONALD ENGEL

*Directly related to this entry are the entries* FUTURE GENERATIONS, OBLIGATIONS TO; ENVIRONMENTAL HEALTH; ENDANGERED SPECIES AND BIODIVERSITY; ENVIRONMENTAL ETHICS; ENVIRONMENTAL POLICY AND LAW; POPULATION ETHICS; *and* POPULATION POLICIES. *For a further discussion of topics mentioned in this entry, see the entries* AGRICULTURE; CLIMATIC CHANGE; ETHICS; FOOD POLICY; HARM; JUSTICE; LIFESTYLES AND PUBLIC HEALTH; METAPHOR AND ANALOGY; NATURE; OBLIGATION AND SUPEREROGATION; PATERNALISM; PUBLIC HEALTH; RESPONSIBILITY; UTILITY; *and* VALUE AND VALUATION. *Other relevant material may be found under the entries* LAW AND MORALITY; TAOISM; *and* TECHNOLOGY.

## Bibliography

AYRES, ROBERT U. 1991. *Eco-Restructuring: The Transition to an Ecologically Sustainable Economy.* Fontainebleau, France: INSEAD.

BERGER, PETER. 1976. *Pyramids of Sacrifice: Political Ethics and Social Change.* Garden City, N.Y.: Anchor/Doubleday.

BRAIDOTTI, ROSI; CHARKIEWICZ, EWA; HAUSLER, SABINE; and WIERINGA, SASKIA. 1994. *Women, the Environment and Sustainable Development: Towards a Theoretical Synthesis.* London: Zed and INSTRAW.

BROOKS, HARVEY. 1992. "The Concepts of Sustainable Development and Environmentally Sound Technology." *ATAS Bulletin* 7:19–24.

COBB, JOHN B., JR. 1992. *Sustainability: Economics, Ecology, and Justice.* Maryknoll, N.Y.: Orbis.

CORSON, WALTER H. 1994. "Changing Course: An Outline of Strategies for a Sustainable Future." *Futures* 26, no. 2:206–223.

DALY, HERMAN E.; COBB, JOHN B., JR.; and COBB, CLIFFORD W. 1989. *For the Common Good: Redirecting the Economy Toward Community, the Environment, and a Sustainable Future.* Boston: Beacon Press.

DE LA COURT, THIJS. 1990. *Beyond Brundtland: Green Development in the 1990s.* New York: New Horizons.

ENGEL, J. RONALD, and ENGEL, JOAN GIBB, eds. 1990. *Ethics of Environment and Development: Global Challenge, International Response.* Tucson: University of Arizona Press.

ESTEVA, GUSTAVO. 1992. "Development." In *The Development Dictionary: A Guide to Knowledge as Power,* pp. 6–25. Edited by Wolfgang Sachs. London: Zed.

FRANKE, RICHARD W., and CHASIN, BARBARA H. 1992. *Kerala: Development Through Radical Reform.* New Delhi: Promilla.

GOULET, DENIS. 1989. *Incentives for Development: The Key to Equity.* New York: New Horizons.

———. 1990. "Development Ethics and Ecological Wisdom." In *Ethics of Environment and Development: Global Challenge, International Response,* pp. 36–49. Edited by J. Ronald Engel and Joan Gibb Engel. Tucson: University of Arizona Press.

INTERNATIONAL CHAMBER OF COMMERCE. 1991. *The Business Charter for Sustainable Development.* Paris: Author.

INTERNATIONAL UNION FOR THE CONSERVATION OF NATURE AND NATURAL RESOURCES (IUCN); UNITED NATIONS ENVIRONMENTAL PROGRAMME (UNEP); and WORLD WILDLIFE FUND (WWF). 1980. *World Conservation Strategy.* Gland, Switzerland: IUCN.

———. 1991. *Caring for the Earth: A Strategy for Sustainable Living.* Gland, Switzerland: IUCN.

JACOBS, PETER, and MUNRO, DAVID A., eds. 1987. *Conservation with Equity: Strategies for Sustainable Development.* Gland, Switzerland: IUCN.

KIDD, CHARLES V. 1992. "The Evolution of Sustainability." *Journal of Agricultural and Environmental Ethics* 5, no. 1: 1–26.

LÉLÉ, SHARACHCHANDRA M. 1991. "Sustainable Development: A Critical Review." *World Development* 19, no. 6: 607–621.

LUDWIG, DONALD; HILBORN, RAY; and WALTERS, CARL. 1993. "Uncertainty, Resource Exploitation, and Conservation: Lessons from History." *Science* 260, no. 5104: 17, 36.

MARIEN, MICHAEL. 1992. "Environmental Problems and Sustainable Futures." *Futures* 24, no. 8:731–757.

NATIONAL COMMISSION ON THE ENVIRONMENT. 1993. *Choosing a Sustainable Future: The Report of the National Commission on the Environment.* Washington, D.C.: Island Press.

NORGAARD, RICHARD B. 1988a. "The Rise of the Global Exchange Economy and the Loss of Biological Diversity." In *Biodiversity,* pp. 206–211. Edited by Edward O. Wilson and Frances H. Peter. Washington, D.C.: National Academy Press.

———. 1988b. "Sustainable Development: A Co-evolutionary View." *Futures* 20, no. 6:606–619.

PINCHOT, GIFFORD. 1910. *The Fight for Conservation*. New York: Doubleday, Page.

RISSER, PAUL G.; LUBCHENCO, JANE; and LEVIN, SIMON A. 1991. "Biological Research Priorities—a Sustainable Biosphere." *BioScience* 41, no. 9:625–627.

ROME, ALEXANDRA; PATTON, SHARYLE; and LERNER, MICHAEL, eds. 1992. *The Peoples' Treaties from the Earth Summit*. Bolinas, Calif.: Commonweal Sustainable Futures Group, Common Knowledge Press.

SACHS, WOLFGANG, ed. 1993. *Global Ecology: A New Arena of Political Conflict*. London: Zed.

SAGOFF, MARK. 1994. "Biodiversity and Agenda 21: Ethical Considerations." In *Proceedings from the Conference on the Ethical Dimensions of the United Nations Programme on Environment and Development, January, 1994, at the United Nations, New York*, pp. 289–300. Edited by Donald A. Brown. Harrisburg, Pa.: Earth Ethics Research Group Northeast.

SCHMIDHEINY, STEPHAN. 1992. "The Business of Sustainable Development." *Finance and Development* 29, no. 4:24–27.

SHIVA, VANDANA. 1988. *Staying Alive: Woman, Ecology and Development*. London: Zed.

SLOCOMBE, D. SCOTT; ROELOF, JULIA K.; CHEYNE, LIRONDEL C.; TERRY, SUSAN NOALANI; and OUDEN, SUZANNE DEN, eds. 1993. *What Works: An Annotated Bibliography of Case Studies of Sustainable Development*. Sacramento, Calif.: International Center for the Environment and Public Policy.

TRZYNA, THADDEUS C., ed. 1994. *Indicators of Sustainability*. Sacramento, Calif.: International Center for the Environment and Public Policy.

TURNER, R. KERRY, and PEARCE, DAVID W. 1990. *The Ethical Foundations of Sustainable Economic Development*. London: International Institute for Environment and Development.

UNITED NATIONS. 1993. *Agenda 21: The United Nations Programme of Action from Rio*. New York: U.N. Department of Public Information.

WARREN, KAREN J. 1994. "Eco-feminism and Agenda 21." In *Proceedings from the Conference on the Ethical Dimensions of the United Nations Programme on Environment and Development, January, 1994, at the United Nations, New York*, pp. 321–338. Edited by Donald A. Brown. Harrisburg, Pa.: Earth Ethics Research Group Northeast.

WESTON, BURNS H.; FALK, RICHARD A.; and D'AMATO, ANTHONY A., eds. 1980. *Basic Documents in International Law and World Order*. St. Paul, Minn.: West.

WORLD COMMISSION ON ENVIRONMENT AND DEVELOPMENT [BRUNDTLAND COMMISSION]. 1987. *Our Common Future*. Oxford: Oxford University Press.

# SWEDEN

*See* MEDICAL ETHICS, HISTORY OF, *section on* EUROPE, *subsection on* CONTEMPORARY PERIOD, *article on* NORDIC COUNTRIES.

# SWITZERLAND

*See* MEDICAL ETHICS, HISTORY OF, *section on* EUROPE, *subsection on* CONTEMPORARY PERIOD, *article on* GERMAN-SPEAKING COUNTRIES AND SWITZERLAND.

# T

## TAOISM

Taoism is an ancient and multifaceted element of traditional Chinese culture. Its origins and scope are debated by modern scholars, Chinese and Western alike. Most understand "Taoism" in terms of the naturalistic thought seen in ancient texts like those of Lao-tzu (the *Tao te ching*) and Chuang-tzu (see Lau, 1982; Graham, 1981). But to others, "Taoism" denotes primarily a religious tradition that emerged around the second century C.E. and has endured to the present (Seidel, 1990; Robinet, 1991, 1993). Specialists today generally employ a comprehensive approach, interpreting both of those elements as aspects of a broad and inclusive cultural tradition, interwoven both historically and thematically (Schipper, 1993).

Taoism may be characterized as a holistic worldview and ethos, including a variety of interrelated moral and religious values and practices. Taoism lacks any coherent conceptual structure, so there have never been any "Taoist positions" regarding ethics or any other issues. Yet, most segments of the tradition share certain assumptions and concerns. One is an assumption that human reality is ultimately grounded in deeper realities; humans are components of a cosmos, a harmonious universe in which all things are subtly but profoundly interrelated (Kirkland, 1993). Taoism is devoted to the pursuit of greater integration with the cosmos, in social as well as individual terms. Taoists vary widely in their understandings of how that integration is best expressed and pursued.

The first section of this entry outlines the elements of classical "Lao-Chuang" Taoism, and the history, teachings, and practices of the much-misunderstood "Taoist religion." The subsequent exploration of the Taoist moral life focuses upon (1) the ideals of refinement (*lien*) and "fostering life"; (2) the ideals of balance and harmony; and (3) the issue of death. Throughout, one should bear clearly in mind that many issues that are considered central in contemporary bioethical debate are completely alien to the traditional Taoist worldview. Taoists not only lacked the concepts of "good" and "evil," but they were simply never interested in arguments over "right or wrong" on any terms. One should thus beware assuming that contemporary issues could ever be translatable into Taoist terms.

### The Taoist heritage

**Classical themes.** In the ancient texts *Lao-tzu* and *Chuang-tzu*, integration with the cosmos is generally expressed in terms of returning to the natural rhythm or flow of life—to the Tao, an impersonal reality that constitutes simultaneously the source of the cosmos, the subtle structures of the cosmos in its pristine state, and the salutary natural forces that—in that pristine state—maintain all things in a natural and healthy alignment. In "Lao-Chuang" Taoism, all the world's problems are attributed to humanity's digression from the Tao, particularly to a loss of proper perspective upon the nature of reality. The goal of Lao-Chuang Taoism is to regain that perspective and thereby return to the original integration with the natural world and its constituent forces and processes. The eponymous Lao-Chuang texts are vague about the means to be employed in achieving that end. Later Lao-Chuang writings (e.g., in texts like the *Kuan-tzu* and *Huai-nan-tzu*) present a more detailed analysis of the human constitution, and suggest specific spiritual and physiological practices to reintegrate the individual and realign him or her with the natural forces of the cosmos (Roth, 1991). Suffice it to note that all such theory assumes none of the dichotomies of mind/matter or body/spirit that underlie much of Western medicine and moral theory. Moreover, it is a mistake to assume (as do most in twentieth-century Asia and the West) that Taoism was essentially individualistic: the basic Lao-Chuang writings (most notably the *Tao te ching*) often addressed broader problems of human society in both moral and political terms. The later Taoist tradition is generally an extension of the ideals and values seen in these earlier writings.

**The Taoist religious tradition: New perspectives.** Until recently, virtually all educated people dismissed postclassical Taoism (often misnamed "popular Taoism") as a mass of disreputable superstitions created and perpetuated by the ignorant masses. Such was certainly *not* the case. The problem is that before the 1970s, few intellectuals, Chinese or Western, had any firsthand knowledge of later Taoism, in terms of either its modern practice or its historical tradition. As scholars began serious analysis of the Taoist texts preserved in the massive collection known as the *Tao-tsang*, and researched the roles that Taoism played in traditional Chinese history and society, they started to develop a far different perspective, though this new perspective has yet to reach the educated public.

Until the 1980s, religious Taoism was often said to have been focused on individual practices intended to confer longevity and/or physical immortality. The pursuit of physical longevity did exist in China from early times, but it is wrong to associate such pursuits with "religious Taoism."

> Western scholars generally have placed emphasis on certain practices or crafts that they suppose have been particularly "Taoist," notably the quest for physical immortality, breath control, techniques of sexual union, herbalism, dietetics, and alchemy. In such a view, though, as in the question of doctrine in general, there is some ambiguity between what is specifically Taoist and what is simply Chinese. (Strickman, 1980, pp. 1044–1045)

Extensive research has generally demonstrated that such practices have little or no intrinsic connection to the traditions of religious Taoism.

**The evolution of the Taoist religion.** The Taoist religion has been compared to a river formed by the confluence of many streams. Its origins lie in the Han dynasty (206 B.C.E.–221 C.E.). During that period, Chinese intellectuals (like the Confucian theorist Tung

Chung-shu) were seeking a comprehensive explanation for worldly events. From such roots, imperial advisers called *fang-shih* produced a series of sacred texts that culminated in the *T'ai-p'ing ching*, which is generally regarded as the first Taoist scripture. According to the *T'ai-p'ing ching*, ancient rulers had maintained an "ambience of Grand Tranquillity" (*t'ai-p'ing*) by observing *wu-wei* (nonaction)—a behavioral ideal of avoiding purposive action and trusting instead to the world's natural order (the Tao). When later rulers meddled with the world, the "Grand Tranquillity" was disrupted. Now, the scripture says, one must return to the Tao by looking within oneself. The text provides specific directions for pursuing union with the Tao, including moral injunctions and instructions for meditation, as well as recommendations for enhancing one's health and longevity through hygienic practices (such as breath control), medicine, acupuncture, and even music therapy. The focus of the *T'ai-p'ing ching* is thus upon providing the people with practical advice for reintegrating with the natural order (Kaltenmark, 1979).

In late Han times, the *T'ai-p'ing ching* helped inspire several social movements. One was led by Chang Tao-ling, who claimed to have received a divine mandate to replace the now-effete Han government with a new social order. Claiming the mantle of "Celestial Master," Chang and his heirs oversaw a religious organization in which male and female priests healed the sick by performing expiatory rituals. This organization, generally called "Celestial Master Taoism," was based on the idea that a healthy society depended upon the moral, physical, and spiritual health of all its members.

In the fourth century C.E., northern China was invaded by peoples from the northern steppes, and the leaders of the Celestial Master movement fled south. There they found a rich indigenous religious culture centered upon the pursuit of personal perfection through ritual activity. Unlike the Celestial Master tradition, the religion of southern China took little interest in ideals of a healthy society: its focus was almost exclusively upon the individual. Modern writers, Chinese and Western, have often mistakenly cited certain of its texts (like the *Pao-p'u-tzu* of the maverick Confucian Ko Hung) as representative of religious Taoism. In so doing, they have completely neglected the rich heritage of the *T'ai-p'ing ching* and most of the subsequent Taoist tradition.

The fourth century C.E. was a period of rich interaction among such diverse traditions, and there were two new developments, both of which occurred as the result of revelations from celestial beings. The first, known as the Shang-ch'ing (Supreme Purity) revelation, was received from angelic beings called "Perfected Ones" who dwelt in distant heavens of that name. The Perfected Ones revealed methods by which the diligent practitioner could ascend to their heavens, particularly visualizational meditation (Robinet, 1993). But Shang-ch'ing Taoism also subsumed the older southern pursuit of personal perfection through alchemy, a transformative spiritual process expressed in chemical terms. Alchemy, often misrepresented as a "typical" element of religious Taoism, actually arose quite independently, though it was embraced by certain Shang-ch'ing Taoists as a practice thought to elevate the aspirant's spiritual state for eventual ascent to the heavens (Strickmann, 1979). What the alchemical tradition shared with Taoism was a vital concern with self-perfection based on an assumption that the individual's being is a unified whole. For exceptional aspirants, alchemy provided secret knowledge that permitted control of the forces of the cosmos that inhere within the constitution of the individual. Outsiders often misunderstood the whole undertaking as a pursuit of physical longevity. But within Taoism, alchemy was actually a method of moral and spiritual self-reinfement: through proper knowledge and action, one could pare away the grosser elements of one's being and eventually ascend to a higher plane of existence. Nonetheless, alchemy was, for most, a purely theoretical interest. The "average" Taoist practiced meditation and morality, and in later ages Taoists discarded the theory of "external alchemy" in favor of "inner alchemy"—a meditative pursuit of reunion with the Tao that employed the language of alchemy metaphorically.

The Shang-ch'ing revelations were immediately followed by a quite different set of revelations, known by the term Ling-pao (Numinous Treasure). Ling-pao Taoism is distinguished by (1) elements influenced by Mahāyāna Buddhism, and (2) a renewed concern with the human community. Ling-pao scriptures (such as the *Tu-jen ching*, "Scripture for Human Salvation") tell of a great cosmic deity—a personification of the Tao—who is concerned to save humanity. By ritual recitation of the scripture, one may participate in its salvific power. In the fifth century, the Ling-pao tradition was refocused by Lu Hsiu-ching, who reconfigured its ritual activities and formulated a new set of liturgies that continue to influence contemporary Taoist practice. A central liturgy is the *chiao*, a lengthy series of rituals that renew the local community by reintegrating it with the heavenly order. Other liturgies, called *chai*, had diverse aims. One was designed to prevent disease by expiating moral transgressions through communal confession. Another labored for the salvation of deceased ancestors. A third was intended to forestall natural disasters and reintegrate the sociopolitical order with the cosmos. Through these liturgies, Taoism incorporated ritual frameworks from all segments of society, from the imperial court to the local village, and unified them through the activity of priests (*tao-shih*), some of whom were women (Kirkland, 1991a).

"Liturgical Taoism" soon became central to life at all levels of Chinese society. Admiring emperors sought to bolster their legitimacy by associating with Taoist masters, and by having them perform liturgies for the sake of state and society. During the T'ang dynasty (618–906 c.e.), cultural leaders in every field associated with such masters, and were deeply influenced by Taoist religious, artistic, and literary traditions. Prominent Taoists like Ssu-ma Ch'eng-chen not only maintained the liturgical tradition but also refined the meditative practices that had always been central to the Taoist spiritual life (Engelhardt, 1987). In addition, certain Taoists became known for their achievements as physicians.

The social prominence of liturgical Taoism changed drastically during the twelfth and thirteenth centuries c.e., when China was again invaded by northern peoples. The foreign rulers often suspected religious organizations of fostering rebellious activities, so Chinese who sought social or political advancement began to dissociate themselves from such organizations. Hence, in late imperial China, liturgical Taoism became divorced from the elite segments of society, and endured primarily among the less affluent and less educated (Kirkland, 1992). The broadly based, ecumenical Taoist tradition of T'ang times dissipated, to be replaced by new, smaller sects. One of the earliest examples was Ch'ing-wei Taoism: founded by a young woman about 900, it introduced "thunder rites," by which a priest internalized the spiritual power of thunder to gain union with the Tao, then healed illnesses. In T'ien-hsin Taoism, founded by a twelfth-century scholar, priests healed mental illness by drawing spiritual power from stars. The most traditional of the new sects was T'ai-i Taoism, which stressed ritual healing and social responsibility, and was popular with some rulers, including the Mongol Khubilai Khan. None of those sects had much lasting influence. One that did endure was Cheng-i (Orthodox Unity) Taoism, which flourished under imperial patronage from the eleventh to eighteenth centuries and is still practiced in Taiwan. It preserves traditional liturgies, adding rituals for exorcism and personal protection. None of the new sects that arose during the "Taoist reformation" was in any way concerned with the pursuit of immortality. Rather, priests of all those sects ministered to the community by healing and performing other ritual services.

Modern Taoism has maintained the pursuit of individual self-perfection through meditation. Earlier Taoist meditation took a variety of forms. But from the eleventh century on, most Taoist meditation was couched in terms of "inner alchemy." Employing terminology from ancient Lao-Chuang texts, "inner alchemy" aims at self-perfection through cultivating "spirit" (*shen*) and "vital force" (*ch'i*) (Robinet, 1989). These practices were embraced in Ch'üan-chen (Complete Perfection) Taoism, a monastic movement founded in the twelfth century. Ch'üan-chen institutions flourished into the twentieth century, as did some of its teachings on self-perfection through meditation.

## The ethical dimensions of Taoism

Many accounts of Taoism lead one to question whether there is—or could be—such a thing as a Taoist ethic, suggesting quite incorrectly that Taoist values were intrinsically egocentric. In fact, all segments of the Taoist tradition fostered a personal ethic, and most segments taught a social ethic as well. At times, in fact, it is clear that Taoism assumed a universalistic ethic that extended not only to all humanity but also to the wider domain of all living things (Kirkland, 1986). These values were not borrowings from Confucianism or Buddhism, but a natural extension of fundamental elements of the Taoist worldview, rooted in the ancient heritage of the *Tao te ching* and the *T'ai-p'ing ching*. That worldview was interwoven with an ethos that encouraged individuals and groups to engage in activities intended to promote the healthy integration of the individual, society, nature, and cosmos.

### The moral life: Ideals of refinement and "fostering life."

The Taoist view of personal identity and human values contrasts sharply with that of Confucianism. Confucians understand humans to be innately distinct from and superior to all other forms of life, because of humans' social inclinations and moral consciousness. Taoism, by contrast, locates the value of humanity not in what separates it from the rest of the natural world but in what humans share with the rest of the world. A constant if not universal goal of Taoism is to propel the individual's attention to ever higher and broader perspectives, to move as far as possible not only beyond the isolated concerns of the individual but also beyond the socioculturally defined concerns of the unreflective. The Taoist goal is not to ignore socioculturally defined concerns but to transcend them.

For that reason, despite all its insistence upon restoring harmony with the natural order, Taoism is not consistent with the activist tendencies of modern environmentalism. No Taoist of any persuasion ever embraced goal-directed action as a legitimate agency for solving problems. The *Tao te ching* in fact implies that, contrary to appearances, nature is ultimately more powerful than all human endeavor, and that if humans will refrain from taking any action, however well-intentioned, nature itself will inevitably rectify any problems.

Taoists insist that we must focus our concern upon ourselves, seeking (re)integration with the deeper realities of the cosmos through a process of personal refinement (*lien*). In some of Lao-Chuang Taoism, that process at times appears so rarefied that it involves no more than altered perceptions: one learns to reject conventional "truths" in pursuit of a deeper state of awareness. But most later Taoists understand the process of refinement as a more comprehensive undertaking, involving a transformation or sublimation of one's physical reality as well. Such "biospiritual" ideals are often couched in terms of the imperative of "fostering life" (*yang-sheng*). Some writers have identified *yang-sheng* with physiological practices designed to enhance individual health and prolong physical life. But in the Taoist context, at least, the term connotes much more:

> Indeed, the very idea of life or health, including as it does both physical and spiritual dimensions, evokes an archaic aura of religious meaning—that the fullness of life is supranormal by conventional standards—and symbolically is closely linked with a generalized Taoist notion of the mystic and religious, individual and social, salvational goal of reestablishing harmony with the cosmic life principle of the Tao. (Girardot, 1978, p. 1631)

Within the Taoist worldview, *yang-sheng* presupposed a personal ethic of moral and spiritual cultivation (Kirkland, 1991b). That ethic, moreover, assumed a dedication not only to the perfection of the individual self but also to reestablishment of a broader, universal harmony.

The term *yang* means "to foster, nourish, *or* care for." Thus the *Tao te ching* sometimes presents the Tao in imagery that suggests a loving parent who exerts no control, and oft-overlooked passages encourage altruistic attention to the needs and interests of others (Kirkland, 1986). In that context, *yang-sheng* can be interpreted as selfless concern with fostering others' lives as well as one's own.

> In fact, rather than being promoted by a Confucian sense of social service, hospitals, orphan care, and community quarantine procedures were linked to the activities of the Taoist and Buddhist monasteries during the Six Dynasties period. . . . The root of this concern for community health care would seem to be most strongly influenced by the Buddhist idea of universal compassion (*karuna*), but in Taoism this idea could be interpreted as an aspect of the selfless kindness and concern for human health extended to all persons in the practice of *wu-wei*. (Girardot, 1978, p. 1636)

Medieval Taoist literature abounds in stories of exemplary men and women who earned recognition—and, on occasion, the boon of immortality—by secretly performing compassionate acts, particularly for people and animals disdained by others (Kirkland, 1986; Cahill, 1990). Such values have sometimes been attributed to Buddhist influence, but they are actually rooted in elements of the ancient Taoist worldview. The Taoist ethos started with the individual, and redirected his or her attention to a broader life context: from body to spirit, from self to community, from humanity to nature. In addition, it presented the would-be Taoist with a moral responsibility to live for a purpose greater than oneself.

Taoist conceptions of history, humanity, and cosmos also undercut some of the paternalistic tendencies so common in other traditions, including Confucianism.

Human lives are to mirror the operation of the Tao, which contrasts markedly with Western images of God as creator, father, ruler, or judge. The Tao is not an external authority, nor a being assumed to possess a moral right to control or intervene in the lives of others. Moreover, the *Tao te ching* commends "feminine" behaviors like yielding, as explicitly opposed to "masculine" behaviors of assertion, intervention, or control. There is thus little temptation for a Taoist to "play God," whether in medicine, government, or law.

**The moral life: Ideals of balance and harmony.**  While Taoism did not create the ideals of balance and harmony, it embraced them to an extent unequaled by other traditions. A fundamental Taoist assumption, applicable to any facet of life, was that disorder is a result of imbalance, whether physical or spiritual, individual or social. Physical illness was generally understood as an indicator of what might be called a biospiritual imbalance within the individual. In many presentations of Chinese medicine, disease is explained as a result of a misalignment of *ch'i*, the natural life force (which eludes the distinction of "body" from "spirit"). In the minds of the peasantry, such misalignment was often understood as the result of moral misdeeds, and some Taoists who were anxious to involve the common people incorporated such ideas into their writings and practices. But in a broader theoretical context, the imbalances that result in disease might better be attributed to a kind of natural entropy. Ancient Chinese thought assumed that the present state of the world represents a degeneration from an earlier state of universal peace and harmony. The goal of life for Confucians and Taoists alike was to restore that original harmony. Certain Taoists took a profound interest in the problem of restoring the harmony of individuals through treating physical maladies (Girardot, 1978). But disease and healing were never understood in purely materialistic terms, and the goal of medicine was never simply the alleviation of physical suffering. Like healers in many traditional cultures, Taoists of most periods assumed that all physical symptoms remit when one restores the biospiritual integrity of the individual and reestablishes a state of balance and harmony with the deeper realities of life. Consequently, some Taoists worked to restore health through therapeutic ritual activity (Strickmann, 1985).

Restoring harmony, however, was never a purely individual matter, for the Taoist any more than for the Confucian. Just as a physical disorder was understood as resulting from a biospiritual imbalance within the individual, so sociopolitical disorder was generally understood as resulting from a biospiritual imbalance on a larger scale. Taoists and Confucians of classical times and the later imperial period felt a responsibility to rectify that imbalance, to play a managerial role in restoring *T'ai-p'ing*, "Grand Tranquillity." *T'ai-p'ing* connoted

a well-ordered society, both in universal terms and in terms of the local community. But it was not merely a political concept:

> It was a state in which all the concentric spheres of the organic Chinese universe, which contained nature as well as society, were perfectly attuned, communicated with each other in a balanced rhythm of timeliness, and brought maximum fulfillment to each living being. (Seidel, 1987a, p. 251)

Taoist priests of all periods assumed a special responsibility to tend to the spiritual dimensions of upholding *T'ai-p'ing*, complementing the real and symbolic activities of the emperor and local magistrate. Until Mongol times, that understanding of the role of the Taoist priest was accepted at all levels of society, and emperors frequently relied upon Taoist priests to provide both advice and ritual support in keeping state and society in harmony with the cosmos.

The Taoist concern with balance and harmony extended to participation in religious activities. While the *Tao te ching* had commended "feminine" behavioral models, the early Taoist religious community offered participation to women, apparently on an equal basis with men. Though it is not clear how often women performed the same priestly functions as men, medieval texts describe women's spirituality in terms that make it only subtly distinguishable from that of men (Cahill, 1990; Kirkland, 1991a). The marginalization of liturgical Taoism after the twelfth century coincided with a more general diminution of opportunities for women throughout Chinese life, and from then on, few women appear in the Taoist tradition.

Taoist attitudes toward sexuality were quite vague. Taoists never articulated any specific sexual ethic. Aside from Confucian moralists, few Chinese regarded sexuality as morally problematic, and most regarded it as a valuable component of human life. Some Taoists took an interest in reproductive forces as the most readily accessible manifestation of the natural forces of the cosmos. The imagery of "inner alchemy" was sometimes applied to those forces, resulting in biospiritual practices aimed at total sublimation and concomitant personal perfection. Particularly in later centuries, some men and women focused their efforts at self-transformation upon the physical or metaphorical transformation of sexual forces. But once again, it is questionable whether such activities ought to be called specifically "Taoist," for they have little in common with the activities of any of the liturgical Taoist organizations.

**Taoist attitudes toward death.**  One of the most intensely debated issues in modern discussions of Taoism is that of its attitude(s) toward death. The controversy stems from some interpreters' insistence that religious Taoists struggled to *avert* death, while the earlier Lao-Chuang Taoists had espoused an *acceptance* of death as a natural conclusion to the cycle of life. There is evidence to support that interpretation, but there are also passages in the *Tao te ching* and other Lao-Chuang texts that suggest the possibility of obviating death and the desirability of attaining a deathless state. A natural conclusion would be that "religious Taoism" focused upon those passages, and set about devising practical methods of attaining such a state. But while none can dispute the commonness of texts describing such methods, it is again questionable whether they can be considered representative of "religious Taoism." It should be noted that the most famous proponent of the pursuit of immortality—the fourth-century Ko Hung—actually repudiated the Taoist tradition. On the other hand, the architects of the Taoist liturgical tradition seldom even alluded to immortality as a desirable goal.

Taoists of all periods would be puzzled by the insistence of modern Western medicine that the prevention of human death transcends all other concerns. To Taoists, the reality of one's life extends far beyond the biological activity of one's body, and extending the latter *for its own sake* would hardly seem even desirable. The Taoist goal is always harmony with the deeper dimensions of life, and in those terms a medical model that defines "life" in strictly biological terms seems perverted.

In reality, Taoist attitudes toward death are hardly reducible to any clear, unequivocal proposition. But one may safely affirm that a pursuit of immortality for its own sake—that is, a search for some trick that would obviate the death event—was never a Taoist goal (Kirkland, 1991b). Rather, Taoists consistently pursued a state of spiritual perfection. Frequently, they expressed that state of perfection as a state that was not subject to death. Chinese literature (by no means specifically Taoist) is replete with stories of *hsien*—wondrous male and female beings who live outside the realm of ordinary life and death. Taoist writers sometimes employed such imagery to suggest the final fruits of spiritual development. Some writings suggest that rare individuals underwent a transformation that merely simulated death (Robinet, 1979). But one must beware mistaking metaphor for reality (Bokenkamp, 1989). When read carefully, most Taoist writings actually present a "postmortem immortality"; that is, a deathless state can indeed be achieved, but biological death remains a necessity (Strickmann, 1979; Seidel, 1987b). Taoist attitudes toward death thus remain a paradox.

**Conclusion.** Though some Taoist writings do present moral injunctions, Taoism never developed any real ethical code, for such an idea makes little sense in a Taoist context. For instance, since there was no divine Lawgiver, Taoists never developed an ethic conceived as obedience to divine authority. Taoists of various periods did accept the existence of divinities, and some Taoist writings incorporated popular concepts of a heavenly hierarchy that dispenses posthumous rewards and punishments. But acceptance of such beliefs was never considered mandatory, and most Taoist literature lacks such ideas.

Similarly, Taoists lacked the notion that the individual—or even the human species—is an independent locus of moral value. In fact, Lao-Chuang Taoism can easily be read as a concerted effort to disabuse humans of the absurd notions of self-importance that most people tacitly embrace as natural and normal. Hence, the very concept of "rights"—for individuals or groups, humans or animals—makes no sense in Taoist terms.

Taoism might appear to embody a virtue ethic. Indeed, the term *te* in the title of the *Tao te ching* is generally translated "virtue." But the Taoist perspective is quite distinct from the virtue ethic developed by Confucians like Mencius. Mencius clearly articulated virtues like *jen* (benevolence), and insisted that proper cultivation of such virtues would result in the perfection of individual, family, society, and state. Much of Taoism seems to suggest a similar model, with the substitution of *te* for *jen*. But though Mencius attributed human moral impulses to a natural inheritance from "Heaven," Lao-Chuang Taoists frequently criticized most Confucians as seeking answers to life's issues in terms that were excessively humanistic. Confucians often seem ambivalent concerning the relevance or even the existence of transhuman realities. And it was upon precisely such realities that Taoism centered itself.

To understand the moral dimensions of Taoism, one must understand the "vague and elusive" concept of the Tao—transcendent yet immanent, divine yet inherent in humanity and all of nature. Most important, since the Tao never acts by design, Lao-Chuang Taoists ridicule the notion that good could result from conscious evaluation of possible courses of action. Such deliberate "ethical reflection," they argue, blinds one to the natural course of action, which is the course that one follows when living spontaneously, without the arrogant and destructive imposition of rationality and intentionality.

The ethical dimensions of Taoism are thus real but subtle. Since Taoists never embraced normative expressions of any kind, to perceive the ethical dimensions of Taoism, one must peer deeply and carefully into the entire tradition, extrapolating from a plethora of sources from different segments of a highly diverse tradition. In doing so, one forms the impression that to live a proper Taoist life is to live in such a way that one restores and maintains the world's holistic unity. The Taoist life involves dedication to a process of self-refinement, which is considered one's natural contribution to the health and well-being of both nature and society. In a sense, to be a Taoist is to accept personal responsibility for taking part in a universal healing, doing one's part to restore the health and wholeness of the individual, society, nature, and cosmos.

RUSSELL KIRKLAND

*Directly related to this entry is the entry* MEDICAL ETHICS, HISTORY OF, *section on* SOUTH AND EAST ASIA, *subsection on* CHINA. *For a further discussion of topics mentioned in this entry, see the entries* ACTION; BUDDHISM; CONFUCIANISM; DEATH, *article on* EASTERN THOUGHT; ENVIRONMENT AND RELIGION; *and* ETHICS, *article on* RELIGION AND MORALITY. *Other relevant material may be found under the entries* ALTERNATIVE THERAPIES; ANIMAL WELFARE AND RIGHTS, *article on* ETHICAL PERSPECTIVES ON THE TREATMENT AND STATUS OF ANIMALS; HUMAN NATURE; NATURE; VALUE AND VALUATION; *and* VIRTUE AND CHARACTER.

## Bibliography

BOKENKAMP, STEPHEN R. 1989. "Death and Ascent in Ling-pao Taoism." *Taoist Resources* 1, no. 2:1–20.

CAHILL, SUZANNE. 1990. "Practice Makes Perfect: Paths to Transcendence for Women in Medieval China." *Taoist Resources* 2, no. 2:23–42.

ENGELHARDT, UTE. 1987. *Die klassische Tradition der Qi-Übungen: Eine Darstellung anhand des Tangzeitlichen Textes Fuqi jingyi lun von Sima Chengzhen.* Wiesbaden: Franz Steiner.

GIRARDOT, NORMAN J. 1978. "Taoism." In vol. 4 of *Encyclopedia of Bioethics*, pp. 1631–1638. Edited by Warren T. Reich. New York: Macmillan.

GRAHAM, ANGUS C. 1981. *Chuang-tzu: The Seven Inner Chapters and Other Writings from the Book Chuang-tzu.* London: Allen & Unwin.

KALTENMARK, MAX. 1979. "The Ideology of the *T'ai-p'ing ching.*" In *Facets of Taoism*, pp. 19–45. Edited by Holmes Welch and Anna Seidel. New Haven, Conn.: Yale University Press.

KIRKLAND, RUSSELL. 1986. "The Roots of Altruism in the Taoist Tradition." *Journal of the American Academy of Religion* 54, no. 11:59–77.

———. 1991a. "Huang Ling-wei: A Taoist Priestess in T'ang China." *Journal of Chinese Religions* 19:47–73.

———. 1991b. "The Making of an Immortal: The Exultation of Ho Chih-Chang." *Numen* 38, no. 2:214–230.

———. 1992. "Person and Culture in the Taoist Tradition." *Journal of Chinese Religions* 20:77–90.

———. 1993. "A World in Balance: Holistic Synthesis in the *T'ai-p'ing kuang-chi.*" *Journal of Sung-Yuan Studies* 23: 43–70.

KOHN, LIVIA, ed. 1993. *The Taoist Experience: An Anthology.* Albany: State University of New York Press.

LAO-TZU. 1982. *Tao te ching.* Translated by D. C. Lau. Hong Kong: Chinese University of Hong Kong Press.

ROBINET, ISABELLE. 1979. "Metamorphosis and Deliverance from the Corpse in Taoism." *History of Religions* 19, no. 1:37–70.

———. 1989. "Original Contributions of *Neidan* to Taoism and Chinese Thought." In *Taoist Meditation and Longevity Techniques*, pp. 297–330. Edited by Livia Kohn. Ann Arbor: University of Michigan Center for Chinese Studies.

———. 1991. *Histoire du Taoïsme dès origines au XIVe siècle.* Paris: Editions du Cerf.

———. 1993. *Taoist Meditation: The Mao-shan of Great Purity.* Translated by Julian Pas and Norman Girardot. Albany: State University of New York Press.

ROTH, HAROLD D. 1991. "Psychology and Self-Cultivation in Early Taoistic Thought." *Harvard Journal of Asiatic Studies* 51, no. 2:599–650.

SCHIPPER, KRISTOFER M. 1993. *The Taoist Body.* Translated by Karen C. Duval. Berkeley: University of California Press.

SEIDEL, ANNA. 1987a. "T'ai-p'ing." In vol. 14 of *Encyclopedia of Religion*, pp. 251–252. New York: Macmillan.

———. 1987b. "Post-Mortem Immortality; or, The Taoist Resurrection of the Body." In *GILGUL: Essays on Transformation, Revolution and Permanence in the History of Religions*, pp. 223–237. Edited by Shaid Shaked, David Shulman, and Gedaliahu G. Strousma. Leiden: E. J. Brill.

———. 1990. *Taoismus: Die inoffizielle Hochreligion Chinas.* Tokyo: Deutsche Gesellschaft für Natur- und Völkerkunde Ostasiens.

STRICKMANN, MICHEL. 1979. "On the Alchemy of T'ao Hung-ching." In *Facets of Taoism*, pp. 123–192. Edited by Holmes Welch and Anna Seidel. New Haven, Conn.: Yale University Press.

———. 1980. "Taoism, History of." In *New Encyclopaedia Britannica, Macropedia*, vol. 17, pp. 1044–1050. Chicago: Encyclopaedia Britannica.

———. 1985. "Therapeutische Rituale und das Problem des Bösen im frühen Taoismus." In *Religion und Philosophie in Ostasien*, pp. 185–200. Edited by Gert Naundorf, Karl-Heinz Pohl, and Hans-Hermann Schmidt. Würzburg: Königshausen und Neumann.

# TEACHING OF BIOETHICS OR MEDICAL ETHICS

*See* BIOETHICS EDUCATION.

# TEAMS, HEALTH-CARE

A health-care team is two or more health professionals (and, when appropriate, other lay or professional people) who apply their complementary professional skills to accomplish an agreed-upon goal. Coordinated, comprehensive patient care is the primary goal of most teams. Other goals may include education of health professionals, patients, or families; community outreach; advocacy; abuse prevention; family support; institutional planning; networking; and utilization review in hospitals. The team approach to patient care has been viewed as a means of building and maintaining staff morale, improving the status of a given profession (for example, nurses and allied health professionals may become team collaborators with the physician rather than working under the physician), or improving institutional efficiency.

Some teams are ongoing, such as a psychiatric care team, home visit team, ventilator patient care team, child development team, or rehabilitation team. Such teams may be responsible for following the person throughout the entire process of health-care interventions, including diagnosis, goal setting and planning, implementation, evaluation, follow-up, and modification of goals for the patient. Other teams form around an event (for example, a disaster plan team or organ transplant team), or focus on a single function, such as discharge planning or the initiation of renal dialysis. Some teams are undisciplinary; others are multidisciplinary, and may include lay people.

Though taken for granted today, a team approach to health care has appeared only recently in many places where Western medicine is practiced. The development of team approaches in the United States reflects the history of that development in North America and Europe as well. In the first period, between World War I and World War II, a multiprofessional approach appeared that later developed into the team model. Major sources of impetus included the proliferation of medical specialties, an increase in expensive, complex technological interventions, and the ensuing challenge of providing a coordinated and comprehensive approach to patient care management. A second period of development occurred between the 1950s and the 1980s, when teamwork became the norm: health care became increasingly hospital-based, enabling a large corps of health professionals in one place to minister to the patient. In addition, new professional groups were generated in the belief that health care should be attentive to patients' social as well as physical well-being. The third period, which continues to the present, has focused on the appropriate goals and functions of the health-care team and evaluation of the team's effectiveness (Brown, 1982).

Ethical issues regarding teams arise in four major areas: challenges arising from the team metaphor itself; the locus of authority for team decisions; the role of the patient as team member; and mechanisms for fostering morally supportable team decisions.

## The team metaphor

It is generally agreed that the health-care team idea and rhetoric arose from assumptions about sports teams and military teams (Nagi, 1975; Erde, 1982). This metaphor is not completely fitting because the health-care team is not in competition with another team. However, it is fitting insofar as members experience their affiliation as entailing "team loyalty," a moral obligation to other members and to the team itself. They may believe that they have voluntarily committed themselves to a type of social contract requiring a member not only to perform maximally but also to protect team secrets, thereby promoting a tendency for cover-ups or protection of weaker members. In the military team, obedience to and trust in the leader is an absolute.

A troubling ethical conflict arises when the member's moral obligation of faithfulness to other team members or "captain" does battle with moral obligations to the patient. This may manifest itself in questions of whether to cover up negligence or a serious mistake by some or all of the team. Overall, holding peers morally accountable for incompetence or unethical behavior may be made more difficult by the team ideal. Therefore, teams must foster rules that require and reward faithfulness to patient well-being, and balance and value of team membership with that of maintaining high ethical standards.

Feminist analyses of bureaucratic structures and bioethical issues highlight a related ethical challenge. The team metaphor entails assumptions about relationships, rules, and "plays" that often exclude women from full participation because their childhood and later socialization did not prepare them for this "game" and its insiders' rhetoric. Noteworthy is the sports or military team ethos of ignoring the personal characteristics of fellow team members (within limits), provided each person is technically well suited to carry out assigned functions. Many women find it almost impossible to function effectively with team members whom they judge as morally deplorable, no matter the latter's technical skills; for such women, the relationships among and integrity of team members is as important as the external goal (Harragan, 1977).

Sometimes a further breakdown of communication and effectiveness accrues because of the team leader's allegiance to scientific rigor and specificity at the expense of subjective attentiveness to caring. Since many team leaders are physicians, on multidisciplinary teams the problems may become interpreted as pointing to serious differences in orientation between physicians and other health-care professionals (addressed in the next section). Whatever its cause, marginalization of some team members results in team dysfunction.

## Locus of authority for decision making

Roles involve ongoing features and conduct appropriate to a situation, and create expectations in the self and others regarding that conduct. Each role has an identity and boundaries, giving rise to the question of whose role carries the authority for team decision making (Rothberg, 1985). The challenge applies to both unidisciplinary and multidisciplinary teams but is highlighted in multidisciplinary ones, particularly those involving physicians and other health professionals. Traditionally the physician was the person in authority by virtue of his or her office. The team metaphor reinforces the nonmovable locus of authority vested in one who holds such office (for example, "captain").

At the same time, the team metaphor created expectations of more equality among members based on competence to provide input. Each member becomes an authority on the basis of professional expertise instead of office, and should be in a position to provide leadership at such time as expertise indicates it. In ethical decisions regarding patient care, the question of authority must be viewed in terms of who should have the morally authoritative voice. Technical expertise does not automatically entail ethical expertise. In both types of decision-making situations, the locus of authority is movable.

Clarification of role identity and boundaries helps to create reasonable expectations and mitigate this type of conflict regarding locus of authority (and concomitant locus of accountability) regarding team decisions (Green, 1988). A further complication arises, however, because teams usually have several members. A critical question regarding such collective decision making is whether team decisions are the sum of individual members, with accountability allocated only to the individuals, or whether a team itself can be regarded as a moral agent (Pellegrino, 1982). Lively debate continues regarding this topic (Abramson, 1984; Newton, 1982; Green, 1988).

Sometimes teams have difficulty coming to consensus about the appropriate course of action. The moral responsibility of the team members is to assure that further role clarification, further attempts at consensus building, and other collective decision-making mechanisms are instrumental only to maximizing patient well-being (or any other appropriate goal of teamwork). Negotiation strategies must be built into the team process so that the authority of any one or several members, or even the team as a whole, does not govern at the cost of the competent, compassionate decision geared to the appropriate ends of that team's activities.

## The patient as team member

There is much discussion about whether and in what respect patients/clients and their families are members of health-care teams. The doctrine of informed consent and its underlying legal and ethical underpinnings dictate that patients and families should have input into decisions affecting themselves and their loved ones. At the same time, much of the team's work proceeds without direct involvement of patients and families. Some have argued that a primary care orientation places the patient as focus and arbiter of the care, and that present team practices fall short of that essential condition (Smith and Churchill, 1986). Others argue that conceptually a primary care approach is consistent with the goals of good teamwork (Barnard, 1987).

## Moral education for teams

The team ideal provides a widely used model for effective and efficient patient care. Ethical issues are an inherent part of clinical decision making. In preparation for facing ethical issues the team can (1) develop a common moral language for discussion of the issues; (2) engage in cognitive and practical training in how to articulate feelings about pertinent ethical issues; (3) clarify values to uncover key interests among team members; (4) participate in common experiences upon which to base workable policies; and (5) refine a decision-making method for the team to use (Thomasma, 1981).

It appears that team approaches to a wide variety of health-care issues and events will continue to develop and grow. The emergence of ethics committees as a type of team approach focusing explicitly on ethical decisions should help further in these deliberations.

RUTH B. PURTILO

*For a further discussion of topics mentioned in this entry,* see the entries ALLIED HEALTH PROFESSIONS; AUTONOMY; FIDELITY AND LOYALTY; MEDICINE AS A PROFESSION; NURSING AS A PROFESSION; PATIENTS' RESPONSIBILITIES; PROFESSIONAL–PATIENT RELATIONSHIP, *article on* ETHICAL ISSUES; RESPONSIBILITY; *and* WOMEN, *section on* WOMEN AS HEALTH PROFESSIONALS, *article on* CONTEMPORARY ISSUES. *Other relevant material may be found under the entries* AUTHORITY; CLINICAL ETHICS; FEMINISM; *and* MEDICINE, ART OF.

## Bibliography

ABRAMSON, MARCIA. 1984. "Collective Responsibility in Interdisciplinary Collaboration: An Ethical Perspective for Social Workers." *Social Work in Health Care* 10, no. 11:35–43.

BARNARD, DAVID. 1987. "The Viability of the Concept of a Primary Health Care Team: A View from the Medical Humanities." *Social Science and Medicine* 25, no. 6:741–746.

BROWN, THEODORE. 1982. "An Historical View of Health Care Teams." In *Responsibility in Health Care,* pp. 3–22. Edited by George J. Agich. Philosophy and Medicine, vol. 12. Boston: D. Reidel.

ERDE, EDMUND. 1982. "Logical Confusions and Moral Dilemmas in Health Care Teams and Team Talk." In *Responsibility in Health Care,* pp. 193–214. Edited by George J.

Agich. Philosophy and Medicine, vol. 12. Boston: D. Reidel.

GILLIGAN, CAROL. 1982. *In a Different Voice: Psychological Theory and Women's Development.* Cambridge, Mass.: Harvard University Press.

GREEN, WILLARD. 1988. "Accountability and Team Care." *Theoretical Medicine* 9:33–44.

HARRAGAN, BETTY L. 1977. *Games Mother Never Taught You: Corporate Gamesmanship for Women.* New York: Warner.

NAGI, SAAD Z. 1975. "Teamwork in Health Care in the United States: A Sociological Perspective." *Milbank Memorial Fund Quarterly* 53:75–81.

NEWTON, LISA H. 1982. "Collective Responsibility in Health Care." *Journal of Medicine and Philosophy* 7, no. 1:11–21.

PELLEGRINO, EDMUND D. 1982. "The Ethics of Collective Judgments in Medicine and Health Care." *Journal of Medicine and Philosophy* 7, no. 1:3–10.

PURTILO, RUTH B. 1988. "Ethical Issues and Teamwork: The Context of Rehabilitation." *Archives of Physical Medicine and Rehabilitation* 69, no. 5:318–326.

ROTHBERG, JUNE. 1985. "Rehabilitation Team Practice." In *Interdisciplinary Team Practice: Issues and Trends*, pp. 19–41. Edited by Pedro J. Lecca and John S. McNeil. New York: Praeger.

SMITH, HARMON L., and CHURCHILL, LARRY R. 1986. *Professional Ethics and Primary Care Medicine: Beyond Dilemmas and Decorum.* Durham, N.C.: Duke University Press.

THOMASMA, DAVID. 1981. "Moral Education in Interdisciplinary Teams." *Prospectus for Change* 6, no. 5:1–4.

# TECHNOLOGY

## I. HISTORY OF MEDICAL TECHNOLOGY

Medical technologies are objects, directed by procedures, that are applied against the hazards of illness. The object is the tangible dimension of technology. The procedure is the focused and standardized plan that guides the use of the object according to defined purposes.

Some medical technologies are more object-embedded. In them the tangible portion is the principal functional component. The X ray, artificial kidney, and penicillin are examples. Others technologies are more procedure-embedded. Their main function is to organize facts, individuals, and/or other technologies. Examples are the medical record, hospital, and surgical procedures. Indeed, the common synonym for the surgical procedure, the operation, connotes actions that are related as parts in a series.

It is important to distinguish technologies from another medium through which actions are taken in medicine—techniques. Medical techniques are procedures mediated through the human senses rather than through objects. Examples are percussion, pulse-feeling, and psychoanalysis. This perspective on medical technology will be used in this essay.

## Technology, nature, and ethics

The works of the Hippocratic corpus, a group of essays on medical theory and therapy written between the fifth and third centuries B.C.E., analyze the relation between nature and the agents of the medical art, from the viewpoints of effectiveness and ethics.

The ancient Greek concepts of health and illness were based on a theory postulating four humors or basic elements of the body: blood, phlegm, yellow bile, and black bile. In health, these were in a stable equilibrium. Illness occurred when one or more of these humors increased or decreased and thus changed their proportional relation. This change caused an instability of the equilibrium state synonymous with health, and the breakdown produced illness. Nature—the force that inclined the humors toward remaining in or returning to the proportional relations of the healthful state—was viewed as the most powerful agent of healing. The purpose of the medical art was to assist nature to reestablish the proportional relationship of health among the humors.

Works in the Hippocratic corpus cautioned physicians against misapplying medical means. Such behavior constituted an offense that could harm both the patient and the reputation of medicine. In the essay "The Art," the following observation is made:

> For in cases where we may have the mastery through the means afforded by a natural constitution or by an art, there we may be craftsmen, but nowhere else. Whenever therefore a man suffers from an ill which is too strong for the means at the disposal of medicine, he surely must not even expect that it can be overcome by medicine. (Hippocrates, 1923a, p. 203)

To exceed the rational limits of the means of medicine was to commit the sin of hubris.

The technology of Greek doctors was relatively simple. They used ointments, compresses, bandages, surgical instruments, simple and compound drugs, and bloodletting in moderation. They used the techniques of history taking, visual observation, and palpation to learn the circumstances of illness, and prescribed diets, bathing, and exercise to maintain health and combat illness.

The Greeks also recognized that the manner in which physicians dressed, approached the bedside, and discussed illness with a patient could influence their success at healing by producing help and avoiding harm, and thus had an ethical meaning. Accordingly, attention to the effects of the physician as a person on the patient as a person became a significant aspect of Greek medical practice. The physician is told "to have at his command a certain ready wit, as dourness is repulsive both to the healthy and the sick." When coming into the sickroom, doctors should consider their "manner of sitting, reserve, arrangement of dress, decisive utterance, brevity of speech." The doctor was to perform all duties "calmly and adroitly, concealing most things from the patient while you are attending him," lest such revelations cause the patient to take "a turn for the worse" (Hippocrates, 1923b, pp. 291–299).

The Hippocratic Greek physicians recognized that appropriate applications of technology required a searching analysis of its capabilities, of the ethical canons that should guide its use, and of the relation between technology and nature in treating patients. Consideration of these three factors was the significant contribution of Greek civilization to the use of medical technology.

## Anatomy and specialization

The content of the technologies used in medical practice did not change appreciably for two thousand years. Indeed, the Hippocratic works and other Greek texts, in Latin translations, formed the core of medical learning in Europe through the Middle Ages.

As the sixteenth century began, however, a growing interest in firsthand exploration of nature, and learning and questioning the authority of tradition, created what we call the Renaissance, generating a perspective that would eventually exert a profound influence on the development and use of technology in medicine. Although the study of the structural composition of the body through anatomic dissection was thwarted by cultural, social, and religious constraints against dismemberment, Renaissance scientific and artistic interest in the body's physical makeup overcame these restrictions and encouraged its exploration.

The leading figure in this movement was Andreas Vesalius, a physician and professor at Padua, who in 1543 published *De humani corporis fabrica.* In it the structure of the body was analyzed in detail and portrayed through illustrations that were far in advance of any previous work. Its illustrations, the work of a still unknown Renaissance artist, were startling in their beauty and detail. In contrast, the typical anatomical illustrations of the day were inaccurate and crude outlines, with organs drawn in more as symbols than as representations. Vesalius corrected over two hundred errors in the work that had been the standard, authoritative text in use for almost fifteen hundred years. Written by the Greek doctor Galen in the second century, it re-

flected typical restrictions on human dissection, for its content was based on animal dissection (mainly pigs and apes) extrapolated to human structure.

Vesalius' book, devoted to the normal anatomy of the body, fostered within medicine an interest in bodily structure, particularly in the changes it underwent when attacked by illness. During the next two hundred years, physicians examined bodies and wrote texts commenting on the pathological transformation of anatomic structure. These efforts were brought together in a 1761 text by the Italian physician Giovanni Battista Morgagni, *The Seats and Causes of Diseases Investigated by Anatomy.* The work's principal objective was to demonstrate that the symptoms of illness in the living were determined by the structural changes produced within the body by disease. Morgagni demonstrated this relation through a tripartite analysis of cases. Typically, he began by reporting on the clinical course of an illness experienced by a patient who eventually died. This was followed by the autopsy findings. Then came a synthetic commentary in which he connected clinical and autopsy results.

Morgagni asserted that through anatomic examination, particular diseases could be recognized by their telltale footprints on the landscape of the body. As the title of Morgagni's work suggests, the author believed that diseases had "seats" in the body, and that they were expressed through characteristic disruptions of the body's fabric in discernible sites. This perspective ran directly counter to that prevailing under the humoral theory of illness, dominant since Hippocratic times.

Anatomy, beginning in the sixteenth century, when it departed from this whole-body perspective, focused the doctor's vision on the search for sites in the body where a change in structure had occurred. The leading question for anatomists and the physicians who adopted their outlook was "Where is the disease?" This question and viewpoint paved the way for the modern specialization of medicine, beginning in the nineteenth century and undergirded by a new technology. It justified a retreat by the doctor from patients as individuals to aspects of their anatomy, giving rise to the practice of having different physicians for the eyes, heart, kidneys, and other organs and organ systems.

## Technology and the nineteenth century

With the anatomic ideology firmly established, the nineteenth century became one of the great centuries for medicine, a time of significant advance and change fueled largely by technologic innovation.

The transformation of diagnosis by technology was one of the century's most important features. The symbol and initiator of this change was a simple instrument used to enhance the conduction of sound, the stethoscope. Its transforming effect was as much caused by the new relationship it generated between physicians and patients as by the new information it provided. Before the stethoscope, the evidence that physicians acquired about illness came mostly from two sources: the visual inspection of the motions and surface of the body, and the story told by the patient of the events, sensations, and feelings that accompanied the illness. It was this encounter with the life of the patient that was at once enlightening, troubling, and engaging for physicians.

The patient's story provided significant diagnostic evidence that often determined the doctor's judgment. But physicians expressed concern about the authenticity of this evidence, which usually could not be confirmed. Who could know if a patient really heard a buzzing in the ears? Diagnosis was prone to the distortions of memory and whim. For all of its evidentiary faults, however, the narrative of the patient's journey through illness connected the doctor with the life of the patient.

The stethoscope challenged the place of the narrative of illness. It was introduced into practice through 1819 treatise (*De l'auscultation médiate*), written by the inventor of the stethoscope, the French physician René Laennec. Laennec claimed that physicians who placed their ear to one end of the foot-long wooden tube that was the first stethoscope and the other end to the chest of a patient, would hear sounds generated by the heart and lungs indicative of health or disease within them. He demonstrated through autopsy evidence that a particular sound perceived in the chest corresponded to a particular lesion within its anatomic structure. He asserted that his technology enabled physicians to diagnose illness not only precisely but often without the help of other symptoms. Doctors need depend on no one else. They could be scientifically self-reliant. The findings of their own senses, extended by a simple instrument, were adequate to reach diagnostic judgments.

This technological advance reduced the significance of the patient's narrative. Why should physicians painstakingly acquire this story and its subjective and unverifiable verbal evidence, if they could use more objective sonic evidence they gathered themselves? With the stethoscope, physicians stepped back from the lives of patients. They began to engage patients through the anatomic and physiologic signs detected by their instruments.

Other simple technologies to extend the doctor's senses into the body, such as the ophthalmoscope (1850), the clinical thermometer (1867), and the sphygmomanometer (1896), were introduced during the nineteenth century. By the century's end physicians had become skillful diagnosticians, seekers of physical clues they used to deduce the source of their patients' troubles. The doctor's black bag contained the technologies to

explore the body physically and to obtain evidence that greatly improved diagnostic accuracy. It was, in fact, through witnessing great skill in the analysis of physical evidence by one of his instructors, Joseph Bell, that a physician-in-training, Arthur Conan Doyle, was led to create the fictional character Sherlock Holmes.

Still, therapy remained limited. In the 1860 address to the Massachusetts Medical Society, Oliver Wendell Holmes, Harvard professor of anatomy, proclaimed: "I firmly believe that if the whole materia medica, *as now used*, could be sunk to the bottom of the sea, it would be all the better for mankind,—and all the worse for the fishes" (Holmes, 1883, p. 203).

The only major bright spot to emerge in the nineteenth century on the therapeutic side of medicine was in surgery. Radical change in the ability of surgeons to perform the dangerous and delicate work of cutting into the body occurred through two separate innovations, one introduced in 1846 and the other in 1867. At the beginning of the nineteenth century, pain had become so inseparably linked with surgical incision that several reports of an anesthetic effect produced by nitrous oxide and ether were disregarded by practitioners. Surgical pain was dealt with by efforts to shorten its presence. Techniques of rapid surgery were developed, with some surgeons capable of detaching a limb in minutes. The conclusive demonstration (in a surgical procedure for a tumor of the neck) at the Massachusetts General Hospital in 1846 of the ability to control operative pain through use of ether, was made by the American Dentist William Morton, who administered the ether. It ameliorated the trauma of surgery for patient and surgeon alike, but cutting into the cavity of the body still was limited by infection.

To control infection, insight was needed into the causal role of bacteria. Joseph Lister, a British surgeon, wrote a paper in 1867 in which he described eleven operations on compound fractures of the limbs in which nine patients recovered without amputation, one required it, and one died. These startling results were made possible by treating the operating space—wound, instruments, surgeon's hands, and air—with the antiseptic carbolic acid. In 1882, the German scientist Robert Koch published a paper that proved through rigorous experiments the causal link between the tubercle bacillus and tuberculosis—a disease that at the time was responsible for about one out of seven deaths in Europe. This essay established the pivotal role played by bacteria in infection. It not only gave further impetus to the practice of antiseptic surgery and liberated surgeons, no longer thwarted by pain or infection, to perform extensive operations within the body cavity. It also produced a new workshop for surgery and all of medicine—the hospital.

# The technologies of twentieth-century medicine

The origins of the hospital reside in military hospitals put up by Roman soldiers on their routes of march, and hospices established early in the history of Christianity to care for the homeless, travelers, orphans, the hungry, and the sick. These multiple activities gradually became divided among separate institutions, one of which was the hospital. It flourished greatly through the medieval period but began a decline afterward, due to diminished church support of its activities.

By the nineteenth century the hospital's medical role was restricted. It was a place for those who could not afford either to call a physician or surgeon to the house for treatment or to employ servants to administer needed bedside care at home. There were two kinds of medicine: home care for the well-to-do and hospital care for the indigent. Hospitals were dangerous places. Infections could rage through them, killing large numbers of patients and making work there dangerous for staff. Hospitals were also feared for the moral dangers said to be posed to women and children by the rough patients they housed.

New technologies transformed the hospital medically and socially. Surgery could no longer be done on kitchen tables at home: it required an antiseptic environment, sterilized instruments, and a staff of skilled nurses for the aftercare of patients undergoing more extensive procedures than were possible in the past.

As the twentieth century dawned, diagnosis and therapy of nonsurgical disease could not be readily done in the home with technology carried in a doctor's bag. diagnostic technology now entered a new phase of development. The simple instruments to extend the senses of the physicians were being replaced by sensing machines too large and expensive to be housed anywhere but in hospitals.

This new technology automatically recorded the data of illness, leaving the reading of its results to the doctor. The X ray, discovered in 1895; the ward laboratory, with its microscopes and chemical tests of the body fluids, which came together as a hospital space in the early 1900s; and the electrocardiograph, introduced in 1906, all converted medical diagnosis from a personal act to a scientific event. The physician leaning over the bedside, at least physically connected to the patient through the stethoscope and similar technologies, became an increasingly anachronistic image as the twentieth century wore on. The physician holding an X ray up to light, studying it, was more in keeping with physicians' growing self-image as scientists. Where was the patient? There was less need for personal medical encounters; the best evidence available to medicine was increasingly not what the patient said, nor what the physician sensed, but what the pictorial or graphic image reported.

As it entered this new technologic phase, medicine required a location within which patients, the increasingly specialized medical staff, and technology could be brought together. The hospital became that place. Its success was dramatic. While there were about four hundred hospitals in the United States in 1875, by 1909 the number grew to over four thousand, and by 1929 surpassed six thousand. No longer shunned but sought by communities, the hospital became the workshop of medicine. By the mid-twentieth century not only patients and technology but also doctors' offices were placed in hospitals. Home care and the house call, no longer adequate as means to apply new medical knowledge, were disappearing as the hospital, perhaps the quintessential technology of the twentieth century to organize medical care, enfolded medicine.

Several other innovations critical to the functions of hospitals and medicine were in place by the mid-twentieth century. One—having integrative influence like the hospital—was the technology of organizing the data of medicine—the medical record. It was fundamentally reformed in the 1920s by the work of the American College of Surgeons (Reiser, 1991). In an era of growing specialization, not only among physicians but also among nurses and the technical experts needed to run the hospital and its machines (there were over two hundred separate health-care specializations by the mid 1970s), communication was of great importance. How to learn what each had done? Through the record, which was the main agent of synthesis in medicine. In its pages the thoughts and actions of a diverse staff were recorded.

But for all its integrative significance, the medical record remains a problem. It shows the results of the information explosion. These data literally burst the confines of the chart. Hundred-page records abound. They contain the details of medical care, but their order often makes following the course of an illness, or locating a particular bit of information, difficult and frustrating. Innovations such as the unit record (having all hospital encounters of a patient recorded in a single place rather than dispersed through separate charts in each clinic); the problem-oriented record (ordering medical data problems—physical, psychologic, or social—rather than by data source, such as putting laboratory data in one place, X-ray data in another); and the computerized record have yet to solve the problem of what to do with the avalanche of technologic evidence.

Another critical innovation available by mid-century was antibiotics. The mass production of penicillin in 1944 (it had been discovered by Alexander Fleming in 1928) inaugurated the antibiotic era in medicine. Antibiotic drugs flowed from the laboratories of the pharmaceutical industry, finally breaking the hold of bacterial illness. Penicillin was called a wonder drug when it was introduced. Given the drug, a patient gravely ill with meningitis or pneumonia would be up and about and home in a week. Not only was it fast-acting and fully curative, but it was safe and cheap. It was commonly thought that penicillin would be the first innovation of a pharmaceutical revolution to produce not only antibacterial drugs but also drugs to deal as effectively with other human ailments. However, the symbol of medicine in the second half of the twentieth century would not be penicillin but a machine that made its debut in the mid-1950s.

The artificial respirator had a long history, dating back to the mid-nineteenth century, when rudimentary forerunners were fashioned to deal mainly with the respiratory crisis of drowning. A tank respirator introduced by Philip Drinker and Charles McKhann in 1929, which used negative-pressure techniques to secure respiration, became the "iron lung" that sustained victims of poliomyelitis. Its effectiveness was variable, and its use was complicated. But by the mid-1950s, using new machines based on positive-pressure technology, clinicians had a far better means of dealing with diseases and accidents that threatened lives through respiratory failure.

Initially, this machine was intended to assist critically ill persons by temporarily sustaining a vital physiologic function and giving them time to recover. For the first time in medical history, physicians acquired a technology that, allied to other advances in nursing, monitoring, and drug therapy, and all brought together by an integrative technique of care embodied in the intensive care unit (ICU), permitted the long-term sustenance of desperately ill people who had no chance of recovery. Now families and medical staff waited by ICU beds, where the main signs of life were not manifest in the expressions or movements of the patient but in the mechanical sounds, motions, and readouts of the new machinery of rescue.

### Ethical issues in applying medical technologies

As families and medical staff assimilated the consequences of the life-support technology represented by the artificial respirator that could prolong dying or life without cognition, they reached out to the ethical traditions of religion, medicine, and society for help (Pius XII, 1958, pp. 501–504). Physicians particularly began to see that the ethical problems to be solved in these crises were as great as or greater than the technical problems of treatment. How to decide whether in a hopeless case to remove the technology that maintained the per-

son's life? On what values should this judgment be based, and who should decide?

Other machines developed in this period posed a similar mix of ethical and technical issues. The artificial kidney was created as a device for acute, intermittent dialysis by Willem Kolff in The Netherlands in 1944. However, it was introduced as a clinically usable machine in the early 1960s in Seattle, Washington, by Belding Schribner. He added an arteriovenous shunt that allowed long-term access to it and made continuing hemodialysis possible. The limited number of machines and personnel to run them led to moral agonizing over developing criteria for selection. Someone had to choose which of the thousands of individuals in the United States having chronic renal failure and able to benefit from dialysis would gain access to a technology that could save their lives. Thirteen years after the machine's introduction, American society decided how to resolve this crisis. In 1973, U.S. congressional legislation provided funds to provide dialysis to all who required it.

Technologies such as the artificial kidney and the respirator have been criticized as offering expensive but partial solutions to fundamental problems of biologic breakdown. The American physician Lewis Thomas calls them "halfway technologies," because they represent only a partial (halfway) understanding of a biologic puzzle that, once solved, will do away with the expense and the disadvantages of such therapies (Thomas, 1977, p. 37).

The extraordinary and growing expense of the health-care system that followed the development of such technologies may be reduced when biomedical research produces comprehensive biologic answers to problems such as organ failure. But in the twentieth century, we have acquired few such complete technologies. One group, already mentioned, is penicillin and other antibiotics, which offer total solutions, that also are inexpensive and rapidly acting, to the problems of bacterial infection. A second generic complete technology is the vaccine. Those invented to prevent smallpox (first introduced in the eighteenth century) and poliomyelitis (developed in the mid-1950s) have in the twentieth century eradicated the first disease and almost wholly contained the second.

The emerging field of genetic research promises fundamental solutions to a host of disorders, with the prospect of their early detection and correction. Finally, the growing ability to visualize the basic structures of the body through endoscopes and computer-driven imaging machines such as the MRI and PET scans provides diagnostic knowledge facilitating the use of therapeutic technologies that promise complete cures. Indeed, genetic and imaging technologies have taken the anatomic concept of illness to its ultimate terminus. To the question "Where is the disease?" the answer now can be "In this particular gene!"

## Conclusion

Technologies, history shows, can be imperative: We may be impelled to use the capacities they provide us without adequate reflection on whether they will lead to the humane goals of medical care. The ancient Greeks understood this issue. They recognized that technologic means must be used in consonance with articulated, ethically informed ends. Their example remains worth following.

STANLEY JOEL REISER

*Directly related to this article are the other articles in this entry:* PHILOSOPHY OF TECHNOLOGY, *and* TECHNOLOGY ASSESSMENT. *Also directly related is the entry* HEALTH-CARE RESOURCES, ALLOCATION OF. *For a further discussion of topics mentioned in this article, see the entries* ARTIFICIAL HEARTS AND CARDIAC-ASSIST DEVICES; ARTIFICIAL ORGANS AND LIFE-SUPPORT SYSTEMS; DEATH, DEFINITION AND DETERMINATION OF, *article on* CRITERIA FOR DEATH; GENETIC ENGINEERING, *article on* HUMAN GENETIC ENGINEERING; HEALTH AND DISEASE, *article on* HISTORY OF THE CONCEPTS; HOSPITAL, *articles on* MEDIEVAL AND RENAISSANCE HISTORY, *and* MODERN HISTORY; MEDICAL ETHICS, HISTORY OF, *section on* EUROPE, *subsection on* ANCIENT AND MEDIEVAL, *article on* GREECE AND ROME; PHARMACEUTICS, *article on* PHARMACEUTICAL INDUSTRY; PROFESSIONAL–PATIENT RELATIONSHIP, *article on* HISTORICAL PERSPECTIVES; *and* SURGERY. *For a discussion of related ideas, see the entries* MEDICAL INFORMATION SYSTEMS; NARRATIVE; *and* SCIENCE, PHILOSOPHY OF. *See also the* APPENDIX (CODES, OATHS, AND DIRECTIVES RELATED TO BIOETHICS), SECTION II: ETHICAL DIRECTIVES FOR THE PRACTICE OF MEDICINE, OATH OF HIPPOCRATES.

## Bibliography

HIPPOCRATES. 1923a. "The Art." In Vol. 2 of *Hippocrates*, pp. 191–217. 4 vols. Translated by William H. S. Jones. Cambridge, Mass.: Harvard University Press.

———. 1923b. "Decorum." In Vol. 2 of *Hippocrates*, pp. 279–301. 4 vols. Translated by William H. S. Jones. Cambridge, Mass.: Harvard University Press.

HOLMES, OLIVER WENDELL. 1883. "Currents and Counter Currents in Medical Science." In his *Medical Essays*, pp. 173–208. 2d ed. Boston: Houghton Mifflin.

KOCH, ROBERT. 1886. "The Etiology of Tuberculosis." In *Recent Essays by Various Authors on Bacteria in Relation to Disease*, pp. 1–66. Edited by W. Watson Cheyne. London: New Sydenham Society.

LAENNEC, RENÉ. 1821. *A Treatise on Diseases of the Chest*. Translated by John Forbes. London: T. & G. Underwood.

LISTER, JOSEPH. 1867. "On the Antiseptic Principle in the Practice of Surgery." *Lancet* 2:353–356.

MORGAGNI, GIOVANNI BATTISTA. 1960. *The Seats and Causes of Diseases Investigated by Anatomy*. Translated by Benjamin Alexander. New York: Hafner.

NIGHTINGALE, FLORENCE. 1863. *Notes on Hospitals*. 3d ed., rev. London: Longman, Green, Longman, Roberts, & Green.

PIUS XII. 1977. [1958]. "The Prolongation of Life." In *Ethics in Medicine: Historical Perspectives and Contemporary Concerns*, pp. 501–504. Edited by Stanley Joel Reiser, Arthur J. Dyck, and William J. Curran. Cambridge, Mass.: MIT Press.

REISER, STANLEY JOEL. 1978. *Medicine and the Reign of Technology*. New York: Cambridge University Press.

———. 1991a. "The Clinical Record in Medicine. Part I: Learning from Cases." *Annals of Internal Medicine* 114, no. 10:902–907.

———. 1991b. "The Clinical Record in Medicine: Part II: Reforming Content and Purpose." *Annals of Internal Medicine* 114, no. 11:980–985.

THOMAS, LEWIS. 1977. "On the Science and Technology of Medicine." In *Doing Better and Feeling Worse: Health in the United States*, pp. 35–46. Edited by John H. Knowles. New York: W. W. Norton.

VESALIUS, ANDREAS. 1980. [1543]. *De humani corporis fabrica*. Stuttgart: Medicina Rara.

## II. PHILOSOPHY OF TECHNOLOGY

Philosophy of technology aspires to comprehensive reflection on the making and using of artifacts. Medicine is increasingly defined not just by the character of its human interactions (physician–patient relationships) or professional expertise (knowledge of illness and related therapies) or its end (health), but also by the type and character of its instruments (from stethoscope to high-tech imaging devices) and the construction of special human-artifact interactions (synthetic drugs, prosthetic devices). Indeed, the physician–patient relationship, medical knowledge, and the concept of health are all affected by technological change. There is even debate about whether the term "artifact" should include nonmaterial as well as material human constructions, in which case all of the above might well be interpreted as technologies. From either perspective, medicine and the issues of bioethics fall within the purview of the philosophy of technology.

## Historical development

Philosophy of technology as a distinct discipline originated with the publication of Ernst Kapp's *Grundlinien einer Philosophie der Technik* (1877), the first book to be entitled a "philosophy of technology." A left-wing Hegelian contemporary of Karl Marx, whose thought includes important analyses of human-machine systems, Kapp left Germany in the mid-1800s to become a pioneer and "hydrotherapist" on the central Texas frontier. Returning to Europe two decades later, he elaborated a general theory of technology as "organ projection"—from the hammer as extension of the fist to railway and telegraph as extensions of the circulatory and nervous systems—thereby promoting analysis of the philosophical-anthropological foundations of technology.

Another major formative figure was Friedrich Dessauer, whose *Philosophie der Technik* (1927) and *Streit um die Technik* (1956) reflect his experience as the inventor of deep penetration X-ray therapy. For Dessauer the philosophical core of technology is the act of invention, for which he sought to provide a Kantian analysis of transcendental preconditions. Dessauer's argument that the fact inventions work shows how inventors depend on insight into a supernatural realm of "pre-established solutions" to technical problems raises basic epistemological and metaphysical issues.

José Ortega y Gasset and Martin Heidegger, two major philosophers of the twentieth century, also contributed texts dedicated to the theme of technology. Ortega's "Meditación de la técnica" (1939) presents technical activity as a means for realizing some supernatural human self-conception, and modern technology as generalized knowledge of how to create such means. Ortega thus pushes anthropological reflection to new depths. Heidegger's "Die Frage nach der Technik" (1954) argues that both traditional technics or craft and modern technology are forms of truth, revealing different aspects of Being. Modern technology in particular is a "challenging" and "setting-upon" that reveals Being as "resource"—that is, the world as a reservoir of materials subject to indefinite human manipulations. In this argument Heidegger likewise carries epistemological and metaphysical reflection well beyond Kantian terms.

Lewis Mumford, Jacques Ellul, Herbert Marcuse, Jürgen Habermas, and Michel Foucault have made further contributions to the development of philosophy of technology from the perspective of social theory. Mumford (1934) focuses attention on technological materials and processes as major elements in the historical development of modern civilization. Ellul (1954) argues that the pursuit of technical efficiency is the defining characteristic of the contemporary world, which constitutes a milieu distinct from the natural and social milieus that preceded it. For Ellul, just as the Hebrew-Christian tradition once demythologized the two earlier milieus, now it called upon to demythologize technology.

Marcuse (1964) and Habermas (1968) have debated the character of technology as ideology. Foucault (1988) views all technologies and sciences as masking power manipulations, and develops a special analysis of technologies as historical transformations and determinations of the self. Such ideas exercise continuing influence in debates over the extent to which technology is properly conceived as an autonomous determinant of human affairs (see Winner, 1986) or as a social construction (see Feenberg, 1991). Such debates in turn influence fundamental orientations with regard to practical questions about the assessment and control of technology that find expression in such applied fields as medical ethics, environmental ethics, engineering ethics, and computer ethics.

Ortega and Heidegger are leading figures in the Continental or phenomenological tradition in the philosophy of technology. Further analyses of phenomenological inspiration can be found in the work of Don Ihde (1979) on human-technics interactions and of Albert Borgmann (1984) on the political-cultural implications of contemporary technological formations.

A different, equally strong tradition in the philosophy of technology is constituted by Anglo-American analytic reflection on artificial intelligence (AI). Here questions center on the extent to which brains are computers and thinking processes can be modeled (see, e.g., Simon, 1969; Dreyfus, 1972). In contrast to the phenomenological tradition, the Anglo-American analysis of AI exhibits considerable interactions with biomedical theory of neurological processes and, to a lesser extent, with biomedical practice.

## Theoretical perspectives

Throughout its diverse strands, philosophy of technology, like philosophy generally, includes theoretical and practical issues, from epistemology and metaphysics to ethics and politics, all of which can helpfully inform bioethics. Comprehensive understanding nevertheless grows out of partial understandings. The making and using of artifacts involve not only the artifacts themselves but also technological knowledge, technological activity, and technological volition. Theoretical analyses can thus conveniently be described by referencing tendencies to interpret technology in one of four primary forms.

**Technology as object.**    The theory that identifies technology with particular artifacts, such as tools, machines, electronic devices, or consumer products, is the commonsense view. Initially it involves a classification of artifacts into different types, according to their own internal structures, different kinds of human engagement, impacts on the environment, or other factors. Mumford, for instance, distinguishes utilities (roads, electric power networks), tools (artifacts under immediate human power and guidance), machines (nonhuman power with immediate human guidance), and automatons (nonhuman power and no immediate human guidance).

Taking a different tack, Borgmann argues a distinction between things and devices. An example of a thing, in Borgmann's special sense, is a traditional fireplace, which engages a variety of human activities ranging from cutting wood to cooking food, functions in a clearly understandable manner, and is an explicit center of daily life. By contrast, a device, such as a heat pump, simply makes available some commodity (hot and cold air) by nonobvious processes and disappears into a background of quotidian activities. The device is a special instance of what Heidegger called a "resource."

Ihde, in a different but equally provocative manner, distinguishes embodiment and hermeneutic relations between humans and their instruments. Embodiment relations experience the world through instruments, as exemplified by eyeglasses, which disappear into and become an unconscious part of the experience of seeing. In hermeneutic relations, by contrast, the instrument itself—for instance, a camera—becomes part of the world with which one engages; a user consciously focuses on the operation and interpretation of this instrument. Both Borgmann's and Ihde's distinctions obviously provide frameworks within which to interpret the myriad tools and instruments of high-technology medicine.

**Technology as knowledge.** Etymologically, however, the word "technology" implies not objects but "knowledge of *techne*," or craft skill. Epistemological analyses of such knowledge distinguish between knowing how (intuitive skill) and knowing that (propositional knowledge). The transition from premodern technics to modern technology can thus be argued as defined by the development of propositional knowledge about *techne* through the unification of technics and science.

This theory of modern technology as applied science is particularly influential among scientists and engineers, and has been given detailed philosophical exposition by Mario Bunge (1967). For Bunge, modern technology develops when the rules of prescientific crafts, originally discovered by trial-and-error methods, are replaced by the "grounded rules" or technological theories. Technological theories can be formulated by applying either the content or the method of science to technical practices. The former application takes preexisting scientific knowledge (e.g., fluid dynamics) and adapts it under certain boundary conditions to formulate an engineering science (aerodynamics). The latter uses the methods of science to formulate distinctive engineering analyses of human-machine interactions, such as operations research and decision theory.

Medicine can readily be incorporated within such an epistemological analysis. Prior to the nineteenth century, most medical practice relied on rule-of-thumb experience. But twentieth-century medicine has involved the progressive grounding of medical practice in the sciences of anatomy and physiology as well as the development of such distinctive fields as epidemiology and biomedical engineering. Indeed, José Sanmartín (1987), for instance, analyzes genetic engineering exactly as an embedding of techniques in scientific theory.

**Technology as activity.** The transformation of some technics (such as medicine) into an applied science is not, however, simply an epistemic event. As Foucault (1963) argues, for example, modern medicine "is made possible as a form of knowledge" by the reorganization of hospitals and new kinds of medical practices. This emphasis on technology as activity or a complex of activities is characteristic of social theory. Ellul's "characterology of technique" and analysis of the central role played by the rational pursuit of technical efficiency in the economy, the state, and what he terms "human techniques" (ranging from education to medicine) is another case in point, as are the Marxist and neo-Marxist analyses of Marcuse, Habermas, and Andrew Feenberg.

The emphasis on technology as activity has roots in Max Weber's observation that there are techniques of every conceivable human activity—from artistic production and performance to mass manufacturing and bureaucratic organization—even education, politics, and religion. One classic problem for social theorists is to explain the character and limits of "technicalization"—that is, the movement from traditional societies, in which techniques are situated within and delimited by nontechnical values, to modern societies, in which techniques are increasingly evaluated solely in technical terms. In traditional societies, for example, animals can be eaten only if butchered in a ritually prescribed manner; in modern societies animal slaughter is largely subject to calculations of efficiency.

Efficiency can also be conceived in economic terms and applied at micro or macro levels. The former is typical of analyses internal to business corporations (including hospitals and clinics); the latter, of social assessments of technology. In regard to technology assessments especially, there arise questions of the limits of technicalization and possible alternative forms of technical institutions (see Feenberg, 1991), as well as of responsible agency and risk.

**Technology as volition.** A fourth element in the interrelationship of knowledge, object, and activity is that of volition. The human activity of making and using artifacts depends not only on knowledge but also on volition. Indeed, it can be argued that volition is even more important in this respect than knowledge, that is, that human action can be ignorant but not unwilled.

The philosophical analysis of volition distinguishes between volition in the weaker senses of wishing, hoping, longing, and desiring, and the stronger or more decisive intending and affirming. Volition in the second or stronger senses is constituted by self-reflective identification with some particular wish, hope, or desire that takes on the character of a project. Ortega, Mumford, and Frederick Ferré (1988) argue that technology is essentially a matter of volition in one or more of these senses. According to Ferré, for instance, technology is grounded in "the urge to live and to thrive." For Ortega, technology is based in the willed attempt at a worldly realization of some specific self-image. For Mumford, technology in a distinctive sense emerges when human beings subordinate their traditional polytechnical activities of craft, religious ritual, and poetry to the monotechnical pursuit of physical power—something that first happened about five thousand years ago in Egypt, with the construction of the pyramids by means of large, rigid, hierarchical social organizations that he terms "megamachines."

Defining technology in terms of volition makes possible the perception of broad historical continuities more than does a focus on the elements of knowledge or object or even activity. It is inherently more believable that the "will" to fly was coeval with human existence than that technical knowledge of how to fly, flying machines, or the human performance of flying or flying-like actions have existed from time immemorial. Such an approach once again has immediate implications for the interpretation of medicine. If medicine is interpreted primarily as grounded in volition, then it is inherently more believable that there exists a fundamental continuity between premodern and modern medicines.

Nevertheless, one of the most sustained critiques of modern medicine is precisely that as volition, it is fundamentally different from all previous kinds of medicine. Ivan Illich's *Medical Nemesis* (1976) argues that modern medicine arises from a basic "social commitment to provide all citizens with almost unlimited outputs." Indeed, the nemesis of rising iatrogenic disease is a direct result of "our contemporary hygienic hubris," which can be reversed only "through a recovery of the will to self-care." In the 1990s, however, Illich becomes critical of the idea of self-care when it serves as an ideological support for what has been termed "health fascism."

## Practical perspectives

Not theoretical analysis, however, but ethical and political concerns predominate in philosophy of technology. Ethics has from its beginnings in the West involved at least marginal considerations of technology. Aristotle's *Nicomachean Ethics*, for instance, in passing identifies *techne* as an intellectual virtue. More than two thousand years later Immanuel Kant distinguished moral and technical imperatives. But in line with such marginal attention, from Plato and Aristotle to the Renaissance,

technology was widely accepted as properly subject to ethical constraints. From the Renaissance to the Enlightenment, by contrast, traditional restraints were effectively replaced with an ethical commitment to the unfettered pursuit of technology for what Francis Bacon called "the relief of man's estate." It is precisely this modern commitment, along with its subsequent questioning in response to a series of increasingly prominent problems, that frames the contemporary prominence of ethical issues in the philosophy of technology.

**Alienation.**    Historically, the first problem of modern technology involved the industrial revolution and alienation. At the basis of modern technological making lies a belief that the world as it is given does not provide a suitable home for human beings; humanity must construct a home for itself. The problem is that human beings do not immediately find themselves at home in the worlds they technologically create. The resulting alienation is especially problematic to the extent that it is grounded in attempts to overcome alienation.

The two most extensive critiques of technological alienation are Romanticism and socialism. The Romantic critique, an early version of which appears in Jean-Jacques Rousseau's *Discourse on the Sciences and the Arts* (1750), focuses on how technology alienates the individual from feelings and sentiments, as manifested in relationships with nature, the past, or other human beings. This is caused, according to the Romantic argument, by a one-sided development of rationality. Romanticism thus perceives technology as an extension of reason and proposes to enclose it within a larger affective life.

By contrast, in the socialist critique of alienation, Marx, like Kapp, explicitly conceives technology as a human organ projection. Marx thus focuses on the separation of human beings from control over the tools and products of their labor, as manifested in an economy based on money and the "fetishism of commodities." In response, socialism argues for a comprehensive restructuring of society to promote worker control of the means of production.

In biomedical practice the use of technological instruments and rationalized systems of diagnosis raises the issue of alienation in the form of questions about the depersonalization of health-care techniques and organizations. Responses can exhibit characteristically Romantic or socialist features. Exemplifying Romanticism are proposals to situate diagnostic techniques within a more humanistic framework, perhaps one of beautiful buildings and a pleasant environment. Exemplifying a socialist response might be arguments for the promotion of patient autonomy by granting patients more direct control over their own health-care institutions.

**Warfare.**    A second ethical problem has centered on technology and war. There are two basic theories about the relationship between war and technology: First, technological weapons make war so horrible that it becomes unthinkable; rational self-interest leads to deterrence of their use. Second, human beings will always tend to miscalculate their self-interests and go to war; weapons production must therefore be limited, and a higher ideal of global human unity promoted.

Prior to World War I, naive versions of the first theory largely supported the pursuit of technology. The trauma of the war contributed to pessimistic criticisms of technological civilization and led to emphasis on the second theory. This pessimistic critique, coupled with idealist attempts at world government, failed to avoid World War II and a technological practice of genocide, the invention and use of the atomic bomb, and a subsequent Cold War spread of nuclear weapons. As a result, much more sophisticated versions of deterrence policy were developed in alliance with management and decision theories. Advanced technological weapons development projects also stimulated science and technology policy and management studies, while the practice of nuclear deterrence was subject to extended moral criticism. One of the more idealistic criticisms argues that human unity and peace, which in the past could remain as moral exhortations, have now become necessities, lest human beings obliterate themselves from the face of the planet. In this argument the rational self-interest of the first theory appears to merge with the idealism of the second.

Prospects for social and genetic engineering call forth similar arguments between pragmatic deterrence management and idealistic delimitation. The progressive refinements of conditioning techniques and sophisticated drug therapies create behavior-control technologies of immense potential power. Developments in recombinant DNA technology and the Human Genome Project offer opportunities to extend this power to the biological creation of human life. As Sanmartín has pointed out, this attack on the vagaries of human nature can be seen as developing new technologies for the prevention of "social diseases" such as war.

**Technology and social change.** Concerns about the relatively specific issues of alienation and warfare have been complemented by more general analyses of the causal relations and patterns of interaction that obtain between technology and social change. Such analyses include bottom-up case studies of changes related to bureaucracy, urbanization, work (from mass production to automation to customized production), leisure and mobility, secularization, communications (from telephone and radio to television and computer), and medical technologies, as well as top-down theoretical reflections on the same dimensions of social life and on the social order as a whole. Within both approaches it is common to find descriptions of disorder between technology and society brought about by technological change along with arguments for addressing such disorder by means of some intellectual and/or volitional adaptations.

In the period between the two world wars, for instance, William F. Ogburn's *Social Change* (1922) described a "cultural lag" between technological development and social adaptation across a variety of indicators, and argued for a more intelligent appropriation of technology. A decade later Henri Bergson's *Two Sources of Morality and Religion* (1932) argued that the vices of industrial civilization as a whole could be corrected only by what he termed a "supplement of soul" that is at once ascetic (against luxuries) and charitable (for eliminating inequalities).

To stress the need for intellectual or rational adaptations is no doubt more characteristic of advanced industrial society, with its concomitant large-scale educational institutions and activities. The kind of piecemeal social engineering advocated by John Dewey and Karl Popper, and the many theories of economic rationality from Pareto efficiency to risk–benefit analysis, and of postindustrial organization from Daniel Bell to Habermas, likewise advocate effective increases in the rational control of modern technology. By contrast, a follower of Bergson such as Ellul argues that technology has become a kind of totalitarian milieu that requires comprehensive demythologizing. Others suggest the need for expansions of affective sensibility. Some theories of postmodern culture exhibit certain affinities with this approach.

With regard to increasing rationality, Kristin Shrader-Frechette (1991) has drawn an explicit parallel between the requirements of informed consent in the practice of medically risky procedures and the general societal adaptation to technological change. With regard to affective responses to technological change, the work of Illich is illustrative.

**Pollution and the environmental crisis.** Perhaps even more demanding of attention than warfare, and adding a new dimension to analyses of technological change, are problems associated with environmental pollution and global climate transformation. The environmental crisis has obvious and fundamental impacts on human health and safety, and thereby on biomedicine. Indeed, outside medical ethics, perhaps the single most intensively explored area of applied philosophy is that of environmental ethics.

Beyond intensified self-interest, environmental change has engendered the new science of ecology and extended ethical concern both temporally (for future generations) and ontologically (for nonhuman entities). As analyzed by Hans Jonas (1979), this extension is grounded in "the altered nature of human action" brought about by the "novel powers" of modern technology. Although all human life requires some technical activity, not until the advent of modern scientific technology did the technical power to create become so explosive as to be capable of fundamentally transforming nature and the future of the human condition. On the basis of this power there arises what Jonas terms an "imperative of responsibility" to "ensure a future."

Jonas explicitly argues the application of this principle of responsibility in the field of bioethics. Applications might also be adumbrated for other discussions in environmental ethics, such as those that distinguish shallow versus deep ecology movements and argue the rights of nature understood as wilderness. Could one not, for instance, distinguish a shallow versus a deep bioethics? Would it not be possible to argue, against excessive medical intervention, a defense of wildness in biology?

**Engineering ethics.**    A second well-developed field of applied ethics with potential implications for the medical dimensions of bioethics is that of engineering ethics (see Martin and Schinzinger, 1989). Here a basic shift has taken place in the interpretation of the primary responsibility of the professional engineer—from loyalty to a company or client (patterned after the ethics of the medical and legal professions) to responsibility to public health, safety, and welfare. Could this shift, resting on a recognition of engineering as social experimentation, have implications for new understandings of professional medical obligation? Is it not the case that technological medicine is, as much as the treatment of individual patients, to some extent a social experiment? If so, then the engineering ethics defense of the rights and role of the whistle-blower might well have analogous applications in the biomedical field.

**Computers and information technology.**    A third well-developed area of applied ethics deals with computers. One defining book in this field was written by a computer scientist (see Weizenbaum, 1976) and based on Mumford's philosophical anthropology of the human as a polyvalent being for whom calculating is only a very small part of thinking and a limited dimension of technics. Key issues in the philosophical analysis of computers concern the degree to which human thinking can be modeled by computers and the extent to which human beings should properly rely on computer programs, especially in areas such as weapons. Subsequent development, as summarized by Deborah Johnson (1985), has emphasized issues of individual privacy and corporate security, the formulation of ethical codes for computer professionals, and liabilities for the malfunctioning of computer programs. The computerization of medical practice calls for the application of such reflection to many aspects of high-tech medical diagnosis and treatment.

**Development and diversity.**    The ambiguities of technology in developing countries, together with reassessments of the impacts of advanced technological transformations in relation to women and ethnic minorities, especially in the United States and Europe, raise new issues regarding the abilities of scientific technology to accommodate true diversity. On the one side, there are questions of equity. In advanced technological countries, technological power and affluence are not equally shared between men and women and among different ethnic communities. Nor does there appear to be equality of opportunity among advanced and developing countries. On the other side, technological development tends to set up national and international economic orders that homogenize personal and world cultures. Distinctions among markets and ways of life are subsumed within the financial structures of transnational corporations and global communications systems. This paradox of inequity and homogenization poses a fundamental challenge to both reflection and action.

Attempts to address this challenge can be found in the alternative technology movement, arguments regarding the ethics and politics of development, and in diverse feminist contributions to the philosophy of technology (as collected, for instance, in Rothschild, 1983). Feminist critiques of technology, for instance, emphasize both the need for equity and the threats of homogenization. Technologies of the workplace are to a large extent sexually differentiated; those of the home are designed and used in ways that confirm masculine and feminine roles. But technological culture creates images of androgynous liberation while medical procedures diminish the experiences of gendered bodies. In the face of this paradox, what some feminists argue is the need for a new theory and practice of technology itself, a truly alternative technology, one that transforms both its masculine biases and its characteristically modern commitments. The ideals and pursuit of alternative medicines can be interpreted as concrete attempts to achieve such a goal.

## Conclusion

Successive technological problems have provoked a series of ethical analyses and moral responses. Reflections on these problems and their emerging responses, because they have been focused on a particular technology, have tended to remain isolated from each other and untested by generalization. Philosophies of technology that have attempted to bridge such particularities, and that include a substantial role for bioethics, can be found in the work of Jonas, Sanmartín, Gilbert Hottois (1990), and Friedrich Rapp (1990).

Complementing such work, problems addressed by the varied discussions of practice have been approached from within a variety of ethical frameworks, among which are natural-law theory, deontologism, and consequentialism. With natural-law theory, one tends to assess technological change in terms of its harmony with some given lawful order perceived in nature. With deontological theory the emphasis is on evaluating the rightfulness and wrongfulness of technological change in accord with some inner criteria of the action. With consequentialism there is an effort to look to the goodness or badness of future results that flow from some particular technology. Each such ethical framework can exhibit selective affinities with different basic theoretical conceptions of technology.

Environmental ethics, for instance, tends to be distinguished by criticisms of technologies that do not harmonize with preexisting natural order. The emphasis here is easily placed on human activity, with nonhuman realities taking on special moral significance. Computer ethics, by contrast, tends to put forth deontological principles about the wrongness, for instance, of the invasion of privacy. Such an ethics emphasizes human intention or volition with respect to technology. Finally, technology policy studies are likely to stress the evaluation of technologies in terms of results, and thus to call attention to the physical consequences of technological decisions. Here the issue of risk becomes a special challenge to the accepted cost-benefit calculus typical of consequentialist analysis.

The suggestive character of such relationships points toward the need for a more systematic pursuit of the philosophy of technology in ways that integrate epistemological, metaphysical, ethical, and political analyses. They also indicate the opportunities for more extended interactions between general philosophies of technology and the issues of biomedical ethics, interactions that have the potential for deepening and increasing the fruitfulness of both.

CARL MITCHAM

*Directly related to this article are the other articles in this entry:* HISTORY OF MEDICAL TECHNOLOGY, *and* TECHNOLOGY ASSESSMENT. *Also directly related are the entries* SCIENCE, PHILOSOPHY OF; MEDICINE, PHILOSOPHY OF; *and* NATURE. *For a further discussion of topics mentioned in this article, see the entries* ALTERNATIVE THERAPIES; GENOME MAPPING AND SEQUENCING; HUMAN NATURE; METAPHOR AND ANALOGY; *and* WARFARE, *article on* CHEMICAL AND BIOLOGICAL WARFARE. *This article will find application in the entries* BIOMEDICAL ENGINEERING; BIOTECHNOLOGY; ENVIRONMENTAL ETHICS; *and* REPRODUCTIVE TECHNOLOGIES.

## Bibliography

For more extensive introductions to philosophy of technology, see Friedrich Rapp (1978), Carl Mitcham (1980), and Frederick Ferré (1988), which can be complemented with the collections of readings by Carl Mitcham and Robert Mackey (1972) and Friedrich Rapp (1974). The most important serials are *Research in Philosophy and Technology* (1978–present) and *Philosophy and Technology* (1981–present). There is also a "Philosophy of Technology" monograph series from Indiana University Press (1990–present). For bibliography, consult Carl Mitcham and Robert Mackey, *Bibliography of the Philosophy of Technology* (Chicago: University of Chicago Press, 1973; paperback reprint with author index, Ann Arbor: Books on Demand, 1985), and supplements that have appeared in *Research in Philosophy and Technology*.

BERGSON, HENRI. 1932. *Les deux sources de la morale et de la religion.* Paris: F. Alcan. Translated by Ruth Ashley Audra, Cloudesley S. H. Brenton, and William H. Carter under the title *The Two Sources of Morality and Religion.* London: Macmillan, 1935.

BORGMANN, ALBERT. 1984. *Technology and the Character of Contemporary Life: A Philosophical Inquiry.* Chicago: University of Chicago Press.

BUNGE, MARIO. 1967. "Action." In *The Search for Truth,* pp. 121–150. Vol. 2 of his *Scientific Research.* Berlin: Springer-Verlag. Translated into Spanish by Manuel Sacristán Luzón under the title *La investigación científica: Su estratégia y su filosofía.* Barcelona: Ariel, 1969.

———. 1985. "Technology: From Engineering to Decision Theory." In *Life Science, Social Science, and Technology,* pp. 219–311. Part 2 of *Philosophy of Science and Technology,* vol. 7 of his *Treatise on Basic Philosophy.* Boston: D. Reidel.

DESSAUER, FRIEDRICH. 1927. *Philosophie der Technik: Das Problem der Realisierung.* Bonn: Friedrich Cohen. 2d enl. ed., *Streit um die Technik.* Frankfurt am Main: J. Knecht, 1956.

DREYFUS, HUBERT L. 1972. *What Computers Can't Do: A Critique of Artificial Reason.* New York: Harper & Row. Rev. ed., *What Computers Can't Do: The Limits of Artificial Intelligence.* New York: Harper & Row, 1979. 2d rev. ed., *What Computers Still Can't Do: A Critique of Artificial Reason.* Cambridge, Mass.: MIT Press, 1992.

ELLUL, JACQUES. 1954. *La technique; ou, l'enjeu du siècle.* Paris: Armand Colin. 2d rev. ed. Paris: Economica, 1990. Translated by John Wilkinson under the title *The Technological Society.* New York: Alfred A. Knopf, 1964.

———. 1977. *Le système technicien.* Paris: Calmann-Lévy. Translated by Joachim Neugroschel under the title *The Technological System.* New York: Continuum, 1980.

———. 1988. *Le bluff technologique.* Paris: Hachette. Translated by Geoffrey W. Bromiley as *The Technological Bluff.* Grand Rapids, Mich.: W. B. Eerdmans, 1990.

FEENBERG, ANDREW. 1991. *Critical Theory of Technology.* New York: Oxford University Press. Carries forward the ideas of Marx, Marcuse, and Habermas.

FERRÉ, FREDERICK. 1988. *Philosophy of Technology.* Englewood Cliffs, N.J.: Prentice-Hall.

FOUCAULT, MICHEL. 1963. *Naissance de la clinique: une archéologie du regard médical.* Paris: Presses universitaires de France. Translated by A. M. Sheridan Smith under the title *The Birth of the Clinic: An Archeology of Medical Perception.* New York: Pantheon, 1973.

———. 1988. *Technologies of the Self: A Seminar with Michel Foucault.* Edited by Luther H. Martin, Huck Gutman, and Patrick H. Hutton. Amherst: University of Massachusetts Press. This late work should be read in light of *Naissance de la clinique*.

HABERMAS, JÜRGEN. 1968. *Technik und Wissenschaft als "Ideologie."* Frankfurt am Main: Suhrkamp. Translated by Jeremy J. Shapiro as the last three essays in *Toward a Rational Society: Student Protest, Science, and Politics*. Boston: Beacon Press, 1970.

HEIDEGGER, MARTIN. 1954. "Die Frage nach der Technik." In his *Vorträge und Aufsätze*, pp. 13–44. Pfullingen: Günther Neske. Translated by William Lovitt under the title "The Question Concerning Technology." In *The Question Concerning Technology and Other Essays*. San Francisco: Harper & Row, 1977.

HOTTOIS, GILBERT. 1984. *Le signe et la technique: La philosophie à l'épreuve de la technique*. Paris: Aubier. Contains the general philosophy of technology upon which Hottois's bioethics is based.

———. 1990. *Le paradigme bioéthique: Une éthique pour la technoscience*. Brussels: De Boeck.

IHDE, DON. 1979. *Technics and Praxis*. Boston: D. Reidel.

———. 1990. *Technology and the Lifeworld: From Garden to Earth*. Bloomington: Indiana University Press. Extends the reflection initiated by *Technics and Praxis*.

ILLICH, IVAN. 1973. *Tools for Conviviality*. New York: Harper & Row. A more general statement of his philosophy of technology.

———. 1976. *Medical Nemesis: The Expropriation of Health*. New York: Pantheon.

JOHNSON, DEBORAH G. 1985. *Computer Ethics*. Englewood Cliffs, N.J.: Prentice-Hall.

———, ed. 1991. *Ethical Issues in Engineering*. Englewood Cliffs, N.J.: Prentice-Hall.

JOHNSON, DEBORAH G., and SNAPPER, JOHN W., eds. 1985. *Ethical Issues in the Use of Computers*. Belmont, Calif.: Wadsworth.

JONAS, HANS. 1979. *Das Prinzip Verantwortung: Versuch einer Ethik für die technologische Zivilisation*. Frankfurt am Main: Suhrkamp. Translated by Hans Jonas and David Herr under the title *The Imperative of Responsibility: In Search of an Ethics for the Technological Age*. Chicago: University of Chicago Press, 1984.

———. 1985. *Technik, Medizin und Ethik: Zur Praxis des Prinzips Verantwortung*. Frankfurt am Main: Insel. A practical application of his general philosophy of technology.

KAPP, ERNST. 1877. *Grundlinien einer Philosophie der Technik: Zur Entstehungsgeschichte der Kultur aus neuen Gesichtspunkten*. Braunschweig: G. Westermann.

MARCUSE, HERBERT. 1964. *One-Dimensional Man: Studies in the Ideology of Advanced Industrial Society*. Boston: Beacon Press.

MARTIN, MIKE W., and SCHINZINGER, ROLAND. 1989. *Ethics in Engineering*. 2d ed. New York: McGraw-Hill.

MITCHAM, CARL. 1980. "Philosophy of Technology." In *A Guide to the Culture of Science, Technology, and Medicine*, pp. 282–363. Edited by Paul T. Durbin. New York: Free Press. The paperback reprint, 1984, has a slightly revised bibliography.

MITCHAM, CARL, and MACKEY, ROBERT, eds. 1972. *Philosophy and Technology: Readings in the Philosophical Problems of Technology*. New York: Free Press. Paperback reprint, 1983. The paperback has an updated, annotated bibliography.

MUMFORD, LEWIS. 1934. *Technics and Civilization*. New York: Harcourt Brace.

———. 1967. *Technics and Human Development*. Vol. 1 of *The Myth of the Machine*. New York: Harcourt Brace Jovanovich. An extended critique of the definition of the human being as a tool-using animal.

———. 1970. *The Pentagon of Power*. Vol. 2 of *The Myth of the Machine*. New York: Harcourt Brace Jovanovich. Analyzes the closed circle of technological rationality.

OGBURN, WILLIAM F. 1922. *Social Change with Respect to Culture and Original Nature*. New York: Viking.

ORTEGA Y GASSET, JOSÉ. 1939. "Meditación de la técnica." In his *Ensimismamiento y alteración*, pp. 55–157. Buenos Aires: Espasa-Calpe. Collected in vol. 5 of *Obras completas*, pp. 313–371. Madrid: Alianza, 1946.

RAPP, FRIEDRICH J. 1978. *Analytische Technikphilosophie*. Freiburg: Karl Alber. Translated as *Analytical Philosophy of Technology*. Boston Studies in the Philosophy of Science, vol. 63. Boston: D. Reidel, 1981.

———. 1982. "Philosophy of Technology." In vol. 2 of *Contemporary Philosophy: A New Survey*, pp. 361–412. Edited by Guttorm Floistad. The Hague: Martinus Nijhoff.

———, ed. 1974. *Contributions to the Philosophy of Technology: Studies in the Structure of Thinking in the Technological Sciences*. Boston: D. Reidel.

———, ed. 1990. *Technik und Philosophie*. Düsseldorf: VDI Verlag. A cooperative overview with contributions by Rapp, Alois Huning, Ernst Oldemeyer, Hans Lenk, and Walther Ch. Zimmerli.

ROTHSCHILD, JOAN, ed. 1983. *Machina ex Dea: Feminist Perspectives on Technology*. New York: Pergamon. Includes twelve representative articles.

SANMARTÍN, JOSÉ. 1987. *Los nuevos redentores: Reflexiones sobre la ingeniería genética, la sociobiología y el mundo feliz que nos prometen*. Barcelona: Anthropos.

SHRADER-FRECHETTE, KRISTIN S. 1991. *Risk and Rationality: Philosophical Foundations for Populist Reforms*. Berkeley: University of California Press.

SIMON, HERBERT A. 1969. *The Sciences of the Artificial*. Cambridge, Mass.: MIT Press. 2d enl. ed., Cambridge, Mass.: MIT Press, 1991.

WEIZENBAUM, JOSEPH. 1976. *Computer Power and Human Reason: From Judgment to Calculation*. New York: W. H. Freeman.

WINNER, LANGDON. 1977. *Autonomous Technology: Technics-out-of-Control as a Theme in Political Theory*. Cambridge, Mass.: MIT Press.

———. 1986. *The Whale and the Reactor: A Search for Limits in an Age of High Technology*. Chicago: University of Chicago Press. A key chapter is "Do Artifacts Have Politics?" pp. 19–39.

## III. TECHNOLOGY ASSESSMENT

Technology assessment (TA) is the multidisciplinary evaluation of the impacts of a technical process, substance, project, or method, such as renal dialysis. Its goal is to discover and predict the harmful and beneficial risks and consequences of some agricultural, biological, chemical, electronic, industrial, or medical technology, and therefore to provide a sound basis for developing public policy regarding it. A key component of TA is the evaluation of social, ethical, and environmental impacts likely to be associated with a technology; an environmental impact assessment is one part of a TA.

Technology assessment, in an informal sense, has been practiced since ancient times, when the Mesopotamians charged their priests with determining the consequences of their technological activities. Although neither technology nor assessment is new, recent scientific discoveries have increased both the importance and the scope of TA. Thomas Jefferson, for example, once remarked that the greatest service that can be rendered any country is to add a useful plant to its culture. Ever since the discovery of recombinant DNA technology in the early 1970s, biotechnology has been an essential tool of inventors doing exactly what Jefferson proposed: adding new plants designed to improve the world's health, food supply, and environment. New plants and microorganisms have been patented since 1980, raising a host of legal, economic, safety, social, political, and ethical problems.

As Jefferson might have foreseen, new biological and medical technologies have brought both benefits and risks. In the life sciences, for example, researchers have developed genetically engineered microbial pesticides that they hope will provide fewer risks and greater benefits than the older chemical pesticides. Other scientists have praised the benefits of hormones (such as bovine somatotropin) used to stimulate milk production in dairy cattle, while animal-rights activists have publicized the stress and disease the hormones allegedly cause in the cattle. Environmentalists have charged that using biological techniques to clean up oil spills stimulates algal blooms and eutrophication, although they recognize the value of controlling the spills. Even as they enjoy the benefits of the world's most advanced medical technologies, proponents of patient rights likewise have argued that doctors have used computed tomography (CT), mammography, and electronic fetal monitoring, for example, in risky ways that raise real doubts as to both their efficacy and their safety (U.S. Congress, 1978; Jennett, 1986). Despite the benefits of the U.S. medical "technocopia," its costs include driving up health-care prices and frequent use of technologies that are sometimes ill suited to the patient (Donaldson and Sox, 1992).

Evaluations of biomedical technologies and environment-related projects are often inadequate because they require one to ascertain, ahead of time, what *present* actions are desirable, given possible *future* impacts. Even experts do not know what the future holds. In the absence of this knowledge, their forecasts are often little

more than "guesstimates." Assessors in the 1870s, for instance, were seriously troubled when they projected that levels of horse manure would reach unmanageable proportions in the cities of the twentieth century. They did not know that invention of the automobile would solve the problem.

Evaluation of proposed technological projects is also difficult, not only because information is frequently inadequate to make good policy, but also because the analysis requires coordinating the skills of experts in the natural sciences, social sciences, and humanities: "Quality assessment requires the artful blending of the quantitative and the qualitative, of the objective and the subjective, and of science and politics. It is a form of philosophical reflection on the large-scale, unintended consequences of technology" (Porter et al., 1980, p. 255).

## The institutionalization of TA

In 1966, U.S. Representative Emilio Daddario, who later became the first director of the U.S. Office of Technology Assessment (OTA), introduced the phrase "technology assessment." Most TA (in the formal sense) in the United States began after 1969, when Congress passed the Technology Assessment Act and created the OTA. Governed by a board of six senators and six representatives, evenly divided between the two political parties, the OTA and its technical staff perform technology assessments and authorize their performance by consulting firms and research groups. Through agencies like the National Science Foundation and regulatory bodies such as the Food and Drug Administration, the Nuclear Regulatory Commission, and the Environmental Protection Agency, the U.S. government also buys TA capability by means of contracts and grants.

Outside the United States, countries such as Sweden, Japan, and the United Kingdom probably have the widest range of TA activities. In Sweden, assessment is conducted by the Secretariat for Future Studies under the Office of the Prime Minister. Many Japanese TA's are accomplished by the (government) Science and Technology Agency, but public participation in assessment activities and policymaking is minimal. France has shown more interest than any other country outside the United States in establishing a national office of assessment and has used the U.S. OTA as a model. Likewise, the U.S. National Institutes of Health program has served as a model for health TA in many nations. Although most TA activity throughout the world takes the form of environmental impact analyses of specific technological proposals, assessment is rapidly becoming more sophisticated and more widespread. TA activities are currently taking place in areas such as Indonesia, Ghana, Egypt, Mexico, and many Third World countries (U.S. Congress, 1984; Goodman and Baratz,

1990). The success of TA efforts in various nations, however, is quite different and often depends on the presence of a critical mass of basic scientific research (Gelijns and Halm, 1991).

To the extent that government-financed attempts at TA are inadequate in scope, purpose, funding, or methodology, the danger exists that unguided and self-directed technology may either falter or injure the public. If technology is not assessed and managed properly, it can undermine democratic institutions, disjoin societal power and responsibility, and cause what Langdon Winner terms "reverse adaptation," a situation in which technology is treated as the end of progress rather than the means to it (Winner, 1977).

## The components of TA

Generally TA may take any one of the following forms: (a) project assessment, which focuses on the risks and impacts of a particular, localized undertaking, such as field-testing a bioengineered pesticide at a specific site; (b) problem-oriented assessment, which addresses means of solving a specific societal problem, such as whether to allow donors to sell organs for transplant; and (c) technology-oriented assessment, which examines a new technology, such as ultrasound, and analyzes the risks and consequences it will impose on society and the environment. Technology-oriented assessment is the form of TA that is broadest in scope, and project assessment is the most limited.

TA typically includes at least ten components: (1) a problem definition; (2) a technology description; (3) a technology forecast; (4) a social description; (5) a social forecast; (6) an impact identification; (7) an impact analysis, including a risk assessment; (8) an impact evaluation, including a risk evaluation; (9) a policy analysis; (10) a communication of results. The first of these ten components involves defining the scope and depth of the assessment and identifying the "parties at interest" to the project—those persons likely to gain or to lose as a result of particular impacts. With respect to biomedical technologies, for example, prospective patients are one group of gainers or losers, whereas industries developing the particular technology are the most obvious members of the set of gainers.

The second component of TA is a thorough description of the technology—for example, gene splicing—being evaluated. At the next stage, the assessors attempt to anticipate the character and timing of changes in the technology, so as to reveal factors such as likely future cost savings, new applications, and possible future scientific breakthroughs. At the fourth stage of TA work, assessors attempt to represent the most plausible future configurations of society and to project possible changes in it. Such configurations might include whether gov-

ernment covers basic costs of medical technologies, like renal dialysis, and how innovation in these technologies might be affected by private, rather than government, health insurance (Gelijns, 1992). Given such projections, assessors attempt at the fifth stage of TA to provide a social forecast involving both the technology being assessed and the type of society in which it is likely to be used. In the case of renal dialysis, for example, assessors might forecast that the technology will undergo significant innovations in countries where government support of science is strong, but that such innovation will not be a function of whether private or public funders cover medical costs. At the sixth stage of TA, assessors attempt to identify both direct and higher-order impacts of the proposed project or technology. For example, one direct impact of patenting genes could be the reduced flow and exchange of both information and germ plasm from private companies to universities (U.S. Congress, 1989).

At the seventh stage, the interdisciplinary TA team studies the likelihood and magnitude of the various risks and consequences identified during work on the previous assessment component. Here expertise essential to particular disciplines plays a great role. Epistemologists may use risk assessment to determine the health and safety risks associated with some technology. Economists may employ cost-benefit analysis to investigate certain financial impacts, while philosophers may use ethical analysis to evaluate the equity of various distributions of risks and benefits, and psychologists may employ psychometric surveys to analyze possible social consequences. The next step in the assessment—and one of the most important—is to use these multidisciplinary analyses to determine the significance of the various impacts, relative to the technology and to societal goals. After they evaluate the relevant impacts, assessors at the ninth stage compare options for implementing technological developments and for dealing with their consequences. On the basis of this analysis, they may or may not make explicit policy recommendations. Finally, at the last stage, the TA team determines ways in which the results of its study can be communicated to persons or groups most likely to gain or lose from the technology.

Each of the ten steps of TA is accomplished by a multidisciplinary assessment team. Such a team evaluating a particular CT scanner, for example, might include a radiologist, a health physicist, a biophysicist, an attorney, an ethicist, a psychologist, a political scientist, an economist, and a systems analyst. Because a good assessment must search out not only the impacts of a particular project but also the interactions among them, members of the team must work, in an interdisciplinary as well as an individual mode, on particular substudies related to their individual fields of expertise.

## TA methodology

Despite the importance of reliable TA, there are no universally accepted techniques associated with it. One reason there is no uniform TA methodology is that each technology must be evaluated, in part, on the basis of its societal acceptability. Although science underlies technology and provides the fundamental knowledge for it, assessors ordinarily evaluate a technology as successful, acceptable, or desirable for quite different reasons than they evaluate a scientific theory. Scientific theories are usually assessed on the basis of fairly well-established criteria for their *truth*, for example, simplicity and explanatory or predictive power. Technological inventions, on the other hand, are judged in the context of the *purpose* for which they are used—for example, employing bioengineered crops to increase agricultural productivity. Their success must be evaluated, in part, on the basis of ethical analysis of their goals and consequences.

In general, the methods typically employed in TA are of three types: analytical, empirical, and synthetic. *Analytical* methods employ formal models from which one deduces insights about the problem at hand; they utilize little raw data. For example, one analytical method might include use of a computer simulation to predict the dispersion of a bioengineered organism throughout an agricultural system (Levin and Strauss, 1991). *Empirical* methods begin with information gathering and inductively build models to explain or to predict impacts. Some important empirical methods include opinion surveys and trend extrapolation. *Synthetic* methods combine the analytical and the empirical approaches so that models are based on empirical information, and data gathering is structured by the preexisting models. Economic forecasting and cost-benefit analysis (CBA) are two important synthetic methods often used in TA.

Analytic methods are generally used in studies whose problems are well defined conceptually. Empirical methods tend to be employed when the assessment problem is well defined and when data are available concerning it. Synthetic methods are often used for more complex problems that frequently are ill defined and for which complete data are not available.

CBA often dominates technology-related decision making because the problems addressed by TA typically are neither clearly defined nor those for which adequate data are available, rendering analytical and empirical assessment methods inappropriate. Another reason is that private industry and the profit motive often drive technological development. For example, the impetus for using advances—such as recombinant DNA technology to produce lymphokines used to treat disease (U.S. Congress, 1987)—is often in private biotech firms. Because

of their emphasis on profitability, the key component of industry-based TAs is almost always CBA.

## The role of ethical analysis in TA

Although evaluation of economic impacts is largely the task of economists, assessors from different disciplines also must play a significant role in evaluating other impacts. One component of this evaluation is ethical analysis of the presuppositions in, and consequences following from, the conclusions reached at each step of the TA. Frequently the ethical dimensions of the ten assessment components are ignored, often because of limited public participation in assessment activities. Little has been written on the role of ethics in assessment, in part because TA sometimes has been viewed erroneously as a purely technical study (see Shrader-Frechette, 1985, 1991).

Because the risks and consequences of various technologies—from genetically engineered microbial pesticides to CT scanning of the brain—rarely fall only on those who benefit from them or primarily on those who are able to assess them technically, TA must include an element of public evaluation. Apart from *what* particular risks are, laypersons (and especially potential technological victims and beneficiaries) have the right to determine *whether* they wish to accept those risks. Whether technological risks and consequences are acceptable is largely a matter of ethics, and in matters of ethics the public has a major role to play. Persons trained to do ethical, legal, social, political, and historical analysis likewise have a key role in TA because all TA takes place in a social, political, and ethical context that itself must be evaluated and because so many of the major questions posed by medical and biological technologies are ethical problems.

The social and ethical problems TA addresses focus on both general and specific questions. Some of the general normative questions include whether a particular technology ought to be implemented and promoted, and what values and disvalues the technology might support. In other words, general ethical questions in TA often address either our vision of what society should be or how humans ought to live as a result of technological developments. The more specific ethical questions in TA include such issues as the following: Does informed consent of tissue and organ donors in biomedical and biological work require disclosure of the prospect of commercial gain? Would creation of a market system in biological materials, such as certain tissues, threaten equal distribution of scarce biotechnological resources? Do the current procedures for field-testing engineering organisms threaten potential victims' due-process rights? Do persons have a right to protection against carcinogens to which they might be exposed without their consent? Do some newer medical technologies—for example, in vitro fertilization—threaten respect for persons or the sacredness of life? These and other specific ethical issues are at the heart of much technological controversy.

Analysis of ethical issues is of special importance in TA for at least three reasons. First, given the inconsistent, unnecessary, or unethical uses of technology, it is important to understand the logic and the potential fallacies characteristic of alternative arguments about the ethics of proposed assessment policies and projects. Second, it is also important to analyze specific moral concepts, such as consent, freedom, and equity. Although clarity about moral concepts is not sufficient to resolve difficult ethical matters, it often is a necessary condition for dealing with the ethical issues raised by a given technology. Third, because all TA is performed within a given social, political, and ethical context, it is important to evaluate the ethical theories—such as utilitarianism, egalitarianism, and libertarianism—that might underlie the desire to implement a particular technology or the consequences following from it.

Apart from which ethical theory, or which view of justice or equity, is correct, it is important to know the implications and presuppositions of each theory, their relationship to different technologies, and the various objections that can be brought against these theories, because various ethical assumptions are often implicit in a given view of technology or in the methods used in TA. For example, many philosophers have criticized CBA, a widely used assessment technique, for its allegedly utilitarian presuppositions. Whether or not one agrees that CBA includes such presuppositions or that they are questionable, ethicists on the TA team need to recognize them if they are present, to point out their significance, and to describe and evaluate them and the alternatives to the methods containing them. While the skills of ethicists may not be sufficient to resolve the ethical quandaries generated by technology-related controversy, nevertheless, greater clarity, the avoidance of logical fallacies, a better understanding of moral theories and concepts, and a critical examination of alternative ethical arguments on policy matters usually provide a more comprehensive TA.

## Strengths and weaknesses of TA

Perhaps the most significant contribution of TA is that it can provide a systematic framework for evaluating technologies prior to their implementation by industry and their regulation by government. Without such a framework, institutionalized through agencies like the OTA, significant technical impacts probably would not be assessed. Instead, industry would likely introduce new technologies, such as digital subtraction angiography (DSA), largely on the basis of its ability to profit from

them. First commercially available in 1980, DSA uses an intravenously injected contrast medium to provide computer imaging of changes in the structure of blood vessels. Although it is less invasive, less risky for the patient, and cheaper than conventional angiography, the quality of the DSA image is often not as good as that of the conventional image (International Conference, 1988). Without TA, there might be considerable pressure to use either conventional or DSA angiography technology purely on the basis of which was more economical for the hospital or the patient. Doing a TA on DSA, however, revealed impacts associated with many other issues, including patient consent, the reliability of the diagnosis, the risk of the procedure, and the trade-offs between quality and cost-effectiveness in medical imaging.

TA also forces both experts and government officials to pay attention to all sides of an issue and to a diverse range of impacts. Hence, TA is an important vehicle for unbiased policymaking, for providing needed information to potential beneficiaries and victims of various technologies, and for reducing public and patient risks associated with medical, chemical, physical, and biological techniques.

Weaknesses associated with TA are typically either the product of experts' failure to use it in as objective and comprehensive a way as possible or the result of the shortcomings of its component methods, such as CBA or probabilistic risk assessment (PRA) (Levin and Strauss, 1991; Fiksel and Covello, 1986). Failures to employ TA in a comprehensive and unbiased way have occurred, for example, when assessors evaluating contraceptive technologies exhibited male bias in overemphasizing control of the female, rather than the male, reproductive system. Other TA biases occur even before specific assessment techniques are used, when scientists and policymakers decide which of many medical technologies, for example, among genetic "superdrugs," have the highest priority for assessment (Donaldson and Sox, 1992). Most TA biases occur after the formal TA process has begun, however, when experts ignore important cultural, economic, and social impacts (such as differences between developed and developing nations) or assume that impacts of a given technology will be the same in different countries. For example, some population experts have assumed that the widespread availability of contraceptive technologies will have similar impacts in developing nations (where there is often little desire to restrict births) and in developed countries (where there is frequently great desire to restrict births).

A more general form of bias in TA has been the tendency to underestimate the importance of cultural, ethical, political, and social impacts—such as high-technology medicine's limiting patient consent or due-process rights—and instead to focus merely on the physical and economic consequences associated with a particular technology. Because the intended effect of a technology is rarely the only impact it has on persons and on the environment, the real challenge of TA is to anticipate unintended higher-order consequences arising from a particular project and how these consequences affect our duties to subsequent generations and our goals for the future.

Because TA includes use of methods such as PRA and CBA, it often falls victim to some of the same difficulties as these two techniques. PRA is typically subject to criticism because the risk probabilities associated with a biomedical hazard, for example, often are uncertain, forcing assessors to use largely subjective, and therefore controversial, risk estimates; also, those who perform PRA frequently reduce possible impacts to injuries and fatalities, and thus ignore the larger ethical, social, political, and legal aspects of risk. Practitioners of CBA and PRA often employ utilitarian value judgments, discount the future, ignore distributive equity, or assess only market costs and benefits associated with particular technologies (Shrader-Frechette, 1985, 1991). For example, many CBAs of high-technology medicine emphasize the cost per case and the associated benefits (of renal dialysis, for instance), but they ignore the aggregate economic effects (of increasing use of expensive medical technologies) on the welfare of the health-care system as a whole (Jennett, 1986).

One way to guard against such difficulties is to guarantee that a variety of members of the public—not merely whites, males, representatives of developed nations, or industry spokespersons—help to evaluate the technology. More generally, we can improve TA by recognizing that potential victims and beneficiaries of a particular technology have a voice in assessment (Shrader-Frechette, 1985, 1991; Goodman and Baratz, 1990). Often their concerns are quite different from those of persons who use the technology or profit from it. For example, when experts evaluate surgery for removal of the gallbladder, they are frequently negative about use of laparoscopic technology because of its association with higher rates of bile-duct injury than standard "open" surgery. Gallstone patients, however, are more positive in assessing laparoscopic technology because of the shorter hospital stay associated with it and the less disfiguring scars (Gelijns, 1992).

Another solution to the difficulties facing TA is to employ extensive peer review, taking care to determine the degree to which policy conclusions are sensitive to different populations at risk and to alternative assessment descriptions, methodologies, and evaluations. As Leon Kass put it, biomedical research and technology are too important to the larger society to be left entirely to experts (U.S. Congress, 1987).

KRISTIN SHRADER-FRECHETTE

*Directly related to this article are the other articles in this entry:* HISTORY OF MEDICAL TECHNOLOGY, *and* PHILOSOPHY OF TECHNOLOGY. *Also directly related are the entries* ENVIRONMENTAL POLICY AND LAW; HEALTH-CARE FINANCING; HEALTH-CARE RESOURCES, ALLOCATION OF, *article on* MACROALLOCATION; *and* PUBLIC POLICY AND BIOETHICS. *The topics in this article will find application in the entries* GENOME MAPPING AND SEQUENCING; *and* KIDNEY DIALYSIS. *For a discussion of ethical analysis, see the entry* CLINICAL ETHICS, *article on* ELEMENTS AND METHODOLOGIES. *For a discussion of cost–benefit analysis, see the entry* UTILITY. *Other relevant material may be found under* PUBLIC HEALTH.

## Bibliography

BURKHARDT, JEFFREY. 1988. "Biotechnology, Ethics, and the Structure of Agriculture." *Agriculture and Human Values* 5, no. 3:53–60.

COATES, JOSEPH F. 1971. "Technology Assessment: The Benefits . . . The Costs . . . The Consequences." *Futurist* 5, no. 6:225–231.

DONALDSON, MOLLA S., and SOX, HAROLD C., eds. 1992. *Setting Priorities for Health Technology Assessment: A Model Process*. Washington, D.C.: National Academy Press.

FIKSEL, JOSEPH R., and COVELLO, VINCENT T., eds. 1986. *Biotechnology Risk Assessment: Issues and Methods for Environmental Introductions*. New York: Pergamon.

GELIJNS, ANNETINE, ed. 1992. *Technology and Health Care in an Era of Limits*. Washington, D.C.: National Academy Press.

GELIJNS, ANNETINE, and HALM, ETHAN A., eds. 1991. *The Changing Economics of Medical Technology*. Washington, D.C.: National Academy Press.

GOODMAN, CLIFFORD, and BARATZ, SHARON R., eds. 1990. *Improving Consensus Development for Health Technology Assessment: An International Perspective*. Washington, D.C.: National Academy Press.

INTERNATIONAL CONFERENCE ON ECONOMICS OF MEDICAL TECHNOLOGY. 1988. *The Economics of Medical Technology: Proceedings of an International Conference.* (1985; Valkenburg, Limburg, Netherlands). Edited by Frans F. H. Rutten, Stanley Joel Reiser, and L. M. J. Groot. New York: Springer-Verlag.

JACKSON, DAVID A., and STICH, STEPHEN P., eds. 1979. *The Recombinant DNA Debate*. Englewood Cliffs, N.J.: Prentice-Hall.

JENNETT, BRYAN. 1986. *High Technology Medicine: Benefits and Burdens*. New ed. New York: Oxford University Press.

KRIMSKY, SHELDON. 1982. *Genetic Alchemy: The Social History of the Recombinant DNA Controversy*. Cambridge, Mass.: MIT Press.

LEVIN, MORRIS A., and STRAUSS, HARLEE S., eds. 1991. *Risk Assessment in Genetic Engineering*. New York: McGraw-Hill.

OMENN, GILBERT S., and COLWELL, RITA R., eds. 1988. *Environmental Biotechnology: Reducing Risks from Environmental Chemicals Through Biotechnology*. New York: Plenum.

PERPICH, JOSEPH G., ed. 1986. *Biotechnology in Society: Private Initiatives and Public Oversight.* New York: Pergamon.

PORTER, ALAN L.; ROSSINI, FREDERICK A.; CARPENTER, STANLEY R.; and ROPER, ALAN T. 1980. *A Guidebook for Technology Assessment and Impact Analysis.* New York: North Holland.

SASSON, ALBERT. 1988. *Biotechnologies and Development.* Paris: United Nations Educational, Scientific, and Cultural Organization.

SHRADER-FRECHETTE, KRISTIN S. 1985. *Science Policy, Ethics, and Economic Methodology: Some Problems of Technology Assessment and Environmental-Impact Analysis.* Boston: Kluwer.

———. 1991. *Risk and Rationality: Philosophical Foundations for Populist Reform.* Berkeley: University of California Press.

SRINIVASAN, MANGALAM, ed. 1982. *Technology Assessment and Development.* New York: Praeger.

SWAIN, MARGARET S., and MARUSYK, RANDY W. 1990. "An Alternative to Property Rights in Human Tissue." *Hastings Center Report* 20, no. 5:12–15.

U.S. CONGRESS. OFFICE OF TECHNOLOGY ASSESSMENT. 1978. *Assessing the Efficacy and Safety of Medical Technologies.* Washington, D.C.: Author.

———. 1984. *Commercial Biotechnology: An International Analysis.* OTA-BA-218. Washington, D.C.: Author.

———. 1987. *Ownership of Human Tissues and Cells.* Vol. 1 of *New Developments in Biotechnology.* OTA-BA-337. Washington, D.C.: Author.

———. 1988. *Field-Testing Engineering Organisms.* Vol. 3 of *New Developments in Biotechnology.* OTA-BA-350. Washington, D.C.: Author.

———. 1989. *Patenting Life.* Vol. 5 of *New Developments in Biotechnology.* OTA-BA-370. Washington, D.C.: Author.

WALTERS, LEROY. 1978. "Technology Assessment." In vol. 4 of *Encyclopedia of Bioethics,* pp. 1650–1654. Edited by Warren T. Reich. New York: Macmillan.

WARMBRODT, ROBERT D. 1991. *Biotechnology: Risk Assessment, January 1986–February 1991.* Quick Bibliography series. Beltsville, Md.: National Agricultural Library.

WINNER, LANGDON. 1977. *Autonomous Technology: Technics-out-of-Control as a Theme in Political Thought.* Cambridge, Mass.: MIT Press.

# TELEOLOGICAL ETHICS

See ETHICS, *article on* NORMATIVE ETHICAL THEORIES. *See also* ETHICS, *article on* TASK OF ETHICS; UTILITY; *and* VIRTUE AND CHARACTER.

# TESTING AND SCREENING

See GENETIC TESTING AND SCREENING; HEALTH SCREENING AND TESTING IN THE PUBLIC-HEALTH CONTEXT; *and* OCCUPATIONAL SAFETY AND HEALTH, *article on* TESTING OF EMPLOYEES.

# THAILAND

See MEDICAL ETHICS, HISTORY OF, *section on* SOUTH AND EAST ASIA, *article on* SOUTHEAST ASIAN COUNTRIES.

# THEOLOGICAL ETHICS

See ETHICS, *article on* RELIGION AND MORALITY.

# THERAPEUTIC RELATIONSHIP

See PROFESSIONAL–PATIENT RELATIONSHIP.

# TOBACCO

See SUBSTANCE ABUSE, *article on* SMOKING.

# TORTURE AND THE HEALTH PROFESSIONAL

See PRISONERS, *article on* TORTURE AND THE HEALTH PROFESSIONAL.

# TOXIC WASTE

See HAZARDOUS WASTES AND TOXIC SUBSTANCES.

---

# TRAGEDY

"Tragedy" refers both to a literary tradition and to human experience. Literary tragedy identifies experiences of such extreme suffering and fearful choice as to expose the vulnerability of a community's framework of values and principles. Medicine, which constantly confronts such experiences, has been described as a "tragic profession" (Hauerwas et al., 1977). In medicine and bioethics, the idea of tragedy occurs in discussions ranging from "who lives and who dies" when medical resources are scarce to how one responds appropriately and compassionately to the severely ill and the dying.

## The tradition of tragedy

When we say that some experience or event is "tragic," we do not usually mean that it precisely fits the form of a tragic story. Often we simply wish to express horror, pity, or our inability to comprehend. Even so, literary tragedy is a source for many of the terms, concepts, and sensitivities through which we respond to suffering and moral ambiguity. To call something "tragic" is to apply a category received from a tradition of literature and commentary that begins with Greek epics and dramas and develops significantly in the Renaissance and Modern periods.

Tragedy resists definition. Several Greek tragedies end happily, so not even "a bad outcome" can be said to be the common feature. Nevertheless, Aristotle's definition in terms of action and its effect on the audience remains useful. To paraphrase him, a tragic drama represents a person's serious actions or choices that lead mistakenly or unwittingly to great misfortune and that the audience witnesses with compassion and horror. Another aspect of Greek tragedy should be noted: Between the action onstage and the audience, the misfortune is witnessed by a chorus. The chorus sometimes participates in the suffering, and it always provides a bridge to the audience. The chorus may articulate thoughts and emotions that the actions evoke, and may thereby help the audience confront painful limits of understanding. Aristotle and the Greek plays, then, identify three elements explored by tragedy: suffering, choice, and the limits of understanding.

**Suffering.**    The practices of medicine and ethics are obviously hedged by suffering and death and by different personal, cultural, and professional understandings of these realities. Like other forms of drama and narrative (including biography and autobiography), tragedy probes misfortune concretely, especially in contexts where the interpersonal complications of suffering become very difficult to communicate or "justify" in moral or religious terms. Illness and caring for the ill, insofar as these experiences cannot be comprehended solely by medical explanations and ethical theory, may be illuminated by other forms of expression. Tragedy calls attention to the kinds of stories patients, healers, and communities tell when they must endure or witness severe suffering and unwelcome choices.

**Choice.**    Medicine creates exceedingly troublesome choices. The most extreme of these may confound the classical imperative to "do no harm." Choices arising from scarce resources (e.g., organs for transplant, medical supplies in times of war or famine) may create crises of just distribution. Medical research can create dangerous conflicts of purpose, as when advancing medical knowledge is confused with offering therapy to patients. Other choices risk extending life beyond reasonable expectations of "quality of life." For some, such choices may involve "moral tragedy"—that is, a ruinous conflict between important values, such as respecting personal autonomy versus benefiting the common good. This view of moral tragedy was articulated by Hegel: tragedies depict a fearful collision between two otherwise justifiable values or principles.

**Limits of understanding.**    Those who practice medicine confront situations that compel difficult choices and baffle their capacities to understand, control, and restore. They encounter limits in understanding both disease processes themselves and "illness" as a complex experience involving the whole web of a person's relationships. Medical ethics encounters similar limits of discernment, due in part to the competing, fragmentary, and possibly incommensurate moral frameworks present in a pluralistic culture (MacIntyre, 1975). Literary tragedy teaches that these limits of understanding are an inevitable part of the relations that exist among patients, caregivers, and the public.

To say that tragedy is a tradition means that in Western culture it provides some of the paradigms we use to understand suffering and the choices that suffering presents us. The elements and language of tragedy sometimes appear in bioethical discourse quite explicitly, and may shape intuitions and considered judgments—as in these illustrations:

Two law professors write of how society invariably disguises the "tragic choices" it makes in respect to health hazards and scarce resources, choices that contradict widely held principles and cherished values (Calabresi and Bobbitt, 1978).

A moral philosopher tells of an intelligent, mature sixteen-year-old who becomes quadriplegic as a result of an auto accident. After coming to understand her limitations and possibilities, she desires to be discharged. The hospital staff hesitates, knowing she wishes to be killed by her willing older brother. The philosopher calls her case "truly tragic" (B. Brody, 1988).

A psychiatrist puzzles over his patient, a history professor who since high school has deliberately induced serious illnesses in himself. These episodes solicit the attentions of his mother, who has long blamed him for a crippling stroke she suffered during his birth. His illnesses are both punishing and self-punishing. They temporarily reconcile him with his mother and give him a sense of control and revenge. After making some progress, he quits therapy and resumes his former pattern. The psychiatrist calls this story "deeply tragic" in light of the patient's "indwelling, self-defeating psychic forces" (Kleinman, 1988, p. 19).

A Protestant ethicist, discussing criteria for withdrawing life support from brain-dead patients, takes note of the "tragic 'vegetable' cases whose respiration and hearts continue naturally" and so fall outside the criteria (Ramsey, 1970, p. 90n). These references suggest that tragedy in life has as much to do with those who witness and reflect on suffering and moral choice, in the manner of a Greek chorus, as with the suffering and choices themselves.

Literary tragedy is best defined not in terms of what it is but what it does. Tragedies inquire and explore.

They probe baffling disjunctions between a culture's picture of the way things are and its vision of how life should be lived. They "test the limits" of a culture's moral expectations, according to James Redfield (1975). Their plots put heroes and communities under stress and thereby test the limits of their virtues and norms; they thus invite audiences to reflect on their values and their limits. When Aristotle stated in the *Poetics* that tragedy creates in the audience a "cleansing," or *catharsis*, of pity and fear, he may have meant that as a tragic drama comes to closure, the audience *learns* (Nussbaum, 1986; Ricoeur, 1984; Redfield, 1975). "Learning" is the purpose and pleasure that Aristotle considered proper to all art.

### Tragic suffering

In Greek tragedy, the chorus often attends to expressions of physical and mental pain that border on the inarticulate. Elaine Scarry (1985) suggests that because consciousness of physical pain is so interior, it is nearly impossible to communicate. Pain resists clear language. Sophocles' isolated, wounded hero Philoctetes "utters a cascade of *changing* cries and shrieks that in the original Greek are accompanied by an array of formal words (some of them twelve syllables long), but that at least one translator found could only be rendered in English by the uniform syllable 'Ah' followed by variations in punctuation (Ah! Ah!!!)" (Scarry, 1985, p. 5). Of the Greek tragedies, *Philoctetes*—though atypical in its sudden happy ending—is often credited with exploring the complex ties binding the ill with those who give them care and with a public whose caring attitude may be questioned.

Philoctetes, en route to the Trojan war, unwittingly violates a sacred precinct and receives a terrible snakebite. His shipmates abandon him on a barren island, because his stinking wound and grotesque cries are intolerable. There he languishes as the play begins. His exile has been viewed as a metaphor for the stigmatization of the sick and the dying (H. Brody, 1987; Leder, 1990). Severe illness can threaten the structures of community, purpose, and personal dignity that shape an individual's character, and the island is a scene of social and spiritual isolation. It threatens to reduce Philoctetes from embodied, civilized person to sheer body, whose lonely routine of survival is almost bestial. When his pain is unbearable, he sometimes begs for amputation, even death; at other times he is desperate for friendship and home. Yet the ill also have their gifts (Wilson, 1947). A seer has foretold that only the magic bow of Philoctetes can win the Trojan war, and wily Odysseus and young Neoptolemus have come to take it, by either deceit or persuasion.

Greek tragedy originates in sacred festivals, and its heroes often undergo rites of passage whereby, in isolation, they are transformed. Severe illness has been viewed analogously: Even when surrounded by the activity of caring persons, one who is very sick becomes isolated from normal tasks and relationships. Identity may become inchoate, and whatever the outcome, one's life is irreversibly changed, toward either death or rebirth (May, 1991). Philoctetes is by vocation a warrior-hero, but pain and isolation have eroded his character; his wound now constitutes much of his identity and he refuses even to consider being reconciled with Odysseus. The sight of Philoctetes arouses pity, but the chorus eventually finds his preoccupation with suffering dismaying and blames him for his indignity. When Neoptolemus informs him of a cure available at Troy, he still refuses, unable to imagine life on new terms.

Suffering can also be a rite of passage for those who provide care; they, too, may be transformed, for better or worse. With Neoptolemus, the orphaned son of Achilles, it is for the better. Though an idealist, he agrees to trick Philoctetes out of his bow in order to end the war. But this further violates the Greek code of hospitality, already broken when Philoctetes was abandoned. So Neoptolemus is disturbed, and as he trades stories with Philoctetes, his conscience is stung. He comes to see him as a father figure, whose eventual trust revives Neoptolemus' own character. He vows to stand beside Philoctetes, come what may. Their new friendship, however, is insufficient to persuade Philoctetes to be reconciled with Odysseus, fight at Troy, and be cured by the physicians there. Only another, the god Heracles, appearing from the underworld, can persuade him, because once, as a mortal, Heracles too suffered unbearable pain and received mercy from Philoctetes. In return, Heracles gave him the extraordinary bow. Thus, Philoctetes is persuaded to risk healing and undertake more struggles.

The "case" of Philoctetes explores features of suffering that contextualize the choices and dilemmas encountered in tragedy. The first is suffering's isolating, nearly unsharable character. Understanding becomes possible only when Philoctetes manages to recount his story and only when it is heard by those whose own histories have prepared them for understanding. Second, Philoctetes's suffering bears on the destinies of many Greeks and Trojans. While Greek tragedies do favor public figures of mythic proportions, they nonetheless explore how suffering is always interwoven with the lives of others. Third, the complex events of this drama put at risk the frames of reference of individuals and communities. Certainly Philoctetes' own world has been shattered. But society is also at the point of rupture. Events threaten both the code of hospitality—the mutual obligations of hosts and guests—and the survival of two peoples, the Greeks and the Trojans. Last, though *Philoctetes* ends well, it need not have. Nothing makes its discoveries of friendship, persuasion, and renewal necessary. Their accomplishment is as contingent as the original snakebite was.

## Tragic choices and dilemmas

Insofar as it may "test the limits of culture" (Redfield, 1975), literary tragedy may be interpreted differently from other cultural and ethical perspectives. Christian views, for instance, tend either to interpret tragedy in terms of the destructive effects of sin or to reject tragedy as fatalistic denial of human responsibility for evil. But tragedy can also be read to show the complications of moral choice. What is inescapable in Greek tragedy is the awful burden of contingency in human affairs. The plays explore how people come to act, feel, and understand when terribly constrained. It has been said that one task of ethics is to reduce the ways that luck confounds our abilities to foster virtue, discern right actions and relationships, and pursue good ends. While ethics seeks to provide reasoned frameworks for the inchoate aspects of our lives, tragedies explore how principles can conflict and virtues fail (Nussbaum, 1986). Tragedy is primarily about the moral complexity of certain choices in the context of contingency and suffering, not about guilt or innocence.

According to Aristotle, tragic suffering is not necessarily the consequence of bad choices. Tragic protagonists are acted on as much as they act. Their actions, however, can compound suffering and may be relatively innocent or culpable. The best plots, Aristotle argued, concern reasonably good persons who come to grief, not because of their wickedness but because of some great *hamartia*—which may be translated as "mistake," "error of judgment," or "missing the mark." Aristotle had in mind a serious action that goes awry for any number of reasons, including lack of alternatives and ignorance about ramifications. In some tragedies, culpable fault does lead to misfortune, as when social or ritual boundaries are arrogantly transgressed. But often, as in *Oedipus Rex*, evident moral liabilities do not by themselves explain why misfortune comes. Philoctetes' failing character is more the result of suffering than its cause. In other tragedies, persons and communities discover their choices constrained by rivalries, gender conflicts, war, or pestilence. When heroes are hedged by fate or contingency or their judgments clouded by turmoil, they may act and come to ruin. Whether or not they are responsible for misfortune, they are nonetheless held accountable; that is, in the midst of suffering, they must give account.

In medicine, as in tragedy, harm may come from errors, some culpable and some unavoidable. People are finite and fallible, insufficiently knowledgeable and insufficiently virtuous to conquer every contingency. Errors occur because of chance or the limits of medical knowledge, and from misjudgment or negligence; these can sometimes be difficult to distinguish (Cassell, 1977). Further, medicine treats individuals who, as particular human beings, cannot adequately be understood by general laws and conditions (Gorovitz and MacIntyre, 1976). Medical errors occur necessarily and are not in themselves tragic; but when they are compounded by other errors or are hidden to ruinous effect, they become analogous to tragedy. The inevitability of error raises questions about our expectations of medicine and law to alleviate and compensate suffering. When caregivers, patients, and society seek to specify culpable fault in every "bad outcome," they in effect deny the inherent chanciness of life and harm the efficient delivery of health care. Conversely, those who ignore culpability—as when professionals conspire to "protect" one another from legitimate grievances—deny both the inevitability and the moral complexity of error.

Tragedy explores not only error but also choices structured by the moral life itself. In *Philoctetes*, we glimpse the classic debate between utilitarians and deontologists. Odysseus appeals to the common good in justifying the deception of Philoctetes, while Neoptolemus insists that a binding imperative has been violated. In their commitments to paramount principles, both utilitarians and deontologists are sometimes said to deny the possibility of tragedy; in any conflict, a clear moral course should be apparent. Rigorous utilitarians, in always seeking to maximize the good for the greatest number, may minimize the significance of misfortune or moral ambiguity. Rigorous deontologists, in applying a single categorical imperative, preclude genuine moral dilemmas. "Neither theory," writes Stanley Hauerwas, "can countenance the idea of moral tragedy—that is, the possibility of irresolvable moral conflict" (Hauerwas, 1983). Alternatively, one could say that tragedy looks different from these perspectives. Rule utilitarians might well acknowledge that sometimes rules intractably conflict. Deontologists might distinguish "the tragic" from "the wrong"; if one's maxim is "Let truth be told though the heavens fall," it would indeed be tragic if the heavens fell.

Medical ethics has been driven by "hard cases" or dilemmas frequently called tragic. A moral dilemma arises when someone "morally ought to do X and morally ought to do Y, but . . . is precluded by circumstances from doing both" (Beauchamp and Childress, 1989, p. 4). Whether to withdraw nourishment from a patient in a persistent vegetative state may become such a dilemma if viewed as a hard choice between preserving human life and easing human suffering. So also if society must choose between funding heart transplants for the few and basic medical care for the many.

For a situation to pose a genuine moral dilemma, both alternatives must involve moral claims. A conflict between moral obligation and self-interest might be a "personal" or "practical" but not "moral" dilemma, though these may be hard to distinguish in actual cases. Especially in light of Hegel's view of tragedy as a clash of justifiable ends, it is possible to define moral tragedy in terms of dilemmas. Moral dilemmas do not always carry the extreme losses associated with tragedy. But people caught in them can find their integrity, the whole texture of their identity and relationships of responsibility, falling into ruin.

> In a tragic ethical dilemma, a person is forced to act contrary to an ethical demand of such high priority that the consequences will be calamitous no matter how the person chooses. They may include destruction or corruption of the good person's character and thereby involve shattering the fragile goodness painfully acquired over the course of a lifetime. (Quinn, 1989, p. 179)

To ethicists who recognize a plurality of principles, none paramount, life may be seen as thoroughly "dilemmatic."

**The "dirty-hands" dilemma.**    Jean-Paul Sartre, in a play about a resistance group's compromising political choices in Nazi-occupied Europe, identified a type of moral dilemma, the problem of "dirty hands." It entails the necessary and willing acceptance of serious moral guilt—or, in Western religious terms, "sin"—in order to seek greater good or avoid greater evil. The agent accepts such guilt knowingly and regretfully (Walzer, 1978). Neoptolemus agonizes over whether to deceive Philoctetes or abandon the Greeks to an endless war. One can imagine some physicians cooperating with their nation's civil defense provisions and others refusing. Both believe cooperation would embroil them in the evil of making war "acceptable," while their refusal would effectively abandon future patients. They accept that in neither way can they avoid doing some evil for the sake of some good.

The idea of "dirty hands" enlarges the relevance of moral tragedy for medicine, especially when the focus is on social responsibility and accountability. Some who write of the hard choices created by science and technology demand that society own up to the disguised interests, violated principles, or "Faustian bargains" that are inevitable when new and powerful capabilities are advanced (Calabresi and Bobbitt, 1978; Lowrance, 1985). Such capabilities include nuclear energy, genetics, and organ transplantation. When vital means and resources like magic bows, cadaver organs, or clean water are limited, all the available choices may incur moral guilt and even bode violence and loss of life.

However, the "dirty hands" dilemma is but a type of tragic choice, in which responsibility becomes clearly specifiable. Literary tragedy is especially concerned with the obscurity of moral responsibility. In respect to vital resources, for example, scarcity may be caused by nature, chance, prior choices that may or may not have been culpable, or some combination. One strives, of course, to resolve such conflicts justly and benevolently; but the remedies, like the "God committees" once used to screen renal dialysis candidates, may produce tragic dilemmas of their own.

## Limits of tragic understanding

Some have argued that only an ethics of virtue, which concerns how character is formed in respect to community, can effectively respond to tragedy; that is, a community's traditions help create the moral skills (virtues) needed to navigate passages through calamitous suffering and hard choice. Modern society, lacking a shared moral framework, finds it difficult to respond to tragedy. In the classical world, strangers were to be accommodated hospitably—that is, as guests or hosts. Odysseus breaks this code, Neoptolemus upholds it, both presume it. But where such moral traditions are not presumed, strangers are treated only as strangers. Emergency rooms must be forced by law, not shared values or beliefs, to accept the uninsured critically ill. Regarding medicine as a commodity or contractual service, fragmented by specialization, creates distance between physicians and patients and may contribute to a litigious climate of distrust. The moral life, then, requires serious attention to the traditions that do function in society, and to the moral skills supported by those traditions.

For Hauerwas and others, moral tragedy arises, in part, from the natural contingencies and finiteness of human life (Hauerwas et al., 1977). Seeing such issues as suicide, abortion, and euthanasia as tragic signifies, first, that we should not be deceived that there are comfortable solutions to the dilemmas they pose. Awareness of tragedy probably "solves" no formal moral question; rather, it encourages us to view the irresolvable character of some moral problems truthfully. Nor should we be deceived that the virtues will suffice: A virtuous intention may become blinding, or the practice of a moral skill may yet bring about harm (Barbour, 1984). Second, we should examine tragic dilemmas in light of "who we are," not merely "what we should do." Hauerwas argues that in the biblical traditions, among others, life has high but not ultimate value. There is no absolute "right to life" or absolute autonomy of persons, but there is a strong commitment toward openness to the future, to valuing children and the elderly, to seeing life as a gift, to promoting care and trust. For Hauerwas, seeing tragedy in light of these commitments creates very strong presumptions against suicide, abortion, and euthanasia (Hauerwas, 1983; Hauerwas et al., 1977).

However, cultural and religious traditions are best seen as providing frameworks for reflecting on choices and commitments; they do not determine the choices themselves or the outcome of debates about them. James M. Gustafson, for example, offers a virtue-related Christian ethic that is cognizant of tragedy but differs from the one Hauerwas proposes. For Gustafson, tragedy means not only remembering but significantly rethinking "who we are," especially insofar as the contingencies of nature are concerned. Recognizing tragedy may mean regretfully assenting to some choices at certain times, such as suicide or abortion, that others would resist (Gustafson, 1984).

The virtues of the tragic hero (e.g., courage, practical intelligence, awareness of finitude) are laudable in medicine but do not resolve certain long-standing disputes. For instance, how one understands tragedy might bear on one's principles for allocating scarce lifesaving medical resources. The very idea of the tragic hero, in whose excellence the community at large depends, might favor allocating such resources not randomly but based on a high consideration for a patient's likely productivity and benefit to society. But tragic suffering and contingency, in which all persons are universally at risk and their value to others incalculable, leads some to advocate using contingency itself—through lotteries or "first come, first served" criteria—as a primary principle for selecting "who shall live when not all can live" (Childress, 1970; Kilner, 1990).

The virtues often recommended in bioethical discussions of tragedy are those of the tragic chorus. The chorus is not necessarily wise; it offers few profound or rescuing insights. The chorus, rather, listens and remembers. It attends, fearfully and often compassionately, to the stories of those who greatly suffer. Kathryn M. Hunter describes a twenty-eight-year-old man, insulin dependent, hospitalized in a persistent vegetative state, with no prospect of recovery. He lacks family, friends, and recorded wishes to guide his care. Among the nurses, some remember him from earlier diabetes treatments; they feel they know him and are disturbed "to think about abandoning him." Hunter recommends in such cases a reflective process among all those caring for the particular patient, modeled on the Greek chorus. These "management rounds" would not decide treatment or substitute for necessary legal or ethical consultations. The caregivers would, as far as possible, reconstruct the patient's story and recount their own quandaries in respect to the patient. They would create "for the moment a sense of community, because, unaided by a family, the staff must act both for the patient

and for society without knowing which side of the question either would favor" (Hunter, 1985, pp. 717, 718).

The tradition of tragedy asks medical ethics to give attention to the mutuality of participants in the circles of illness, healing, and understanding. Patients and caregivers come with complex, richly laden stories. A more nuanced understanding of the cultural and interpersonal aspects of illness and healing will not resolve all ethical quandaries, but it may deepen appreciation for the whole range of relationships that exist in medicine. If all people share in the tragic character of suffering and moral choice, though not in a common understanding of it, our attentions to that fact can at least sometimes promote honesty, trust, and care.

LARRY D. BOUCHARD

*Directly related to this entry are the entries* VIRTUE AND CHARACTER; PROFESSIONAL–PATIENT RELATIONSHIP; MEDICINE, ART OF; *and* PAIN AND SUFFERING. *For a further discussion of topics mentioned in this entry, see the entries* AGING AND THE AGED, *article on* THEORIES OF AGING AND LIFE EXTENSION; BODY; DEATH, ATTITUDES TOWARD; HEALTH AND DISEASE; RESPONSIBILITY; *and* VALUE AND VALUATION. *Other relevant material may be found under the entries* BIOETHICS; CARE; DEATH; DEATH AND DYING: EUTHANASIA AND SUSTAINING LIFE, *articles on* HISTORICAL ASPECTS, *and* ETHICAL ISSUES; ETHICS; HARM; LIFE, QUALITY OF; *and* MEDICAL MALPRACTICE.

## Bibliography

BARBOUR, JOHN D. 1984. *Tragedy as a Critique of Virtue: The Novel and Ethical Reflection.* Chico, Calif.: Scholars Press.

BEAUCHAMP, TOM L., and CHILDRESS, JAMES F. 1989. *Principles of Biomedical Ethics.* 3d ed. New York: Oxford University Press.

BRODY, BARUCH A. 1988. *Life and Death Decision Making.* New York: Oxford University Press.

BRODY, HOWARD. 1987. *Stories of Sickness.* New Haven, Conn.: Yale University Press.

CALABRESI, GUIDO, and BOBBITT, PHILIP. 1978. *Tragic Choices.* New York: W. W. Norton.

CASSELL, ERIC J. 1977. "Error in Medicine." In *Knowledge, Value, and Belief,* pp. 295–309. Edited by H. Tristam Engelhardt, Jr., and Daniel Callahan. Hastings-on-Hudson, N.Y.: Hastings Center.

CHILDRESS, JAMES F. 1970. "Who Shall Live When Not All Can Live?" *Soundings* 53:339–355.

GOROVITZ, SAMUEL, and MACINTYRE, ALASDAIR C. 1976. "Toward a Theory of Medical Fallibility." *Journal of Medicine and Philosophy* 1, no. 1:51–71.

GUSTAFSON, JAMES M. 1984. *Ethics from a Theocentric Perspective.* 2 vols. Chicago: University of Chicago Press.

HAUERWAS, STANLEY. 1983. *The Peaceable Kingdom: A Primer in Christian Ethics.* Notre Dame, Ind.: University of Notre Dame Press.

HAUERWAS, STANLEY; BONDI, RICHARD; and BURRELL, DAVID
B. 1977. *Truthfulness and Tragedy: Further Investigations in
Christian Ethics.* Notre Dame, Ind.: University of Notre
Dame Press.

HUNTER, KATHRYN MONTGOMERY. 1985. "Limiting Treatment
in a Social Vacuum: A Greek Chorus for William T." *Archives of Internal Medicine* 145, no. 4:716–719.

KILNER, JOHN F. 1990. *Who Lives? Who Dies? Ethical Criteria
in Patient Selection.* New Haven, Conn.: Yale University
Press.

KLEINMAN, ARTHUR. 1988. *The Illness Narratives: Suffering,
Healing, and the Human Condition.* New York: Basic
Books.

LEDER, DREW. 1990. "Illness and Exile: Sophocles' *Philoctetes.*"
*Literature and Medicine* 9:1–11.

LOWRANCE, WILLIAM W. 1985. *Modern Science and Human
Values.* New York: Oxford University Press.

MACINTYRE, ALASDAIR C. 1975. "How Virtues Become Vices:
Values, Medicine and Social Context." In *Evaluation and
Explanation in the Biomedical Sciences,* pp. 97–111. Edited
by H. Tristram Engelhardt, Jr., and Stuart F. Spicker.
Dordrecht, Netherlands: D. Reidel.

MAY, WILLIAM F. 1991. *The Patient's Ordeal.* Bloomington: Indiana University Press.

NUSSBAUM, MARTHA C. 1986. *The Fragility of Goodness: Luck
and Ethics in Greek Tragedy and Philosophy.* New York:
Cambridge University Press.

QUINN, PHILIP L. 1989. "Tragic Dilemmas, Suffering Love,
and Christian Life." *Journal of Religious Ethics* 179, no.
1:151–183.

RAMSEY, PAUL. 1970. *The Patient as Person: Explorations in
Medical Ethics.* New Haven, Conn.: Yale University Press.

REDFIELD, JAMES M. 1975. *Nature and Culture in the "Iliad":
The Tragedy of Hector.* Chicago: University of Chicago
Press.

RICOEUR, PAUL. 1984. Vol. 1 of *Time and Narrative.* Translated
by Kathleen McLaughlin and David Pellauer. Chicago:
University of Chicago Press.

SCARRY, ELAINE. 1985. *The Body in Pain: The Making and Un-
making of the World.* New York: Oxford University Press.

WALZER, MICHAEL. 1978. "Political Action: The Problem of
Dirty Hands." In *Private and Public Ethics: Tensions Between Conscience and Institutional Responsibility,* pp. 96–
124. Edited by Donald G. Jones. New York: Edwin
Mellen.

WILSON, EDMUND. 1947. *The Wound and the Bow: Seven Studies in Literature.* New York: Oxford University Press.

# TRANSPLANTATION

See ORGAN AND TISSUE TRANSPLANTS. See also ORGAN
AND TISSUE PROCUREMENT; and XENOGRAFTS.

# TREATMENT REFUSAL

See DEATH AND DYING: EUTHANASIA AND SUSTAINING
LIFE, article on ETHICAL ISSUES; PATIENTS' RIGHTS; and
RIGHTS, article on RIGHTS IN BIOETHICS.

# TRIAGE

Triage is the medical assessment of patients to establish
their priority for treatment. When medical resources are
limited and immediate treatment of all patients is impossible, patients are "sorted" in order to use the resources most effectively. The process of triage was first
developed and refined in military medicine, and later
extended to disaster and emergency medicine.

In recent years, it has become common to use the
term "triage" in a wide variety of contexts where decisions are made about allocating scarce medical resources.
However, "triage" should not be confused with more
general expressions such as "allocation" or "rationing"
(Childress, 1983). Triage is a process of screening patients on the basis of their immediate medical needs and
the likelihood of medical success in treating those needs.
Unlike the everyday practice of allocating medical resources, triage usually takes place in circumstances of
temporary crisis requiring quick decisions about the critical care of a pool of patients. Generally, these decisions
are controlled by utilitarian considerations.

## History

Baron Dominique Jean Larrey, Napoleon's chief medical
officer, is credited with organizing the first deliberate
plan for classifying military casualties (Hinds, 1975).
Larrey was proud of his success in treating battle casualties despite severe scarcity of medical resources. He insisted that those who were most seriously wounded be
treated first, regardless of rank. Although there is no record of Larrey's using the term "triage," his plan for sorting casualties significantly influenced later military
medicine.

The practice of systematically sorting battle casualties first became common during World War I. It was
also at this time that the term "triage" entered British
and U.S. military medicine from the French (Lynch et
al., 1925). Originally, "triage" (from the French verb
*trier,* "to sort") referred to the process of sorting agricultural products such as wool and coffee. In military medicine, "triage" was first used both for the process of
prioritizing casualty treatment and for the place where
such screening occurred. At the *poste de triage* (casualty
clearing station), casualties were assessed for the severity
of their wounds and the need for rapid evacuation to
hospitals in the rear. The emphasis was on determining
need for immediate treatment and the feasibility of
transport.

The following triage categories have become standard, even though terminology may vary:

1. *Minimal.* Those whose injuries are slight and require
little or no professional care.

2. *Immediate.* Those whose injuries, such as airway obstruction or hemorrhaging, require immediate medical treatment for survival.

3. *Delayed.* Those whose injuries, such as burns or closed fractures of bones, require significant professional attention that can be delayed for some period of time without significant increase in the likelihood of death or disability.

4. *Expectant.* Those whose injuries are so extensive that there is little or no hope of survival, given the available medical resources.

First priority is given to those in the "immediate" group. Next, as time and resources permit, care is given to the "delayed" group. Little, beyond minimal efforts to provide comfort care, is given to those in the "expectant" category. Active euthanasia for "expectant" casualties has been considered but is almost never mentioned in triage proposals (British Medical Association, 1988). Those in the "minimal" group are left to take care of themselves until all other medical needs are met.

From the beginning, the manifest reason for such sorting was maximum utility. One early text on military medicine advised, "The greatest good of the greatest number must be the rule" (Keen, 1917, p. 13). Over the years, however, it became clear that this utilitarian principle could be interpreted in different ways. The most obvious meaning was that of limited medical utility. The good to be sought was saving the greatest number of casualties' lives.

But the principle could also be construed to mean doing the greatest good for the military effort. When interpreted this way, triage could produce very different priorities. For example, it was sometimes proposed that priority be given to the least injured in order to return them quickly to battle (Lee, 1917). An oft-cited example of the second use of the utilitarian principle for triage occurred during World War II (Beecher, 1970). Commanders of U.S. forces in North Africa had to decide how to use their extremely limited supply of penicillin. The choice was between battle casualties with infected wounds and soldiers with gonorrhea. The decision was made to give priority to those with venereal disease, on the grounds that they could most quickly be returned to battle preparedness. A similar decision was made in Great Britain to favor members of bomber crews who had contracted venereal disease, because they were deemed most valuable to the continuation of the war effort (Hinds, 1975).

As military triage has evolved during the twentieth century, the goal of maintaining fighting strength has increasingly become the dominant, stated goal. In the words of two surgeons, "Traditionally, the military value of surgery lies in the salvage of battle casualties. This is not merely a matter of saving life; it is primarily one of returning the wounded to duty, and the earlier the better" (Beebe and DeBakey, 1952, p. 216).

The nuclear weapons used at the end of World War II introduced unprecedented destructive power. In the nuclear age, triage plans have had to include the possibility of overwhelming numbers of hopelessly injured civilians. In earlier days, it was not uncommon to plan for one or two thousand casualties from a single battle. Now, triage planners must consider the likelihood that a single nuclear weapon could produce a hundred times as many casualties or more. At the same time a single blast could destroy much of a community's medical capacity. Such probabilities have led some analysts to wonder if triage would be a realistic expectation following a nuclear attack (British Medical Association, 1983).

Triage has moved from military into civilian medicine in two prominent areas: the care of disaster victims and the operation of hospital emergency departments. In both areas, the categories and many of the strategies of military medicine have been adopted.

The necessity of triage in hospital emergency departments is due, in part, to the fact that a number of patients needing immediate emergency care may arrive almost simultaneously and temporarily overwhelm the hospital's emergency resources. More often, however, the need for triage in hospital emergency departments stems from the fact that the majority of patients are waiting for routine care and do not have emergent conditions. Thus, screening patients to determine which ones need immediate treatment has become increasingly important. Emergency-department triage is often conducted by specially educated nurses using elaborate methods of scoring for severity of injury or illness (Purnell, 1991; Gilpin and Nelson, 1991; Wiebe and Rosen, 1991).

## Ethical issues

The traditional ethic of medicine obligates health-care professionals to protect the interests of patients as individuals and to treat people equally on the basis of their medical needs. These same commitments to fidelity and equality have, at times, been prescribed for the treatment of war casualties. For example, the Geneva Conventions call for medical treatment of all casualties of war strictly on the basis of medical criteria, without regard for any other considerations (International Committee of the Red Cross, 1977). However, this principle of equal treatment based solely on medical needs and the likelihood of medical success appears to have had little or no effect on triage in military medicine. In triage, as generally practiced, health-care professionals think of patients in aggregates and give priority to goals such as preserving military strength; loyalty to the individual patient is set aside in order to accomplish the most good or prevent the most harm. The good that might be accomplished for one must be weighed against what the same amount of effort and resources could do for others. The tension between keeping faith with the individual patient and the utilitarian goal of seeking the greatest good for the greatest number is the primary ethical issue arising from triage.

Triage generates a number of additional ethical questions. To what extent are the utilitarian goals of military or disaster triage appropriate in the more common circumstances of allocating everyday medical care, such as beds in an intensive care unit? If some casualties of war or disaster are categorized as hopeless, what care, if any, should they be accorded? Should their care include active euthanasia? Should health-care professionals join in the triage planning for nuclear war if they are morally opposed to the policies that include the possibility of such war (Leaning, 1988)?

Triage is a permanent feature of contemporary medical care in military, disaster, and emergency settings. As medical research continues to produce new and costly therapies, it will be tempting to import the widely accepted principles of triage for decisions about who gets what care. Indeed, whenever conditions of scarcity necessitate difficult decisions about the distribution of burdens and benefits, the language and tenets of medical triage may present an apparently attractive model. This is true for issues as far from medical care as world hunger and population control (Hardin, 1980; Hinds, 1976). The moral wisdom of appropriating the lessons of medical triage for such diverse social problems is doubtful and should be carefully questioned. Otherwise, utilitarian considerations characteristic of triage may dominate issues better addressed in terms of loyalty, personal autonomy, or distributive justice.

GERALD R. WINSLOW

*Directly related to this entry are the entries* UTILITY; *and* JUSTICE. *This entry will find application in the entry* WARFARE, *article on* MEDICINE AND WAR. *For a further discussion of topics mentioned in this entry, see the entries* DEATH AND DYING: EUTHANASIA AND SUSTAINING LIFE, *article on* HISTORICAL ASPECTS; HEALTH-CARE RESOURCES, ALLOCATION OF, *article on* MICROALLOCATION; *and* WARFARE, *articles on* NUCLEAR WARFARE, *and* CHEMICAL AND BIOLOGICAL WARFARE.

## Bibliography

BEEBE, GILBERT W., and DEBAKEY, MICHAEL E. 1952. *Battle Casualties: Incidence, Mortality, and Logistic Considerations.* Springfield, Ill.: Charles C. Thomas.

BEECHER, HENRY K. 1970. "Scarce Resources and Medical Advancement." In *Experimentation with Human Subjects*, pp. 66–104. Edited by Paul A. Freund. New York: George Braziller.

BRITISH MEDICAL ASSOCIATION. 1983. *The Medical Effects of Nuclear War.* Chichester, U.K.: John Wiley and Sons.

———. 1988. *Selection of Casualties for Treatment After Nuclear Attack: A Document for Discussion.* London: Author.

BURKLE, FREDERICK M. 1984. "Triage." In *Disaster Medicine: Application for the Immediate Management and Triage of Civilian and Military Disaster Victims*, pp. 45–80. Edited by Frederick M. Burkle, Jr., Patricia H. Sanner, and Barry W. Wolcott. New Hyde Park, N.Y.: Medical Examination.

CHILDRESS, JAMES F. 1983. "Triage in Neonatal Intensive Care: The Limitations of a Metaphor." *Virginia Law Review* 69:547–561.

GILPIN, D. A., and NELSON, P. G. 1991. "Revised Trauma Score: A Triage Tool in the Accident and Emergency Department." *Injury: The British Journal of Accident Surgery* 22, no. 1:35–37.

HARDIN, GARRETT. 1980. *Promethean Ethics: Living with Death, Competition, and Triage.* Seattle: University of Washington Press.

HINDS, STUART. 1975. "Triage in Medicine: A Personal History." In *Triage in Medicine and Society: Inquiries into Medical Ethics*, pp. 6–22. Edited by George R. Lucas, Jr. Houston: Institute of Religion and Human Development.

———. 1976. "Relations of Medical Triage to World Famine: A History." In *Lifeboat Ethics: The Moral Dilemmas of World Hunger*, pp. 29–51. Edited by George R. Lucas, Jr., and Thomas W. Ogletree. New York: Harper and Row.

INTERNATIONAL COMMITTEE OF THE RED CROSS. 1977. "Geneva Conventions: Protocol I, Additional to the Geneva Conventions of 12 August 1949, Relating to the Protection of Victims of International Armed Conflicts (1977)." In *Encyclopedia of Human Rights*, pp. 637–659. Edited by Edward Lawson. New York: Taylor and Francis.

KEEN, WILLIAM W. 1917. *The Treatment of War Wounds.* Philadelphia: W. B. Saunders.

KILNER, JOHN F. 1990. *Who Lives? Who Dies?: Ethical Criteria in Patient Selection.* New Haven, Conn.: Yale University Press.

LEANING, JENNIFER. 1986. "Burn and Blast Casualties: Triage in Nuclear War." In *The Medical Implications of Nuclear War*, pp. 251–283. Edited by Fredric Solomon and Robert Q. Marston. Washington, D.C.: National Academy Press.

———. 1988. "Physicians, Triage, and Nuclear War." *Lancet* 2, no. 8605:269–270.

LEE, ROBERT I. 1917. "The Case for the More Efficient Treatment of Light Casualties in Military Hospitals." *Military Surgeon* 42:283–286.

LYNCH, CHARLES; FORD, J. H.; and WEED, F. W. 1925. *Field Operations: In General View of Medical Department Organization.* Vol. 8 of *The Medical Department of the United States Army in the World War.* Washington, D.C.: U.S. Government Printing Office.

O'DONNELL, THOMAS J. 1960. "The Morality of Triage." *Georgetown Medical Bulletin* 14, no. 1:68–71.

PURNELL, LARRY D. 1991. "A Survey of Emergency Department Triage in 185 Hospitals." *Journal of Emergency Nursing* 17, no. 6:402–407.

RUND, DOUGLAS A., and RAUSCH, TONDRA S. 1981. *Triage.* St. Louis, Mo.: Mosby.

VICKERY, DONALD M. 1975. *Triage: Problem-Oriented Sorting of Patients.* Bowie, Md.: Robert J. Brady.

WIEBE, ROBERT A., and ROSEN, LINDA M. 1991. "Triage in the Emergency Department." *Emergency Medicine Clinics of North America* 9, no. 3:491–503.

WINSLOW, GERALD. 1982. *Triage and Justice.* Berkeley: University of California Press.

# TRUST

## Trust between patients and providers

Trust between patients and providers is a central topic for bioethics. Consider the trust (or distrust) involved when someone contemplates major surgery: First of all, there is the relation between the surgeon and patient. The patient needs from the physician both a high level of competence (both judgment and skill) and a concern for the patient's well-being. For health-care professionals to behave in a responsible or trustworthy way requires both technical competence and moral concern—specifically, a concern to achieve a good outcome in the matter covered, which is sometimes called "fiduciary responsibility," the responsibility of a person who has been entrusted in some way. The moral and technical components of professional responsibility have led sociologist Bernard Barber to speak of these as two "senses" of trust (Barber, 1983). However, if the patient trusts the surgeon, it is not in two senses; the patient trusts the surgeon simply to provide a good, or perhaps the best, outcome for the patient. To fulfill that trust, the surgeon needs to be both morally concerned for the patient's well-being (or at least health outcome) and technically competent.

Because the exercise of professional responsibility characteristically draws on a body of specialized knowledge that is brought to bear on the promotion or preservation of another's welfare, to trust someone to fulfill a professional responsibility is to trust that person to perform in a way that someone outside that profession cannot entirely specify, predict, or often even recognize. In drawing attention to this point, Trudy Govier says that trust is "open-ended" (Govier, 1992). The point is not captured in the frequent suggestion that trust is necessary because the trusting party cannot control or monitor the trusted party's performance. It would do the patient little good to have full prescience of all the events in the operation, or even the ability to guide the surgeon's hand, unless the patient also happened to be a surgeon. Although a typical patient might be able to recognize some acts of gross malpractice, such as being stitched up with foreign bodies left inside, the patient would not know the implications of most of what

he or she saw and would have no idea of how to improve the surgeon's performance. For this reason, from the point of view of the patient, there are no good alternatives to having trustworthy professionals. There are no good alternatives in these circumstances because the patient must rely on the discretion of the practitioner.

Philosophers like John Ladd (1979) and legal theorists like Joel Handler (1990) have drawn attention to the role of discretion in many areas of professional practice. They have argued that because of the role of discretion, the criteria for morally responsible practice cannot be specified in terms of rules or rights alone. The centrality of discretion makes it all the more difficult to separate competence (having adequate knowledge and skill) and moral elements (exercising sufficient concern for the client's well-being) in the professional's behavior.

The provider—in this case the surgeon—also must trust the patient. At a minimum, the surgeon depends on the patient to disclose all information relevant to the case so as to minimize the risks of unexpected events in the operating room. If the patient disappoints the surgeon and does not disclose all relevant information, the negative consequence for the surgeon is, at most, to impair the surgeon's professional performance. The disappointment does not carry a risk of death or disability for the surgeon. The difference in the severity of risk is one of the many aspects of a trust relationship that is counted as a difference of power in that relationship. The lesser severity of consequence for the provider—in this case the surgeon—can obscure the mutuality of trust in the patient–provider relationship.

When the provider is a nurse or physical therapist rather than a surgeon, the provider's central tasks often require an understanding of the patient's experiences, hopes, and fears. Although some nursing, such as the work of the surgical nurse who assists in the operating room, does not depend on an understanding of the patient's experience, most nursing does. Postsurgical nursing care is a good example. This care typically includes motivating the patient to do things such as coughing and breathing deeply in order to reduce the risk of postoperative lung infection. These acts are often quite uncomfortable. Such nursing requires an understanding of the individual patient's state of mind and the ability to motivate the patient—the ability to inspire confidence and hope in patients.

**Changing the standards of the patient–provider relationship.** When sociologist Talcott Parsons put forward his influential theory that professionals function as trustees, or in a "fiduciary" capacity (Parsons, 1951), the standard for the so-called fiduciary aspects of the relationship between patients and physicians was that the provider furthered the patient's well-being by being entrusted to make medical decisions in the best interests of that patient.

The doctrine of informed consent for medical procedures was adopted only gradually over the next two decades as a check on provider discretion. This doctrine has been implemented to require informed consent only for a very circumscribed set of procedures. To treat competent persons against their will is considered battery, in legal terms. Therefore, there is a foundation in law for the prohibition of forced or nonconsensual treatment of all types. In practice, however, information is often given only for major procedures, and practitioners tend to assume consent for lesser interventions, including most medical tests. Although patient-oriented practitioners will offer an explanation of why they are ordering a particular test, others will explain only when explicitly asked. For procedures other than surgery, formal requests for consent are rare unless there is a significant risk of death or severe disability from the procedure.

Furthermore, most patients are well informed only about the risk of death or significant permanent injury in circumstances in which informed consent is legally or institutionally mandated. Significant risk—such as becoming temporarily psychotic as a result of the trauma of open-heart surgery, as a result of intensive-care procedures, or from the sleep deprivation that often results from those procedures—is rarely disclosed to patients. The rationale for not telling a patient about to have bypass surgery or enter intensive care is that the risk will seem so shocking that the patient will refuse needed care.

Although the standard of informed consent is enforced by law and institutional practice only for certain risks of major procedures, the U.S. President's Commission for the Study of Ethical Problems in Medicine and Biomedical and Behavioral Research (President's Commission) has urged that the informed-consent standard be replaced by another, more comprehensive standard, the standard of "shared decision making."

The President's Commission's 1982 report, *Making Health Care Decisions*, advocated such a shift, which would presumably apply to most significant health-care decisions. The rule of informed consent requires only the recognition of the patient's right of veto over the alternatives that the provider has presented to the patient. In contrast, shared decision making requires participation of the patient in setting the goals and methods of care and, therefore, in formulating the alternatives to be considered. This participation requires that patients and practitioners engage in complex communication, which the practitioners have a fiduciary responsibility to foster. This new standard is particularly appropriate for a pluralistic society, in which the responsible provider may have an idea of the patient's good that is significantly different from the patient's own idea.

The responsibility to foster shared decision making requires significant skill on the part of medical professionals in understanding patients of diverse backgrounds and in fostering communication with them in difficult circumstances—circumstances in which their communication may be compromised by fear and pain as well as by a lack of medical knowledge. Although some physicians, notably primary-care providers, have sought the skills to fulfill the responsibility to foster such communication, this responsibility is not one that medical education prepares physicians to accept.

**Implementing the fiduciary standard.** Ironically, although the fiduciary responsibility in health care has often been viewed primarily as the responsibility of physicians, as was noted above, it is other classes of providers, especially nurses, who are educated in a way that prepares them to understand patients' experience. Although there is much to recommend the new fiduciary standard in health care, its realization requires either a major change in medical education or a change in the relations among members of the health-care team, so that those who are prepared to oversee and foster shared decision making have the authority to do so. Without such changes, the trust that one's health care will be shaped by one's own priorities and concerns is not well founded.

In many cases, distrust of either individual providers or medical institutions has been warranted, especially for women, people of color, and the poor, whose experience has often been discounted or who have been viewed as less rational or less competent than white males. Annette Dula argues that historical events, from the Tuskegee syphilis study to the experience with screening for sickle-cell carrier trait, confirm that trust of the health-care system on the part of African-Americans is often not warranted (Dula, 1992). The problem is one of the need not only for assurance but also for evidence that the former conditions no longer prevail.

Many poor or uninsured people have not even had a significant patient-provider relationship; when they are able to obtain health care, it is often with a provider whom they see in only a single clinical encounter. It is therefore impossible to establish a trusting relationship that would serve the patient's health interest. If society is obliged to provide decent health care for its citizens, this failure of the health-care system is a betrayal of trust not by individual providers but by society and its health-care institutions.

## Trust and family members

Trust among family members is at least as important an issue for health care as is trust in the provider-patient relationship. The trustworthiness of parents and guardians to decide the care of children and other dependent family members is widely discussed, and trust among family members is beginning to receive more attention in connection with the writing of living wills and health proxy statements. The issues of the competence of family members to give various forms of care or to make technical decisions, and the sufficiency of their concern for the patient's well-being, parallel those issues for providers. The matter is further complicated by the phenomenon of psychological denial that interferes with decision making about the health care of a person who is important in one's own life. Denial, as well as incompetence or lack of commitment to the patient's welfare, may compromise a person's decisions or care when the health or life of a close friend or relative is gravely threatened. Therefore, warranted trust in family members to provide or decide one's care requires confidence not only in their competence and in their concern for one's well-being but also in their psychological ability to come to terms with the situation.

## Other areas of trust in health care

There is also the question of the public's trust in a class of professionals, which is distinct from the question of the public's concern that, should they become clients of these professionals, their interests will be well served. For example, Sissela Bok (1978) has examined the concern about the trustworthiness of lawyers, not by their clients but by the public. Of particular concern is lawyers' commitment to keep the crimes of their clients confidential, even certain ongoing or planned crimes. The public believes that lawyers should not violate usual ethical norms for the sake of their clients' interests. The corresponding issue in health care is the fear that providers will, in protecting patient confidentiality, put the public health or the safety of individuals at undue risk. The question of ethical criteria for breaking confidentiality is regularly discussed, especially in the case of a sexually transmitted disease or a patient intent on harming another person. However, there is no widespread public concern that health-care providers may be going so far in protecting patient confidentiality that they are derelict in protecting the public.

In addition to the public's trust of providers, the trust or distrust of medical technology is often a significant factor. The risk is particularly salient in the case of artificial organs, joints, and other body parts. In place of the components of competence and concern of a trusted provider, the qualities required of a technology to warrant trust are its performance (it performs the function it was designed to perform) and its relative safety (it is relatively unlikely to cause accidents or to have other injurious side effects). Of course, with such life-critical technologies as artificial organs, the performance issue is itself a safety issue.

There are many aspects of the health-care system on which patients rely but which most rarely consider. Many people become fully aware of their trust only when that trust is disappointed. A case in point is the discovery that research misconduct occurred in a major breast cancer study. The belated revelation of misconduct made patients aware of their trust in medical research.

## The morality of trust

Although Sissela Bok has discussed trust as a moral resource since the 1970s, the question of the morality of trust relationships—the question of the circumstances under which, from a moral point of view, one ought to trust—was not explicitly discussed until Annette Baier's 1986 essay, "Trust and Anti-Trust." Two earlier essays were important in laying the foundation for this major turn in the discussion. In 1984, Ian Hacking provided a devastating assessment of the use of game theory to understand moral questions, such as the Prisoner's Dilemma, which will be discussed below. Baier herself argued in 1985 for broadening the focus in ethics from obligations and moral rules to the subject of who ought, as a moral matter, to be trusted and when. As Kathryn Addelson points out, Baier's change of focus establishes a general perspective on ethical legitimacy that is shared by all—both the powerful and those whom society labels "deviant"—rather than privileging the perspective of those who make, instill, and enforce moral rules (Addelson, 1994).

Baier's general account of the morality of trust illuminates the strong relation between the trustworthy and the true. A trust relationship, according to Baier, is decent to the extent that it stands the test of disclosure of the premises of each party's trust (Baier, 1986). For example, if one party trusts the other to perform as needed only because the truster believes the trusted is too timid or unimaginative to do otherwise, disclosure of these premises will tend to insult the trusted party and give him or her an incentive to prove the truster wrong. Similarly, if the trusted party fulfills the truster's expectations only through fear of detection and punishment, disclosure of these premises may lead the truster to suspect that the trusted would betray the trust, given an anonymous opportunity to do so.

Although explicit discussion of moral trustworthiness is relatively recent, both professional ethics and the philosophy of technology have given considerable attention to the concept of responsibility. Since being trustworthy is key to acting responsibly in a professional capacity, or to being a responsible person if one considers responsibility a virtue, the literature on responsibility provides at least an implicit discussion of many aspects of the morality of trust, much of which is relevant to the subject of trust in health care.

## Conceptual relationships

Trust involves both confidence and reliance. Annette Baier argues that if we lack other options, we may continue to rely on something even when we no longer trust it (Baier, 1986). Similarly, we may have confidence in something, or confidence in our expectations concerning it, without relying on it. To rely only on what we can trust is a fortunate circumstance.

Niklas Luhmann (1988) urges a different distinction between confidence and trust, suggesting that "trust" be used only when the truster has considered the alternatives to trusting. Such use is incompatible with unconscious trust, a phenomenon to which Baier draws attention. Luhmann's discussion of the distinction between trust and confidence highlights the element of risk in trusting. Risk or vulnerability does characterize situations in which trust is necessary, in contrast to situations in which one's control of the outcome makes trust unnecessary. However, the element of risk taking in trust is captured in the notion of reliance when trust is understood as confident reliance. Being vulnerable in one's reliance does not require that one have considered the alternatives, if any, to such reliance.

Although one often trusts people, their intentions and goodwill, there is also trust in mere circumstances or events: One may trust that a taxi will come along shortly, even if no taxi has been ordered, without believing anything about another person's reliability in providing a taxi.

The risk taken in trusting does leave the truster liable to disappointment (or worse), whether that trust is of persons or events. But only when trust is in other people, and not merely in the events involving them, can one be let down by them. Suppose that a person is awakened every weekday by another person's calling for a neighbor. If the first person has come to rely on being awakened, but one day the other person does not come for the neighbor or does so quietly, the first person's expectations will be disappointed. But the person will not have been disappointed or let down by the one who usually picks up the neighbor. To be disappointed by another person, that person must at least be aware of doing or not doing the act in question. Here the person doing the calling for the neighbor is not aware of waking up the first party, much less of being trusted to do it. As Baier mentions (1986), it is possible for there to be trust of which the trusted person is unaware, and so one might let down another without being aware of letting that person down.

Niklas Luhmann (1979) has shown how trust simplifies human life by endowing some expectations with assurance. To consider all possible disappointments, defections, and betrayals by those on whom we rely, the possible consequences of those disappointments, and any actions that one might take to prevent those disappointments or change their effect is prohibitively costly in terms of time and energy. Trust reduces that burden.

## The literature on trust

Sociologists like Bernard Barber (1983) and Luhmann (1979, 1988) have written on many facets of the notion of trust, and legal theorists have reflected on the distinct, though related, notion of a legal trust. Until the 1980s, however, the explicit attention given to the common notion of trust, or confident reliance, in Anglo-American philosophy was largely in relation to such questions as how the "prisoners" in the so-called Prisoner's Dilemma might solve their problem of assurance with regard to one another's behavior so as to cooperate in achieving a mutually beneficial outcome. (In the Prisoner's Dilemma, each of two prisoners will receive a light sentence if neither confesses to a crime, and a more severe sentence if both confess; but if one confesses and the other does not, the latter will be freed, but the former will receive the most severe sentence of all. Without assurance about each other's behavior, and in spite of knowing that both would be better off if neither confesses, both are likely to confess and be less well off.)

Recent literature on trust has examined trust in a variety of different social circumstances, involving a wide range of objects and systems, persons in a wide variety of roles, and matters in which they might be trusted or distrusted. For example, some writers focus on cases of the breakdown of trust in war, under the influence of the Mafia, or in some other extreme situation. Differences in the domain of application of the notion of trust lead to an unusually wide range of estimates of its character and importance. They also lead to disparate distinctions between trust and such notions as reliance, faith, vulnerability, and confidence, as well as to different conclusions about the moral value and the moral risks associated with trust.

Those who write about trust in a market context often take economic rationality—according to which each person simply seeks to maximize his or her goals by the most efficient means—as their model. They then often regard trust as a way of coping with "imperfect rationality," understood as uncertainty about the facts or about one another's behavior, and how to estimate the consequences for the achievement of one's goals. The economic model of rationality is not readily applicable in considerations of ethics because it was designed to avoid consideration of values other than efficiency, and it treats moral considerations as nonobjective "personal preferences." Where a market context is assumed, the relatively minor risk of being a "sucker" is likely to be mentioned as a barrier to trust. (See, for example, Dasgupta, 1988.) In discussions of trust among family members or between nations (Bok, 1990a), much more is recognized to be at stake.

Feminists like Trudy Govier argue that attention to trust relationships will bring attention to other relationships, such as those between parents and children, that have been neglected when contracts are the focus of attention. Such relationships, however, together with the features of trust that are prominent in them, continue to be ignored in much of the literature on trust. For example, Geoffrey Hawthorn mentions a parent's nonegoistic motives toward his or her child, only to turn immediately to "more ordinary" instances of nonegoistic motives (Hawthorn, 1988).

Bernard Williams (1988), who begins his own essay with a discussion of the Prisoner's Dilemma, argues that the problem of how nonegoistic motivation is to be encouraged and legitimated does not have a general solution. He argues that the problem of trust or cooperation is not one that can be solved in a general way at the level of decision theory, social psychology, or the general theory of social institutions. To ensure cooperation in a given situation requires an understanding of the ways in which the people in that situation are motivated. Williams believes that solutions to the problem of cooperation are found only for particular historically shaped societies, rather than for society in general. He argues that investigating the sorts of combinations of motivations that make sense in that society might lead to a general perspective on the problems of cooperation in such a society. However, as he says, "there is no one problem of cooperation: the problem is always how a given set of people cooperate" (1988, p. 13). Those whose cooperation is of the greatest interest in bioethics are patients, their families, the health-care providers, and the policymakers who shape the health-care system.

CAROLINE WHITBECK

*Directly related to this entry are the entries* FIDELITY AND LOYALTY; *and* PROFESSIONAL–PATIENT RELATIONSHIP. *For a further discussion of topics mentioned in this entry, see the entries* BENEFICENCE; CONFIDENTALITY; FAMILY; HEALTH AND DISEASE, *article on* THE EXPERIENCE OF HEALTH AND ILLNESS; INFORMED CONSENT; MEDICAL MALPRACTICE; PATIENTS' RESPONSIBILITIES; PATIENTS' RIGHTS; PRIVACY AND CONFIDENTIALITY IN RESEARCH; PRIVACY IN HEALTH CARE; PRIVILEGED COMMUNICATIONS; RESPONSIBILITY; *and* RISK. *Other relevant material may be found under the entries* CARE; MEDICAL EDUCATION; MEDICINE, ART OF; NURSING, THEORIES AND PHILOSOPHY OF; OBLIGATION AND SUPEREROGATION; TEAMS, HEALTH-CARE; *and* VIRTUE AND CHARACTER.

## Bibliography

ADDELSON, KATHRYN. 1994. *Moral Passages: Notes Toward a Collectivist Ethics.* New York: Routledge.

BAIER, ANNETTE. 1985. "What Do Women Want in a Moral Theory?" *Nous* 19, no. 1:53–63. Reprinted in her *Moral Prejudices: Essays on Ethics.* Cambridge, Mass.: Harvard University Press, 1994.
———. 1986. "Trust and Antitrust." *Ethics* 96, no. 2:232–260. Reprinted in her *Moral Prejudices: Essays on Ethics,* pp. 95–129. Cambridge, Mass.: Harvard University Press, 1994.
———. 1993. "Trust and Distrust of Moral Theorists." In *Applied Ethics: A Reader,* pp. 131–142. Edited by Earl R. Winkler and Jerrold R. Coombs. Oxford: Basil Blackwell.
———. 1994a. *Moral Prejudices: Essays on Ethics.* Cambridge, Mass.: Harvard University Press.
———. 1994b. "Sustaining Trust." In her *Moral Prejudices: Essays on Ethics,* pp. 152–182. Cambridge, Mass.: Harvard University Press.
———. 1994c. "Trust and Its Vulnerabilities." In her *Moral Prejudices: Essays on Ethics,* pp. 130–151. Cambridge, Mass.: Harvard University Press.
———. 1994d. "Trusting People." In her *Moral Prejudices: Essays on Ethics,* pp. 183–203. Cambridge, Mass.: Harvard University Press.
BALOS, BEVERLY, and FELLOWS, MARY LOUISE. 1991. "Guilty of the Crime of Trust: Nonstranger Rape." *Minnesota Law Review* 75, no. 3:599–618.
BARBER, BERNARD. 1983. *The Logic and Limits of Trust.* New Brunswick, N.J.: Rutgers University Press.
BENNER, PATRICIA E. 1984. *From Novice to Expert: Excellence and Power in Clinical Nursing Pratice.* Menlo Park, Calif.: Addison-Wesley.
BENNER, PATRICIA E., and WRUBEL, JUDITH. 1989. *The Primacy of Caring: Stress and Coping in Health and Illness.* Menlo Park, Calif.: Addison-Wesley.
BOK, SISSELA. 1978. *Lying: Moral Choice in Public and Private Life.* New York: Pantheon.
———. 1990a. *A Strategy for Peace: Human Values and the Threat of War.* New York: Pantheon.
———. 1990b. "Can Lawyers Be Trusted?" *University of Pennsylvania Law Review* 138, no. 3:913–933.
DASGUPTA, PARTHA. 1988. "Trust as a Commodity." In *Trust: Making and Breaking Cooperative Relations,* pp. 49–72. Edited by Diego Gambetta. Oxford: Basil Blackwell.
DULA, ANNETTE. 1991. "Toward an African-American Perspective on Bioethics." *Journal of Health Care for the Poor and Underserved* 2, no. 2:259–269.
———. 1992. "African Americans and Mistrust of the Medical Community." Address given at Harvard Medical School, Cambridge, Mass., November 1992.
GAMBETTA, DIEGO, ed. 1988. *Trust: Making and Breaking Cooperative Relations.* Oxford: Basil Blackwell.
GOOD, DAVID. 1988. "Individuals, Interpersonal Relations, and Trust." In *Trust: Making and Breaking Cooperative Relations,* pp. 31–48. Edited by Diego Gambetta. Oxford: Basil Blackwell.
GOVIER, TRUDY. 1992. "Trust, Distrust, and Feminist Theory." *Hypatia* 7, no. 1:16–33.
HACKING, IAN. 1984. "Winner Takes Less." *New York Review of Books* 31:17–21.
HANDLER, JOEL F. 1990. *Law and the Search for Community.* Philadelphia: University of Pennsylvania Press.

HARDIN, RUSSELL. 1991. "Trusting Persons, Trusting Institutions." In *Strategy and Choice*, pp. 185–209. Edited by Richard Zeckhauser. Cambridge, Mass.: MIT Press.

———. 1992. "The Street Level Epistemology of Trust." *Analyse und Kritik* 14:152–176.

HAWTHORN, GEOFFREY. 1988. "Three Ironies in Trust." In *Trust: Making and Breaking Cooperative Relations*, pp. 111–126. Edited by Diego Gambetta. Oxford: Basil Blackwell.

LADD, JOHN. 1980. "Legalism and Medical Ethics." In *Contemporary Issues in Biomedical Ethics*, pp. 1–35. Edited by John W. Davis, C. Barry Hoffmaster, and Sarah Shorten. Clifton, N.J.: Humana.

———. 1982. "The Distinction Between Rights and Responsibilities: A Defense." *Linacre Quarterly* 49 (May): 121–142.

LAMMERS, STEPHEN. 1985. "Some Ethical Issues in the End-Stage Renal Disease Program." *Weaver Information and Perspectives on Technological Literacy* 3, no. 2:4–5.

LUHMANN, NIKLAS. 1979. *Trust and Power.* New York: John Wiley & Sons.

———. 1988. "Familiarity, Confidence, Trust: Problems and Alternatives." In *Trust: Making and Breaking Cooperative Relations*, pp. 94–107. Edited by Diego Gambetta. Oxford: Basil Blackwell.

MacINTYRE, ALASDAIR. 1984. "Does Applied Ethics Rest on a Mistake?" *Monist* 67, no. 4:498–513.

MITCHAM, CARL. 1987. "Responsibility and Technology: The Expanding Relationship." In *Technology and Responsibility*, pp. 3–39. Edited by Paul T. Durbin. Philosophy and Technology no. 3. Boston: D. Reidel.

PARSONS, TALCOTT. 1951. *The Social System.* Glencoe, Ill.: Free Press.

PELLEGRINO, EDMUND D.; VEATCH, ROBERT M.; and LANGAN, JOHN T. 1991. *Ethics, Trust, and the Professions: Philosophical and Cultural Aspects.* Washington, D.C.: Georgetown University Press.

RICH, ADRIENNE C. 1979. "Women and Honor: Some Notes on Lying (1975)." In her *On Lies, Secrets and Silence: Selected Prose, 1966–1978*, pp. 185–194. New York: W. W. Norton.

U.S. PRESIDENT'S COMMISSION FOR THE STUDY OF ETHICAL PROBLEMS IN MEDICINE AND BIOMEDICAL AND BEHAVIORAL RESEARCH. 1982. *Making Health Care Decisions: A Report on the Ethical and Legal Implications of Informed Consent in the Patient-Practitioner Relationship.* 3 vols. Washington, D.C.: U.S. Government Printing Office.

WILLIAMS, BERNARD. 1988. "Formal Structures and Social Reality." In *Trust: Making and Breaking Cooperative Relations*, pp. 3–13. Edited by Diego Gambetta. Oxford: Basil Blackwell.

# TRUTH-TELLING

*See* INFORMATION DISCLOSURE.

# TURKEY

*See* MEDICAL ETHICS, HISTORY OF, *section on* NEAR AND MIDDLE EAST, *article on* TURKEY.

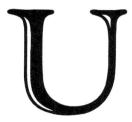

# UNETHICAL RESEARCH

See RESEARCH, UNETHICAL.


# UNITED KINGDOM

See MEDICAL ETHICS, HISTORY OF, section on EUROPE, subsection on CONTEMPORARY PERIOD, article on UNITED KINGDOM.


# UNITED STATES

See MEDICAL ETHICS, HISTORY OF, section on THE AMERICAS, articles on COLONIAL NORTH AMERICA AND NINETEENTH-CENTURY UNITED STATES, and UNITED STATES IN THE TWENTIETH CENTURY.


## UNORTHODOXY IN MEDICINE

*The following is a revision and update of the first-edition entry "Orthodoxy in Medicine" by Martin Kaufman.*

Unorthodoxy in medicine is defined as practices that are not accepted as correct, proper, or appropriate or are not in conformity with the beliefs or standards of the dominant group of medical practitioners or laypersons in a society. Individual healers who persist in engaging in these activities despite the disapproval and opposition of members of the dominant group may be classified as "unorthodox practitioners." The use here of the terms "orthodox" and "unorthodox" serves neither to condemn nor to condone but rather to help explain the relationship between those who fall into one category of practitioners and those who do not.

Orthodox physicians can be differentiated on the basis of their education, whether low-grade, acceptable, or superior; on the basis of skills, whether minimal, ordinary, or extraordinary; and on the basis of their practice, whether specialist or generalist. The point is that however differentiated from each other, orthodox physicians collectively share certain ways of apprehending phenomena and diagnosing and handling problems, and they maintain certain standards of conduct—all of which binds them together. In short, they may be regarded as being part of a professional community in that they speak the same language, rely on the same general pool of knowledge, share certain beliefs and values, and strive for common goals.

It is not possible to say the same thing for the general category of unorthodox medical practitioners. Though they may be differentiated according to training, skill, and type of practice, they do not constitute a distinct community. In fact, they represent a heterogeneous population promoting disparate beliefs and practices that vary considerably from one movement or tradition to another and form no consistent or complementary body of knowledge. This is not to imply that there are no similarities or social, political, and intellectual ties among them. However, the only fundamental characteristic they share is their alienation from the dominant medical profession. As a whole, unorthodox medicine has no real corporate identity, although within each movement or tradition a great deal of consensus may be observed.

Throughout modern Western history, ethical questions about unorthodox practice have been raised principally by the orthodox medical community. For example, in the United States, when the profession sought to organize on a local and state level in the early nineteenth century, one of the chief priorities of the leaders of this movement was to define who should be considered a "regular" versus a "nonregular" practitioner and, once having done so, to determine what actions regular physicians should take against those violating the norms of orthodox medicine.

### The AMA's "consultation clause"

On a national level, the American Medical Association (AMA), formed in 1846, quickly adopted a Code of Ethics, which contained a so-called consultation clause declaring that no one can be considered a regular practitioner, or a fit associate in consultation, whose practice is based on an exclusive dogma, to the rejection of the accumulated experience of the profession and of the aids actually furnished by anatomy, physiology, pathology, and organic chemistry.

The most articulate spokesman for the AMA code was a Connecticut physician named Worthington Hooker, whose book *Physician and Patient* (1849) was the first systematic treatise on medical ethics by an American. Much of his book is concerned with sectarian practitioners. Sectarian medicine constitutes one form of unorthodox practice consisting of individuals who band together around a set of deviant health beliefs and establish their own medical schools, journals, associations, and hospitals. In the United States, the most prominent examples have been homeopathy, eclecticism, Thomsonianism, and physio-medicalism, which flourished in the nineteenth century, and osteopathy and chiropractic in the twentieth century.

Against these sectarians, Hooker gave five major reasons for supporting the AMA code's "consultation clause"—themes that found recurring expression by its advocates throughout the nineteenth century and into the twentieth. Hooker argued, first, that the belief system of sectarian healers was alien to the accumulated experience of the profession; second, that their practices were dangerous to their patients; third, that their education was inferior to that of regular practitioners; fourth, that their social behavior did not conform to that expected of gentlemen; and, fifth, that any association with these healers both legitimized the irregular and lowered the status of the regular profession before the public.

Scientific medicine, argued Hooker, was based on observation and experience. To understand disease, one needed to carefully record symptoms, determine the cause of the problem by gathering as much evidence as possible, weigh variations and circumstances peculiar to the individual patient, and consider all relevant factors in the case before deciding on a course of therapy. With respect to medical treatment, he said, the type and content of intervention should be based on the known and predictable physiological effects of the dosages of the drugs used. Sectarians, however, framed their whole approach to disease on theory rather than observation. They were rationalists who took a few observations and expanded these findings into an all-encompassing system to explain all problems in terms of disease causation, diagnosis, and therapy. Samuel Thomson (1796–1843) launched the Thomsonian movement on the belief that all disease was due to "obstructed perspiration" and that heat had to be restored to the body. Under this logic, all therapy was directed at opening up the pores.

Samuel Hahnemann (1755–1843), the founder of homeopathy, believed in treating all patients by creating short-lived artificial illnesses that would closely mimic the effects of actual diseases and somehow substitute for them. He argued that a drug that would produce symptoms in a well person would cure the same symptoms in a sick person and that the smaller the dose, the more powerful the medicine. He also maintained that almost all chronic diseases were produced by Psora, or "the itch" (Hahnemann, 1849). According to Hooker, such dogmas were the antithesis of scientific thinking. How, he asked, could an ethical physician practice or associate himself with one who subscribed to these exclusive and ridiculous notions?

As Thomsonianism and homeopathy were based on unscientific thinking, Hooker maintained that practitioners who embraced these systems posed a danger to their patients because they subjected the sick to theories that went against the accumulated knowledge of the profession. Furthermore, the distinctive therapies these sectarians utilized, independent of the dogma they rested on, posed grave risks. In the case of Thomson and his followers, their regimen of vomiting and sweating for all patients caused needless suffering and death. As for the homeopaths, given that the infinitesimal doses of their drugs did not physiologically harm their patients, critics like Hooker argued that they did no good and prevented or delayed the sick from receiving remedies that had value.

Hooker considered sectarians as well as other unorthodox practitioners to be "quacks." Quacks operated on unfounded theories and used highly dubious treatments. But the quack label was extended to social behavior as well. They were not gentlemen who subscribed to common rules of etiquette and proper professional behavior but unprincipled rogues, many of whom intentionally fooled the public to earn a livelihood. They were boastful pretenders who publicly ridiculed the practices and skills of regular physicians while making exaggerated claims in the press and elsewhere of the individual prowess or benefits of their systems.

## The consultation clause in action

In the years following the appearance of Hooker's book, the AMA began to enforce the consultation clause. In the mid-1850s, all affiliated local and state societies were required to adopt the entire code in their own constitutions, and some began to hold trials and remove from membership physicians who were caught consulting with irregulars. In addition, regular medical societies used the consultation clause as the basis for actively opposing sectarian practitioners' gaining access to hospitals supported by public funds, opposed the right of sectarians to serve on boards of health, and blocked their acceptance as military physicians and surgeons. In the minds of those who supported the consultation clause, all these actions were consistent with the goals of protecting the public's health.

Not surprisingly, sectarian practitioners had a different view of the motives of the code's supporters. They postulated three reasons why the AMA opposed them: first, they were getting better results than the regulars, which made orthodox physicians look bad; second, orthodox physicians were dogmatically committed to their own "system," which resulted in their branding everything they did not believe in as quackery; and, third, the ethical concerns of the regulars were merely a smokescreen for their desire to restrict economic competition.

At the time the consultation clause was adopted, many orthodox physicians were still practicing what was later called "heroic medicine," which consisted of employing powerful remedies in large doses. For "inflammatory" diseases, copious and repeated bleedings were not uncommon. Calomel, a form of mercury and a strong cathartic, was often used as a standard procedure to "clean out the system" in most diseases. Unfortunately, mercury is not readily excreted from the body, and many Americans of the era suffered the cumulative systemic effects of mercury poisoning, including the rotting of bones and the loss of teeth.

Even after the Civil War, when orthodox medicine turned away from depletive therapeutics to drugs given to "strengthen" the system, the widespread professional use of alcohol and narcotics meant that orthodox medicine occasionally posed significant dangers to the recovery of patients. Under homeopathy, its chief competitor during this era, the patient merely had to suffer the disease, rather than the combination of the illness and the methods used to treat the illness. Consequently, homeopathic and other sectarian healers' claims of better

results appear, in retrospect, to have had a basis in fact, independent of the validity of the philosophical and scientific arguments used to justify their therapeutic management. Thus, orthodox physicians' continuing ethical concern that unorthodox physicians "necessarily" do harm to patients is not generally supported by recent historical research.

The mixed results of the consultation clause—in addition to the fact that many otherwise regular physicians were ignoring it—was a major reason why some orthodox practitioners in the last quarter of the nineteenth century sought to modify or abolish the proscription. Another was the ethical dilemma of AMA members who wished to subscribe to the code and found themselves in situations where they were called to help a person in need and found that an irregular healer was still on the case. Should a desperately ill person, they inquired, be put in the position of having to discharge the other physician before the regular could step in? And what should the regular practitioner do if the patient refused? Which was more important to an ethical physician, a sense of personal dignity and the dignity of the profession or helping to save the life of the patient?

## Assimilating the unorthodox

In addition, over the years, the actual educational background of some sectarian practitioners as well as their practice patterns were changing, making the characterization of the irregular as an unprincipled quack more difficult to apply successfully. Homeopaths and eclectics (who substituted botanical remedies for chemical drugs) as well as the regulars were all affected by the growing scientific knowledge of the time. The advances in pathology, physiology, and bacteriology were changing the way each practitioner thought about disease. With respect to therapeutics, the type of drugs used and their dosages were coming closer together. With these changes in progress, a growing number of regulars questioned the validity of the consultation clause. Some AMA members argued that by sharing fellowship with homeopaths and eclectics, orthodox physicians could accelerate the positive steps that members of these movements had already taken. In 1903, the AMA changed its code to allow fellowship with "other" physicians who had renounced sectarianism, a change that led to the eventual assimilation of these competing movements.

In the twentieth century, orthodox medicine began a new cycle of battles with two new systems based on spinal manipulation: osteopathy, originated by Andrew Taylor Still (1828–1917), and chiropractic, founded by Daniel David Palmer (1845–1913). As osteopathic physicians, or D.O.s (doctors of osteopathy), incorporated the diagnostic and therapeutic tools utilized by M.D.s and raised their educational standards, they too became recognized by the AMA in the 1960s as acceptable colleagues, although many osteopathic physicians still resist complete assimilation. Chiropractors, on the other hand, who still center their activities on the spinal column, used federal antitrust laws in the 1980s to force the AMA to end ethical restrictions on its members' ability to consult with them.

While the aforementioned debate has perhaps as much to do with "medical etiquette" as it does with "medical ethics," it is significant that during the whole period in which sectarian movements and orthodox medicine have battled each other, the issue of whether it was "ethical" for patients themselves to undergo treatment by an unorthodox practitioner was seldom raised. Even orthodox physicians did not directly challenge a person's right to obtain whatever type of advice or treatment he or she desired, even though they certainly tried to limit patients' options by having the state either prohibit or restrict the activities of all but orthodox practitioners.

There have, however, been exceptions. Resorting to unorthodox practitioners or treatments has been directly challenged when individuals are suspected of being mentally incompetent and particularly when minors are not receiving orthodox care because of the religious or philosophical beliefs of their parents. While some ethicists, like H. Tristram Engelhardt, Jr., argue for wide parental latitude in a "minimalist" state, and unilaterally support the parental right to make health-care decisions for their children (Engelhardt, 1986), the courts have long supported the state's efforts to require parents to have their children receive orthodox care when permanent physical damage can result or, alternatively, for the state to become guardian of such endangered children when parents refuse. Nevertheless, if judges can be convinced that orthodox treatment has but a slim hope of benefiting the child, or that the risks of such orthodox treatment are serious enough to raise legitimate doubts in parents about subjecting their children to these procedures or regimens, courts may allow parents to pursue an alternative course.

NORMAN GEVITZ

*Directly related to this entry is the entry* ALTERNATIVE THERAPIES. *For a further discussion of topics mentioned in this entry, see the entries* AUTONOMY; HEALING; HEALTH AND DISEASE; LICENSING, DISCIPLINE, AND REGULATION IN THE HEALTH PROFESSIONS; MEDICINE, PHILOSOPHY OF; MEDICINE AS A PROFESSION; *and* PUBLIC HEALTH, *article on* PHILOSOPHY OF PUBLIC HEALTH. *Other relevant material may be found under the entry* VALUE AND VALUATION.

## Bibliography

BYNUM, WILLIAM F., and PORTER, ROY, eds. 1987. *Medical Fringe and Medical Orthodoxy, 1750–1850.* London: Croom Helm.

COOTER, ROGER, ed. 1988. *Studies in the History of Alternative Medicine.* Basingstoke, U.K.: Macmillan.

ENGELHARDT, H. TRISTRAM, JR. 1986. *The Foundations of Bioethics.* New York: Oxford University Press.

GEVITZ, NORMAN. 1982. *The D.O.'s: Osteopathic Medicine in America.* Baltimore: Johns Hopkins University Press.

———. 1989. "The Chiropractors and the AMA: Reflections on the History of the Consultation Clause." *Perspectives in Biology and Medicine* 32, no. 2:281–299.

———. 1991. "Christian Science Healing and the Health Care of Children." *Perspectives in Biology and Medicine* 34, no. 3:421–438.

HAHNEMANN, SAMUEL. 1849. *Samuel Hahnemann's Organon of Homeopathic Medicine.* 3d U.S. ed. Translated by Constantine Hering. New York: William Radde.

HOOKER, WORTHINGTON. 1849. *Physician and Patient; or, A Practical View of the Mutual Duties, Relations, and Interests of the Medical Profession and the Community.* New York: Baker & Scribner.

KAUFMAN, MARTIN. 1988. "Homeopathy in America: The Rise and Fall and Persistence of a Medical Heresy." In *Other Healers: Unorthodox Medicine in America,* pp. 99–123. Edited by Norman Gevitz. Baltimore: Johns Hopkins University Press.

PALMER, DANIEL DAVID, and PALMER, BARTLETT JOSHUA. 1906. *Science of Chiropractic.* Davenport, Iowa: Palmer School of Chiropractic.

ROTHSTEIN, WILLIAM G. 1972. *American Physicians in the Nineteenth Century: From Sects to Science.* Baltimore: Johns Hopkins University Press.

STILL, ANDREW TAYLOR. 1908. *Autobiography of Andrew T. Still.* Kirksville, Mo.: Author.

WARNER, JOHN HARLEY. 1986. *The Therapeutic Perspective: Medical Practice, Knowledge, and Identity in America, 1820–1885.* Cambridge, Mass.: Harvard University Press.

YOUNG, JAMES HARVEY. 1992. *American Health Quackery.* Princeton, N.J.: Princeton University Press.

# URUGUAY

*See* MEDICAL ETHICS, HISTORY OF, *section on* THE AMERICAS, *article on* LATIN AMERICA.

# UTILITARIANISM

*See* ETHICS, *articles on* NORMATIVE ETHICAL THEORIES, *and* TASK OF ETHICS; *and* UTILITY.

# UTILITY

The concept of utility in bioethics raises questions about both its meaning and measurement and its normative requirements for moral choice. Although associated most prominently with the utilitarian ethics of Jeremy Bentham (1748–1832) and John Stuart Mill (1806–1873), philosophical discourse on utility ranges back to Epicurus (341–270 B.C.E.) and can be found in the work of philosophers of moral sentiment, such as David Hume (1711–1766), who observed that "utility, in all subjects, is a source of praise and approbation; . . . it is a foundation of the chief part of morals, which has a reference to mankind and our fellow creatures" (Hume, 1948, p. 221). However, interpretations of utility as a moral concept and moral norm are diverse. This entry explores conceptions of utility in moral philosophy, moral theology, and public policy and illustrates its normative relevance for bioethics.

## Philosophical interpretations

The ethics of Bentham and Mill reflect one dominant philosophical understanding of utility, the "happiness" theory (Brandt, 1982). Bentham considered utility to be a primary source for legal and social reform, and even, as illustrated by the title of his major theoretical work, *An Introduction to the Principles of Morals and Legislation* (1789), as a guide for use by legislators. On the basis of an understanding that human nature is governed by the "two sovereign masters" of pleasure and pain, Bentham defined utility as "that property in any object, whereby it tends to produce benefit, advantage, pleasure, good, or happiness . . . or . . . to prevent the happening of mischief, pain, evil, or unhappiness to the party whose interest is considered" (1789, p. 12). The principle of utility (or the "greatest happiness" or "greatest felicity" principle) is the moral and political expression of psychological hedonism: We ought to approve and do, or disapprove and refrain from doing, actions according to their promotion of pleasure and happiness.

Mill's view of utility, itself integrated with liberal political reform and social activism in such areas as education and the status of women, is likewise related to a conception of human nature. As articulated in his classic essay *Utilitarianism* (1863), since human beings desire to realize happiness through their actions, utility or the greatest happiness principle is necessarily the standard of morality. Mill requires a moral agent to be a "disinterested and benevolent spectator" with respect to his or her own happiness relative to that of other persons. This ethic of disinterested benevolence allowed Mill to propose a harmony between secular and sacred morality:

Christian teachings on the Golden Rule and loving one's neighbor as oneself express the ideal perfection of utilitarian morality (Mill, 1971). This convergence of utility and love finds expression in contemporary bioethics in the writings of Joseph Fletcher (1966) and R. M. Hare (1981).

Mill offered a substantive critique of Bentham's concept of utility regarding the content of pleasure. Bentham's "felicific calculus" proposed that the value of a pleasure will vary according to features of intensity, duration, certainty, nearness, fecundity (the prospect that a pleasure or pain will be followed by sensations similar in kind), purity, and the number of persons affected. These features emphasize the quantity of pleasure, as expressed in Bentham's aphorism: "Quantity of pleasure being equal, pushpin is as good as poetry" (Monro, 1967, p. 283). Mill differentiated pleasures as more or less valuable according to qualitative features; thus the pleasures of the "higher faculties"—intellect, feelings, imagination, moral sentiments—are more desirable than the "lower" bodily or sensual pleasures. For Mill, qualitative content of utility meant, "It is better to be a human being dissatisfied than a pig satisfied; better to be Socrates dissatisfied than a fool satisfied" (Mill, 1863, p. 20). The primacy of the pleasures of mind over those of body could be validated, according to Mill, by the preferences of persons who had experienced both.

The core feature of contemporary expositions of the "desire" theory of utility resides precisely in an appeal to personal preferences (Brandt, 1982). Since people typically express desires for various conditions, including happiness or pleasure, the desire theory is necessarily broader and more pluralistic in content than the happiness concept of utility. Indeed, while hedonistic theories of utility are often criticized for infringing on personal self-determination for the sake of overall social welfare, the desire theory instead stresses a convergence between the principles of utility and respect for autonomy.

However, defining "utility" by the satisfaction of preferences risks a lack of discrimination with regard to which preferences should be satisfied. A pure desire or preferentialist theory—"pure" in that no restrictions are imposed on what would count as a morally reasonable preference—seems to treat all preferences as morally equal and leaves moral agents without a standard by which to differentiate unreasonable, bad, or fanatical preferences (such as satisfaction derived from abuse or torture of another, or from racial or ethnic bigotry). The plausibility of preference utility requires that we distinguish between what is desired (which is agent-specific) and what is desirable (which may be agent-neutral). Thus, pure preferentialism may be revised along the lines of some form of "idealized" or "corrected" preferentialism. John C. Harsanyi, for example, distinguishes between a person's manifest or actual preferences and his or her true preferences, as corrected by sufficient factual information for a decision, careful reasoning, and the capacity for rational choice. Harsanyi would also exclude "antisocial preferences"—such as sadism, envy, resentment, and malice—from considerations of social utility (Harsanyi, 1982).

Similarly, R. M. Hare has articulated a concept of utility constituted by "perfectly prudent" preferences, which is derived from a logical property of morality, the universalizability of preferences. Universalizability requires that we apply the same principles to others and to ourselves in similar situations. The moral agent is to ask: "What do I prefer should happen to me were I placed in the same position as that other person, with his or her preferences?" (Hare, 1986, p. 640). Hare derives from the universalizability thesis a moral requirement of impartiality toward the good of all others, which he claims unites Christian, Kantian, and utilitarian ethics.

This form of corrected preferentialism is also embedded in the two levels of moral thinking Hare believes we engage in (Hare, 1981). A first level is composed of rules and principles that we intuitively rely on in our everyday moral choices. However, this intuitive level is inadequate because it does not specify which principles and rules should be adopted as moral guidelines, nor does it indicate how conflicts between principles are to be resolved. Moral agents must then resort to a second level of critical thinking, in which such questions are resolved by direct application of utility. At this second level, human beings approximate the reasoning processes of "archangels," a metaphor that is closely related to Mill's ideal of the disinterested and benevolent spectator. The two related levels of moral thinking establish procedural restrictions on pure preferentialism and overcome the problem of accommodating evil preferences. While bad desires should be accorded equal consideration with other preferences, the utility of satisfying the desires of a sadist or racist will be outweighed, Hare maintains, by the disutility produced in the frustration of the desires and preferences of victims.

The problem of corrected preferentialism is that there may be little correspondence between actual and true or perfectly prudent preferences. The frustration of actual preferences by policies based on corrected preferentialism itself creates disutility. Moreover, though corrected preferentialism gives us the preferences people would have under conditions of sufficient information and reflection, excluding or discounting some preferences assumes there are certain preferences people ought to have. In short, corrected preferentialism presupposes that, in some instances, people do not know what is in their own good.

## Theological correlations

The philosophical debate over utility resonates in theological discussions of the principle of proportionality. The concept of "mixed teleology" has been invoked by some contemporary theologians in the Roman Catholic tradition to describe a vision of the moral life constituted primarily in terms of goals and ends. That is, human beings ought to pursue certain basic goods—for example, life, health, family life and raising children, knowledge, friendship, aesthetic experience—that are fundamental to well-being. This understanding of human nature permits the pursuit of more basic values than does hedonistic utilitarianism, but it is also more restrictive than forms of preference utilitarianism, as these basic goods of human well-being designate the preferences people ought to have.

In Roman Catholic moral theology, proportionality can assume two related but distinct senses (Finnis, 1983). First, proportionality may refer to the "fittingness" or "appropriateness" of a chosen means to the ends sought. The good of knowledge, for example, requires that we make choices about the normative and descriptive content of our readings, conversations, or observations. Second, proportionality refers to the balancing of goods and evils in assessing the consequences of action. This second sense is exemplified in traditional reasoning about the rule of double effect. Stemming from a principle of biblical morality—that we should never do evil that good might result (that is, the ends do not justify *all* means)—the rule of double effect justifies moral choices in which four conditions are met: (1) the act is morally good or indifferent; (2) the moral agent intends good effects or results; (3) evil effects of an action are not a means to the good; and (4) there is a favorable proportion or balance of good and evil results. This reasoning has been invoked in cases of justified fetal deaths, refusals of life-sustaining treatment, and collateral damage (civilian deaths) in warfare.

Some theologians consider proportionality compatible with virtually exceptionless moral norms and limit its application to conflicts of the goods necessary for human flourishing—for example, a conflict between prolonging life and relieving suffering. In such quandaries, the promotion of one good (relief of suffering) may risk infringing another good (prolongation of life) but can be considered justifiable if based on proportionate reason. Other theologians extend the domain of proportionality beyond conflict situations and suggests a moral analogue between utility and proportionality.

Scholars such as John Finnis have sharply criticized this more expansive scope of proportionality, known as "proportionalism," on several grounds that mirror philosophical debates over utility in ethics. Proportionality, he claims, can only direct fitting decisions between means and ends; it cannot inform commitments to basic goals in the first place. The content of proportionality thus depends on a substantive view of human flourishing. Moreover, Finnis believes that basic human goods are "incommensurable"—that is, they cannot be compared. The outcome orientation of proportionalism also neglects intrinsic moral wrongs (Finnis, 1983).

## Economic interpretations and applications

The concept of utility has played a significant role in contemporary theories of economic and social policy. As Peter J. Hammond suggests, "The whole study of welfare economics is founded more or less explicitly on utilitarian ideas," as reflected in principles of social welfare function, efficiency, and effectiveness (Hammond, 1982, p. 85). Several reasons account for the economic appropriation of utility. Since explicit appeals to utility emerged in a historical context of reform of social institutions, utility has an embedded tradition of policy change. Any utilitarian moral theory also presumes a model of calculated decision making that seems to cohere well with theories of rational choice that view people as acting in ways that seek to maximize their interests over time. Finally, the desire interpretation of utility gives content to the economic ideal of "consumer sovereignty." The utility consequences to individuals, aggregated for the society as a whole, offer a standard for preferring one policy to another on questions of social welfare. On broad issues of income redistribution and taxation or the allocation of scarce resources within medicine, utility may be measured through formal techniques of cost-benefit, cost-effective, or risk-benefit analysis. Objections to such methods often invoke questions about the distribution of costs, risks, and benefits among various groups.

A major question in economic applications of utility is how a method may move from delineating individual preferences to evaluating social welfare functions. Given the constraints of limited information that individuals experience in expressing preferences among policy options, including uncertainty about the comparative outcomes of the options, economic theorists no less than philosophers seem willing to concede that actual preferences can be mistaken and require modification. This, in turn, has prompted critiques of the ideal of consumer sovereignty similar to those directed against corrected preferentialism.

Even if the preference utility for a given individual can be constructed, the question of its social significance remains. Some method for making interpersonal comparisons of utility is required to maximize social welfare. Designating universalizability of preferences and impar-

tiality as methodological conditions enables some approaches to propose collective preferences; others rely on an assumption of identical individuals to validate interpersonal comparisons. Determining social utility by outcomes nonetheless must be sensitive to matters of process and representation. Social priorities in treating diseases, for example, may differ with the comparative weights given to the preferences of current sufferers, those of nonsufferers who are imagining the condition, and those of researchers who have studied the disease and those it afflicts (Loomes and McKenzie, 1989).

The tensions between utility as an economic principle, the ideal of consumer sovereignty, and methods of interpersonal comparisons are exemplified in debates over the valuing of life as part of cost-benefit analysis. A conventional approach to calculating a value for life is that of discounted future earnings (DFE), which considers the average age of death of persons killed by a certain disease or accident and then computes the expected future income of the person had he or she lived a normal lifespan. The future earnings are then discounted, since income earned today could be invested and is thus worth more than anticipated income. The DFE method has been sharply criticized as not reflecting an "individual's utility loss from death," which is not only economic but existential, and for underestimating a societal value for life. Moreover, DFE suggests that society should give greater priority to programs favoring young adult white males on the grounds that, given the perpetuation of current earning patterns, they can be expected to earn more income in comparison with, for example, women or the elderly (Rhoads, 1980).

An alternative approach, willingness to pay (WTP) for risk reduction, is essentially the economic expression of preference utilitarianism. WTP assumes that consumer preferences are the best guide for public policy, and valuing life on a WTP method reflects the aggregate of individual preferences regarding risk assumption/avoidance divided by the number of preventable deaths anticipated due to risk-averse behaviors. Even some proponents, however, deem WTP an insufficient guide to public policy, which should be informed by equality, equitable distribution, and the symbolic significance of the sanctity of life. In addition, some critics challenge the proposed connection between individual preferences and the valuation of life for social policy purposes.

The concept of preference utility is also embedded in a method, the quality-adjusted life year (QALY), which seeks to measure both life expectancy and quality of life according to community ethical values. The moral and economic rationale for the QALY method is the preference of a rational person for a healthier, though shorter, life over a longer life accompanied by extensive morbidity and disability. QALYs may be used at a microlevel to assess alternative therapies for a particular patient or at a macrolevel to set social priorities in allocating health-care resources.

At the level of clinical decision making, the QALY method has been challenged as a result of empirical studies indicating that personal preferences about health status can undergo dramatic variations over time and circumstance. The preference value of relief from anginal pain, for example, "may depend not only on how disabled and distressed [persons] feel at that moment, but may also be influenced by the perception of how their present health state will affect their future health" (Loomes and McKenzie, 1989, p. 303). In the area of personal health choices, this exemplifies a problem that may be characteristic of preference utilitarianism generally—namely, an assumption of temporal stability in priorities given to desires and preferences (Brandt, 1982).

The use of QALYs for macroallocation decisions has drawn criticism on much the same grounds as the methods for valuing life. Some critics, for example, claim that the QALY method prioritizes life units rather than the lives of people and thus violates principles of equal concern and respect for individual preferences (Harris, 1987). Moreover, a policy of maximizing QALYs will tend to bias health priorities in favor of younger generations, who would receive more life years from comprehensive neonatal and pediatric care than the elderly would from geriatric care. Harris therefore finds ageism embedded in QALYs and extends his concerns to sexism and racism. The question is whether the values QALYs seek to promote, such as efficiency, quality of life, and collective benefits, can be affirmed without violating other central ethical principles. This issue has assumed immense practical significance in debates over rationing health care, especially since certain rationing proposals have explicitly adopted the QALY method in setting health-care priorities.

### Utility and bioethics

Contemporary bioethics can neither live without utility nor live with utility as the primary moral principle. Utility is frequently portrayed as a specification of the normative principle of beneficence and considered a "balancing" principle in assessing harms and benefits (Beauchamp and Childress, 1989). Several issues in bioethics display the necessity and the limits of utility.

The principle of utility is embedded in debates over social priorities for health care. This is prominently displayed in the controversial Oregon Health Plan of 1993, which grew out of a 1987 decision by the state legislature to reallocate Medicaid funds from rescue care (thirty-four organ transplants) to preventive health services for

1,500 pregnant women and children from low-income families. The legislature subsequently sought to provide a guaranteed package of basic health services for all citizens through a process of Medicaid reform and rationing. This process culminated in a prioritized list of 688 condition and treatment pairs, with a funding cutoff after service 568. A dominant factor in determining the priority of a health condition was the impact of its related treatment on quality of life. These judgments in turn relied on a modified QALY method that incorporated citizens' preferences for health-care outcomes and measured changes in quality of life as net benefits realized from treatments (Hadorn, 1991). The social necessity of setting health-care priorities has not, however, muted critics' objections that any explicit rationing policy should be adopted as a last resort only after administrative inefficiencies have been remedied and should also embody fair representation of health-care preferences and equitable distribution toward the poor.

Questions of utility have also loomed large in debates about rationing scarce resources. Widespread consensus exists about the appropriateness of medical utility, which requires scarce resources to be rationed according to criteria of need and probability of benefit. However, disagreement exists about the moral acceptability of social utility, which selects recipients on the basis of their contributions (prospective or retrospective) to social welfare (Rescher, 1969). Other writers claim that the use of social utility methods denies equality of opportunity and allows social utility only under conditions of extreme community emergency, such as a natural catastrophe, in which treating injured medical personnel first would permit many other people to receive treatment more quickly. The emergency proviso would be an exception to a rule of equal opportunity only under normal conditions. However, the increasing pressures that individual choices for health care create on social resources and capacities will continue to make utility a necessary principle in bioethics, even if at times it must be limited by justice and respect for persons.

COURTNEY S. CAMPBELL

*Directly related to this entry are the entries* ETHICS, *article on* NORMATIVE ETHICAL THEORIES; *and* ECONOMIC CONCEPTS IN HEALTH CARE. *For a discussion of related ideas, see the entries* AUTONOMY; BENEFICENCE; *and* JUSTICE. *For a further discussion of topics mentioned in this entry, see the entries* DOUBLE EFFECT; ETHICS, *article on* RELIGION AND MORALITY; HARM; HEALTH CARE, ALLOCATION OF; LIFE, QUALITY OF, *article on* QUALITY OF LIFE IN HEALTH-CARE ALLOCATION; PAIN AND SUFFERING; RISK; *and* VALUE AND VALUATION.

# Bibliography

BARROW, ROBIN. 1991. *Utilitarianism: A Contemporary Statement*. Brookfield, Vt.: Edward Elgar.

BEAUCHAMP, TOM L., and CHILDRESS, JAMES F. 1989. *Principles of Biomedical Ethics*. 3d ed. New York: Oxford University Press.

BENTHAM, JEREMY. 1982. [1789]. *An Introduction to the Principles of Morals and Legislation*. Edited by James H. Burns and Herbert L. A. Hart. New York: Methuen.

BRANDT, RICHARD B. 1982. "Two Concepts of Utility." In *The Limits of Utilitarianism*, pp. 169–185. Edited by Harlan B. Miller and William H. Williams. Minneapolis: University of Minnesota Press.

FINNIS, JOHN. 1983. *Fundamentals of Ethics*. Washington, D.C.: Georgetown University Press.

FLETCHER, JOSEPH F. 1966. *Situation Ethics: The New Morality*. Philadelphia: Westminster.

HADORN, DAVID C. 1991. "Setting Health Care Priorities in Oregon: Cost-Effectiveness Meets the Rule of Rescue." *Journal of the American Medical Association* 265, no. 17:2218–2225.

HAMMOND, PETER J. 1982. "Utilitarianism, Uncertainty, and Information." In *Utilitarianism and Beyond*, pp. 85–102. Edited by Amartya K. Sen and Bernard A. O. Williams. Cambridge: At the University Press.

HARE, R. M. 1981. *Moral Thinking: Its Levels, Method, and Point*. Oxford: At the Clarendon Press.

———. 1982. "Utilitarianism and Moral Theory." In *Utilitarianism and Beyond*, pp. 23–38. Edited by Amartya K. Sen and Bernard A. O. Williams. Cambridge: At the University Press.

———. 1986. "Utilitarianism." In *Westminster Dictionary of Christian Ethics*, pp. 640–643. Edited by James F. Childress and John Macquarrie. Philadelphia: Westminster.

HARRIS, JOHN. 1987. "QALYfying the Value of Life." *Journal of Medical Ethics* 13, no. 3:117–123.

HARSANYI, JOHN C. 1982. "Morality and the Theory of Rational Behaviour." In *Utilitarianism and Beyond*, pp. 39–62. Edited by Amartya K. Sen and Bernard A. O. Williams. Cambridge: At the University Press.

HUME, DAVID. 1948. [1751]. "An Enquiry Concerning the Principles of Morals." In *Hume's Moral and Political Philosophy*. Edited by Henry D. Aiken. New York: Hafner.

LOOMES, GRAHAM, and MCKENZIE, LYDIA. 1989. "The Use of QALYs in Health Care Decision Making." *Social Science and Medicine* 28, no. 4:299–308.

MILL, JOHN STUART. 1971. [1863]. *Utilitarianism*. Edited by Samuel Gorovitz. Indianapolis, Ind.: Bobbs-Merrill.

MILLER, HARLAN B., and WILLIAMS, WILLIAM H., eds. 1982. *The Limits of Utilitarianism*. Minneapolis: University of Minnesota Press.

MONRO, DAVID H. 1967. "Jeremy Bentham." In *Encyclopedia of Philosophy*, pp. 280–285. Edited by Paul Edwards. New York: Macmillan.

MOORE, GEORGE EDWARD. 1966. [1903]. *Principia Ethica*. Cambridge: At the University Press.

O'CONNELL, TIMOTHY E. 1978. *Principles for a Catholic Morality*. New York: Seabury.

PENZ, G. PETER. 1986. *Consumer Sovereignty and Human Interests*. Cambridge: At the University Press.

RESCHER, NICHOLAS. 1969. "The Allocation of Exotic Medical Lifesaving Therapy." *Ethics* 79, no. 3:173–186.

RHOADS, STEVEN E. 1980. "How Much Should We Spend to Save a Life?" In *Valuing Life: Public Policy Dilemmas*, pp. 285–311. Edited by Steven E. Rhoads. Boulder, Colo.: Westview.

RILEY, JONATHAN. 1988. *Liberal Utilitarianism: Social Choice Theory and J. S. Mill's Philosophy*. Cambridge: At the University Press.

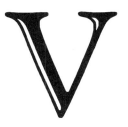

# VALUE AND VALUATION

Though values are integral to human experience, it is only in modern societies that they have gained an explicit place in ethics. In traditional societies, values generally operate as components of the common culture that are taken for granted. Their moral discourse focuses on the rules that define primary human obligations and on notions of moral excellence. Values first acquire ethical importance where individuals have wide choices about how they are to live their lives. These choices lead to a plurality of value perspectives whose competing claims may appear to express little more than subjective preferences. The challenge to ethics, then, is to devise ways of assessing values critically in relation to normative moral discourse.

In European civilizations, wide value choices were first opened up by the rise of capitalism and of liberal democratic states. In this context, value considerations are never far removed from market dynamics or from basic principles of human liberty. Although class and status factors bar many from the benefits of these modern social formations, their impact on human life remains pervasive, compelling us for the sake of social order to accommodate various value orientations.

## The concept of values

We take note of the realities in our world that matter to us. Values are concepts we use to explain how and why various realities matter. Values are not to be confused with concrete goods. They are ideas, images, notions. Values attract us. We aspire after the good they articulate. We expect to find our own good in relation to what they offer.

Because values are linked to realities we experience, they have an objective reference. They disclose features in our everyday world to which we attach special importance. Positive values are balanced by disvalues. Disvalues express what we consider undesirable, harmful, or unworthy about particular phenomena. They identify realities that we resist or strive to avoid. Virtually everything we experience has valuative significance: objects, states of affairs, activities, processes, performances, relational networks, and so on.

Values are linked to acts of valuation (Scheler, 1973). For every value that appears, there is a corresponding valuative orientation (Husserl, 1970). This orientation may not be fully self-conscious; still less is it an expression of critical judgment. It is, nonetheless, the subjective basis for the appearance of values. Without valuing subjects, there can be no such thing as values.

In an elemental sense, values are disclosed by feelings (Ricoeur, 1966). Explicit value language comes later, if at all. How do I know that health is good? I know because I feel good when I am healthy. The positive feeling signals the presence of value. How do I know that a performance of Shakespeare's *Hamlet* is good? Even an informed aesthetic judgment has an affective basis: I was moved by it. In being moved, I apprehend value. My primal awareness of value becomes explicit as I identify the features in a phenomenon that draw me to it. Human languages furnish a rich vocabulary for conversations about values.

The correlation between values and valuative acts does not imply that values are purely subjective or that they are merely secondary embellishments of empirical fact. On the contrary, the notion of an empirical reality devoid of all valuative meaning is itself an abstraction. As our perceptions disclose an object's reality, so our affections disclose its worth (Ricoeur, 1966). By means of perceptions and affections, we apprehend facets of the realities we encounter. Apart from corresponding acts of consciousness, however, nothing whatever can appear.

### Values and human needs

Values are intimately related to human needs and desires (Niebuhr, 1960; Ogletree, 1985; Ricoeur, 1966). We value realities that satisfy basic needs and fulfill deeply felt aspirations. We associate disvalues with realities that threaten or diminish human well-being. Human well-being is only part of the story. With a growing environmental consciousness, value discussions embrace non-human life forms as well, perhaps creaturely well-being as a whole. Human life then gains its value within a natural world that has intrinsic worth. Religious communities honor a world-transcending center of values from which all lesser values derive their significance.

There are as many kinds of values as there are regions of experience where we distinguish good or bad, better or worse, beneficial or harmful: sensory values, organic values, personal values, interpersonal values, social values, cultural values, and spiritual values (Scheler, 1973). Social values can be differentiated into economic, political, legal, associational, and familial subsets. Cultural values embrace religious, moral, cognitive, and aesthetic interests (Parsons, 1969). The formal value types all contain values and disvalues. Notions of creaturely well-being are implied if not stated.

### Value issues in biomedical practice

Virtually all kinds of values figure in biomedical practice. Organic values are basic: life, health, vigor, bodily integrity. The purpose of medicine is to save lives and to promote healing. Yet the ill and injured are never merely "patients," organisms suffering treatable maladies; they are persons with dignity who have their own life plans (May, 1991; Ramsey, 1970). Personal values, therefore, qualify organic values. Patients as persons may in no case be subjected to medical procedures without informed consent. Ideally, they participate actively in their own healing.

Organic values are inherently problematic. Our impulses press us to strive for life, strength, and agility. Yet these strivings are limited by our vulnerability to illness,

injury, disability, and, finally, certain death. Modern medicine inclines us to define the limits of organic life not as natural features of finitude but as problems to be solved. This tendency requires us to make value judgments about the boundaries of medical intervention. Medical practices inattentive to these boundaries can deprive the dying of the personal space they need to achieve closure in their life pilgrimages.

At this point, organic values are qualified by more encompassing value commitments. Such commitments can help us to accept life's limits, acknowledge goods more noble than our own survival, and endure sufferings and disappointments with grace and wisdom. Life, death, health, and illness are never purely physiological; they are moral and spiritual as well. Health care must also have moral and spiritual as well as physiological dimensions (Cousins, 1979; May, 1991; Nelson and Rohricht, 1984).

Professional and economic values intersect medical practice in similar ways. Physicians have specialized knowledge that equips them to provide socially valued services. They enjoy social status as professionals who maintain standards for medical practice. In this role, they are public guarantors of prized social values (May, 1983). Physicians in the United States offer services for fees, primarily through third-party payments. Accordingly, medical practice is also a market transaction, and physicians are businesspeople with economic interests. The stake in economic values qualifies professional devotion to patient well-being.

The organization of health care profoundly conditions its operative values. Modern medicine requires sophisticated technologies affordable only to large medical centers. These institutions, usually constituted as corporations, dominate medical practice in the United States. The technologies they use are typically produced and supplied by global corporations. The income they receive derives largely from corporate employee-benefit plans and from insurance firms that service them. Health-related industries have become a major component of the economy, perhaps inappropriately overriding the legitimate claims of other social goods. Powerful economic and political interests support the continued growth of medical enterprises with little regard for wider social ramifications.

Because the desire for quality medical services is urgent, intense public debate surrounds federal policies that bear upon the organization, regulation, and funding of health care. The struggle is to determine appropriate government roles for the oversight and financing of biomedical activities. In this struggle, conflicting political values intersect health-care practices as public actors respond to constituent interests.

Similar sociocultural analyses could be directed to the roles played in the health-care system by values resident in families, religious communities, research institutes, medical colleges, the legal system, the media, and the arts. Ethical studies of the intersection between biomedical practices and social processes uncover a volatile mix of conflict-laden value issues.

## Fluidity of values

Values are not only pervasive but also fluid. Any concrete experience harbors many values and disvalues, none of which is definitive or self-contained. Illness can be a physical malady, a ruthless disruption of personal plans, an economic disaster, an opportunity for self-discovery, a moment of human bonding, an occasion for medical virtuosity, or a case study in biomedical research (May, 1991). Each of these meanings captures some of the values that belong to a particular experience. As attention shifts, one set of values continually flows into another.

Our terminology for values is similarly fluid. The word "health" can be used descriptively; it also identifies an important value. "Justice" can designate a basic moral principle; it can refer equally to a value worthy of promotion in social arrangements. The term "objective" may characterize "value-free" inquiry, but it also designates a cognitive value.

Because of their fluidity, values resist schematic classification. Attempts to construct comprehensive value schemes do, however, have heuristic significance. They heighten awareness of the range of our valuative connections with our world, and they stimulate reflections on what belongs to human well-being (Hartmann, 1932; Perry, 1926; Scheler, 1973).

## Moral values

Within the value field, we can isolate a subset of moral values. Moral values cluster around personal identity, interpersonal relationships, and the makeup of groups, associations, social institutions, whole societies, and even the global community (Scheler, 1973). Numerous values—dignity, integrity, mutual respect, loyalty, friendship, social cohesion, fairness, stability, effectiveness, inclusiveness—are moral in import. Anthropocentric values are supplemented and corrected by the moral claims of animals and, more broadly, by the moral claims of the environment, a self-sustaining ecosystem. Even religious devotion to the divine life has moral dimensions, for the faithful are obliged to honor God as the final bearer of value.

Moral values enjoy precedence within the value field because they identify the basic loci of all valuing experience—that is, valuing subjects in relationship. Where moral values are secure, we can cultivate a wide array of values. Where moral values are in danger, all values are at risk.

Even so, in our responses to concrete cases we regularly rank some nonmoral values above specifically moral ones. Faced with a health emergency, our regard for life itself, an organic value, surpasses normal preoccupations with human dignity, a moral value. We do what we can to save a life! At the same time, we know that life as such is but one value among many. Prolonging human life can never, therefore, be the primary goal.

Similarly, human beings can often best advance their own good through value commitments that transcend specifically moral considerations. Cognitive, aesthetic, and especially spiritual values finally stand "higher" than moral values in most value schemes because they bestow significance on existence in its travail and woe. Yet these values still require for their realization valuing subjects who are bearers of moral value.

We normally discuss moral values in terms of rights and duties. Rights identify claims that others properly make on us. These claims intersect our value-oriented projects and disclose our duties. A physician's professional judgment about a course of therapy is subject to the patient's informed consent. The abortion debate hinges on differing assessments of fetal rights against a pregnant woman's right to choose.

Duties consist of obligations and prohibitions. Obligations specify what we must do no matter what else we might also hope to accomplish. Hospital emergency rooms must treat seriously injured persons regardless of whether they can pay, offering such care as a part of normal operations. Prohibitions specify what we must not do regardless of larger objectives. We must not use human beings as research subjects without their consent no matter how important the research may be.

It is for the sake of moral values that basic rights and duties are binding. We may set such mandates aside only when extraordinary measures are required to safeguard the values they protect. For the sake of human dignity, physicians are normally obliged to do all they reasonably can to sustain the lives of their patients. Precisely for the sake of human dignity, however, this obligation loses its force when further medical interventions would only prolong the dying process.

## Values and human action

Value awareness gains practical importance in terms of action (Ricoeur, 1966). We adopt courses of action that promise results favoring our prized values; we act to inhibit developments that endanger our values. Values guide decision making, disposing us to choose one course of action over another. We justify our decisions in terms of the values they are designed to promote.

Matters do not always turn out as we expect. We may lack the skill, the power, the influence, or the knowledge to achieve our objectives. In medical practice, few surprises follow the skilled application of routine therapies proven to be effective for treating particular ills. Physicians do not stay within safe territory, however. They regularly confront medical problems that they cannot diagnose with confidence and for which there are no known clinical responses with assured results. Medical outcomes frequently fall short of human hopes. They include side effects whose disvalues outweigh desired values. "Side effects" belong to action consequences even when they do not reflect our intentions.

When our actions affect the actions of others, uncertainty increases. Other people may not react as we expect. They may misunderstand our intentions or respond carelessly. We may misread their value commitments. Perhaps the relevant network of human interactions is so vast and complex that it surpasses what we can grasp. Here, too, the outcomes may not fit our values. Prediction is most reliable for highly routine actions with widely understood purposes. It is least reliable for novel initiatives, such as new directions in policy.

Because we cannot fully control or predict the consequences of our actions, the fit between actions and values is inexact. This inexactness carries over into value assessments. We may readily name the values that attach to desired outcomes. Before we can evaluate a course of action, however, we have to consider the uncertainties. We have to weigh the disvalues that could accompany significant miscalculations.

Considerations of value differ from discussions of duty by virtue of the inexact fit between values and action. Duty refers not to the likely outcomes of actions but to actions as such, which are largely in our power. It specifies ground rules that order human activity. In general, we may pursue a larger vision of the good only within constraints set by these ground rules. In its early stages, biomedical ethics properly gave precedence to the delineation of basic moral duties.

The fit between values, action, and action consequences remains close enough, however, that values must figure in the ethical examination of action. I am accountable to myself and others not simply for the conformity of my actions to rules that define my duties but also for values and disvalues that reside in the results of my actions. In decision making, I project the likely outcomes of actions I am considering and I weigh probabilities that qualify my projections. I also bring into view risks of unpleasant surprises. Practical reflection on values depends on substantial knowledge of the social dynamics that structure action.

## Values in society and culture

In traditional societies, the most crucial value issues are largely settled. To be viable, a society requires a shared set of reasonably cohesive values. This shared value cluster composes the society's moral identity. It is expressed in many ways within the common culture: public rituals, speeches, novels, paintings, school textbooks, standard histories, and scholarly investigations.

Modern societies with market economies and liberal democracies are not able to sustain comprehensive value syntheses. At best, they promote what John Rawls calls a "thin" theory of the good—that is, elemental goods that all are presumed to need and want whatever else they might also desire (Rawls, 1971). Within the framework of basic goods, such societies host a multiplicity of concrete value orientations, reflecting the diverse priorities of individuals and groups within the society.

Some question whether we can sustain even a "thin" theory of the good without a widely shared, substantive value synthesis fostered in basic social institutions (MacIntyre, 1984). The disintegration of traditional cultural values tends to undermine interest in the common good. Private preoccupations with individual advantage and "interest group" politics then displaces public discourse about the good of the society as a whole. Likewise, political battles are fought without the restraints of civility necessary to social order. Value theory becomes urgent when basic values are in dispute. Its task is not only to advance critical investigations of persistent value disputes but also to show how various value streams within a pluralistic society can contribute to the good of all.

## Critical reflection on values

The scrutiny of values has four crucial layers: (1) the reflective identification of our operative values; (2) assessments of the fit between these operative values and considered judgments about creaturely well-being; (3) analyses of value relations in order to identify compatible and incompatible values sets; and (4) imaginative constructions of value syntheses capable of ordering life priorities in personal, communal, and social contexts.

The investigation of values begins with description. We seek to become self-conscious about the values we prize, taking note of value commitments ingrained in stable life patterns and ongoing institutional involvements. The descriptive task is informed by historical studies of normative traditions and of social developments leading to current practices. As we make our operative values explicit, we are often stimulated to reorder our priorities. We recognize that existing arrangements do not reflect our convictions about what matters most in life.

The relation that values have to basic human needs suggests a second step in value studies. British utilitarians and American pragmatists sought to test our presumptive values by empirical investigations (Bentham, 1948; Dewey, 1931). Their aim was to discover life practices and value attachments that truly accord with primary human needs. Much human-science research functions as value inquiry of this sort, shedding light on value patterns that tend to promote human well-being in contrast to those that finally prove dysfunctional. Historical, philosophical, and theological reflections can also inform such inquiry. For ethics, the challenge is to clarify the contributions empirical studies can make to the critical assessment of values and to incorporate those contributions into constructive philosophical and religious thought.

The third step is an analysis of value relations. Not all values are compatible with one another, at least not in practical terms. We cannot both affirm free speech and shield people from all offensive public expressions. We cannot protect the environment without constraining market freedoms. Likewise, we cannot guarantee everyone health care that fully utilizes the most advanced medical technologies while also controlling aggregate health-care costs. Critical thought examines values in terms of their fit with one another. It dramatizes the necessity of choices among different sets of values. We bypass some values and endure relative disvalues for the sake of value combinations that reflect considered priorities.

The crucial step in the critical study of values is the imaginative construction of coherent value syntheses capable of guiding action. Because modern societies harbor a multiplicity of value perspectives, attempts to determine value priorities take place in several contexts.

Individuals develop a mature moral identity by clarifying the connections and priorities that order personally cherished values. Value syntheses are no less vital for families, special-interest associations, and religious bodies. These collectives gain moral, and perhaps religious, identity through shared value commitments. Organizations that give concrete form to economic, legal, political, and cultural institutions are themselves more effective when they make their defining values explicit.

Coherent sets of values are not easily achieved or sustained. They enjoy the greatest authority when they emerge as critical appropriations and transformations of normative value traditions within contemporary life settings. Because of the complexity of experience, value syntheses can never fully overcome areas of ambivalence or wholly resolve internal strains. Within limits, we can accommodate value conflicts that we acknowledge and honor. Such conflicts may even stimulate creativity.

Within comprehensive value syntheses, value priorities normally run in two contrary directions. Elemental sensory, organic, and economic values enjoy priority over higher political, cultural, and spiritual values in the sense that they furnish the conditions necessary to the appearance of the higher values. Political, cultural, and spiritual values enjoy priority over more basic sensory, organic, and economic values in the sense that they bestow meaning and significance on the more elemental values. Moral values play the mediating role because they identify the loci of value experience. These contrasting modes of priority can shed light on concrete values conflicts.

## Public value syntheses

A basic value of modern societies is the protection of private spaces for people to pursue diverse visions of the good. Social cohesion rests, then, on minimal agreements that allow individuals and groups to live together in their diversity. In the United States, the prevailing value synthesis combines liberal democratic principles and principles of free-market capitalism. Enduring controversies concern the nature and extent of appropriate government intervention in market processes. Less clearly articulated are images of a greater national community embracing many races, cultures, and religions. The latter images are countered by persisting patterns of racism, ethnocentrism, and religious intolerance.

In biomedical ethics, the most urgent challenge is to form a public value synthesis that can guide health-care reform. Though difficult disputes remain, there is considerable agreement that a good system will guarantee basic care for all, maintain acceptable standards of quality, foster an active partnership between patients and physicians, take account of the defining values of those who give and receive care, sustain advanced biomedical research, hold total costs to manageable levels, and protect contexts for personal preferences and individual initiatives in delivering and receiving care. These values—especially the contention that all people must have access to basic medical services—all have important moral dimensions.

Any workable system will include value trade-offs. It will require a reexamination of standards of quality care, a balance between health-care needs and other social goods, and a workable mix of economic incentives and government regulations that maintains discipline within the system while allowing space for individual initiatives. Any system will also confront limits. Moral creativity requires imaginative responses to limits in the promotion of creaturely well-being.

Because of the subtleties involved, bioethics cannot easily incorporate notions of value and valuation into deliberations about basic human duties. Yet values pervade human experience. They even shape our perceptions of the obligations and prohibitions that set constraints on our actions. As we examine more comprehensively the moral issues that reside in biomedical practice, the more we will discover the necessity of systematic value assessments. Critical value studies will tend as well to force a shift in the dominant structure of moral reasoning, from the linear logic of the syllogism to the more nuanced process of weaving multiple value considerations together into an illuminating pattern of moral understanding. While the resulting judgments may appear less precise and decisive, they will probably be more true to life.

THOMAS W. OGLETREE

*For a further discussion of topics mentioned in this entry, see the entries* ACTION; INTERPRETATION; LIFE; LIFE, QUALITY OF; *and* RIGHTS. *This entry will find application in the entries* ANIMAL WELFARE AND RIGHTS, *article on* ETHICAL PERSPECTIVES ON THE TREATMENT AND STATUS OF ANIMALS; HEALTH-CARE RESOURCES, ALLOCATION OF; HEALTH AND DISEASE; MEDICINE, ART OF; RESEARCH METHODOLOGY, *article on* CONCEPTUAL ISSUES; *and* UTILITY. *For a discussion of related ideas, see the entry* ETHICS. *Other relevant material may be found under the entry* BIOETHICS.

## Bibliography

BENTHAM, JEREMY. 1948. *An Introduction to the Principles of Morals and Legislation.* Edited by Laurence J. LaFleur. New York: Hafner.

COUSINS, NORMAN. 1979. *Anatomy of an Illness As Perceived by the Patient: Reflections on Healing and Regeneration.* New York: W. W. Norton.

DEWEY, JOHN. 1931. *Philosophy and Civilization.* New York: Minton, Balch.

HARRON, FRANK; BURNSIDE, JOHN W.; and BEAUCHAMP, TOM L. 1983. *Health and Human Values: A Guide to Making Your Own Decisions.* New Haven, Conn.: Yale University Press.

HARTMANN, NICOLAI. 1932. *Ethics.* Vol. 2, *Moral Values.* Translated by Stanton Coit. New York: Allen & Unwin.

HUSSERL, EDMUND. 1970. *The Crisis of European Sciences and Transcendental Phenomenology: An Introduction to Phenomenological Philosophy.* Translated by David Carr. Evanston, Ill.: Northwestern University Press.

MACINTYRE, ALASDAIR. 1984. *After Virtue.* 2d ed. Notre Dame, Ind.: University of Notre Dame Press.

MAY, WILLIAM F. 1983. *The Physician's Covenant: Images of the Healer in Medical Ethics.* Philadelphia: Westminster.

———. 1991. *The Patient's Ordeal.* Bloomington: Indiana University Press.

NELSON, JAMES B., and ROHRICHT, JO ANNE SMITH. 1984. *Human Medicine: Ethical Perspectives on Today's Medical Issues.* Rev. ed. Minneapolis: Augsburg.

NIEBUHR, H. RICHARD. 1943. *Radical Monotheism and Western Culture.* New York: Harper & Row.

OGLETREE, THOMAS W. 1985. *Hospitality to the Stranger: Dimensions of Moral Understanding.* Philadelphia: Fortress.

PARSONS, TALCOTT. 1969. *Politics and Social Structure.* New York: Free Press.

PERRY, RALPH BARTON. 1926. *The General Theory of Value: Its Meaning and Basic Principles Construed in Terms of Interest.* Cambridge, Mass.: Harvard University Press.

RAMSEY, PAUL. 1970. *The Patient as Person: Explorations in Medical Ethics.* New Haven, Conn.: Yale University Press.

RAWLS, JOHN. 1971. *A Theory of Justice.* Cambridge, Mass.: Harvard University Press.

RICOEUR, PAUL. 1966. *Freedom and Nature: The Voluntary and the Involuntary.* Translated by Erazim V. Kohák. Evanston, Ill.: Northwestern University Press.

SCHELER, MAX. 1973. *Formalism in Ethics and Non-Formal Ethics of Values: A New Attempt Toward the Foundation of an Ethical Personalism.* 5th rev. ed. Translated by Manfred S. Frings and Roger L. Funk. Evanston, Ill.: Northwestern University Press.

VEATCH, ROBERT M. 1991. *The Patient–Physician Relation: The Patient as Partner.* Bloomington: Indiana University Press.

# VEGETARIANISM

*See* ANIMAL WELFARE AND RIGHTS, *article on* VEGETARIANISM.

# VENEZUELA

*See* MEDICAL ETHICS, HISTORY OF, *section on* THE AMERICAS, *article on* LATIN AMERICA.

# VETERINARY ETHICS

Veterinary medicine, as the distinctive medical discipline we know today, emerged during the nineteenth century as an adjunct to agriculture. Animals were valued for the food or fiber they provided or for the work they performed, and the veterinarian's role in society was to keep the animals healthy so they could serve people's needs. Even after anticruelty laws had become widespread by the late 1800s, and the horse doctor became the dog doctor with the growth of companion animal practice in the mid-twentieth century, the veterinarian's ethic remained unexamined and substantive ethical issues officially unacknowledged.

Unlike medical doctors, whose engaging of ethical issues can be traced back to Hippocrates, veterinarians did not have a historic tradition of professional ethics to draw on. Until the late 1970s, the field of veterinary ethics focused primarily on issues of business etiquette and professional relations. The Code of Ethics of the American Veterinary Medical Association (AVMA) addressed such areas as referrals to other veterinarians and whether it was "ethical" to have a large insert for one's practice in the Yellow Pages. Social changes, such as the emergence of the animal-welfare/rights movement and its impact on public consciousness, helped catalyze consideration of the complex of ethical concerns that face the veterinarian.

Two people acted as gadflies to the profession in this important period: Michael W. Fox, a veterinarian with the Humane Society of the United States, and Bernard E. Rollin, a philosopher at Colorado State University. Fox and Rollin published articles in influential journals (Fox, 1983b; Rollin, 1978, 1983) that pointed out the need for systematic examination of the ethical concerns of the veterinary profession. Fox also wrote letters to the *Journal of the AVMA* on this theme (Fox, 1983a). In 1978, Rollin inaugurated the first regular, required, full-term course in veterinary ethics at the Colorado State University College of Veterinary Medicine. Both Fox and Rollin wrote books on animal welfare and rights. Rollin, in addition, had taught and published in human medical ethics, and he was sensitive to the differences between the problems of human medical ethics and those of veterinary medical ethics. In particular, owing to his extensive work in the moral status of animals, Rollin was aware that veterinary medicine had not yet addressed its moral obligation to animals. By the end of the 1980s, veterinary interest in the ethics of the profession had developed enough to warrant publication of a textbook on the subject by Jerrold Tannenbaum of Tufts University (Tannenbaum, 1989).

## The veterinary oath and its moral dilemmas

When the veterinarian graduates from veterinary school, he or she is administered the veterinarian's oath, which includes a promise "to use my scientific knowledge and skills for the benefit of society through the protection of animal health, the relief of animal suffering, the conservation of livestock resources, the promotion of public health, and the advancement of medical knowledge" (see the Appendix, Volume 5). The veterinarian is immediately faced with a fundamental ethical dilemma: to whom does he or she owe primary loyalty, the owner or the animal? In a 1978 article, Rollin used the examples of a pediatrician and a car mechanic to illustrate the two possible choices. When the repairs on a car are more costly than the car's value, the owner can simply tell the mechanic to "junk" it or not do the repairs; there is no such choice in a necessary surgery or treatment of a child (Rollin, 1978). The pediatrician is ethically (and legally) obligated to act as advocate of the child's well-being. On the other hand, the basic current legal status of animals is that they are property, although their sentient qualities have been the basis of limited protection provided by so-called welfare laws (in the United States, primarily local anticruelty ordinances and federal laboratory animal laws).

In addition to the responsibilities they have to the animal and the owner, veterinarians must weigh practice judgments in light of the needs of society in general ("public health"), peers, and themselves as well. As the oath also states, "I will practice my profession conscientiously, with dignity, and in keeping with the principles of veterinary medical ethics. I accept as a lifelong obligation the continual improvement of my professional knowledge and competence" (Appendix, Volume 5). In the face of often conflicting interests of animal, owner, society, profession, and self, the individual veterinarian is often presented with situations that require complex ethical judgments (Rollin, 1988). The traditional minimalistic animal ethics proscribing cruelty, from which anticruelty laws derived, are not adequate to mid-twentieth-century uses of animals such as confinement agriculture or testing and research, which were not matters of cruelty yet caused significant suffering in pursuit of profit and scientific knowledge (Rollin, 1981). In seeking a new animal ethic, society began to apply the notion of rights, which protect human nature from being submerged for the sake of general welfare, to animals in order to protect their fundamental interests as dictated by their nature (or "telos"). The veterinarian came to be considered a natural animal advocate. As society elevated to the status of animals by applying a rights ethic, the status and effectualness of the veterinarian began to increase (Rollin, 1983).

## Laboratory-animal legislation: Effect on the profession

One area—laboratory-animal medicine—has had its ethical obligations to animals articulated by law because of societal concern for animal welfare. Before the 1985 Amendment to the Animal Welfare Act, which originated as a Colorado state bill written by Rollin and others, and the National Institutes of Health Reauthorization Act of 1985, which turned animal use "guidelines" into regulations, researchers enjoyed carte blanche in the use of animals. The pursuit of knowledge, or "advancement of medical knowledge," had completely trumped consideration of animal pain, suffering, or distress, and laboratory-animal veterinarians were relegated to the role of keeping animals in good enough shape to serve their research purposes. The legislation that was passed in 1985, as well as the original Animal Welfare Act of 1966 and other amendments to that act, was a direct result of societal response to well-publicized atrocities in research and testing activities and the correlative demand for assurance that animals' interests were protected.

Laboratory-animal veterinarians, because of animal-protective legislation, now fulfill the most unambiguous role of all veterinarians regarding animal well-being: They are obligated by law to act as animal advocates, to assure that pain and suffering do not occur or are minimized by proper medication, that proper animal care is provided, and that humane euthanasia is performed. The veterinarians are aided by Institutional Animal Care and Use Committees, which review research or testing protocols for humane considerations before studies may commence and provide regular monitoring of facilities.

### Small-animal-practice concerns

Although the role of the veterinarian has been defined by society in law for the laboratory-animal veterinarian, this has not occurred in other areas of veterinary medicine in which owner interest and animal interest may conflict. The small-animal veterinarian is often faced with ethical decisions based on these conflicts. Examples include cosmetic or behavior-altering surgery and orthodontic intervention for cosmetic reasons. In general, these procedures could be considered in the interests of the animal only if the animal were afflicted with a condition that was causing or was likely to cause it pain or distress. Dewclaw removal—dewclaws can catch and tear when dogs run through rough terrain—or repair of malocclusions like base-narrow lower canines, in which the offending tooth or teeth can drive into the upper palate, can easily be justified as in the animal's interest. Cosmetic surgery that causes the animal to conform to standards of style (e.g., ear cropping) or surgery that is used to curb "objectionable" behavior (e.g., declawing of cats, devocalizing of dogs) can be viewed as causing pain and distress to the animal for frivolous human reasons. Likewise, straightening teeth that are functional to provide a perfect bite for the show dog could be considered unnecessary.

Many veterinarians refuse to do purely cosmetic surgery, and consequently they lose clients. Other small-animal veterinarians believe they owe their major loyalty to the owner. They may argue that providing the service of cosmetic surgery enhances the animal's value, emotional as well as monetary, to the owner. Still other veterinarians will provide behavior-altering surgeries, such as declawing, after first pursuing, with an owner, honest attempts at retraining or other options. They may justify their actions by saying that the owner would otherwise get rid of the pet or that they are fostering the continuation of a rewarding relationship for both pet and owner.

Surgically neutering (spaying or castrating) dogs and cats to prevent sexual behaviors and overpopulation of pets is well accepted by North American society, but (especially for dogs) is largely rejected in other countries in favor of owner responsibility in administering contraceptives and controlling pets. Many small-animal veterinarians readily neuter cats and dogs, assuming that the discomfort of the surgery is of less import than the enhancement of the desirability of the pet to the owner (the elimination of objectionable sexual behavior, for instance) and the elimination of the chance of unwanted pregnancies; in addition, there are health advantages to neutering.

### Some equine-practice concerns

The equine veterinarian is under similar tension, only more so. Lameness is the most frequent complaint of horse owners, as the horse's usefulness requires a smooth and efficient gait. The equine veterinarian is often pressured to provide painkilling medication or surgery to cut the nerves to the feet of race or performance horses because of lameness. In some respects this is a compassionate action, as the animal is rendered fully or relatively free of pain. However, there are cases in which eliminating painful sensations may cause the animal to use and seriously injure a limb. Pressures to administer performance-enhancing drugs, or to look the other way when objectionable training techniques may be used, may be severe for equine veterinarians. Veterinarians may also be called on to perform purely cosmetic surgery, such as tail docking or tail "breaking" for an artificially high tail carriage. Unfortunately, horses are generally of little entertainment or economic value if they do not "go sound," or conform to an ideal of beauty.

### A look at food-animal medicine

Food-animal veterinarians have always been placed in a position of tension between the interests of animals and the interests of producers. In traditional agriculture, which prevailed as an "extensive" (as opposed to "intensive") endeavor until the mid-twentieth century, the tension was mitigated to some extent because producers generally did well economically only if they provided for the health and welfare of their individual animals. With the rise of confinement agriculture, however, new considerations have entered into the picture, and producers can prosper—in fact, may make the most profits—even if numerous individual animals suffer from poor health or die. For instance, feedlots may utilize diets that cause digestive and liver disease in a certain percentage of animals, but that loss will be more than compensated economically by the weight gain in the remaining animals. Furthermore, the use of antibiotics, vaccines, growth promoters, etc., have permitted selectivity in meeting animal needs and the separation of economic productivity from animal well-being. Animals can thus suffer in areas not related to economic productivity, yet producers can do well. Since the advent of intensive agriculture, veterinary concern for individual animals has tended to be replaced by a "herd health" philosophy to serve the livestock industry.

In confinement operations, a certain death loss is expected from the animals, whether from contagious or so-called production diseases, which are caused by handling, artificial environments, selective breeding, population density, or nutrition in the operation. Veterinary care in confinement operations usually covers only animals that are expected to recover without costing more in money and labor than the animals' market value. In sheep feedlots, a common daily chore is picking up dead or moribund animals. Discovering which animals are sick, separating them from their group, and treating or euthanizing them is often considered too expensive to support. In complete confinement houses for swine, animals are fed antibiotics because respiratory disease is so prevalent owing to high ammonia levels. To combat fighting in tight quarters among feeder pigs, their tails are amputated so the animals cannot wound each other by tail biting. Mastitis and footrot in dairy cattle are production diseases caused by the enforcement of high milk yields while the cattle are maintained on dirt lots. The average dairy cow is worn out and culled in four or five years, less than half of the expected useful lifetime fifty years ago.

Agrarian values of husbandry have been abandoned in much of present-day agriculture, affecting how the veterinarian may conduct his or her profession, because whereas a small farmer once maintained a modest lifestyle by caring for a few individual animals, a corporation now looks at profit margin only. Even in the more traditional agricultural activity of cattle ranching, economic considerations militate against veterinarians' controlling the pain of such activities as branding, dehorning, and castration. Thus the modern food-animal veterinarian faces a variety of conflicts arising out of tension between economic considerations on the one hand and animal health and welfare considerations on the other.

### The veterinarian and euthanasia

Even if the veterinarian's inclination is to act as an animal advocate, he or she may be thwarted by the owner's wishes, because of the legal status of animals as chattel or property. Occasionally a veterinarian is faced with a situation in which a pet is suffering without hope of recovery, as in terminal cancer, but where euthanasia is not an option because an owner refuses to authorize it. Many veterinarians quietly euthanize such animals as a humane act in spite of its illegality; but a more direct approach, utilized by veterinarians who often deal with death and the consequent grief of owners, is to discuss the inevitable with clients beforehand and exercise a humane ethic by requesting the clients to agree to euthanasia if certain clinical signs, like unremitting pain or inability to eat, arise.

A more common delay of euthanasia occurs when a food animal is kept alive despite suffering to maximize income. This scenario is most often seen in large, commercial operations, where, for instance, a sow with a fractured leg or a cow with a cancerous eye could be kept alive without expensive treatment until parturition or weaning of offspring. It is interesting to note that the laboratory-animal veterinarian is required by law to euthanize when faced with hopeless animal suffering, while the private practitioner is hamstrung by laws of private property in situations that do not constitute cruelty under the law.

The most obvious and rewarding use of euthanasia—killing without causing pain or distress—is to end an animal's suffering due to unremitting illness or fatal injury. However, there are other uses of euthanasia, such as end points for research, humane slaughter for meat, and humane killing of unwanted pets by pounds, shelters, or veterinarians. The AVMA Panel on Euthanasia periodically updates and publishes its report on euthanasia. The report examines methods of killing and labels as unacceptable those that cause animals to suffer. For instance, the report accepts an overdose of anesthetic, which causes an animal to become unconscious before dying, but condemns an overdose of paralytic drug, which causes motor and respiratory paralysis and suffocation in an alert animal.

Many small-animal veterinarians are confronted with requests for "convenience" euthanasia—euthanasia of healthy pets for owners who have rejected the implied contract of care they incurred when they acquired the pet. Some veterinarians avoid these ethical dilemmas by refusing categorically to perform any "convenience" euthanasia, even though they know that the owner may choose a nonhumane alternative, such as abandonment. Others accept such animals on the condition that they be allowed to find a home for the animal as an alternative to euthanasia; this route obviously requires time, effort, and probably expense on the part of the veterinarians but helps to satisfy their obligation to the animal.

Accepting an animal for euthanasia, and then not performing it, however, is a breach of contract and indefensible on legal grounds. One interesting dilemma that has challenged equine veterinarians is insurance companies' requirement that expensive horses be euthanized if they are rendered unfit by accident or illness for an insured purpose (e.g., racing, breeding, or showing) even if these animals are otherwise capable of a pain-free, or even useful, existence. When enormous sums of money are at stake, consideration of the animal's interests tends to disappear.

### Veterinarians and anticruelty laws

Animal cruelty laws are notoriously lax. Most allow conviction only in cases of purposeful abuse, and in any case generally result in insignificant fines. However, the veterinarian may be able to make a difference in the lives of animals by reporting and testifying in animal abuse cases. Reporting a client for battering his dog or starving his horses or other stock, when all efforts at education and persuasion are exhausted, may be the only means of protecting animals. In taking a stand as an animal advocate, the veterinarian may experience a loss of clientele and income, thereby placing personal interest in conflict with animal and client interests.

### The veterinarian's obligation to society

The veterinarian's obligation to society can also be the occasion for conflicts relating to self or business interests. The most straightforward example may be the protection of society from contaminated animal-source foods. Hormonal and medicinal additives to feed, or treatments of individual animals with medications, can result in residues in meat and milk. These products, if allowed for food animals, have government-mandated withdrawal times before slaughter or milking. Sometimes products used in animal production are not approved for any food animal administration. Yet because of poor planning, inattention to withdrawal times, or attempt to defraud, producers may send contaminated animals or their products to market. The underlying motive is usually profit. If a veterinarian discovers that a producer is feeding an illegal additive, or if, for example, a heifer is sent to slaughter before the withdrawal time of the penicillin she was given, the food-animal veterinarian has a public-health obligation—an obligation to society—to report the client despite professional confidentiality concerns. The loss of one client may be the least of the financial impact of such an ethical choice; other potential or actual clients may avoid association with the veterinarian because of fear of also being turned in, as some illegal practices in the food-animal industry may be widespread, especially in a given region.

The laboratory-animal veterinarian's career can be seen as a service to society, in that he or she provides clinical support or scientific information for the advancement of scientific knowledge. Despite his or her legal mandate as animal advocate, the veterinarian may experience personal conflict in areas of pain or disease research; for example, studies that involve the most animal suffering may also provide the most useful information for the betterment of humans and animals alike. The laboratory-animal veterinarian must also come to grips with the fact that virtually all of his or her patients will be killed at the end of a study.

The zoo or wildlife veterinarian serves societal interests in areas of animal conservation and wildlife management. Incarceration, as in a zoo, is not generally in individual animals' interests, but captive breeding programs may be needed to preserve a valued species. Similarly, situations may arise in which a disease is introduced into study animals to determine pathophysiol-

ogy or treatment for that species or similar groups. The use of wild animals in research, especially when capture is a part of the research design, has been severely criticized by animal welfare and rights groups because of unacceptably high numbers of "stress" losses of animals used in the studies.

### Policing the profession: Obligations to peers

The veterinarian, like practitioners in other professions, may have to take an ethical or legal stand regarding the practices of his or her peers—as, for example, when one gives testimony in a malpractice suit. Certainly a person's choice in business practices and commitment to medical standards indicate the quality of his or her moral fiber and loyalty to the profession. It is not unusual for veterinarians to sever professional or personal ties with other veterinarians over professional standards, although it is rare for them to make allegations of malpractice or business malfeasance of other veterinarians. This course is largely left to state boards of veterinary medicine, which respond to complaints by the public. Reluctance to speak out against professional misconduct by other veterinarians is not unique to this profession. A certain degree of prudence must be exercised by professionals to avoid unfairly slandering a colleague without knowing the entire story; for instance, a client's account of a veterinarian's actions may be biased and medically naïve. Many veterinarians also believe that exposing misconduct puts the entire profession in a bad light, even if the public would likely have a positive regard for "policing the ranks." Veterinarians, like other professionals, are allowed a fair amount of leeway in regulating themselves, since they are presumed to know the issues better than laypeople. Failure to self-police can result in loss of autonomy, with rules initiated and governed by people who know little about the profession, such as legislators.

### The veterinarian's obligation to self and personal values

The veterinarian's obligation to self is best fulfilled by examination of and adherence to his or her professional and personal values. Some veterinarians believe the veterinarian's only or major loyalty should be to the animal. Most veterinarians probably enter the profession with a desire to protect animal health and relieve animal suffering, without an understanding of competing interests. A fuzzy or unexamined ethic may lead to compromising professional decisions. Veterinary schools have responded to the need for ethical training in their curricula, with the understanding that veterinary students need intellectual tools to examine their own ethics throughout their professional lives.

## Veterinary ethics today

The profession is by no means monolithic in its attitudes, but the AVMA and other veterinary organizations have gradually begun to take official positions on animal issues. A number of practitioners' organizations, including the American Society of Laboratory Animal Practitioners, the American Association of Bovine Practitioners, the American Association of Equine Practitioners, and some state veterinary organizations, have taken animal-welfare positions or have held symposia or meetings pertaining to issues of concern to them. Advocacy groups, such as the Association of Veterinarians for Animal Rights, have emerged. The Animal Welfare Committee of the AVMA has encouraged the association to take published positions on a variety of companion animal, exhibit and performance animal, research animal, and agricultural animal issues. Although some positions are weak and tentative (mainly on agricultural issues), many are specifically protective (e.g., condemning use of the steel-jawed trap and recommending to the American Kennel Club and breed associations that ear cropping be dropped from standards and that dogs with cropped ears be prohibited from showing). The AVMA also sponsors an annual Animal Welfare Forum, in which veterinary educators, animal advocates, philosophers, and others examine the need for animal-welfare reform within the profession.

Given that the formal articulation and organized study of veterinary ethical issues are new, the field has made a good deal of progress. In the future, we can expect the emergence of more sophisticated treatments of many of the issues we have articulated. With society's expectations that the veterinarian serve as mandated animal advocate (as evidenced by the aforementioned laboratory-animal laws), veterinarians will doubtless be in the forefront of emerging social concerns about animal use and treatment.

M. LYNNE KESEL

*Directly related to this entry are the entries* ANIMAL RE-SEARCH; ANIMAL WELFARE AND RIGHTS, *especially the articles on* DOMESTIC ANIMALS AND PETS, *and* ETHICAL PERSPECTIVES ON THE TREATMENT AND STATUS OF ANIMALS; *and* GENETIC ENGINEERING, *article on* ANIMALS AND PLANTS. *For a further discussion of topics mentioned in this entry, see the entries* HARM; LICENSING, DISCIPLINE, AND REGULATION IN THE HEALTH PROFESSIONS; OBLIGATION AND SUPEREROGATION; RESEARCH, UNETHICAL; RESPONSIBILITY; RIGHTS; VALUE AND VALUATION; *and* WHISTLEBLOWING. *For a discussion of related ideas, see the entry* DEATH AND DYING: EUTHANASIA AND SUSTAINING LIFE, *article on* ETHICAL ISSUES. *Other relevant material may be found under the entries* COMPASSION; ETHICS; MEDICAL CODES AND OATHS, *article on* ETHICAL ANALYSIS; PROFESSION AND PROFESSIONAL ETHICS; *and* VIRTUE AND CHARACTER. *See also the* APPENDIX (CODES, OATHS, AND DIRECTIVES RELATED TO BIOETHICS), SECTION V: ETHICAL DIRECTIVES PERTAINING TO THE WELFARE AND USE OF ANIMALS.

## Bibliography

FOX, MICHAEL W. 1983a. Letter. *Journal of the American Veterinary Medical Association* 182, no. 12:1314–1315.

———. 1983b. "Veterinarians and Animal Rights." *California Veterinarian* 37, no. 1:15.

———. 1984. *Farm Animals: Husbandry, Behavior, and Veterinary Practice.* Baltimore: University Park Press.

ROLLIN, BERNARD E. 1977. "Moral Philosophy and Veterinary Medical Education." *Journal of Veterinary Medical Education* 4, no. 1:180–182.

———. 1978. "Updating Veterinary Medical Ethics." *Journal of the American Veterinary Medical Association* 173, no. 8:1015–1018.

———. 1983. "Animal Rights and Veterinary Medical Education." *California Veterinarian* 37, no. 1:9–15.

———. 1988. "Veterinary and Animal Ethics." In *Law and Ethics of the Veterinary Profession.* pp. 24–48. Edited by James E. Wilson. Yardley, Pa.: Priority.

———. 1991–present. "Veterinary Ethics." *Canadian Veterinary Journal.* A regular feature. Stories of actual ethical dilemmas are contributed by veterinarians to be analyzed by philosopher Rollin; comments by veterinarians and others are presented by the editors.

———. 1992. *Animal Rights and Human Morality.* Rev. ed. Buffalo, N.Y.: Prometheus.

TANNENBAUM, JERROLD. 1989. *Veterinary Ethics.* Baltimore: Williams & Wilkins.

# VIOLENCE

*See* ABUSE, INTERPERSONAL; *and* HOMICIDE.

# VIRTUE AND CHARACTER

"Virtue" is the translation of the ancient Greek *arete,* which meant any kind of excellence. Inanimate objects could have *arete,* since they were assumed to have a *telos,* that is, a purpose. Thus, the *arete* of a knife would be its sharpness. Animals could also have *arete;* for example, the strength of an ox was seen as its virtue. Though an animal could possess *arete,* the Greeks assumed natural potentialities in men and women to be virtues requiring enhancement through habits of skill. Therefore, Aristotle defined virtue as "a kind of second nature" that disposes us not only to do the right thing to gain pleasure from what we do" (Aristotle, 1962, 1105b25–30).

Since there are many things that "our nature" as humans inclines us to do, Aristotle argues, there can be many human virtues. How particular virtues are constituted can vary with different understandings of "human nature" and the different social roles and their correlative skills. Yet the virtues, according to Aristotle, are distinguished from the arts, since in the latter excellence lies in results. In contrast, for the virtues it matters not only that an act itself is of a certain kind, but also that the agent "has certain characteristics as he performs it; first of all, he must know what he is doing; secondly, he must choose to act the way he does, and he must choose it for its own sake; and in the third place, the act must spring from a firm and unchangeable character" (Aristotle, 1962, 1105a25–30).

The word *hexis*, which Aristotle uses for "character," is the same word that denotes the habitual dispositions constitutive of the virtues. Character, therefore, indicates the stability that is necessary so that the various virtues are acquired in a lasting way. Character is not simply the sum of the individual virtues; rather, it names the pattern of thought and action that provides a continuity sufficient for humans to claim their lives as their own (Kupperman, 1991). However, the material form associated with character may vary from one society to another. Therefore any definition of virtue, the virtues, and character can be misleading because it can conceal the differences between various accounts of the nature and kinds of virtues as well as character.

## The role of virtue in recent moral philosophy

Ancient philosophers as well as Christian theologians, though offering quite different accounts of the virtues, assumed that any account of the well-lived life had to take virtue into consideration. Modern moral philosophy, in contrast, treats virtues—if it treats them at all—as secondary to an ethics based on principles and rules. The attempt to secure an account of morality that is not as subject to variations as an ethics of virtue certainly contributed to this displacement of virtues. The first edition of the *Encyclopedia of Bioethics*, for example, had no entry on virtue or character.

In his widely used and influential introduction to philosophical ethics, William Frankena manifests the approach to ethics that simply assumed that considerations of virtue were secondary. According to Frankena, ethical theory should be concerned primarily with justifying moral terms and clarifying the differences between appeals to duty and consequences. The virtues, to the extent they were discussed by theorists such as Frankena, were understood as supplements to the deter-

mination of right and wrong action. The virtues in such a theory were seen more as the motivational component in more basic principles, such as benevolence and justice. As Frankena put it,

> We know that we should cultivate two virtues, a disposition to be beneficial (i.e., benevolence) and a disposition to treat people equally (justice as a trait). But the point of acquiring these virtues is not further guidance or instructions; the function of the virtues in an ethics of duty is not to tell us what to do, but to insure that we will do it willingly in whatever situation we may face. (Frankena, 1973, p. 67)

Frankena's understanding of the nature and role of the virtues drew on the commonsense view that in order to know what kind of person one ought to be, one needs to know what kind of behavior is good or bad. Unless one knows what constitutes acts of truth-telling or lying, one has no way to specify what the virtue of truthfulness or honesty might entail. Ethical theories were assumed to be aids to help people make good decisions on the basis of well-justified principles or rules. Virtues were secondary for that endeavor.

This account of ethics seemed particularly well suited to the emerging field of bioethics. It was assumed that the task of medical ethics was to help physicians and other health-care providers make decisions about difficult cases created by the technological power of modern medicine. Whether a patient could be disconnected from a respirator was analyzed in terms of the difference between such basic rules as "do no harm" and "always act that the greatest good for the greatest number be done." The case orientation of medical decision making seemed ideally suited to the case orientation of ethical theory exemplified by Frankena.

In their influential book, *Principles of Biomedical Ethics*, Tom L. Beauchamp and James F. Childress retain the structure of ethics articulated by Frankena. Their account of biomedical ethics revolves around the normative alternatives of utilitarian and deontological theories and the principles of autonomy, nonmaleficence, beneficence, and justice. Each of these fundamental principles has correlative primary virtues—that is, respect for autonomy, nonmalevolence, benevolence, and justice—but these "virtues" play no central role. Beauchamp and Childress justify leaving an account of virtue to the last chapter by saying that there are no good arguments for "making judgments about persons independent of judgments about acts or . . . making virtue primary or sufficient for the moral life" (Beauchamp and Childress, 1983, p. 265).

Both philosophers (Pincoffs, 1986) and theologians (Hauerwas, 1985) have challenged the assumption that ethics in general and biomedical ethics in particular should be focused primarily on decisions and principles. It is a mistake, they argue, to separate questions of the rightness or goodness of an action from the character of the agent. To relegate the virtues to the motivation for action mistakenly assumes that the description of an action can be abstracted from the character of the agent. To abstract actions from the agent's perspective fails to account for why the agent should confront this or that situation and under what description. Those who defended the importance of virtue for ethics argued, following Aristotle, that *how* one does *what* one does is as important as what one does.

The renewed interest in the nature and significance of virtue ethics has been stimulated by the work of Alasdair MacIntyre, in particular his book *After Virtue* (1984). MacIntyre's defense of an Aristotelian virtue theory was but a part of his challenge to the presuppositions of modern moral theory. MacIntyre attacked what he called "the Enlightenment project," the attempt to ground universal ethical principles in rationality qua rationality—for example, Kant's categorical imperative (Kant, 1959). MacIntyre agrees that principles and rules are important for ethics, but he rejects any attempt to justify those principles or rules that abstracts them from their rootedness in the historical particularities of concrete communities. The narratives that make such communities morally coherent focuses attention on the virtues correlative to those narratives. For the Greeks, for example, the *Odyssey* acted as the central moral text for the display of the heroic virtues. To separate ethics from its dependence on such narratives is to lose the corresponding significance of the virtues.

MacIntyre's defense of an ethics of virtue is part of his challenge to the attempt to secure agreement among people who share nothing besides the necessity to cooperate in the interest of survival. Enlightenment theories of ethics, MacIntyre argues, falsely assume that an ahistorical ethics is possible; a historical approach tries to justify ethical principles from anyone's (that is, any rational individual's) point of view.

Renewed interest in the ethics of virtue has accompanied a renewed appreciation of the importance of community in ethics. Those commentators who emphasize the importance of community presume that morally worthy political societies are constituted by goods that shape the participants in those societies to want the right things rightly. Therefore ethics, particularly an ethics of virtue, cannot be separated from accounts of politics. Such a politics cannot be reduced to the struggle for power but, rather, is about the constitution of a community's habits for the production of a certain kind of people—that is, people who have the requisite virtues to sustain such a community.

## Bioethics and the ethics of virtue

In the past the practice of medicine was thought to be part of the tradition of the virtues. As Gary Ferngren and Darrel Amundsen observe, "If health was, for most Greeks, the greatest of the virtues, it is not surprising that they devoted a great deal of attention to preserving it. As an essential component of *arete*, physical culture was an important part of the life of what the Greeks called *kalos kagathos*, the cultivated gentleman, who represented in classical times the ideal of the human personality" (Ferngren and Amundsen, 1985, p. 7). It should not be surprising, therefore, that not only was health seen as an analogue of virtue but medicine was understood as an activity that by its very nature was virtuous.

In medical ethics, the "ethics of virtue" approach tends to focus on the doctor–patient relationship. The trust, care, and compassion that seem so essential to a therapeutic relationship are virtues intrinsic to medical care. Medicine requires attention to technical knowledge and skill, which are virtues in themselves; however, the physician must also have a capacity—compassion—to feel something of patients' experience of their illness and their perception of what is worthwhile (Pellegrino, 1985). Not only compassion but also honesty, fidelity, courage, justice, temperance, magnanimity, prudence, and wisdom are required of the physician.

> Not every one of these virtues is required in every decision. What we expect of the virtuous physician is that he will exhibit them when they are required and that he will be so habitually disposed to do so that we can depend upon it. He will place the good of the patient above his own and seek that good unless its pursuit imposes an injustice upon him, or his family, or requires a violation of his own conscience. (Pellegrino, 1985, p. 246)

The importance of virtue for medical ethics has been challenged most forcefully by Robert Veatch. According to Veatch, there is no uncontested virtue ethic. The Greeks had one set of virtues, the Christians another, the Stoics another; and there is no rational way to resolve the differences among them. This is a particularly acute problem because modern medicine must be practiced as "stranger medicine," that is,

> medicine that is practiced among people who are essentially strangers. It would include medicine that is practiced on an emergency basis in emergency rooms in large cities. It would also include care delivered in a clinic setting or in an HMO that does not have physician continuity, most medicine in student health services, VA Hospitals, care from consulting specialists, and the medicine in the military as well as care that is delivered by

private practice general practitioners to patients who are mobile enough not to establish long-term relationships with their physicians. (Veatch, 1985, p. 338)

Virtue theory is not suited to such medicine, Veatch argues, because "there is no reasonable basis for assuming that the stranger with whom one is randomly paired in the emergency room will hold the same theory of virtue as one's self" (Veatch, 1985, p. 339). The ethics of "stranger medicine" is best construed, Veatch contends, on the presumption that the relationship between doctor and patient is contractual. Such a relationship is best characterized by impersonal principles rather than in terms of virtue. The virtues make sense only within and to particular communities, and therefore only within a "sectarian" form of medicine.

Veatch's argument exemplifies what Alasdair MacIntyre calls the Enlightenment project. Yet MacIntyre would not dispute the descriptive power of Veatch's characterization of modern medicine. He thinks medicine is increasingly becoming a form of technological competence, bureaucratically institutionalized and governed by impersonal ethical norms. MacIntyre simply wishes to challenge the presumption that this is a moral advance. Put more strongly, MacIntyre challenges the presumption that such a medicine and the morality that underlies it can be justified in the terms Veatch offers. In particular, he asks, how can one account for the trust that seems a necessary component of the doctor–patient relationship without relying on an ethic of virtue?

Contrary to Veatch, James Drane (1988) and others argue that medicine does not exist within a relationship between strangers, but in fact depends on trust and confidence, if not friendship, between doctor and patient. Ethics, they hold, is not based on principles external to medical care and then applied to medicine; rather, medicine is itself one of the essential practices characteristic of good societies. Medicine thus understood does not need so much to be supplemented by ethical considerations based on a lawlike paradigm of principles and rules; on the contrary, medical care becomes one of the last examples left in liberal cultures of what the practice of virtue actually looks like. Those who work from an ethics of virtue do not come to medicine with general principles justified in other contexts, to be applied now to "medical quandaries"; rather, they see medicine itself as an exemplification of virtuous practices.

Here medicine is understood in the Aristotelian sense, as an activity—that is, as a form of behavior that produces a result intrinsic to the behavior itself (Aristotle, 1962). In MacIntyre's language, medicine is a practice in which the goods internal to the practice extend our powers in a manner that we are habituated in excellence (MacIntyre, 1984). Put simply, the practice of medicine is a form of cooperative human activity that makes us more than we otherwise could be.

MacIntyre's account of practice and Aristotle's account of activity remind us that the kinds of behavior that produce virtue are those done in and for themselves. Thus virtue is not acquired by a series of acts—even if such acts would be characterized as courageous, just, or patient—if they are done in a manner that does not render the person performing the actions just. As Aristotle says, "Acts are called just and self-controlled when they are the kinds of acts which a just and self-controlled man would perform; but the just and self-controlled man is not he who performs these acts, but he who also performs them in the way that the just and self-controlled men do" (Aristotle, 1962, 1105B5–9).

There is an inherently circular character to this account of the virtues that cannot be avoided. We can become just only by imitating just people, but such "imitation" cannot be simply the copying of their external actions. Becoming virtuous requires apprenticeship to a master; in this way the virtues are acquired through the kind of training necessary to ensure that they will not easily be lost. How such masters are located depends on a social order that is morally coherent, so that such people exhibit what everyone knows to be good. Medicine, because it remains a craft that requires apprenticeship, exemplifies how virtue can and should be taught.

William F. May (1992) suggests that the very meaning of a profession implies that one who practices it is the kind of person who can be held accountable for the goods, and corresponding virtues, of that profession. Medicine as a profession functions well to the extent that medical training forms the character of those who are being initiated into that practice. This does not imply that those who have gone through medical training will be virtuous in other aspects of their lives; it does imply, however, that as physicians they will exhibit the virtues necessary to practice medicine.

In *Becoming a Good Doctor: The Place of Virtue and Character in Medical Ethics*, James Drane (1988) suggests that the character of the doctor is part of the therapeutic relationship, and that there is a structure to the doctor–patient relationship that is based on the patient's trust that the physician will do what is necessary to help the patient heal. The physician's task, Drane argues, is not to cure illness but to care for patients, and such care depends on the character of the physician. Drane, in contrast to Robert Veatch, argues that medicine must remain a virtuous practice if it is to be sustained in modern societies.

Paul Ramsey's (1970) insistence that the focus of medicine is not the curing of illness but the care of patients "as persons," can be interpreted as an account of medicine commensurate with an emphasis on the virtues. The particular character of the judgments clinicians must make about each patient is not unlike Aristotle's description of practical wisdom, or *phronesis*. According to Aristotle, ethics deals with those matters that can be other; a virtuous person not only must act rightly but also must do so "at the right time, toward the right objects, toward the right people, for the right reasons, and in the right manner" (1962, 1106B20–23). Similarly, physicians must know when to qualify what is usually done in light of the differences a particular patient presents. From this perspective, medicine is the training of virtuous people so they are able to make skilled but fallible judgments under conditions of uncertainty.

The increasing recognition of the narrative character of medical knowledge (Hunter, 1991) reinforces this emphasis on virtue and character. That the disease entities used for diagnosis are implicit narratives means medicine is an intrinsically interpretative practice that must always be practiced under conditions of uncertainty. Accordingly, patient and physician alike bring virtues (and vices) to their interaction that are necessary for sustaining therapeutic relationships.

## Continuing problems for an ethics of virtue

To construe medicine as a virtue tradition establishes an agenda of issues for investigation in medical ethics. How are the virtues differentiated? Are there some virtues peculiar to medicine? How are different virtues related to one another? How is the difference between being a person of virtue and character, and the possession of the individual virtues, to be understood? Can a person possess virtues necessary for the practice of medicine without being virtuous? Can a person be courageous without being just?

Such questions have been central to the discussion of the virtues in classical ethical theory. For example, Aristotle maintained that none of the individual virtues could be rightly acquired unless they were acquired in the way that the person of practical wisdom would acquire them. Yet one could not be a person of practical wisdom unless one possessed individual virtues such as courage and temperance. Aristotle did not think the circular character of his account was problematic because he assumed that the kind of habituation commensurate with being "well brought up" is the way we were initiated into the "circle."

Yet in what sense the virtues are habits remains a complex question that involves the question of how the virtues are individuated. For Aristotle some of the virtues are "qualities" that qualify the emotions, but not all the virtues are like courage and temperance in that respect. Aristotle's resort to the artificial device of the "mean" for locating the various virtues has caused more problems than it has resolved. These matters are made even more complex by the importance Aristotle gives to friendship in the *Nicomachean Ethics*, where it is treated as a virtue even though it is not a quality but a relation.

The Christian appropriation of the virtues did little to resolve these complex issues. For Saint Augustine the virtues of the pagans were only "splendid vices" insofar as they were divorced from the worship of God. In "Of the Morals of the Catholic Church," Augustine redescribed the fourfold division of the virtues as four forms of love:

> that temperance is love giving itself entirely to that which is loved; fortitude is love readily bearing all things for the loved object; justice is love serving only the loved object, and therefore ruling rightly; prudence is love distinguishing with sagacity between what hinders it and what helps it. The object of this love is not anything, but only God, the chief good, the highest wisdom, the perfect harmony. So we may express the definition thus, that temperance is love keeping itself entire and uncorrupt for God; fortitude is love bearing everything readily for the sake of God; justice is love serving God only, and therefore ruling well all else, as subject to man; prudence is love making a right distinction between what helps it toward God and what might hinder it. (1955, p. 115)

Thomas Aquinas, influenced profoundly by Augustine and Aristotle, provided an extraordinary account of the virtues that in many ways remains unsurpassed. According to Aquinas, charity, understood as friendship with God, is the form of all the virtues. Therefore, like Augustine, he maintained that there can be no true virtue without charity (Aquinas, 1952). Unlike Augustine, however, Aquinas grounded the virtues in an Aristotelian account of human activity, habits, and passions. For Aquinas, therefore, the virtues are dispositions or skills necessary for human flourishing.

Aquinas's account of the virtues does present some difficulties, however. Even though he followed Augustine's (and Plato's) account of the four "cardinal" virtues—prudence, courage, temperance, and justice—neither he nor Augustine successfully argued why these four should be primary. (Aristotle does not single out these four as primary.) Indeed, it is clear from Aquinas's account that he thought of the cardinal virtues as general descriptions that required more specification through other virtues, such as truthfulness, gentleness, friendship, and magnanimity (Aquinas, 1952).

These issues obviously bear on medicine considered as part of the virtue tradition. Are there virtues peculiar to the practice of medicine that require particular cultivation by those who would be doctors? If the virtues are interdependent, can a bad person be a good doctor? Or, put more positively, do the virtues required to be a good doctor at least set one on the way to being a good person? If the Christian claim that the "natural virtues" must be formed by the theological virtues of faith, hope, and charity is correct, does that mean that medicine as a virtue requires theological warrant?

Some of these questions have not been explored with the kind of systematic rigor they deserve. MacIntyre, however, suggests some promising directions. For example, he has argued that practices are not sufficient in themselves to sustain a full account of the individual virtues, their interrelations, or their role in areas such as medicine. Practices must be understood within the context of those goods necessary for the display of a whole human life and within a tradition that makes the goods that shape that life intelligible (MacIntyre, 1984). Those initiated into the practice of medicine, for example, might well have their moral life distorted if medicine as a virtue was not located within a tradition that placed the goods that medicine serves within an overriding hierarchy of goods and corresponding virtues. Yet what such a hierarchy would actually consist of remains to be spelled out.

These matters are made more complex to the extent that those who stand in virtue traditions cannot draw on the distinction between the moral realm and the nonmoral realm so characteristic of Kantian inspired moral theory. Once distinctions between the moral and the nonmoral are questioned, strong distinctions between deontological ethics, consequential ethics, and the "ethics of virtue" are equally questionable. L. Gregory Jones and Richard Vance (1993) argue, for example, that to assume that the virtues are an alternative to an ethics of principles and rules simply reproduces the assumption that there is a distinct realm called "ethics" that can be separated from the practices of particular communities. It was this assumption that led to the disappearance of virtue from modern moral theory.

For example, Aristotle thought that how a person laughed said much about his or her character. Therefore, what we consider matters of personal style and/or etiquette were considered morally significant by the ancients. For the virtues to encompass such matters as part of human character makes problematic the distinction so crucial to modernity—that is, the distinction between public and private morality. Thus, from such a perspective, what physicians do in their "private time" may well prove important for how they conduct themselves morally as physicians.

Equally troubling is the role "luck" plays in an ethics of virtue. For example, Aristotle thought that a lack of physical beauty made it difficult for a person to be happy: "For a man is scarcely happy if he is very ugly to look at, or of low-birth, or solitary and childless" (1962, 1099A35–37). Modern egalitarian sensibilities find it offensive to think that luck might play a role in our being virtuous (Card, 1990), yet the Greeks thought it unavoidable for any account of the virtuous and happy life. Indeed, as Martha Nussbaum (1986) has argued, the very strength the virtues provide create a "fragility" that cannot be avoided. Illness may well be considered part of a person's "luck" that limits the ability to live virtuously. Medicine may thus be understood as the practice that can help restore a person to virtue.

How medicine and an ethics of virtue are understood differs greatly from one historical period to another as well as from one community to another. To the extent that medicine can no longer be sustained as a guild, perhaps it should no longer be construed in the language of the virtues. As Mark Wartofsky asks, "How is benevolence, as a distinctively *medical* virtue, to be interpreted in those forms of the practice where the individual patient is literally seen not as a person but only through the mediation of the records, laboratory reports, or a monitoring of data in a computer network?" (Wartofsky, 1985, p. 194).

Yet many continue to argue that any treatment of medicine that makes the virtues of both physician and patient secondary cannot be a medicine anyone should desire or morally support. Truthfulness, for example, is a virtue intrinsic to the care of patients; without it, whatever care is given, even if it is effective in the short run, cannot sustain a morally healthy relationship between patient and physician. Good medicine requires communication and participation by the patient that can be secured only by the physician's telling the patient the truth as well as the patient's demanding truthful speech. Without such truthful communication, the patient, as Plato argued, is reduced to the status of a slave (Drane, 1988). Ironically, in the name of freedom, the kind of medicine Veatch (1985) envisioned looks like a medicine fit for slaves—admittedly an odd conclusion since Veatch assumes that a contractual relation between physician and patient is the condition for a free exchange. Moreover, even Veatch continues to assume that truth-telling is a virtue necessary for medicine to survive as a practice between strangers.

For his part, Drane raises issues at the heart of any account of the virtues as well as of medicine as a virtue tradition. If it is true that truthfulness is a virtue intrinsic to the practice of medicine, can that virtue conflict with, for example, the virtue of benevolence? Plato and Aristotle assumed the unity of the virtues. Accordingly, the virtues would not conflict with one another if they were rightly oriented to a life of happiness. Aquinas held that the virtues might conflict during the time we are "wayfarers," but not in heaven. Drane resolves the possibility of such conflict by suggesting that medicine requires the truth to be spoken, but benevolently. One may doubt, however, whether this attractive suggestion resolves all questions about the conflict among the virtues, particularly in medical care.

If medicine is to be construed in the tradition of the virtues, the virtues and character of patients must be considered. The very term "patient" suggests a necessary virtue that is closely associated with Christian accounts of the virtues. If we must learn to live our lives patiently, then illness may appear in quite a different light than it does in those accounts of the moral life that have no patience with patience. For example, if suffering is thought to be an occasion to learn better how to be patient, then a medicine of care may be sustainable even when cure cannot be accomplished.

Karen Lebacqz (1985) suggests that the circumstances in which patients find themselves, especially the circumstance of pain and helplessness, can invite them to become accepting and obedient. These traits, which may appear virtuous, may just as likely be vices if they are not shaped by fortitude, prudence, and hope. Lebacqz suggests that these virtues are particularly relevant to the condition of being a "patient," because they provide the skills necessary to respond to illness in a "fitting" manner. No one way of expressing these virtues suits all patients; yet they do provide the conditions for our learning the tasks required in health and illness.

Questions of virtue also relate to issues of justice in the distribution of health care. For if the patient can ask medicine to supply any need abstracted from a community of virtue, then there seems no way to limit in a moral way the demands for medical care. In such a situation, those who have more economic and social power can command more than is due medically, since medicine seems committed to meeting needs irrespective of the habits that created those needs. Liberal political theory has often tried to show how a just society is possible without just people; a "medicine of strangers" may result in a maldistributed medicine.

## Conclusion

There is no consensus about the nature of virtue and/or the virtues that a good person should possess. That should not be surprising: the attempt to introduce the virtues into bioethics has gone hand in hand with an emphasis on the inevitable historical character of ethical reflection. If, as MacIntyre (1984) has argued, the virtues can be described only in relation to a particular tradition and narrative, then the very assumption that a universal account of ethics—and in particular, of medical ethics—is problematic. Yet the very character of medicine as a practice whose purpose is care for the ill

remains one of the richest resources for those committed to an account of the moral life in the language of the virtues.

STANLEY HAUERWAS

*Directly related to this entry are the entries* BENEFICENCE; CARE; COMPASSION; FRIENDSHIP; JUSTICE; NARRATIVE; PATIENTS' RESPONSIBILITIES, *article on* VIRTUES OF PATIENTS; TRUST; *and* ETHICS, *article on* NORMATIVE ETHICAL THEORIES. *For a further discussion of topics mentioned in this entry, see the entries* ACTION; AUTONOMY; EMOTIONS; INFORMATION DISCLOSURE, *article on* ATTITUDES TOWARD TRUTH-TELLING; PROFESSIONAL–PATIENT RELATIONSHIP; RIGHTS; *and* UTILITY. *This entry will find application in the entries* BIOETHICS; MEDICINE AS A PROFESSION; *and* NURSING, THEORIES AND PHILOSOPHY OF. *For further discussion of related ideas, see the entries* CASUISTRY; CONSCIENCE; FEMINISM; FREEDOM AND COERCION; *and* HUMAN NATURE. *Other relevant material may be found in the entry* PRIVILEGED COMMUNICATIONS.

## Bibliography

AQUINAS, THOMAS. 1952. *Summa Theologica.* Translated by the Fathers of the English Dominican Province. Chicago: Encyclopaedia Britannica.

ARISTOTLE. 1962. *Nicomachean Ethics.* Translated by Martin Ostwald. Indianapolis: Bobbs-Merrill.

AUGUSTINE. 1955. Selections from "Of the Morals of the Catholic Church." In *Christian Ethics: Sources of the Living Tradition,* pp. 110–118. Edited by Waldo Beach and H. Richard Niebuhr. New York: Ronald Press.

BEAUCHAMP, TOM L., and CHILDRESS, JAMES F. 1983. *Principles of Biomedical Ethics.* 2d ed. New York: Oxford University Press.

CARD, CLAUDIA. 1990. "Gender and Moral Luck." In *Identity, Character, and Morality: Essays in Moral Psychology,* pp. 199–218. Edited by Owen J. Flanagan and Amelie Oksenberg Rorty. Cambridge, Mass.: MIT Press.

DRANE, JAMES F. 1988. *Becoming a Good Doctor: The Place of Virtue and Character in Medical Ethics.* Kansas City, Mo.: Sheed & Ward.

FERNGREN, GARY B., and AMUNDSEN, DARREL W. 1985. "Virtue in Hell/Medicine in Pre-Christian Antiquity." In *Virtue and Medicine: Explorations in the Character of Medicine,* pp. 3–22. Edited by Earl E. Shelp. Dordrecht, Netherlands: D. Reidel.

FLANAGAN, OWEN J., and RORTY, AMELIE OKSENBERG, eds. 1990. *Identity, Character, and Morality: Essays in Moral Psychology.* Cambridge, Mass.: MIT Press.

FRANKENA, WILLIAM K. 1973. *Ethics.* 2d ed. Englewood Cliffs, N.J.: Prentice-Hall.

HAUERWAS, STANLEY. 1985. *Character and the Christian Life.* 2d ed. Notre Dame, Ind.: University of Notre Dame Press.

HUNTER, KATHRYN MONTGOMERY. 1991. *Doctors' Stories: The Narrative Structure of Medical Knowledge.* Princeton, N.J.: Princeton University Press.

JONES, L. GREGORY, and VANCE, RICHARD P. 1993. "Why the Virtues Are *Not* Another Approach to Medical Ethics: Re-conceiving the Place of Ethics and Contemporary Medicine." In *Religious Methods and Resources in Bioethics,* pp. 203–225. Edited by Paul F. Camenisch. Dordrecht, Netherlands: Kluwer.

KANT, IMMANUEL. 1959. *Foundations of the Metaphysics of Morals, and What is Enlightenment?* Translated by Lewis White Beck. New York: Liberal Arts Press.

KUPPERMAN, JOEL. 1991. *Character.* New York: Oxford University Press.

LEBACQZ, KAREN. 1985. "The Virtuous Patient." In *Virtue and Medicine: Explorations in the Character of Medicine,* pp. 275–288. Edited by Earl E. Shelp. Dordrecht, Netherlands: D. Reidel.

MacINTYRE, ALASDAIR. 1984. *After Virtue: A Study in Moral Theology.* 2d ed. Notre Dame, Ind.: University of Notre Dame Press.

MAY, WILLIAM F. 1992. "The Beleaguered Rulers: The Public Obligation of the Professional." *Kennedy Institute of Ethics Journal* 2, no. 1:25–41.

NUSSBAUM, MARTHA C. 1986. *The Fragility of Goodness: Luck and Ethics in Greek Tragedy and Philosophy.* Cambridge: At the University Press.

PELLEGRINO, EDMUND D. 1985. "The Virtuous Physician, and the Ethics of Medicine." In *Virtue and Medicine: Explorations in the Character of Medicine,* pp. 237–256. Edited by Earl E. Shelp. Dordrecht, Netherlands: D. Reidel.

PELLEGRINO, EDMUND D. and THOMASMA, DAVID C. 1993. *The Virtues in Medical Practice.* New York: Oxford University Press.

PINCOFFS, EDMUND L. 1986. *Quandaries and Virtues: Against Reductivism in Ethics.* Lawrence: University Press of Kansas.

RAMSEY, PAUL. 1970. *The Patient as Person: Explorations in Medical Ethics.* New Haven, Conn.: Yale University Press.

VEATCH, ROBERT M. 1985. "Against Virtue: A Deontological Critique of Virtue Theory and Medical Ethics." In *Virtue and Medicine: Explorations in the Character of Medicine,* pp. 329–346. Edited by Earl E. Shelp. Dordrecht, Netherlands: D. Reidel.

WARTOFSKY, MARK. 1985. "Virtues and Vices: The Social and Historical Construction of Medical Norms." In *Virtue and Medicine: Explorations in the Character of Medicine,* pp. 175–200. Edited by Earl E. Shelp. Dordrecht, Netherlands: D. Reidel.

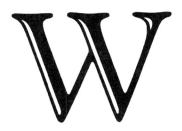

# WARFARE

## I. MEDICINE AND WAR

*This article is based in part on the entry "Warfare" in the first edition of the* Encyclopedia of Bioethics; *Part I ("Medicine and War") of that entry was authored by E. A. Vastyan, and Part II ("Biomedical Science and War") was coauthored by the current author and Mark Sidel.*

Ethical conflicts occur whenever medicine and war intersect. This article discusses four general types of potential ethical conflict: (1) conflict between the military obligation of physicians and other medical personnel to provide care to members of the military force of which they are members and the medical obligation to serve others—such as members of opposing military forces and civilians—who need their care; (2) conflict between the obligation of military medical personnel to "conserve the fighting strength" and the medical obligation to respond to the special needs or rights of individual military personnel under their care, even if such response hinders the "fighting strength"; (3) conflict between "combatant" and "noncombatant" roles for medical personnel; and (4) conflict between the national obligation to serve one's country through service in a military force and the international obligation to prevent war or to prevent specific actions by the military force of one's own country.

The history of physician involvement with military forces is a long one. Homer praised the efforts of the sons of Asclepios in providing surgical care before the gates of Troy (Homer, 1990); and Hippocrates, recognizing the battleground as an important training ground for surgeons, urged that "he who would become a surgeon should join an army and follow it" (Vastyan, 1978, p. 1695).

But physicians and other medical personnel had relatively little to offer military casualties until the eighteenth century. Since then, rapid developments in military weaponry and concurrent advances in medical technology and in techniques for evacuation of casualties have made deployment of medical resources increasingly important to armies and their commanders. To the armies of the czar, for example, Peter the Great brought the *feldsher*, modeled on the *feldscherer* (field barber–surgeon) of the Prussian armies. In the New World, deplorable medical care during the American Revolution caused bitter political conflicts over the management of hospitals and health care for soldiers. The increase in the number of military casualties during the wars of the nineteenth century and the extraordinary increase in both military and civilian casualties during the wars of the twentieth century, together with dramatic improvements in the ability to treat casualties successfully, led to changes in the types of ethical issues that arise and an increase in their number.

## Military obligations versus medical obligations

As a member of the military forces of a nation, the military physician is charged with the mission of protecting the strength of the military force. As a member of the broader medical profession, on the other hand, the physician is generally obligated to care for all the sick and wounded who need his or her services and to set priorities for providing those services on the basis of the urgency and effectiveness of medical need.

Hippocrates, often called "the father of medicine," apparently rejected the principle that physicians have an obligation in war to succor "enemies" as well as "friends." The evidence is found in Plutarch's *Lives*, in a reference to "Hippocrates' reply when the Great King of Persia consulted him, with the promise of a fee of many talents, namely, that he would never put his skill at the service of Barbarians who were enemies of Greece" (Plutarch, 1914, p. 373).

Just before the start of the U.S. Civil War, the American Medical Association (AMA) selected, as the model for a commemorative stone carving for placement in the Washington Monument, then being built in the District of Columbia, the painting *Hippocrates Refuses the Gifts of Artaxerxes*, portraying Hippocrates' dismissal of the emissaries of the king of Persia. The inscription the AMA selected was *Vincit Amor Patriae*, "Love of Country Prevails" (Stacey, 1988).

In a time of "unjustifiable and monstrous rebellion," a phrase used contemporaneously by one of its leaders, the AMA probably meant by its use of the painting and the inscription to applaud the refusal to provide medical services for enemies. Indeed no evidence can be found that in the pre–Civil War United States there was a great deal of sympathy for evenhanded medical care in time of war (Sidel, 1991b).

**Physicians as impartial healers.**   The physician's responsibility to treat those in medical need on both sides did not burn itself into either public or medical consciousness until the late 1860s, in the aftermath of the Crimean War and the U.S. Civil War. Leadership in raising this new consciousness was assumed by nonphysicians: Florence Nightingale, who served as a nurse in Turkey and the Crimea from 1854 to 1856, and Dorothea Dix, whose work in bringing humane care to mental patients in the United States led President Abraham Lincoln to invite her to organize the U.S. Army Nursing Corps and to become the first Superintendent of Nurses in the U.S. Army.

Henri Dunant, a Swiss banker who was an eyewitness at the Battle of Solferino in 1859, organized medical services for the Austrian and French wounded. In 1864, he helped initiate an international conference in Geneva that led to the founding of the International Red Cross and its national affiliates. The conference adopted a Convention for the Amelioration of the Condition of the Wounded and Sick in Armed Forces in the Field. Fourteen signatory nations pledged to regard the sick and wounded, as well as personnel, facilities, and transport for their care, as neutrals on the battlefield. For his efforts, Dunant was awarded the first Nobel Peace Prize.

Two contemporaneous events in the United States influenced future codifications and applications of international law and their bearing on medicine. Francis Lieber, a German-born philosopher-lawyer-historian, was commissioned by the Union Forces in the Civil War to draft a code of conduct for armies in the field. The resultant Lieber Code was promulgated in May 1863 as General Order No. 100 by the Union Army. Closely related to this development was the 1865 trial of Captain Henry Wirz, a physician who served as commandant of the infamous Confederate prison at Andersonville, Georgia. He was charged with a series of offenses alleging inhumane regard for prisoners under his charge. His plea of "superior orders" mitigating the negligence of duty with which he was charged was disallowed, and Wirz was convicted and sentenced to be hanged.

During the eighty years following the first Geneva treaty on treatment of war casualties, three other related international agreements were negotiated in the Hague and in Geneva. The Convention for the Amelioration of the Wounded, Sick, and Shipwrecked Members of Armed Forces at Sea dealt with the care of casualties of naval warfare. The Convention Relative to the Treatment of Prisoners of War regulated the treatment and repatriation of prisoners. The Convention Relative to the Protection of Civilian Persons in Time of War prohibited deportation, taking of hostages, torture, and discrimination in treatment. These three agreements, plus the original Geneva accord, were codified in a single, formal document in Geneva in 1949; together, they are called the Geneva Conventions. Agreed to at that time by sixty nations, the 1949 conventions were declared binding upon all nations according to "customary law, the usages established among civilized people . . . the laws of humanity, and the dictates of the public conscience" ("The Geneva Conventions," 1983).

Under the conventions, medical personnel are singled out for certain specific protections by an explicit separation of the healing from the wounding roles. Medical personnel and treatment facilities are designated as immune from attack, and captured medical personnel are to be promptly repatriated. In return, specific obligations are required of medical personnel:

1. Regarded as "noncombatants," medical personnel are forbidden to engage in or be parties to the acts of war.
2. The wounded and sick—soldier and civilian, friend and foe—must be respected, protected, treated humanely, and cared for by the belligerents.
3. The wounded and sick must not be left without medical assistance, and only urgent medical reasons authorize any priority in the order of their treatment.
4. Medical aid must be dispensed solely on medical grounds, "without distinctions founded on sex, race, nationality, religion, political opinions, or any other similar criteria."
5. Medical personnel shall exercise no physical or moral coercion against protected persons (civilians), in particular to obtain information from them or from third parties.

Such duties are imposed clearly, permitting no exceptions, and given priority over all other considerations. Thus, the Geneva Conventions formalized the recognition that, while professional expertise merits special privileges, it likewise incurs very specific legal as well as moral obligations (Vastyan, 1978). That special role of physicians is now embodied in the public expectations and in the ethical training of doctors in most societies. It is also embedded in the World Medical Association's Declaration of Geneva, which is administered as a "modern Hippocratic Oath" to graduating classes at many medical schools.

There is, however, evidence of deviation from these principles. An example of the erosion of the principle of equal medical care for "enemies" occurred in the United States during the Cold War. The medical society of Maryland and the AMA refused to criticize a Maryland psychiatrist who testified voluntarily before the Un-American Activities Committee of the U.S. House of Representatives in 1960 about information he had obtained in the course of treatment of an employee of the National Security Agency (NSA). His patient, together with another NSA employee with whom the patient had allegedly had a sexual relationship, later defected to the USSR. The psychiatrist, clearly without his patient's permission, provided to the committee information given to him by his patient, and the material was leaked to the press by the committee. To a petition by a group of Maryland psychiatrists and other physicians asking that the psychiatrist be censured, the medical society responded that "the interests of the nation transcend those of the individual" (Sidel, 1961).

## Obligations to enhance military strength versus personnel needs

Military physicians must accept different priorities than do their civilian colleagues (Vastyan, 1974). The primary role of the military physician is expressed in the motto of the U.S. Army Medical Department: "To conserve the fighting strength" (Bellamy, 1988). In describing this role, a faculty member of the Academy of Health Sciences at Fort Sam Houston in 1988 cited as "the clear objective of all health service support operations" the goal stated in 1866 by a veteran of the Army of the Potomac in the U.S. Civil War:

"... [to] strengthen the hands of the commanding general by keeping his Army in the most vigorous health, thus rendering it, in the highest degree, efficient for enduring fatigue and privitation [sic], and for fighting." (Rubenstein, 1988, p. 145)

Principles of triage unacceptable in civilian practice may be required, such as placing first emphasis on patching up the lightly wounded so they can be sent back to battle. For example, "overevacuation" (the presumed excessive transfer of personnel to a safe area rather than back to the military operation) is cited as "one of the cardinal sins of military medicine" (Bellamy, 1988). Violation of patient confidentiality unacceptable in civilian practice may be required. Medical personnel may be required to administer experimental drugs or immunizations to troops without their free and informed consent (Annas, 1992).

## Combatant versus noncombatant roles for medical personnel

Perhaps history's most dramatic attempt to meld these conflicting obligations was made by the Knights Hospitallers of Saint John of Jerusalem, members of a religious order founded in the eleventh century. With a sworn fealty to "our Lords the Sick," the Knights defended their hospitals against "enemies of the Faith," becoming the first organized military medical officers. They were "warring physicians who could strike the enemy mighty blows, and yet later bind up the wounds of that same enemy along with those of their own comrades" (Vastyan, 1978, pp. 1695–1696).

A more recent example of erosion of the distinction between combatant and noncombatant roles was demonstrated in a U.S. Army exhibit at the 1967 AMA Convention. It was entitled "Medicine as a Weapon" and featured a photograph of a Green Beret (Special Forces) Aidman handing medicine to a Vietnamese peasant (Liberman et al., 1968). Dr. Peter Bourne, who had been an Army physician working with the Special Forces in Vietnam, wrote that the primary task of Special Forces Medics was "to seek and destroy the enemy and only incidentally to take care of the medical needs of others on the patrol" (Liberman et al., 1968, p. 303).

In 1967, Howard Levy, a dermatologist drafted into the U.S. Army Medical Department as a captain, refused to obey an order to train Special Forces Aidmen in dermatological skills. He refused specifically on the grounds that the aidmen were being trained predominantly for a combat role and that cross-training in medical techniques eroded the distinction between combatants and noncombatants. For this refusal he was charged with one of the most serious breaches of the Uniform Code of Military Justice: willfully disobeying a lawful order. Tried by a general court-martial in 1967, Levy admitted his disobedience, saying he had acted in accordance with his ethical principles. The physicians who testified for the defense "argued that the political use of medicine by the Special Forces jeopardized the entire tradition of the noncombatant status of medicine" (Langer, 1967, p. 1349). They agreed with Levy that a physician is responsible for even the secondary ethical implications of his acts; that he must not only act ethically himself, but also anticipate that those to whom he teaches medicine will act ethically as well. Although Levy was a medical officer, the court-martial panel did not include a physician. Levy was given a dishonorable discharge and sentenced to three years of hard labor in a military prison. Levy's appeals were not successful (Glasser, 1967; Langer, 1967).

Inside or outside the armed forces, medical personnel may also be involved in war-related research and development, such as work on biological weapons or on the radiation effects of nuclear weapons. In such work, it is said to have been common practice to concentrate physicians into "principally or primarily defensive operations" (Rosebury, 1963). But work on weapons and their effects can never be exclusively defensive, and at times the distinction is quite arbitrary. The question arises whether there is a special ethical duty for physicians (because of their medical obligation to "do no harm") to refuse to participate in such work, or whether in nonpatient-care situations physicians simply share the ethical duties of all human beings (Sidel, 1991a).

The noncombatant role of the physician in military service is an ambiguous one, even if frank combatant activities are eschewed. Military physicians, like all members of the armed forces, are limited by threat of military discipline in the extent to which they can publicly protest what they believe to be an unjust war. The issue of what is a "just war," which has been debated for over two millennia, can be touched on only briefly here

(Seabury and Codevilla, 1989; Walzer, 1977). There are generally held to be two elements in a just war: *jus ad bellum* (when is it just to go to war?), and *jus in bello* (what methods may be used in a just war?). Among the elements required for *jus ad bellum* are a just grievance and the exhaustion of all means short of war to settle the grievance. Among the elements required for *jus in bello* are protection of noncombatants and proportionality of force, including avoiding use of weapons of mass destruction such as chemical, biological, and nuclear weapons and massive bombing of cities. Membership in the armed forces, even in a noncombatant role, usually requires self-censorship of public doubts about the justness of a war in which the armed forces are engaged.

In addition, medical personnel, like other human beings, may consider themselves pacifists. "Absolute pacifism" opposes the use of any force against another human being, even in self-defense against direct, personal attack. The argument underlying this position, for many of its adherents, is that the use of force can only be ended when all humans refuse to use it, and that acceptance of one's own injury or even death is preferable to use of force against another. More limited forms of pacifism, such as "nuclear pacifism," hold that the use of certain weapons of mass destruction in war is never justified, no matter how great the provocation or how terrible the consequences of failure to use them. It has been suggested under the term "maternal pacifism" that women, because of their nurturing roles, have a special responsibility to oppose the use of force (Ruddick, 1989).

When a group is threatened with genocide, as the Nazis attempted in World War II, many who might otherwise adopt a pacifist or limited pacifist position believe that force may be justified. Their shift in position is based on the threat to the very survival of the group, a threat that makes the pacifist argument—that current failure to resist will lead to future diminution in violence—seem untenable.

There is considerable debate whether physicians, because of a special dedication to preservation of life and health, have a special obligation to serve or to refuse to serve in a military effort. That position is made more complex by the physician's role as a military noncombatant. Many military forces nonetheless permit physicians, like other military personnel, to claim conscientious objector status. In the United States, conscientious objection is defined as "a firm, fixed, and sincere objection by reason of religious training and belief to: (1) participation in war in any form, or (2) the bearing of arms." Religious training and belief is defined as "belief in an external power or being or deeply held moral or ethical belief to which all else is subordinate and . . . which has the power or force to affect moral well-being"

(U.S. Department of Defense, 1982). The person claiming conscientious objector status must convince a military hearing officer that the objection is sincere.

## Obligations to serve in war versus to prevent war

As wars kill an increasing percentage of civilians with so-called conventional weapons, and as threats of the use of weapons of mass destruction continue, what form of service is appropriate for the ethical physician? One response was suggested in the late 1930s by John A. Ryle, then Regius Professor of Physic at the University of Cambridge:

> It is everywhere a recognized and humane principle that prevention should be preferred to cure. By withholding service from the Armed Forces before and during war, by declining to examine and inoculate recruits, by refusing sanitary advice and the training and command of ambulances, clearing stations, medical transport, and hospitals, the doctors could so cripple the efficiency of the staff and aggravate the difficulties of campaign and so damage the morale of the troops that war would become almost unthinkable. (Ryle, 1938, p. 8)

During the Vietnam War more than 300 American medical students and young physicians brought Ryle's vision a step closer to reality by signing the following pledge:

> In the name of freedom the U.S. is waging an unjustifiable war in Viet Nam and is causing incalculable suffering. It is the goal of the medical profession to prevent and relieve human suffering. My effort to pursue this goal is meaningless in the context of the war. Therefore, I refuse to serve in the Armed Forces in Viet Nam; and so that I may exercise my profession with conscience and dignity, I intend to seek means to serve my country which are compatible with the preservation and enrichment of life. (Liberman et al., 1968, p. 306)

Ryle's vision is a variation on that of Aristophanes in his comedy *The Lysistrata*, written in 411 B.C.E., just before the probable time of Hippocrates' refusal to treat the Persians (ca. 400 B.C.E.). The title character, an Athenian woman, ends the second Peloponnesian War by organizing the wives of the soldiers of both Athens and Sparta to refuse sexual intercourse with their husbands while the war lasts. The Athenians and Spartans make peace quickly and go home with their wives (Aristophanes, 1979).

Some physicians and other medical personnel have refused to support war by serving in the armed forces. In one of the most dramatic examples, Yolanda Huet-Vaughn, a captain in the U.S. Army Medical Service Reserve, refused to obey an order for active duty in the Persian Gulf. In her statement, she explained:

> I am refusing orders to be an accomplice in what I consider an immoral, inhumane and unconstitutional act, namely an offensive military mobilization in the Middle East. My oath as a citizen-soldier to defend the Constitution, my oath as a physician to preserve human life and prevent disease, and my responsibility as a human being to the preservation of this planet, would be violated if I cooperate. (Sidel, 1991b, p. 102)

The reasons Huet-Vaughn gave for her action were quite different from the reasons given by Levy. Levy refused to obey an order that he believed required him to perform a specific act that would violate the Geneva Conventions; Huet-Vaughn refused to obey an order she believed required her to support a particular war that she felt to be unjust and destructive to the goals of medicine and humanity.

One of the questions Huet-Vaughn's action raises is whether physicians have a special ethical responsibility, in view of their obligation to protect the health and the lives of their patients and the people of their communities, to refuse to support a war they believe will cause major destruction to the health and environment of both combatants and noncombatants (Geiger, 1991; Sidel, 1991b). If a physician considers service in support of a particular war unethical on the grounds of sworn fealty to medical ethics, may—or, indeed, must—that doctor refuse to serve, even if that objection does not quality for formal conscientious objector status? Furthermore, is there an ethical difference if the service is required by the society—as in a "doctor draft"—or if the service obligation has been entered into voluntarily to fulfill an obligation in return for military support of medical training or for other reasons? And is military service indeed a "voluntary obligation" if enlistment, as it is for many poor and minority people, is prodded by lack of educational or employment opportunities or, as for many doctors, by the cost of medical education or specialty training that in other societies would be provided at public expense?

While few physicians are willing or able to take an action such as that taken by Huet-Vaughn, other actions are available to oppose acts of war considered unjust, to oppose a specific war, or to oppose war in general. One is acceptance of a service alternative consistent with an ethical obligation to care for those wounded or maimed without simultaneously supporting a war effort. Opportunities for service in an international medical corps such as Médecins du Monde or Médecins sans Frontieres are limited, but U.S. physicians may wish to demand that their nation redirect some of the billions of dollars it spends annually on preparation for war to the United

Nations or the World Health Organization to help fund an international medical service to treat the casualties of war.

Other physicians may work, as individuals and particularly in groups, to help to prevent war by contributing to public and professional understanding of the nature of modern war, the risks of weapons of mass destruction, and the nature and effectiveness of alternatives to war. Among the groups organized for this purpose are the International Physicians for the Prevention of Nuclear War, whose U.S. affiliate is Physicians for Social Responsibility. If the world is to survive, physicians may need to consider new forms of national service and to contribute in a broader sense to their nation and their planet (Lown, 1986).

In the broader context of medical ethics, it is widely accepted that opposition to war does not permit the ethical physician to refuse medical care to victims of war that he or she is in a position to serve, and that such care does not presume the physician's support of the war being fought. Ethical dilemmas arise when the physician actively supports the war effort by membership in a military medical service or by assigning priority to patient care based on military demands rather than patient needs. These issues and those associated with the role of the physician in peacemaking and peacekeeping, often grotesquely distorted by the fervor that may accompany war and preparation for war, require dispassionate analysis and action in times of peace.

VICTOR W. SIDEL

*Directly related to this article are the other articles in this entry:* PUBLIC HEALTH AND WAR, NUCLEAR WARFARE, CHEMICAL AND BIOLOGICAL WEAPONS, *and* INTERNATIONAL WEAPONS TRADE. *Also directly related is the entry* PRISONERS, *article on* TORTURE AND THE HEALTH PROFESSIONAL. *For a further discussion of topics mentioned in this article, see the entries* CARE; CONFLICT OF INTEREST; CONSCIENCE; JUSTICE; MEDICAL CODES AND OATHS, *article on* ETHICAL ANALYSIS; OBLIGATION AND SUPEREROGATION; *and* TRIAGE. *For a discussion of related ideas, see the entries* CIVIL DISOBEDIENCE AND HEALTH CARE; HEALTH OFFICIALS AND THEIR RESPONSIBILITIES; *and* MILITARY PERSONNEL AS RESEARCH SUBJECTS. *Other relevant material may be found under the entries* INTERNATIONAL HEALTH; PROFESSION AND PROFESSIONAL ETHICS; UTILITY; VALUE AND VALUATION; *and* VIRTUE AND CHARACTER.

## Bibliography

ANNAS, GEORGE J. 1992. "Changing the Consent Rules for Desert Storm." *New England Journal of Medicine* 326, no. 1:770–773.

ARISTOPHANES. 1979. *The Lysistrata.* In Vol. 3 of *Aristophanes,* pp. 6–123. Translated by Benjamin Bickley Rogers. Cambridge, Mass.: Harvard University Press.

BELLAMY, RONALD F. 1988. "Conserve the Fighting Strength." *Military Medicine* 153, no. 4:185–186.

GEIGER, H. JACK. 1991. "Conscience and Obligation: Physicians and Just War." *PSR Quarterly* 1:113–116.

"The Geneva Conventions of 1949." 1983. In *Human Rights Documents: Compilation of Documents Pertaining to Human Rights,* pp. 325–461. Washington, D.C.: U.S. Government Printing Office.

GLASSER, IRA. 1967. "Judgment at Fort Jackson: The Court-Martial of Captain Howard B. Levy." *Law in Transition Quarterly* 4 (Spring):123–156.

HOMER. 1990. *The Iliad.* Translated by Robert Fagles. New York: Viking.

LANGER, ELINOR. 1967. "The Court-Martial of Captain Levy: Medical Ethics v. Military Law." *Science* 156, no. 3780:1346–1350.

LIBERMAN, ROBERT; GOLD, WARREN; and SIDEL, VICTOR W. 1968. "Medical Ethics and the Military." *New Physician* 17, no. 11:299–309.

LOWN, BERNARD. 1986. "Nobel Peace Prize Lecture: A Prescription for Hope." *New England Journal of Medicine* 314, no. 15:985–987.

PLUTARCH. 1914. "Marcus Cato." In Vol. 2 of *Lives,* pp. 302–385. Translated by Bernadotte Perin. Cambridge, Mass.: Harvard University Press.

ROSEBURY, THEODOR. 1963. "Medical Ethics and Biological Warfare." *Perspectives in Biology and Medicine* 6:512–523.

RUBENSTEIN, DAVID A. 1988. "Health Service Support and the Principles of War." *Military Medicine* 153, no. 3:145–146.

RUDDICK, SARA. 1989. *Maternal Thinking: Toward a Politics of Peace.* Boston: Beacon Press.

RYLE, JOHN A. 1938. Foreword to *The Doctor's View of War,* pp. 7–10. Edited by Horace Joules. London: George Allen & Unwin.

SEABURY, PAUL, and CODEVILLA, ANGELO. 1989. *War: Ends and Means.* New York: Basic Books.

SIDEL, VICTOR W. 1961. "Confidential Information and the Physician." *New England Journal of Medicine* 264, no. 22:1133–1137.

———. 1991a. "Biological Weapons Research and Physicians: Historical and Ethical Analysis." *PSR Quarterly* 1, no. 1:31–42.

———. 1991b. "Quid Est Amor Patriae?" *PSR Quarterly* 1, no. 1:96–104.

STACEY, JAMES. 1988. "The Cover." *Journal of the American Medical Association* 260:448.

U.S. DEPARTMENT OF DEFENSE. 1982. Air Force Regulation 35-24. Washington, D.C.: Author.

VASTYAN, E. A. 1974. "Warriors in White: Some Questions About the Nature and Mission of Military Medicine." *Texas Reports on Biology and Medicine* 32, no. 1:327–342.

———. 1978. "Warfare: I. Medicine and War." In vol. 4 of *Encyclopedia of Bioethics,* pp. 1695–1699. Edited by Warren T. Reich. New York: Macmillan.

WALZER, MICHAEL. 1977. *Just and Unjust Wars: A Moral Argument with Historical Illustrations.* New York: Basic Books.

## II. PUBLIC HEALTH AND WAR

Wars have always exacted a severe toll on the public health of civilian populations. Noncombatants have often been the intentional victims of warfare; dramatic examples during the twentieth century include the hundreds of thousands of civilian deaths that resulted from the bombing of Dresden and the nuclear explosions that destroyed Hiroshima and Nagasaki. In addition, war has had severe indirect consequences on public health through the destruction of medical facilities and public utilities and through mass starvation. The Allied blockade of Germany in 1916–1918, the siege of Leningrad in 1941, the war-induced famine in Holland during 1944–1945, and the Nigerian civil war in 1969 caused millions of deaths among the noncombatant populations.

Since 1980, approximately 130 armed conflicts have occurred worldwide; thirty-two of these wars each caused more than 1,000 battlefields deaths (Cobey et al., 1993). Most occurred in Asia, Africa, and Latin America; however, since 1990, three European conflicts—in the former Yugloslavia, Azerbaijan, and Georgia—have caused more than 300,000 deaths.

Civilian populations have increasingly been the intentional target of military actions; shelling of urban centers has been common in Bosnia and Herzegovina, Angola, Lebanon, and Somalia. In addition, modern weapons such as napalm, cluster bombs, and land mines have not discriminated between combatants and innocent civilians. The heavy civilian toll in recent wars is illustrated by the United Nations Children's Fund (UNICEF) estimate that 1.5 million children have been killed in wars since 1980. Only 5 percent of the casualties in World War I were civilians; the proportion rose to 50 percent in World War II, and was estimated to be 80 percent during wars of the 1980s (Grant, 1992).

## Public-health impact of war

**Direct.**    The direct public-health consequences of war include death, injury, sexual assault, disability, and psychological stress. Particularly high civilian death rates have been reported in Angola, Ethiopia, Liberia, Mozambique, Rwanda, Somalia, Southern Sudan, El Salvador, Guatemala, Afghanistan, Cambodia, Tajikistan, and Bosnia and Herzegovina (Zwi and Ugalde, 1991; Toole et al., 1993). Between 1991 and 1993, an estimated 40,000 people died of war-related injuries in just two cities—Mogadishu, Somalia and Sarajevo, Bosnia and Herzegovina. During a relatively brief period of conflict in April 1994, an estimated 500,000 civilians in Rwanda were brutally killed.

Systematic sexual violence directed primarily against women has been documented in many modern wars, notably during the war of independence of Bangladesh, and more recently in the former Yugoslavia, resulting in high incidence of severe psychological trauma, unwanted pregnancies, and sexually transmitted diseases (Swiss and Giller, 1993).

An estimated 100 million mines have been laid by various armed factions in Afghanistan, Angola, Cambodia, El Salvador, Iraq, Mozambique, Somalia, and other war zones, resulting in a global epidemic of deaths, injuries, and disabilities. Approximately one in 360 Cambodians is an amputee, largely due to land mine injuries (Asia Watch, 1991). Land mines are among the most indiscriminate weapons. Although they are ostensibly laid to kill or maim opposing military forces, they more often strike innocent civilians who inadvertently walk on them, frequently many years after their deployment. Since mines are often laid on agricultural land, the indirect economic impact of lost production is enormous.

Immeasurable psychological trauma has been caused by widespread human-rights abuses, including detention, torture, and forced displacement (institutionalized in the former Yugoslavia as "ethnic cleansing"). Since 1980, an estimated 10 million children have been directly affected by the brutality of war, much of it motivated by ethnic, religious, and ideological conflicts (UNICEF, 1992).

**Indirect.**    The indirect public health consequences of war have been mediated by hunger, mass migration, and collapsed health services, especially in impoverished, developing countries where basic services and food reserves are already inadequate. The intentional use of food deprivation as a weapon has become increasingly common (MacCrae and Zwi, 1992). For example, armed factions on all sides have obstructed food aid deliveries in Southern Sudan, resulting in mass hunger and, during 1993, death rates up to fifteen times those reported in nonfamine times. In 1992, widespread looting and banditry deprived millions of Somalis of much-needed food aid. Death rates among displaced persons in the town of Baidoa reached twenty-five times baseline rates (Moore et al., 1993).

Between 1990 and 1993, the global number of refugees and internally displaced persons fleeing war increased from 30 million to 44 million (U.S. Committee for Refugees, 1993). Crude death rates (CDR), defined as the number of deaths per 1,000 population per month (not age-adjusted), among refugees ranged between five and twelve times the death rates in their countries of origin, and CDRs among internally displaced persons were six to twenty-five times baseline rates. Most deaths were caused by preventable conditions such as malnutrition, diarrhea, pneumonia, measles, and malaria (Centers for Disease Control and Prevention [CDC], 1992). High death rates reflect the prolonged period of deprivation suffered prior to displacement, the often inadequate response to humanitarian crises by the international community, and problems of gaining access to provide relief assistance to war-affected communities.

Health facilities have been intentionally destroyed by armed factions in Afghanistan, Angola, Bosnia, Mozambique, and other war-stricken countries. In addition, the high costs of both maintaining military forces and treating war wounded have often led to insufficient funding for basic health services. In the Bosnian province of Zenica, for example, the proportion of surgical cases related to war injuries rose from 22 percent to 78 percent between April and November 1993, resulting in the cessation of almost all preventive health services (Toole et al., 1993).

Perhaps the most significant consequence of war on public health relates to the tremendous cost of preparing for war. Military budgets throughout both the industrialized and developing worlds have diverted precious resources from public-health and other social development programs. Moreover, the destruction of environmental resources, such as water sources, agricultural land, livestock, and housing has had a major impact on public health in numerous countries affected by war.

## Ethical issues

Modern warfare has increasingly involved flagrant violations of the Geneva Conventions related to the protection of civilian persons in time of war (International Committee of the Red Cross [ICRC], 1950). Ethnic cleansing, detention of civilians, summary executions, and torture are clearly illegal under international law. The unrestricted ability of combatants to target civilians is fostered by the officially sanctioned international arms trade. The ICRC, the custodian of the Geneva Conventions, has often been deprived of access to civilians in countries such as Somalia, Sudan, and Bosnia and Herzegovina.

International economic sanctions are often employed to cripple governments engaged in armed conflict. However, these sanctions have often had a greater effect on the health of civilians in those countries than on the policies of the targeted governments. For example, increased death rates among children were documented in Iraq during the period following the 1991 Gulf War (Harvard Study Team, 1991). Economic sanctions against Iraq and the bombing of public utilities during the war contributed to these increased death rates.

International public opinion has increasingly supported the use of force by the United Nations to ensure delivery of humanitarian aid in situations either where governance has completely collapsed (e.g., Somalia and Liberia) or where governments consciously hinder access by relief agencies (e.g., Sudan and Bosnia and Herze-

govina). However, there are no clear guidelines that might promote a consistent deployment of force to achieve humanitarian objectives (Dewey, 1993). The U.N. Charter prohibits interference in the affairs of a sovereign nation, thereby giving more weight to the rights of the state than to individual citizens.

Two contradictory examples from 1992 illustrate the ethnical dilemmas inherent in the use of force to save lives from hunger and disease. In Bosnia and Herzegovina, European soldiers deployed to ensure the safe delivery of humanitarian supplies were powerless to prevent flagrant abuses of human rights committed in their presence (Jean, 1992). In contrast, the international armed contingent, which was originally dispatched to Somalia in late 1992 to ensure the safe delivery of relief supplies, eventually became a party to the internal conflict, leading to battles between U.N. troops and one local armed faction in heavily populated areas of the capital, Mogadishu, with high civilian casualty rates resulting (Brauman, 1993). Thus, well-motivated intervention by the international community may inadvertently increase the risks to the intended beneficiaries.

Decisive action by the international community has often been too late to prevent a high death toll from hunger and disease among affected civilians. Global indifference early in the evolution of humanitarian disasters often reflects lack of information that in turn is a result of selective reporting by the media.

The neutral role and humanitarian responsibilities of health workers in war settings have been clearly defined. Unfortunately, there have been numerous reports of physicians collaborating in acts of torture and other human rights abuses (Geiger and Cook-Deegan, 1993). Once access to an affected area is assured, health personnel have a critical role in accurately documenting the public-health impact of war on civilian populations, thereby acting as effective advocates for prompt and adequate response. Relief programs may pose a difficult choice for health workers, between the provision of individual curative care and the implementation of more effective, community-based programs such as childhood immunization.

## Conclusions

Modern warfare has exacted a devastating toll on civilian populations; high mortality, morbidity, and disability rates have resulted directly from traumatic injuries and indirectly from hunger and mass displacement. Since the end of the Cold War, the potential for a more unified and coherent "international community" has emerged. Currently, the international community's authority and operational capacity rests with the U.N. Security Council and various U.N. agencies where decisions are heavily influenced by governments of the U.N. member states.

The United Nations has a responsibility to monitor carefully the public-health consequences of evolving conflicts and to apply aggressive diplomacy early to seek solutions. When conflicting parties obstruct access to civilians by relief agencies the world needs to respond in a consistent and effective manner. Existing international legal conventions may be inadequate to protect civilians against forced migration and other abuses such as sexual violence. Clearer guidelines on the use of force to deliver humanitarian aid in conflict settings need to be developed. In addition, when economic sanctions are applied against particular sides in a conflict, the international community needs to ensure that humanitarian supplies are exempt.

Relief programs should reflect the real needs of affected populations rather than the availability of surplus commodities in donor countries. Health personnel have a pivotal role in the scientific assessment of public-health needs and the monitoring of health and nutrition trends. Primary prevention is the basic strategy of public health; consequently, in war settings, public-health practitioners need to recognize that primary prevention means stopping the violence, and they should actively explore methods for promoting sustainable peace.

MICHAEL J. TOOLE

*Directly related to this article are the other articles in this entry:* MEDICINE AND WAR, NUCLEAR WARFARE, CHEMICAL AND BIOLOGICAL WEAPONS, *and* INTERNATIONAL WEAPONS TRADE. *For a further discussion of topics mentioned in this article, see the entries* EUGENICS; FOOD POLICY; HEALTH-CARE RESOURCES, ALLOCATION OF; *and* RESPONSIBILITY. *Other relevant material may be found under the entries* HEALTH OFFICIALS AND THEIR RESPONSIBILITIES; HEALTH POLICY, *article on* POLITICS AND HEALTH CARE; INTERNATIONAL HEALTH; *and* PUBLIC HEALTH, *articles on* DETERMINANTS OF PUBLIC HEALTH, *and* PHILOSOPHY OF PUBLIC HEALTH.

## Bibliography

ASIA WATCH. 1991. *Land Mines in Cambodia—The Coward's War, September 1991.* New York: Author and Physicians for Human Rights.

BRAUMAN, RONY. 1993. *Le Crime humanitaire: Somalie.* Paris: Arléa.

CAHILL, KEVIN M., ed. 1993. *A Framework for Survival: Health, Human Rights, and Humanitarian Assistance in Conflicts and Disasters.* New York: Basic Books.

CENTERS FOR DISEASE CONTROL AND PREVENTION (CDC). 1992. "Famine-Affected, Refugee, and Displaced Populations: Recommendations for Public Health Issues." *Morbidity and Mortality Weekly Report* 41 (RR–13):1–76.

COBEY, JAMES C.; FLANAGIN, ANNETTE; and FOEGE, WILLIAM H. 1993. "Effective Humanitarian Aid: Our Only Hope for Intervention in Civil War." *Journal of the American Medical Association* 270, no. 5:632–634.

DEWEY, ARTHUR. 1993. "The Military Role in Emergency Response." In *New Strategies for a Restless World,* pp. 45–50. Edited by Harlan Cleveland. Minneapolis, Minn.: American Refugee Committee.

GARFIELD, RICHARD M., and NEUGUT, ALFRED I. 1991. "Epidemiologic Analysis of Warfare: A Historical Review." *Journal of the American Medical Association* 266, no. 5:688–692.

GEIGER, H. JACK, and COOK-DEEGAN, ROBERT M. 1993. "The Role of Physicians in Conflicts and Humanitarian Crises: Case Studies from the Field Missions of Physicians for Human Rights, 1988–1993." *Journal of the American Medical Association* 270, no. 5:616–620.

GRANT, JAMES P. 1992. *The State of the World's Children, 1992.* New York: Oxford University Press.

HARVARD STUDY TEAM. 1991. "The Effect of the Gulf Crisis on the Children of Iraq." *New England Journal of Medicine* 325, no. 13:977–980.

INTERNATIONAL COMMITTEE OF THE RED CROSS (ICRC). 1950. *The Geneva Conventions of August 12, 1949: Analysis for the Use of National Red Cross Societies.* Geneva: Author.

JEAN, FRANÇOIS. 1992. "The Former Yugoslavia." In *Populations in Danger,* pp. 15–20. Edited by François Jean. London: John Libbey.

MacCRAI, JOANNA, and ZWI, ANTHONY B. 1992. "Food as an Instrument of War in Contemporary African Famines: A Review of the Evidence." *Disasters* 16, no. 4:299–321.

MOORE, PATRICK S.; MARFIN, ANTHONY A.; QUENEMOEN, LYNN E.; GESSNER, BRADFORD D.; AYUB, AXMED Y. S.; MILLER, DANIEL; SULLIVAN, KEVIN M.; and TOOLE, MICHAEL T. 1993. "Mortality Rates in Displaced and Resident Populations of Central Somalia During 1992 Famine." *Lancet* 341, no. 8850:935–938.

SWISS, SHANA, and GILLER, JOAN E. 1993. "Rape as a Crime of War." *Journal of the American Medical Association* 270, no. 5:612–615.

TOOLE, MICHAEL J.; GALSON, STEVEN; and BRADY, WILLIAM. 1993. "Are War and Public Health Compatible?" *Lancet* 341, no. 8854:1193–1196.

TOOLE, MICHAEL, and WALDMAN, RONALD. 1993. "Refugees and Displaced Persons: War, Hunger, and Public Health." *Journal of the American Medical Association* 270, no. 5:600–605.

U.S. COMMITTEE FOR REFUGEES. 1993. *World Refugee Survey, 1993.* Washington, D.C.: Author.

ZWI, ANTHONY, and UGALDE, ANTONIO. 1991. "Political Violence in the Third World: A Public Health Issue." *Health Policy and Planning* 6, no. 3:203–217.

## III. NUCLEAR WARFARE

On August 6, 1945, a single bomb from a U.S. warplane obliterated most of the Japanese city of Hiroshima, killing over 100,000 people, almost all civilians. Three days later, 70,000 more civilians were killed by a single warhead that exploded over the city of Nagasaki.

In the weeks after the bombings, many initial survivors in Hiroshima and Nagasaki began developing medical problems that baffled local physicians—hair loss, hemorrhaging, very low blood cell counts, diarrhea, and infections—now known as the classic manifestations of radiation sickness resulting from a nuclear explosion.

After proposals in the late 1940s to place all nuclear weapons under international control failed, the United States and the Soviet Union—followed later by the United Kingdom, France, and then China—entered an expanding "nuclear arms race" in which the size, number, and different types of nuclear weaponry grew rapidly. Hundreds of nuclear test explosions were conducted, both in the atmosphere and under water, resulting in radioactive exposure of nearby civilians and in the worldwide distribution of radioisotopes including strontium-90, detectable in baby teeth of children in the United States.

Alarmed by the immediate health hazards posed by the testing of nuclear weapons, and also concerned about the long-term effects of radiation on the human gene pool, physicians such as Albert Schweitzer, who had been awarded the 1952 Nobel Peace Prize, joined with scientists and many others in calling for a ban on all nuclear test explosions (Schweitzer, 1958) and for the abolition of nuclear weapons. In 1962, a series of articles describing the medical consequences of thermonuclear war was published in the *New England Journal of Medicine* by a group of physicians who formed a new organization called Physicians for Social Responsibility (PSR) (Sidel et al., 1962). The authors estimated that following a thermonuclear attack on Boston more than two million people would die in the Boston area alone, with 1.5 million citizens injured immediately after the attack. The majority of medical facilities would be destroyed, the disposal of corpses would be difficult or impossible, and the risks of epidemic disease would be high. Given the inability of the medical profession to respond effectively to such devastation, the authors concluded that "physicians, charged with the responsibility for the lives of their patients and the health of their communities, must also explore a new area of preventive medicine, the prevention of thermonuclear war" (Sidel et al., 1962, p. 1144).

A formal argument for medical responsibility with regard to preventing nuclear war was articulated as follows (Cassel and Jameton, 1982):

1. Physicians have a special and central professional responsibility to treat disease and to reduce mortality.
2. A large-scale nuclear war would cause death and illness on a massive and unprecedented scale.
3. Physicians would be unable to intervene effectively in the human injury and death expected in a large-scale nuclear war.
4. Prevention is the only way to reduce mortality where treatment is ineffective.
5. A large-scale nuclear war is possible, or even probable, in the decades ahead.
6. Efforts by physicians could help prevent nuclear war.
7. Therefore, physicians have a central and urgent professional responsibility to help prevent nuclear war.

Many physicians and scientists worked to fulfill this responsibility through participation in the preparation of scholarly reports by organizations such as the World Health Organization (WHO) and the Institute of Medicine (IOM) of the U.S. National Academy of Sciences, summarizing scientific knowledge about the likely effects of nuclear war and identifying previously unsuspected health aspects of nuclear warfare. One report in the mid-1980s concluded that a large-scale nuclear war between the United States and the Soviet Union might result in several hundred million human fatalities from burn, blast, and radiation effects; in addition, climatic change and disruption of energy supplies needed to support agriculture could cause more than one billion deaths in developing countries, thousands of miles from the nuclear explosions themselves (Harwell et al., 1985; Pittock et al., 1985). Computer models of a "nuclear winter," caused by blockage of sunlight by massive injection of smoke into the atmosphere, raised the possibility of human extinction.

In 1981, members of PSR and similar organizations in other countries joined together in a new organization, International Physicians for the Prevention of Nuclear War (IPPNW). IPPNW was awarded the 1985 Nobel Peace Prize for its educational activities, undertaken collaboratively by physicians from the United States, the Soviet Union, and many other nations. In its announcement, the Nobel Committee applauded IPPNW for performing "considerable service to mankind by spreading authoritative information and by creating an awareness of the catastrophic consequence of nuclear warfare. . . . This in turn contributes to an increase in the pressure of public opposition to the proliferation of nuclear weapons. . . . Such an awakening of public opinion . . . can give the present arms limitation negotiations new perspectives and a new seriousness."

## Controversies

During the 1980s, many of the activities of PSR and of IPPNW were considered controversial, both within the medical community and among political and other leaders. Some critics argued that, with sufficient preparation, some significant medical response to nuclear attack was in fact possible, and that limiting professional efforts to prevention was thus irresponsible. Others disagreed about the likelihood of large-scale nuclear war, or about whether efforts by physicians could reduce that likelihood. Even those who accepted the argument as summarized by Christine Cassel and Andrew Jameton (1982) disagreed about the proper activities—ranging from research and education to political advocacy—through which medical responsibility for the prevention of nuclear war should be fulfilled. Although it might be appropriate for physicians to describe and warn of the medical consequences of use of nuclear weapons, as well as of limitations in the capacity of health professionals to respond in the wake of nuclear attack, some argued that physicians should refrain from proposing any specific recommendations—such as a ban on nuclear tests or a freeze on the production of weapons—about how the risk of nuclear war might be reduced (Relman, 1986). Some criticized PSR and IPPNW for "medicalizing" problems—and possible solutions—that were more properly viewed as political, social, or military in nature.

A particularly intense controversy centered on the ethical responsibilities of physicians in making plans for medical care following nuclear attack, especially following a 1982 request from the U.S. Department of Defense that U.S. health-care facilities prepare explicit contingency plans for handling casualties from a possible nuclear war. Some physicians argued that the capacity of the health profession to mitigate the devastation following nuclear attack was so limited that participation by physicians in planning any such response would not only be a waste of professional effort, but also might fuel dangerous misconceptions about the survivability of nuclear war. This might in turn increase the likelihood of such a war. Others argued, however, that just as physicians do not abandon patients in individual clinical care when the odds of success are small but not zero, physicians should not refuse to participate in plans for providing medical care—even of limited effectiveness—to citizens after nuclear attack. In 1988, the British Medical Association published *Selection of Casualties for Treatment After Nuclear Attack: A Document for Discussion*, which reviewed evidence about the health problems that could exist following nuclear attack and emphasized the agonizingly difficult ethical problems that would face physicians in a postattack period. These issues include triage and involvement in active euthanasia, as large numbers of individuals would likely be suffering from severe pain with inadequate analgesics available. To many readers, this stark portrayal of the postattack period was added evidence that physicians should focus exclusively on a preventive approach to ensure that nuclear war would never take place.

Other ethical issues raised in relation to nuclear weapons include abuses of informed consent in experiments done within the United States to assess the effects of plutonium exposure on military personnel and civilians, as well as the failure to provide information for individuals working within the nuclear weapons industry about the risks to their health from occupational exposures. Beginning in the 1990s, the opening of archives both in the former Soviet Union and in the Department of Energy in the United States brought to light the extensive patterns of secrecy prevailing from the 1940s on regarding nuclear testing. These included deception about the conduct of nuclear test explosions (the United States alone exploded more than 200 nuclear warheads unannounced) and misleading information about the size of nuclear arsenals (the former Soviet Union had approximately 20,000 more warheads than had ever been acknowledged). Important information related to the health hazards associated with nuclear weapons production was regularly withheld from public debate and from workers themselves.

The moral arguments physicians posed against the development and possible use of nuclear weapons were formally linked with efforts to address the threat of nuclear war through international law. In May 1993, WHO petitioned the International Court of Justice to issue an advisory opinion on the legality of the use of nuclear weapons in armed conflict. Opponents claimed that this action distorted the health-related work of WHO for political purposes, while supporters argued that it was only the political interests of the nuclear weapons states that led them to attempt to interfere with WHO's legitimate concern about the health risks posed by their nuclear arsenals.

Despite these activities, by the mid-1990s even the fulfillment of all existing political agreements to reduce nuclear weapons by the early twenty-first century would leave arsenals with the explosive force of more than two tons of TNT for each man, woman, and child on earth—the equivalent of more than 500,000 Hiroshima bombs.

LACHLAN FORROW

*Directly related to this article are the other articles in this entry:* MEDICINE AND WAR, PUBLIC HEALTH AND WAR, CHEMICAL AND BIOLOGICAL WEAPONS, *and* INTERNATIONAL WEAPONS TRADE. *For a further discussion of topics mentioned in this article, see the entries* DEATH AND DYING: EUTHANASIA AND SUSTAINING LIFE; INFORMED CONSENT, *article on* CONSENT ISSUES IN HUMAN RESEARCH; OCCUPATIONAL SAFETY AND HEALTH, *article on* ETHICAL ISSUES; RESEARCH, UNETHICAL; *and* TRIAGE. *Other relevant material may be found under the entries* HEALTH OFFICIALS AND THEIR RESPONSIBILITIES; RESPONSIBILITY; *and* VALUE AND VALUATION.

## Bibliography

BRITISH MEDICAL ASSOCIATION. 1988. *Selection of Casualties for Treatment After Nuclear Attack: A Document for Discussion.* London: Author.

CASSEL, CHRISTINE, and JAMETON, ANDREW. 1982. "Medical Responsibility and Thermonuclear War." *Annals of Internal Medicine* 97, no. 3:426–432.

HARWELL, M. A.; HUTCHINSON, T. C.; CRUPPER, W. P., JR.; HARWELL, C. C.; and GROVER, H. D. 1985. *Ecological and Agricultural Effects.* Vol. 2 of *Environmental Consequences of Nuclear War.* SCOPE, no. 28. Chichester, U.K.: John Wiley & Sons.

PITTOCK, A. B.; ACKERMAN, T. P.; CRUTZEN, P. J.; MacCRACKEN, M. C.; SHAPIRO, C. S.; and TURCO, R. P. 1985. *Physical and Atmospheric Effects.* Vol. 1 of *Environmental Consequences of Nuclear War.* SCOPE, no. 28. Chichester, U.K.: John Wiley & Sons.

RELMAN, ARNOLD S. 1986. "The Physician's Role in Preventing Nuclear War." *New England Journal of Medicine* 315, no. 14:889–891.

SCHWEITZER, ALBERT. 1958. *Peace or Atomic War?* New York: Henry Holt.

SIDEL, VICTOR W.; GEIGER, H. JACK; and LOWN, BERNARD. 1962. "The Physician's Role in the Post Attack Period." *New England Journal of Medicine* 266, no. 22:1137–1145.

SOLOMON, FREDERIC, and MARSTON, ROBERT Q., eds. 1986. *The Medical Implications of Nuclear War.* Washington, D.C.: National Academy Press.

WORLD HEALTH ORGANIZATION (WHO). 1984. *Effects of Nuclear War on Health and Health Services: Report of the International Committee of Experts in Medical Services and Public Health to Implement Resolution WHA34.38.* WHO Pub. A36/12. Geneva: Author.

## IV. CHEMICAL AND BIOLOGICAL WEAPONS

The development, production, storage, transfer, use, and even destruction (demilitarization) of chemical and biological weapons (CBW) pose a number of related ethical issues. First, these weapons, like nuclear weapons, are largely indiscriminate in their effects and are generally more effective against vulnerable noncombatants than against combatants; they are therefore known as "weapons of mass destruction," and their use is widely considered to be a violation of the proportionality principle of "just war." Second, these weapons, like nuclear weapons, are the subject of intensive international arms-control efforts involving problems of definition, verification, and enforcement. Third, biomedical scientists and physicians may be called on to participate in research and development on more effective CBW, as well as on methods for defense against them and on treatment of their victims.

## Chemical weapons

Chemical weapons (CW), which have been known since antiquity, are designed to produce direct chemical injury to their targets in contrast to explosive or incendiary weapons, which produce their effect through blast or heat. In the siege of the city of Plataea in 429 B.C.E., for example, the Spartans placed enormous cauldrons of pitch, sulfur, and burning charcoal outside the city walls to harass the defenders. Although nations signing the 1899 Hague Declaration promised not to use CW, during World War I these weapons—including, in order of use, tear gas, chlorine gas, phosgene, and mustard gas—were employed. Overall, 125,000 tons of CW were used during World War I, resulting in 1.3 million casualties. One-quarter of all casualties in the American Expeditionary Force in France were caused by them (Harris and Paxman, 1982; Sidel and Goldwyn, 1966; Sidel, 1989; United Nations, 1969; World Health Organization, 1970.

In 1925, twenty-eight nations negotiated the Geneva Protocol for the "prohibition of the use in war of asphyxiating poisonous or other gases and of all analogous liquids, materials or devices and of bacteriological methods of warfare" (Wright, 1990, p. 368). In fact, however, the Protocol prohibited only the use, not the development, production, testing, or stockpiling, of these weapons. Furthermore, many of the nations ratifying the Protocol reserved the right to use such weapons in retaliation, and the Protocol became in effect a "no first use" treaty with no verification or enforcement provisions. The United States was one of the initial signers, but the U.S. Senate did not ratify the treaty until 1975 (Sidel, 1989; Wright, 1990).

Despite the Protocol, use of CW continued. Italy used mustard gas during its invasion of Abyssinia (Ethiopia), and Japan used mustard and tear gases in its invasion of China. Germany, with its excellent dye and pesticide industries, developed acetylcholinesterase inhibitors known as nerve gases, and the United States and Britain stockpiled CW during World War II; transportation and storage accidents caused casualties (Infield, 1971), but there was no direct military use. Following World War II, CW were used by Egypt in Yemen; mustard and nerve gases were used in the Iran–Iraq war; and Iraq used CW against Kurdish villages in its own territory. CW stockpiles and production facilities in Iraq were ordered destroyed by the United Nations following the 1991 Persian Gulf War. The United States and Russia are known to maintain CW stockpiles, and a number of other countries have either stockpiles or facilities for rapid CW production (Harris and Paxman, 1982; Sidel, 1989).

Troops can be protected against these weapons for limited periods by the use of gas masks and impenetrable garments. Such protective gear, however, reduces the efficiency of troops by as much as 50 percent and damages morale, so use or threat of use of CW may continue to be considered effective against troops. Civilian populations, on the other hand, cannot be adequately protected. Israel, for example, provides every civilian in the country with a gas mask and a self-injectable syringe filled with atropine, a temporary antidote to nerve gas. However, this limited protection is inadequate against weapons such as mustard gas that attack the skin, or against longer-term exposure to nerve gas. Furthermore, poorly trained civilians are likely to injure themselves with equipment like self-injectable syringes (Amitai et al., 1992).

Production of CW has been associated with serious accidents to workers and with high levels of pollution in the production sites and nearby communities. Tests of mustard gas, nerve agents, and psychochemicals, including lysergic acid diethylamide (LSD), during and after World War II involved thousands of military personnel, many of whom subsequently claimed disabilities from the exposure. Records of participation and of effects are so poor that only a small fraction of those who participated can be identified. Even destruction of the weapons is dangerous, since toxic ash is produced by their incineration (Sidel, 1993).

A Chemical Weapons Convention (CWC) that prohibits the development, production, storage, and transfer of these weapons and calls for their demilitarization was approved by the United Nations General Assembly in 1992. It was signed by 136 nations in January 1993, with additional nations continuing to add their signatures; ratification and adoption of implementing legislation are proceeding in the signatory nations. However, many issues, including verification, weapons destruction methods, and penalties for noncompliance, remain to be solved by the Preparatory Commission before the CWC comes into effect.

In the 1960s and 1970s the United States used both tear gas and herbicides in Vietnam. Although most nations that are parties to the Geneva Protocol considered tear gas and herbicides to be CW, and thus prohibited under the provisions of the Protocol, the United States until recently rejected that interpretation (Sidel and Goldwyn, 1966; Sidel, 1989). Many countries use tear gas on a regular basis to quell civil disorders (Hu et al., 1989). The signatories to the CWC have agreed not to use riot-control agents or herbicides as weapons of war.

## Biological weapons

Biological weapons (BW) depend upon the ability of microorganisms to infect and multiply in the attacked organism. In this they differ from toxins, which, as biological products used as chemicals, are covered under CW as well as BW treaties. BW are very hard to defend against and are not as controllable or predictable in their use as are CW (Harris and Paxman, 1982; Geissler, 1986; Sidel and Goldwyn, 1966; Sidel, 1989; United Nations, 1969; World Health Organization, 1970).

The effects of BW were officially summarized by a U.S. government agency in 1959: "Biological warfare is the intentional use of living organisms or their toxic products to cause death, disability, or damage in man, animals, or plants. The target is man, either by causing sickness or death or through limitation of his food supplies or other agricultural resources. . . . Biological warfare has been aptly described as public health in reverse" (U.S. Department of Health, Education, and Welfare, 1959).

BW have been known since antiquity. Persia, Greece, and Rome used diseased corpses to contaminate sources of drinking water. In 1347, Mongols besieging the walled city of Caffa (now called Feodosiya), a seaport on the east coast of the Crimea, began to die of the plague. The attackers threw their comrades' corpses into the besieged city; the defenders, who were Genoans, fled back to Genoa and carried the plague further into Europe. During the French and Indian Wars, Lord Jeffrey Amherst, commander of the British forces at Fort Pitt, gave tribal emissaries blankets in which smallpox victims had slept (Harris and Paxman, 1982; Geissler, 1986).

During World War I, Germany is alleged to have used the equine disease glanders against the cavalries of eastern European countries (Harris and Paxman, 1982, p. 74). According to testimony at the Nuremberg trials, prisoners in German concentration camps were infected during tests of BW. Great Britain and the United States, fearing the Germans would use BW in World War II, developed their own. The British tested anthrax spores on Gruinard Island, off the coast of Scotland; the island remained uninhabitable for decades. The United States developed anthrax spores, botulism toxin, and other agents as BW but did not use them (Bernstein, 1987).

In the 1930s, Japanese troops dropped rice and wheat mixed with plague-carrying fleas from planes, resulting in plague in areas of China that had been previously free of it. During World War II, Japanese laboratories conducted extensive experiments on prisoners of war using a wide variety of organisms selected for possible use as BW, including anthrax, plague, gas gangrene, encephalitis, typhus, typhoid, hemorrhagic fever, cholera, smallpox, and tularemia (Wright, 1990). Unlike the Soviet Union, which in 1949 prosecuted twelve of those involved in this work, the United States never prosecuted any of the participants. Instead, U.S. researchers met with Japanese biological-warfare experts in Tokyo and urged that the experts be "spared embarrassment" so the United States could benefit from their knowledge (Powell, 1981; Williams and Wallace, 1989).

**Difficulties of surveillance.** After World War II development of BW continued. None of the numerous allegations of BW use have been substantiated (or even fully investigated), but it is known that extensive BW testing has been done. In the 1950s and 1960s, for example, the University of Utah conducted secret, large-scale field tests of BW, including tularemia, Rocky Mountain spotted fever, plague, and Q fever, at the U.S. Army Dugway Proving Ground. In 1950 U.S. Navy ships released as simulants (materials believed to be nonpathogenic that mimic the spread of BW) large quantities of bacteria in the San Francisco Bay area to test the efficiency of their dispersal. Some analysts attributed subsequent infections and deaths to one of these organisms. During the 1950s and 1960s, the United States conducted 239 top-secret, open-air disseminations of simulants, involving such areas as the New York City subways and Washington National Airport (Cole, 1988). The U.S. military developed a large infrastructure of laboratories, test facilities, and production plants related to BW. By the end of the 1960s, the United States had stockpiles of at least ten different biological and toxin weapons (Geissler, 1986). A 1979 outbreak of pulmonary anthrax in the Soviet Union is now said to have been caused by accidental release from a Soviet BW factory. Recent disclosures by Russian scientists indicate extensive environmental contamination and medical problems due to CW production ("Russian Experts," 1993).

In 1969 the Nixon administration—with the concurrence of the Defense Department, which declared that BW lacked "military usefulness"—unconditionally renounced U.S. development, production, stockpiling, and use of BW, and announced that the United States would unilaterally dismantle its BW program. In 1972 the Soviet Union, which had urged a more comprehensive treaty including restrictions on CW, ended its opposition to a separate BW treaty. The United States, the Soviet Union, and other nations negotiated the Convention on the Prohibition of the Development, Prevention and Stockpiling of Bacteriological (Biological) and Toxin Weapons and on Their Destruction (BWC). The BWC prohibits—except for "prophylactic, protective and other peaceful purposes"—the development or acquisition of biological agents or toxins, as well as weapons carrying them and means of their production, stockpiling, transfer, or delivery. The U.S. Senate ratified the BWC in 1975, the same year it ratified the Geneva Protocol of 1925. As of 1987, 110 nations had ratified the BWC and an additional twenty-five nations had signed but not yet ratified it (Wright, 1990).

Invoking the specter of possible new biological weapons and unproven allegations of aggressive BW programs in other countries, the Reagan administration initiated intensive efforts to conduct "defensive research," permitted under the BWC. The budget for the U.S. Army Biological Defense Research Program (BDRP), which sponsors programs in a wide variety of academic, commercial, and government laboratories, increased dramatically during the 1980s. Much of this research work is medical in nature, including the development of immunizations and of treatments against organisms that might be used as BW (Piller and Yamamoto, 1988; Wright, 1990).

While research and development of new BW is outlawed by the BWC, it is possible that it will still occur. Novel dangers lie in new genetic technologies, which permit development of genetically altered organisms not known in nature. Stable, tailor-made organisms used as BW could travel long distances and still be infectious, rapidly infiltrate a population, cause debilitating effects very quickly, and be resistant to antibiotic treatment (Piller and Yamamoto, 1988).

### Ethical issues for biomedical scientists

Biologists, chemists, biomedical scientists, and physicians have played important roles in CBW research and development. Fritz Haber, awarded the 1918 Nobel Prize in chemistry for his synthesis of ammonia, is known as the father of Germany's chemical weapons program of World War I. In his speech accepting the Nobel Prize, Haber declared poison gas "a higher form of killing" (Harris and Paxman, 1982). By contrast, during the Crimean War the British government consulted the noted physicist Michael Faraday on the feasibility of developing poison gases; Faraday responded that it was entirely feasible, but that it was inhumane and he would have nothing to do with it (Russell, 1962).

Many scientists who explicitly recognize the ethical conflicts involved in work on weapons argue that a higher ethical principle—the imperative of defending one's country or of helping to curb what is perceived as evil or destructive—permits or even demands participation in such work. Dr. Theodor Rosebury, who worked on BW during World War II, based his participation on his belief that crisis circumstances, expected to pass in a limited time, required that he act as he did. "We were fighting a fire, and it seemed necessary to risk getting dirty as well as burnt," he later wrote (Rosebury, 1963). Rosebury refused any further participation in BW work after the end of the war (Rosebury, 1949).

Other scientists resolved their ethical dilemma by arguing that their work on weapons was designed to reduce the devastation of war. For example, Dr. Knut

Krieger, while working on "nonlethal" CBW in the 1960s, argued that his research would lead to decreased fatalities: "If we do indeed succeed in creating incapacitating systems and are able to substitute incapacitation for death it appears to me that, next to stopping war, this would be an important step forward" (Reid, 1969).

Relevant ethical concerns about "defensive research" on BW by biomedical scientists include content, safety, context, and locus (Lappé, 1990).

**Content.**    The Japanese laboratory established in 1933 to develop BW was called the Epidemic Prevention Laboratory. One of its activities was supplying vaccines for troops bound for Manchuria, but its major work was developing and testing BW (Powell, 1981). Military forces today could conduct research on offensive use of BW under the cover of defensive research, since "offensive" and "defensive" research are inextricably joined in at least some phases of the work (Huxsoll et al., 1989). During the parts of the work in which offensive and defensive efforts are parallel, it is possible that new forms of organisms may be found or developed that would be more effective as biological weapons. The possibility that offensive work on BW is being done in the United States under the cover of defensive work has been denied by the leadership of the BDRP, who point out where the two types of research diverge (Huxsoll et al., 1989). Critics nonetheless raise questions about the ambiguity of BDRP research, arguing that "these efforts are highly ambiguous, provocative and strongly suggestive of offensive goals" (Jacobson and Rosenberg, 1989; Piller and Yamamoto, 1988; Wright, 1990).

**Safety.**    Many analysts believe that CW or BW research, even if truly defensive in intent, may be dangerous to surrounding communities if toxic materials or virulent infectious organisms are accidentally released.

**Context.**    CW or BW research, even if truly defensive in intent, can be viewed by a potential military adversary as an attempt to develop protection for a nation's military forces or its noncombatants against weapons the nation itself might wish to use for offensive purposes, thus permitting that nation to protect its own personnel in a CW or BW first strike. In fact, the military justification for preparing any form of altered organisms is that they are needed for preparation of defenses. It is therefore impossible for adversaries to determine whether a nation's "defensive" efforts are part of preparation for an "offensive" use of weapons.

**Locus.**    These fears are usually based on military sponsorship of "defensive" BW research. Other nations may view with suspicion, even if the research is relatively open, the intense interest of military forces rather than civilian medical researchers in vaccines or treatment against specific organisms. Such fears can help feed a continuing BW arms race.

More generally, concern has been expressed about the militarization of genetic engineering and of biology in general. Characterization of biological weapons as "public health in reverse" may therefore have an even broader and more sinister meaning: the entire field of biology—and particular aspects of it such as the use of human genome research to design weapons to target specific groups—may be in danger of military subversion to destructive ends (Piller and Yamamoto, 1988; Wright, 1990). The imprisonment of a chemist by the Russian government and the revocation of his university diploma for publishing an article describing the development of new, highly toxic CW illustrates the restrictions on scientists engaged in CBW research (Janowski, 1993).

### Ethical issues for physicians

The question that first arises is whether it is constructive to view certain ethical responsibilities as peculiar to the physician's social role. Theodor Rosebury described the response to physician participation in work on BW during World War II: "There was much quiet but searching discussion among us regarding the place of doctors in such work . . . a certain delicacy concentrated most of the physicians into principally or primarily defensive operations." Rosebury goes on to point out that the modifiers "principally" and "primarily" are needed "because military operations can never be exclusively defensive" (Rosebury, 1963). What is seen as the special responsibility of physicians is based largely on an ethical responsibility not to use the power of the physician to do harm (*primum non nocere*). While the Hippocratic oath as written seems to apply to the relationship of the physician to an individual patient, its meaning has been broadened by many to proscribe physician participation in actions harmful to nonpatients.

So far as research on "offensive" weapons of war is concerned, there seems to be a consensus that physicians participate in such research at their ethical peril, even if their country demands it or they think it useful for "deterrence" or other "preventive" purposes. But because of the ambiguity of "defensive" work on BW, the dilemma for the physician is not easily resolved, even for those who believe that "defensive" efforts are ethically permissible.

Some proponents of defensive research on BW have argued that it is entirely ethical—that, in fact, responsibility demands—that physicians work on it. According to this perspective, not only will defenses be needed if such weapons are used against the United States but this work may also be useful in developing protection against naturally occurring diseases (Crozier, 1971; Huxsoll et al., 1989; Orient, 1989). Other analysts take a different position. They believe it unethical for physicians to play a role in military-sponsored BW research because it has a strong potential for intensifying a BW arms race and helping to militarize the science of biology, thus increasing the risk of the use of BW and the destructiveness of their effects if they are used (Jacobson and Rosenberg, 1989; Nass, 1991; Sidel, 1991).

The question is, where on the "slippery slope" of physician participation in preparing for use of BW should physicians draw the line? If physicians engage in civilian-sponsored research on disease control that carries an obligation to report all findings in the open literature, even if the research may have implications for BW, such participation, most analysts agree, cannot be ethically faulted. When, on the other hand, physicians engage in military-sponsored research in which the openness of reporting is equivocal and the purposes ambiguous, it is difficult to distinguish their work ethically from that on the development of weapons.

As noted, the BWC prohibits any "development, production, stockpiling, transfer or acquisition of biological agents or toxins"—except for "prophylactic, protective and other peaceful purposes." The responsibility for government-sponsored medical research for prophylactic, protective, and other peaceful purposes in the United States lies largely with the National Institutes of Health (NIH) and the Centers for Disease Control (CDC). The NIH or the CDC might therefore be given the responsibility and the resources for medical research of this type. The U. S. Army may still want to conduct nonmedical research and development on defense against BW, such as work on detectors, protective clothing, and other barriers to the spread of organisms. Under this proposed division of effort, such research is less likely to be seen as offensive, less likely to provoke a BW race, less likely to pervert the science of biology, and less likely to involve physicians (Sidel, 1989).

A different type of ethical issue related to CBW arose during the Persian Gulf War in 1991. The United States provided protective measures, such as immunization against botulinum toxin and anthrax, for its military forces. Despite the fact that some of these measures were experimental, no informed-consent procedures were used and compliance was often required. Furthermore, these measures were made available to military forces but not to noncombatants in the area (Annas, 1992; Howe and Martin, 1991).

In addition to the ethical dilemmas involved in these decisions, it may be unethical for physicians simply to ignore the issues involved in CBW. One of the greatest dangers of these weapons may be the apathy of the medical profession toward them. The fact that BW are the ones with which physicians may become engaged and the ones about which they have specialized knowledge gives physicians a special responsibility not only to

refuse to work on them but also actively to work to reduce the threat of CBW development or use.

## Conclusion

Physicians and biomedical scientists should support methods for international epidemiologic surveillance to detect the use of BW and to investigate incidents in which use has been alleged after an unexplained disease outbreak (Geissler, 1986; Nass, 1992a, 1992b) and support the Vaccines for Peace Programme for control of "dual-threat" agents (Geissler and Woodall, 1994). Support might also be given for measures to strengthen the BWC by introduction of verification proposals put forth at the 1991 BWC Review Conference (Falk, 1990; Rosenberg and Burck, 1990; Rosenberg, 1993). With regard to chemical weapons, biomedical scientists and physicians might support effective implementation of the 1993 CWC (Smithson, 1993).

More broadly, physicians may wish to explore the connection between CBW and nuclear weapons. It has been argued that the nuclear powers, by refusing to substantially reduce their vast stockpiles of nuclear weapons and by refusing to agree to verifiable cessation of nuclear-weapons testing and production, provoke nonnuclear powers to contemplate development and production of CBW for "deterrence" against nuclear weapons. The U.S. Defense Intelligence Agency reported that "third world nations view chemical weapons as an attractive and inexpensive alternative to nuclear weapons" (U.S. General Accounting Office, 1986; Zilinskas, 1990a, 1990b). There is much physicians can do, for example, through the International Physicians for the Prevention of Nuclear War (the organization that received the 1985 Nobel Peace Prize) and its affiliates in many countries, to reduce the provocation and the proliferation of weapons of mass destruction caused by the continuing nuclear-arms race.

Individual physicians and scientists can add to the awareness of the dangers of CBW by signing the pledge, sponsored by the Council for Responsible Genetics (5 Upland Road, Cambridge, Mass. 02140), "not to engage knowingly in research and teaching that will further development of chemical and biological warfare agents." U.S. physicians also may wish to support legislation to transfer all medical aspects of biological defense from the military to the NIH or the CDC. Physicians may help awaken the medical profession to the dangers of CBW and nuclear weapons by adding a clause to the oath taken by medical students upon graduation from medical school, similar to the oath for medical students in the former Soviet Union, requiring them "to struggle tirelessly for peace and for the prevention of nuclear war" (Cassel et al., 1985, p. 652). The addition might, for example, be worded thus: "Recognizing that nuclear, chemical, and biological arms are weapons of indiscriminate mass destruction and threaten the health of all humanity, I will refuse to play any role that might increase the risk of use of such weapons and will, as part of my professional responsibility, work actively for peace and for the prevention of their use."

VICTOR W. SIDEL

*Directly related to this article are the other articles in this entry:* MEDICINE AND WAR, PUBLIC HEALTH AND WAR, NUCLEAR WARFARE, *and* INTERNATIONAL WEAPONS TRADE. *For a further discussion of topics mentioned in this article, see the entries* CONFLICT OF INTEREST; HARM; PRISONERS, *article on* RESEARCH ISSUES; RESEARCH, UNETHICAL; *and* RESPONSIBILITY. *Other relevant material may be found under the entries* BIOETHICS; BIOMEDICAL ENGINEERING; BIOTECHNOLOGY; HAZARDOUS WASTES AND TOXIC SUBSTANCES; HEALTH OFFICIALS AND THEIR RESPONSIBILITIES; HEALTH POLICY, *article on* HEALTH POLICY IN INTERNATIONAL PERSPECTIVE; INTERNATIONAL HEALTH; JUSTICE; MILITARY PERSONNEL AS RESEARCH SUBJECTS; PUBLIC HEALTH, *articles on* DETERMINANTS OF PUBLIC HEALTH, *and* PHILOSOPHY OF PUBLIC HEALTH; PUBLIC POLICY AND BIOETHICS; TECHNOLOGY, *article on* TECHNOLOGY ASSESSMENT; *and* VALUE AND VALUATION.

## Bibliography

AMITAI, YONA; ALMOG, SHLOMO; SINGER, RAPHAEL; HAMMER, RUTH; BENTUR, YEDIDIA; and DANON, YEHUDE L. 1992. "Atropine Poisoning in Children During the Persian Gulf Crisis: A National Survey in Israel." *Journal of the American Medical Association* 268, no. 5:630–632.

ANNAS, GEORGE J. 1992. "Changing the Consent Rules for Desert Storm." *New England Journal of Medicine* 326, no. 11:770–773.

BARSS, PETER. 1992. "Epidemic Field Investigation as Applied to Allegations of Chemical, Biological or Toxin Warfare." *Politics and the Life Sciences* 11, no. 1:5–22.

BERNSTEIN, BARTON J. 1987. "Churchill's Secret Biological Weapons." *Bulletin of the Atomic Scientists* 43, no. 1: 46–50.

CASSEL, CHRISTINE K.; JAMETON, ANDREW L.; SIDEL, VICTOR W.; and STOREY, PATRICK B. 1985. "The Physician's Oath and the Prevention of Nuclear War." *Journal of the American Medical Association* 254:652–654.

COLE, LEONARD A. 1988. *Clouds of Secrecy: The Army's Germ Warfare Tests over Populated Areas.* Totowa, N.J.: Rowman & Littlefield.

CROZIER, DAN. 1971. "The Physician and Biologic Warfare." *New England Journal of Medicine* 284, no. 18:1008–1011.

FALK, RICHARD. 1990. "Inhibiting Reliance on Biological Weaponry: The Role and Relevance of International Law." In *Preventing a Biological Arms Race,* pp. 241–266. Edited by Susan Wright. Cambridge, Mass.: MIT Press.

GEISSLER, ERHARD, ed. 1986. *Biological and Toxin Weapons Today.* London: Oxford University Press.

GEISSLER, ERHARD, and WOODALL, JOHN P. 1994. *Control of Dual-Threat Agents: The Vaccines for Peace Programme.* New York: Oxford University Press.

HARRIS, ROBERT, and PAXMAN, JEREMY. 1982. *A Higher Form of Killing: The Secret Story of Chemical and Biological Warfare.* New York: Hill & Wang.

HOWE, EDMUND G., and MARTIN, EDWARD D. 1991. "Treating the Troops." *Hastings Center Report* 21, no. 2:21–24.

HU, HOWARD; FINE, JONATHAN; EPSTEIN, PAUL; KELSEY, KARL; REYNOLDS, PRESTON; and WALKER, BAILUS. 1989. "Tear Gas: Harassing Agent or Toxic Chemical Weapon?" *Journal of the American Medical Association* 262, no. 5:660–663.

HUXSOLL, DAVID L.; PARROTT, CHERYL D.; and PATRICK, WILLIAM C. 1989. "Medicine in Defense Against Biological Warfare." *Journal of the American Medical Association* 262, no. 5:677–678.

INFIELD, GLENN B. 1971. *Disaster at Bari.* New York: Macmillan.

JACOBSON, JAY A., and ROSENBERG, BARBARA HATCH. 1989. "Biological Defense Research: Charting a Safer Course." *Journal of the American Medical Association* 262:675–676.

JANOWSKI, PAT. 1993. "Speak No Evil: A Dissident Is Detained for Revealing the Existence of a Powerful Poison Gas." *Sciences* 33, no. 6:4–5.

LAPPÉ, MARC. 1990. "Ethics in Biological Warfare Research." In *Preventing a Biological Arms Race,* pp. 78–99. Edited by Susan Wright. Cambridge, Mass.: MIT Press.

NASS, MERYL. 1991. "The Labyrinth of Biological Defense." *PSR Quarterly* 1:24–30.

———. 1992a. "Anthrax Epizootic in Zimbabwe, 1978–1980: Due to Deliberate Spread?" *PSR Quarterly* 2:198–209.

———. 1992b. "Can Biological, Toxin, and Chemical Warfare Be Eliminated?" *Politics and the Life Sciences* 11: 30–32.

ORIENT, JANE M. 1989. "Chemical and Biological Warfare: Should Defenses be Researched and Deployed?" *Journal of the American Medical Association* 262, no. 5:644–648.

PILLER, CHARLES, and YAMAMOTO, KEITH R. 1988. *Gene Wars: Military Control over the New Genetic Technologies.* New York: Beech Tree.

POWELL, JOHN W. 1981. "A Hidden Chapter in History." *Bulletin of the Atomic Scientists* 37, no. 8:44–52.

REID, ROBERT W. 1969. *Tongues of Conscience: Weapons Research and the Scientists' Dilemma.* New York: Walker.

ROSEBURY, THEODOR. 1949. *Peace or Pestilence: Biological Warfare and How to Avoid It.* New York: Whittlesey House.

———. 1963. "Medical Ethics and Biological Warfare." *Perspectives in Biology and Medicine* 6:512–523.

ROSENBERG, BARBARA HATCH. 1993. "Progress Toward Verification of the Biological Weapons Convention." In *Verification 1993,* pp. 189–196. Edited by J. B. Poole and R. Guthrie. Trowbridge, U.K.: Redmond.

ROSENBERG, BARBARA HATCH, and BURCK, GORDON. 1990. "Verification of Compliance with the Biological Weapons Convention." In *Preventing a Biological Arms Race,* pp. 300–329. Edited by Susan Wright. Cambridge, Mass.: MIT Press.

Russell, Bertrand. 1962. *Fact and Fiction.* New York: Simon and Schuster.

"Russian Experts Say Many Died Making Chemical Weapons." 1993. *New York Times,* December 24, p. A4.

Sidel, Victor W. 1989. "Weapons of Mass Destruction: The Greatest Threat to Public Health." *Journal of the American Medical Association* 262, no. 5:680–682.

———. 1991. "Biological Weapons Research and Physicians: Historical and Ethical Analysis." *PSR Quarterly* 1:31–42.

———. 1993. "Farewell to Arms: The Impact of the Arms Race on the Human Condition." *PSR Quarterly* 3:18–26.

Sidel, Victor W., and Goldwyn, Robert M. 1966. "Chemical and Biological Weapons—A Primer." *New England Journal of Medicine* 274, no. 1:21–27.

Smithson, Amy E., ed. 1993. *The Chemical Weapons Convention Handbook.* Washington, D.C.: Henry L. Stimson Center.

United Nations. 1969. *Chemical and Bacteriological (Biological) Weapons and the Effects of Their Possible Use: Report.* E.69.I.24. New York: Author.

U.S. Department of Health, Education, and Welfare. 1959. *Effects of Biological Warfare Agents: For Use in Readiness Planning.* Washington, D.C.: U.S. Government Printing Office.

U.S. General Accounting Office. 1986. *Chemical Warfare Progress and Problems in Defensive Capability: Report to the Chairman, Committee on Foreign Affairs, U.S. House of Representatives.* GAO/PEMD-86-11.

Williams, Peter, and Wallace, David. 1989. *Unit 731: The Japanese Army's Secret of Secrets.* London: Hodder & Stoughton.

World Health Organization. 1970. *Health Aspects of Chemical and Biological Weapons: Report of a WHO Group of Consultants.* Geneva: Author.

Wright, Susan, ed. 1990. *Preventing a Biological Arms Race.* Cambridge, Mass.: MIT Press.

Zilinskas, Raymond A. 1990a. "Biological Warfare and the Third World." *Politics and the Life Sciences* 9, no. 1:59–76.

———. 1990b. "Terrorism and Biological Weapons: Inevitable Alliance?" *Perspectives in Biology and Medicine* 34, no. 1:44–72.

## V. INTERNATIONAL WEAPONS TRADE

Modern warfare poses a direct and ongoing threat to public health that raises serious ethical issues for medical and scientific professionals. As Richard Rhodes has pointed out, "The scale of public man-made death in modern times is comparable with the scale of death in former times from epidemic disease" (Rhodes, 1988, p. 680). Because the greatest source of man-made death in the second half of the twentieth century stems from the scores of violent conflicts that have been fought on the soil of developing nations, the international traffic in armaments that fuels these wars is a legitimate concern for doctors and scientists, both in their professional capacities and in their roles as citizens.

Since World War II, more than forty million people have died in the more than 125 wars that have been fought in the developing world (Ball, 1991). The vast majority of the weaponry used in these conflicts has been supplied by the industrialized nations. Even in those cases where imported armaments are not used in active conflicts, they exact a heavy toll by diverting public resources from fulfilling unmet needs in health care, nutrition, education, environmental protection, and economic development. From 1978 to 1988, developing nations spent 23 percent more on the purchase of foreign weapons than they received in development aid, resulting in a significant net drain on their already fragile economies (Sivard, 1991). The public-health impacts of wars fought with imported conventional armaments last far beyond the formal conclusion of the conflicts themselves, as disruptions to agriculture, water and sewage systems, and housing patterns increase the incidence of illness and death (International Negotiation Network, 1992).

The greatest economic beneficiaries of the international arms trade are the weapons-producing firms and military establishments of the major supplier nations. Five countries—the United States, France, Russia, the United Kingdom, and China—control more than 85 percent of the global arms trade, which was running at roughly $50 billion per year by the end of the 1980s (O'Hanlon et al., 1992). These five major arms-supplying nations hold the key to the development of any meaningful international system of controlling arms transfers.

The nations of the developing world provide the largest market for armaments, and the leading recipients are concentrated in Asia and the Middle East. In 1992, the top five recipients—Taiwan, Saudi Arabia, Indonesia, Kuwait, and Malaysia—accounted for more than three-quarters of the dollar value of weapons imports to the Third World (Grimmett, 1993). However, these figures do not fully account for the growing black-market trade in light weaponry that is fueling dozens of ethnic and territorial conflicts from Rwanda to Somalia to the former Yugoslavia to Afghanistan (Klare, 1994).

Throughout the Cold War era, despite periodic public protests, the arms trade was by and large treated as a sort of necessary evil of international affairs. Curbing arms sales took a backseat to concerns about controlling and reducing arsenals of nuclear, chemical, and biological weaponry. The Persian Gulf War of 1990–1991 brought about a sea change in public and governmental attitudes regarding the relative urgency of exerting control over the arms trade. This shift stemmed from two principal factors: the destructive power of the conventional armaments used in the conflict and the fact that the majority of nations that intervened to reverse Iraq's invasion of Kuwait had supplied arms to the Iraqi armed forces until the eve of the war (Hartung, 1994).

In light of these developments, the international political debate over the arms trade moved from the question of whether to curb weapons trafficking to the issue of how best to do so. In 1991 alone, the five major arms-supplying nations agreed to common guidelines on transfers of weaponry to regions of potential conflict; the United Nations began to implement a voluntary register that will record major weapons shipments as a means of guarding against destabilizing arms buildups; and officials of the World Bank and the International Monetary Fund began to discuss restricting loans to nations that overspend on armaments. In all, over three dozen nations and twelve international organizations have taken steps to constrain weapons proliferation since the end of the Persian Gulf War (Ionno et al., 1992).

The failure of these governmental initiatives actually to reduce weapons exports has sparked a number of citizen initiatives aimed at prohibiting arms sales to specific regions or under specific circumstances. A number of prominent scientific organizations that have historically been active in debates over nuclear-arms control and disarmament—including International Physicians for the Prevention of Nuclear War, the Federation of American Scientists, and the Pugwash group—have now taken on the issue of the international arms trade as well. Organizations of health professionals such as Physicians for Human Rights and relief organizations such as the International Committee of the Red Cross have applied their special skills and knowledge to the task of documenting the public-health impacts of inhumane weapons such as antipersonnel land mines (Arms Project of Human Rights Watch and Physicians for Human Rights, 1993).

For scientists and physicians concerned about public health and the uses to which the products of science are put, the arms trade is a priority issue that will have to be addressed in the post–Cold War era, just as the U.S.–Soviet nuclear arms race had to be addressed during the era of the Cold War (Sidel, 1989).

WILLIAM D. HARTUNG

*Directly related to this article are the other articles in this entry:* MEDICINE AND WAR, PUBLIC HEALTH AND WAR, NUCLEAR WARFARE, *and* CHEMICAL AND BIOLOGICAL WEAPONS. *For a further discussion of topics mentioned in this article, see the entries* HEALTH-CARE RESOURCES, ALLOCATION OF, *article on* MACROALLOCATION; *and* PUBLIC HEALTH, *article on* DETERMINANTS OF PUBLIC HEALTH. *Other relevant material may be found under the entries* HEALTH OFFICIALS AND THEIR RESPONSIBILITIES; HEALTH POLICY, *article on* POLITICS AND HEALTH CARE; INTERNATIONAL HEALTH; *and* VALUE AND VALUATION.

## Bibliography

ARMS PROJECT OF HUMAN RIGHTS WATCH AND PHYSICIANS FOR HUMAN RIGHTS. 1993. *Landmines: A Deadly Legacy.* New York: Human Rights Watch.

BALL, NICOLE. 1991. *Briefing Book on Conventional Arms Transfers.* Boston: Council for a Livable World Education Fund.

GRIMMETT, RICHARD F. 1993. *Conventional Arms Transfers to the Third World, 1985–1992.* Washington, D.C.: Congressional Research Service, Library of Congress.

HARTUNG, WILLIAM D. 1994. *And Weapons for All.* New York: HarperCollins.

INTERNATIONAL NEGOTIATION NETWORK. 1992. *State of World Conflict Report 1991–1992.* Atlanta: Carter Center of Emory University.

IONNO, SANDRA; LOGAN, COLLEEN; and POWELL, MARK. 1992. *Recent Initiatives to Control the Arms Trade.* Washington, D.C.: British American Security Information Council (BASIC).

KLARE, MICHAEL T. 1991. "Gaining Control: Building a Comprehensive Arms Restraint System." *Arms Control Today* 21, no. 5:9–13.

———. 1994. "The Light Weapons Trade and the International System in the Post–Cold War Era." Paper delivered at conference of *International Trade in Light Weapons,* Academy of Arts and Sciences, Boston, February 24–25.

KLARE, MICHAEL T; ARNSON, CYNTHIA; MILLER, DELIA; and VOLLMAN, DANIEL. 1981. *Supplying Repression: U.S. Support for Authoritarian Regimes Abroad.* Washington, D.C.: Institute for Policy Studies.

LAURANCE, EDWARD J. 1992. *The International Arms Trade.* New York: Lexington Books.

O'HANLON, MICHAEL E; FARRELL, VICTORIA S.; and GLAZERMAN, STEVEN. 1992. *Limiting Conventional Arms Exports to the Middle East.* Washington, D.C.: Congress of the United States, Congressional Budget Office.

RHODES, RICHARD. 1988. "Man Made Death: A Neglected Mortality." *Journal of the American Medical Association* 260, no. 5:686–687.

SIDEL, VICTOR W. 1989. "Weapons of Mass Destruction: The Greatest Threat to Public Health." *Journal of the American Medical Association* 262, no. 5:680–682.

SIVARD, RUTH LEGER. 1991. *World Military and Social Expenditures, 1991.* Washington, D.C.: World Priorities.

STOCKHOLM INTERNATIONAL PEACE RESEARCH INSTITUTE. 1993. *SIPRI Yearbook 1993: World Armaments and Disarmament.* Oxford: Oxford University Press.

# WASTE DISPOSAL, HAZARDOUS

*See* HAZARDOUS WASTES AND TOXIC SUBSTANCES.

# WHISTLEBLOWING IN HEALTH CARE

Whistleblowing entered the English language in the 1960s as a metaphor derived from a referee's use of a whistle to call a foul (Partridge, 1984). It refers to a warning issued by a member or former member of an organization to the public about a serious wrongdoing or danger created or concealed within the organization. Sissela Bok holds that there are three essential elements to whistleblowing (Bok, 1982). The whistleblower (1) dissents from an action or practice within the organization; (2) breaches loyalties by taking the matter outside the organization; and (3) makes an accusation against an individual or individuals in the organization. Whistleblowing is distinguishable from internal dissent or accusation by the use of external vehicles of warning (e.g., the media or government agencies), and from anonymous or secretive leaking of information by the willingness of the whistleblower to be named publicly. Numerous acts of whistleblowing have been documented in business, government, and the professions.

In the health-care arena, whistleblowing incidents have involved public warnings about malfeasance or dangers in patient care, research, and public health. Anyone employed by or associated with an organization may become a whistleblower, but bioethics literature is dominated by discussions of whistleblowing by nurses.

Nurses frequently have inside knowledge about the untoward behavior of doctors, hospitals, and nursing homes. Ethical standards in nursing require loyalty not only to doctors but also to patients. When a doctor harms or threatens to harm patients, and internal means of redress are nonexistent or ineffective, a nurse may feel morally compelled to blow the whistle on the doctor's behavior. An operating room nurse, for example, may know that a surgeon regularly operates under the influence of drugs or alcohol. If established hospital mechanisms for intervention (e.g., quality assurance committee, medical policy committee, the vice-president for nursing) fail to correct the situation, the nurse may find it necessary to alert the state licensing authority, the hospital accrediting agency, or the local newspaper.

Regardless of the outcome for the surgeon, blowing the whistle places the nurse in jeopardy. Nurses' relative lack of power in the health-care system exposes nurse whistleblowers to some of the extreme forms of retaliation that often befall whistleblowers: loss of employment, loss of promotion or demotion, reassignment, blacklisting, accusation of mental instability, harassment, and shunning. In this case, it is easy to imagine that other surgeons at the hospital might refuse to operate with the whistleblowing nurse. This could provoke an undesirable reassignment or termination.

Whistleblowing raises multiple ethical issues, beginning with evaluation of motive. Generally, whistleblowers present themselves as motivated to protect other individuals or society in general; their willingness to step forward publicly is evidence of this honorable motive. Some whistleblowers, however, may be driven by a desire for revenge for real or perceived injustices attributed to the organization, by personal animosities, or by ideology. The accuracy of the charge made by the whistleblower and the fairness of the accusations against individuals are also central ethical considerations. Organizations and individuals can be harmed significantly and often irreparably by public accusations. Retractions or corrections of false or unfair allegations seldom receive the same degree of public attention as the initial accusations.

Even when allegations of wrongdoing or danger are well founded, whistleblowing involves a breach of loyalty. At its best, loyalty is one of the most admirable virtues. Loyalty within organizations creates deeply satisfying personal commitments, fosters relationships of mutual trust, and facilitates collective action. Whistleblowing and fear of whistleblowing can destroy these personal and social goods. Potential whistleblowers should therefore attempt to use methods of redress within the organization before going outside, in spite of the frustrations and delays internal mechanisms can sometimes cause. To minimize the need for whistleblowing, organizations should create effective means for hearing complaints, protecting complainants, and acting expeditiously on valid complaints.

The wrongdoing or danger that prompts whistleblowing must be substantial enough to outweigh the harms produced by breach of loyalty. There must be good reason to believe that public disclosure will end the wrongdoing or avoid the danger at stake. Otherwise, the harms produced by breaching organizational loyalty will not be justified by the prevention of worse harms.

Potential whistleblowers should also assess the personal costs involved, including impact on family and career. Morality requires a reasonable degree of action on behalf of others, but it does not require heroic self-sacrifice. When the potential harm to the whistleblower and his or her family outweighs the harm he or she is trying to correct or avoid, a would-be whistleblower is justified in remaining silent. In many cases, however, it is exceedingly difficult to calculate potential harms. Decisions about whistleblowing must then rely on individual conviction and practical wisdom.

In spite of these cautions, whistleblowers can provide an indispensable service to the public and to their own organizations. External regulation of organizations is inevitably partial and too often after the fact. Organizations can become so resistant to internal criticism that needed reform can be accomplished only by the pressure of external revelations. Courageous disclosures by insiders privy to an organization's private behavior and secrets can spare individuals and the general public significant harms. Ethical analysis of any specific act of whistleblowing involves not only breach of loyalty to the organization but also service rendered on behalf of wider or more significant loyalties. A nurse whistleblower, for example, may find loyalty to a surgeon outweighed by loyalty to patients or loyalty to a hospital's public image outweighed by loyalty to the life and health of those the hospital serves. Organizational loyalties that refuse to recognize the need for these wider and deeper loyalties are blind and can be personally and socially destructive.

Potential whistleblowers should examine their motives, consult with trusted colleagues to confirm key facts, and exhaust all reasonable means of resolving the matter inside the organization. When internal mechanisms for complaint do not exist or are ineffective, individuals considering whistleblowing should determine the legal ramifications, weigh the harms and benefits at stake, and minimize the breach of loyalty if they choose to act. To reduce the need for whistleblowing, organizations should minimize secrecy, create reliable internal mechanisms for redressing complaints, protect those who use these mechanisms, and develop systems for periodic self-assessment throughout the organization.

CHARLES J. DOUGHERTY

*Directly related to this entry are the entries* FRAUD, THEFT, AND PLAGIARISM; FIDELITY AND LOYALTY; TEAMS, HEALTH-CARE; *and* CONFLICT OF INTEREST. *For a further discussion of topics mentioned in this entry, see the entries* MEDICAL CODES AND OATHS, *article on* ETHICAL ANALYSIS; NURSING ETHICS; OBLIGATION AND SUPEREROGATION; *and* PROFESSIONAL–PATIENT RELATIONSHIP, *article on* ETHICAL ISSUES. *Other relevant material may be found under the entries* HEALTH CARE, QUALITY OF; HEALTH OFFICIALS AND THEIR RESPONSIBILITIES; MEDICAL MALPRACTICE; PROFESSION AND PROFESSIONAL ETHICS; *and* VIRTUE AND CHARACTER. *See also the* APPENDIX (CODES, OATHS, AND DIRECTIVES RELATED TO BIOETHICS), SECTION II: ETHICAL DIRECTIVES FOR THE PRACTICE OF MEDICINE.

## Bibliography

BANJA, JOHN D. 1985. "Whistleblowing in Physical Therapy." *Physical Therapy* 65, no. 11:1683–1686.

BOK, SISSELA. 1982. "Whistleblowing and Leaking." In her *Secrets: On the Ethics of Concealment and Revelation.* New York: Pantheon.

DOUGHERTY, CHARLES J.; EDWARDS, BARBA J.; and HADDAD, AMY M. 1990. *Ethical Dilemmas in Perioperative Nursing.* Denver: Association of Operating Room Nurses.

ELLISTON, FREDERICK; KEENAN, JOHN; LOCKHART, PAULA; and VAN SCHAICK, JANE. 1985. *Whistleblowing Research: Methodological and Moral Issues.* New York: Praeger.

FELIU, ALFRED G. 1983. "Thinking of Blowing the Whistle?" *American Journal of Nursing* 83, no. 11:1541–1542.

FIESTA, JANINE. 1990a. "Whistleblowers: Heroes or Stool Pigeons?—Part I." *Nursing Management* 21, no. 6:16–17.

———. 1990b. "Whistleblowers: Retaliation or Protection?—Part II." *Nursing Management* 21, no. 7:38.

GLAZER, MYRON, and GLAZER, PENINA. 1989. *The Whistleblowers: Exposing Corruption in Government and Industry.* New York: Basic Books.

HADDAD, AMY M., and DOUGHERTY, CHARLES J. 1991. "Whistleblowing in the OR: The Ethical Implications." *Today's O.R. Nurse* 13, no. 3:30–33.

KIELY, MARY A., and KIELY, DEIRDRE C. 1987. "Whistleblowing: Disclosure and Its Consequences for the Professional Nurse and Management." *Nursing Management* 18, no. 5:41–45.

KOHN, STEPHEN M., and KOHN, MICHAEL D. 1988. *The Labor Lawyer's Guide to the Rights and Responsibilities of Employee Whistleblowers.* New York: Quorum Books.

MURPHY, ELLEN K. 1989. "Legal Aspects of Whistle-Blowing." *AORN Journal* 49, no. 2:480–484.

PARTRIDGE, ERIC. 1984. *A Dictionary of Slang and Unconventional English.* Edited by Paul Beale. New York: Macmillan.

ROTHROCK, JANE C. 1988. "Whistle-blowing: Is It Worth the Consequences?" *AORN Journal* 48, no. 4:757–762.

U.S. PRESIDENT'S COMMISSION FOR THE STUDY OF ETHICAL PROBLEMS IN MEDICINE AND BIOMEDICAL AND BEHAVIORAL RESEARCH. 1981. *Whistleblowing in Biomedical Research.* Edited by Judith Swazey and Stephen Sher. Washington, D.C.: U.S. Government Printing Office.

# WILDLIFE CONSERVATION AND MANAGEMENT

*See* ANIMAL WELFARE AND RIGHTS, *article on* WILDLIFE CONSERVATION AND MANAGEMENT.

# WITHHOLDING OR WITHDRAWING MEDICAL TREATMENT

*See* DEATH AND DYING: EUTHANASIA AND SUSTAINING LIFE, *article on* ETHICAL ISSUES. *See also* ARTIFICIAL ORGANS AND LIFE-SUPPORT SYSTEMS; *and* INFANTS, *article on* ETHICAL ISSUES.

# WOMEN

## I. HISTORICAL AND CROSS-CULTURAL PERSPECTIVES

A central problem of women's history is that women have been defined by men using concepts and terms based on men's experiences. Such androcentric thought pervades all domains of knowledge. Scholarship in women's studies, developed largely since the late 1960s across a broad range of disciplines, shows that attitudes, customs, laws, and institutions affecting women are grounded in religious and functionalist perspectives according to which "woman" is said to have been created from and after man; has been identified with her sexuality and defined by her sexual function; and has been confined to roles and relationships that are extensions of her reproductive capacity. Alongside this history stands a centuries-old feminist critique that challenges as self-serving and often misogynist the assumptions and intentions of the religions, philosophies, sciences, and familial and political institutions that have shaped the experiences of women in most eras and cultures. Moreover, both the definition of women and its critique reflect a Eurocentric bias that today is the subject of much criticism. This article summarizes the scholarship produced since the mid-1970s by historians of women, reflecting their collective efforts to compensate for ahistorical assumptions and to constitute a written record both more inclusive of the experiences of women and more open to differences of perspective. It assumes that the history of women requires consideration of moral and ethical as well as social, economic, and political issues.

### Women defined

From ancient times it has been customary to define "woman," in relationship to man, as a limited and contingent part of a dimorphic species. Western cultures have placed heavy constraints on female lives, sometimes justifying these constraints by attributing to women, such as Pandora and Eve, responsibility for human misfortunes resulting from their allegedly weaker self-control or greater lasciviousness. Despite the existence of exceptional women in myth and history, most women in most historical societies have been confined to positions of dependency. Ultimately, whether on the basis of their capacity for pregnancy and resulting physical vulnerability or the use of women's fertility in forging relationships of social and economic value, women, like children, have been denied an independent voice. Seen as "lesser men" by the fathers of Western philosophy, women have been viewed as "Other," as not-man, through a discourse in which human being was embodied in the male sex (Beauvoir, 1952).

Deprived of political power and identified with sexual temptation, women have been subject to myriad laws and customs that have at once prescribed and enforced their secondary status. Men have termed women "the sex"; defined them primarily in terms of their sexuality; and, as masters of family and public power, created and staffed the institutions that control female sexuality. In the early fifteenth century, the Italian-born French author Christine de Pizan (1364–ca. 1430) challenged the prevailing androcentric definition of her sex, declaring that the evil attributed to women by learned men existed in men's minds and that, if permitted education, women would become as virtuous and capable as men.

Resistance and rebellion by individual women have a long history; and organized protest, termed "feminism" only since the 1890s, is traceable through a history that is continuous for at least two centuries. However, the condition of women has only occasionally been viewed as a general problem of social justice. The "woman question," as it was phrased in the nineteenth century, was debated as a political, social, and economic, but rarely as a moral issue; women's rights and responsibilities were discussed as matters of expediency. In the great democratic revolutions of the late eighteenth century, the "inalienable rights of man" were not extended to women. Men, as heads of traditional patriarchal families, continued to speak for their dependents, women as well as children. While some Enlightenment philosophers, most notably Theodore von Hippel (1741–1796), had admitted the abstract equality of all human beings, and others, such as the Marquis de Condorcet (1743–1794), advocated women's accession to equal education and to full civic rights, social arrangements nevertheless made it expedient to ignore their claims. Ultimately, most efforts to improve women's status and condition have been justified on grounds of expediency: if women vote, said the suffragists of 1915, war would be less likely; if mothers earned fathers' wages, said the feminists of 1985, fewer children would live in poverty.

Most matters related to women, then, whether intellectual constructs or social institutions, whether constraining or enlarging women's options, whether produced by misogynists or feminists, have rested on utilitarian grounds. Woman, first of all as an individual human being, was rarely the subject of thought or decision; woman as wife and mother or potential mother has been the ideal type. Even for suffragist leaders of the nineteenth and twentieth centuries, the resort to arguments of expediency over considerations of justice or ethics has itself been an expedient (Kraditor, 1965). By the 1990s, however, following two decades of reexamination of all domains of knowledge by scholars in women's studies, feminist theorists began to challenge arguments based on expediency (while sometimes using them as well) and to demand a voice in the discourse through which both knowledge and social institutions are established. Noting injustice in the treatment of women, and the absence of concern about women at the center of most modern and contemporary philosophical systems, they criticize ethical theory itself as a hegemonic expression of the values of a dominant class or gender (Walker, 1992).

It is simpler, and historically has been more effective, to argue the needs of women in terms of their differences from men—their needs as wives and mothers, their concerns with nurturant values, their familial and social responsibilities. Women often do speak "in a different voice," reflecting different moral concerns and material circumstances (Gilligan, 1982). Women have been and remain deeply divided over their own definition of self: as individuals entitled to, and now demanding, equality of treatment with men; or as persons with gender-specific differences and resulting relationships with families, friends, and communities to whom they bear responsibilities that limit individual autonomy and rights. "Equal rights feminists" have been challenged for basing their claims on an abstract concept of personhood that denies female specificity. Rather than buttressing the claims of individualism based in nineteenth-century liberal philosophy (Fox-Genovese, 1991; Pateman, 1987), they should, according to this view, emphasize the need for men as well as women to acknowledge their dependence on and debts to the communities that are essential to their existence.

Furthermore, through failure to emphasize female differences, women may continue to be measured through a single, male-constructed lens that ignores or denigrates female-specific experiences. Yet woman along with man should be the measure of all things—and the universalizing of human experience based only on consideration of dominant cultures should be avoided. Awareness of the dimensions of this "equality vs. difference" question is critical to understanding a wide range of historical and contemporary issues regarding the status of women. Can gender-specific needs of individuals such as pregnant women be acknowledged in law that also supports equality of treatment for all individuals? Can employment preferences be granted to men if, historically, most women have not pursued a given occupation? How should a history grounded in gender distinctions be interpreted (Scott, 1988)?

Scholars today recognize that neither "man" nor "woman" has a single, fixed meaning; cross-cultural and international differences defy simple definition. The concept of separate spheres of human activity labeled public and private, political and personal, society and family, however, has a long history; the reality of women's lives was obscured by these universalizing categories of analysis often used by philosophers, politicians, and professors. As the twenty-first century approaches, historians of women have firmly established the historicity of women, a critical first task. Women's lives, as well as their consciousness, vary, not only by era but also by class, race, age, marital status, region, religion, education, and a host of factors peculiar to individual circumstances. Implicit in this work is a political message: that changes over time past make future change conceivable. Also implicit is an accusation of injustice against a system of societal arrangements that has suppressed women, for the questions raised in this scholarship deal often with omissions, silences, and double standards. This form of scholarship elicits new knowledge and conjectures about human possibilities.

## Women in traditional Western societies

As the story has been reconstructed, women in history have become increasingly visible (Bridenthal et al., 1987). New anthropological studies suggest that women may have enjoyed greater equity with men in prehistorical times (Sanday, 1981). Agrarian economies with relatively little differentiation of tasks allowed for more egalitarian relationships within families; families themselves constituted societies, and participation was not dichotomized by gender, or sex roles. The classical world, with its more advanced economies, and greater wealth and militarism, vested both property rights and citizenship only in men, as heads of households. Separated into family and polity, society became a male world of civic virtue. Relegated to the household, women became men's property, and a double standard of sexuality was constructed to assure female subjection to patriarchal family interests. A woman's honor, and that of her family, was identified with her chastity. The virtue of a woman, said Aristotle, was to obey. Differentiation by class allowed some variation of roles for women; but Plato's philosopher queens aside, no women could claim equal treatment in regard to property, citizenship, marriage, criminal law, or access to social institutions. Women existed to reproduce and to serve men's needs; rights in their progeny were assigned to men.

**Influence of Christianity.**    The spread of Christianity brought new possibilities for women: for some, a role in spreading the new religion; for all, a promise of spiritual equality. Christianity created new opportunities for women's voices to be heard, especially by instituting marriage laws requiring consent and establishing, in some instances, inheritance and property rights for women. Monasteries and convents, while providing shelter for the destitute, also offered education and alternative careers for a small, often highborn, minority. The high Middle Ages saw the foundation of the first universities in the Western world, beginning in 1088 with Bologna, whose famous twelfth-century legal scholar, Gratian, incorporated into his influential study Aristotle's dualistic view of women as passive and men as active, in law as well as reproductive physiology.

This Aristotelian dualism was also advanced by the work of Thomas Aquinas in the thirteenth century; he combined his reading of Aristotle with the Christian view of creation to assert that woman was a "defective and misbegotten" man, assigned by nature to the work of procreation. The rebirth of learning thus gave new life to the hoary tradition of defining women as not-men and for men, in terms of qualities they lacked and services they provided. Renaissance thinkers transmitted across the ages classical Greece's sharp distinction between polity and household. The literature of courtly love notwithstanding, as dynastic power was reconstituted in bureaucratic and political structures, the separation of public and private arenas of human activity increased; and relative to aristocratic men, upper-class women faced new restrictions. Growth of the market economy, however, probably had a more liberating effect on rural and urban women of other classes.

Neither the Renaissance nor the Reformation, both considered watersheds in European history, brought reformed ideas about women to the fore. The advent of Protestantism meant the closing of nunneries that had allowed some women, notably those who could offer a dowry to the church, agency outside marriage. It also deprived all classes of women of the succor of the Virgin Mary and female saints. However, Protestantism did provide some literate women as well as men direct access to the word of God in the Bible. By ending clerical celibacy, it opened opportunities to ministers' wives, and ultimately, especially in the dissenting sects, it allowed women wider participation in church affairs. In the Counterreformation, some Catholic laywomen formed communities through which they provided social services for the poor, ill, and orphaned. Nuns continued to serve as teachers, nurses, and social workers. But Catholics and Protestants alike, following the biblical injunction of Paul, taught women silence in public and subjection to men in private.

**Urban vs. rural experience.**    Controversy over the effects of the Renaissance and Reformation on women's lives continues to fuel debate among historians of women. In an increasingly complex society, generalizations fail to satisfy: some women prospered, enjoyed education by leading humanist scholars such as Erasmus, and wielded power on behalf of dynastic lines. Urban craftsmen's wives shared in domestic production and local marketing of goods, and helped to manage artisanal workshops. City women developed professions of their own, largely in the healing arts, midwifery, and retail establishments, especially those purveying food. But most wage-earning women worked as domestic servants, frequently for a decade before marriage and sometimes for their entire lives; "maid" had become synonymous with "female servant."

However, most women, like most men, lived in rural settings, where all members of the household pooled their labor in a family economy organized to produce the goods and services essential to supporting and reproducing themselves. They lived within households and made essential contributions to the economic survival of their families. Labor needs over the family's life cycle determined the status, residence, and welfare of most people (Tilly and Scott, 1978). Only after centuries-long structural changes in agriculture and industry, in company with a demographic shift that reduced both mortality and fertility, did the employment of female productive capacity generate public debate over a "woman question." Ultimately it was a shift in the location of women's traditional work—especially making cloth and garments—from the household into the factory, and the ensuring restructuring of (especially married) women's economic contribution to the family, that created the conditions for feminist debate. Only then did the question "Should a woman work?" or "Should she have a 'right to work'?" make sense.

**Effects of political and scientific developments.**    In addition to religious reformation and the expansion of commerce and trade, other major trends in the early modern period led to new institutions and novel ideas that affected women's lives and challenged traditional views of women's "nature." Political centralization and the rise of science also meant change in women's lives. According to one recent interpretation, the great witchcraft persecution of the sixteenth and seventeenth centuries reflected not only religious and gender conflict but also efforts to legitimize political authority by exercising new forms of social control over individual behavior (Larner, 1981). Because women's relative physical and economic weaknesses made their recourse to magic power seem plausible, and because their alleged sexual insatiability predisposed them to temptation by the devil, 80 percent of the victims of witch-hunts were female—often older, single, eccentric women lacking male protection.

Ultimately science disproved many misogynist notions about the female body. However, despite studies in embryology challenging the Aristotelian view of women's passivity in reproduction that also buttressed attitudes and customs denying them agency in society, only in the late nineteenth and early twentieth centuries were such classical and false assumptions finally displaced by scientific knowledge.

Although by the eighteenth century the economic, political, and intellectual structures that maintained traditional attitudes and institutionalized age-old practices toward women were subject to a multitude of challenges, time-honored patterns persisted. Just as in the thirteenth century Thomas Aquinas had recapitulated Aristotle, so the influential eighteenth-century philosopher Jean-Jacques Rousseau reinforced belief in woman's role as the helpmate of man. Like Adam's Eve, Rousseau's Sophie, the ideal wife of his ideal citizen, Émile, was created to serve, support, and console the chief actor on the human stage, the man to whom she was legally subject. The Napoleonic Code of 1804, and similar codes of law subsequently promulgated across Europe, required married women to obey their husbands. Voices that demanded inclusion of civil rights for women along with the "Rights of Man"—Condorcet in France, von Hippel in Germany, Mary Wollstonecraft in England—were silenced as the Age of Reason gave way to an Age of Steel. Men alone wrote and signed the new "social contract"; as "natural" dependents, women could not aspire to citizenship.

And yet women increasingly did claim civil rights. Despite the negative examples of Wollstonecraft (dead after childbirth and infamous more for her unconventional lifestyle than for her contributions to radical philosophy), Marie Antoinette, Olympe de Gouges (author of *The Declaration of the Rights of Woman and the Female Citizen,* 1791), and Jeanne Manon Roland (dead on the Jacobins' guillotine, ostensibly for having violated the boundaries of conventional femininity), and despite increasingly restrictive legal codes and an ideology of domesticity that won widespread support across class lines, new philosophic currents, based in the Enlightenment concept of human perfectibility, generated the first organized movements for women's rights.

## Women in transforming societies

Inspired by the French Revolution, women in the nineteenth century began to form groups through which collectively to advocate improved treatment of their sex. By the mid-nineteenth century, organized groups we now call "feminist" were formed in France, England, the United States, Prussia, and even Russia, to challenge women's subject status. The new protest took place in the context of economic as well as political transformation in western and central Europe and the United States. Revolutionary changes in methods of agriculture and transportation, and the rise of an enlarged market economy, industrialization, and urbanization brought profound alteration to family structures and relationships. More young people, including women, could claim and find opportunities for social and geographic mobility and economic independence.

Especially for women, however, escape from the confines of the patriarchal family brought new vulnerabilities (Tilly and Scott, 1978). With female wages far below subsistence levels, a woman alone required assistance, and might trade sex for survival, risking dismissal from employment for her "loose morals" or extreme deprivation if deserted by her male partner.

Social reformers responded, purportedly in women's defense. Not all protesters and reformers called for "equality" for women; few, if any, entertained ideas of identical rights and responsibilities for both sexes. Utopian schemes for the total reconstruction of society aside, debate over the status of women most often focused on ways to "protect" them: to shelter traditional women's work from the intrusion of men; to safeguard women (along with children) from unsafe conditions and/or excessive hours of labor; to secure for women rights to inherited property, their own earnings, and custody of their persons as well as some share in legal authority over their children in cases of divorce. Divorce itself, largely illegal or difficult to obtain before the twentieth century, was one of many reform issues about which women themselves differed, often on the basis of class, religion, or ethnicity.

**Defining feminism.** Emphasis by historians on the woman-suffrage movement, which began as a minority concern within women's groups in the mid-nineteenth century and peaked near the beginning of the twentieth, has obscured not only the larger concerns of women activists but also deep differences within feminist movements. Campaigns for "equal rights," grounded in the assumptions of liberal individualism, became dominant to a greater extent in England and the United States than elsewhere. Contemporary English-language dictionaries tend to define feminism as a movement toward political, social, educational, economic, and legal rights for women equal to those of men. This has been termed "individualistic" feminism (Offen, 1988).

The feminisms of continental Europe in that earlier era, as well as later women's movements in Third World countries, reflected a closer association with the social question—that is, with issues of class and nation—and with family relationships and community ties. This constitutes a "relational" form of feminism. Socialist feminists, while cognizant of women's needs for education and encouragement to participate fully in political struggles in support of class goals, declined to envision as their purpose access to equal—and equally exploitative—conditions with working-class men. Others, including Catholic feminists in large numbers, insisted on improvement of women's status in order to enhance their performance in traditional women's roles and relationships. In some countries, notably the United States, a "century of struggle" for women's rights grew out of religious ferment and the recognition that no subjected person, woman or slave, could be fully responsible to God as a moral being. Nineteenth-century equal-rights feminism and the concurrent movement for "protective legislation" offered contrasting answers to the "woman question."

**Equal but different.** Differentiation between "individualistic" and "relational" forms of feminism heightens current debate over the definition of feminism. It also parallels a major controversy among feminist theorists that cuts to the heart of moral issues regarding women. Must arguments undergirding a political movement on behalf of women—the various forms of feminism—be grounded in the assumption that human beings are identical? If so, equal-rights law can be used to deny pregnant women special insurance and employment benefits. Equality so defined may demand identity of treatment.

Alternatively, to emphasize women's particularity, to focus on sexual differences, may invite legislation (and buttress attitudes) restricting women's options in the guise of acknowledging their special needs. Precisely this argument was long used to justify labor laws that denied many excellent employment opportunities to all women because they required occasional work during evening hours or involved physically demanding tasks. More recently, women workers in potentially hazardous industries have faced coerced sterilization or loss of employment on grounds of their capacity for reproduction. But to deny that women on the basis of their sex constitute a special class can also deprive them of support they may need—for example, in pregnancy. It can even, some argue, destroy the very basis for a political movement in their name and interest.

This "difference versus equality" debate, often in inchoate form, has led to extended conflict over definitions of feminism and feminist demands. It also raises fundamental issues regarding individual rights, family responsibilities, and the prerogatives of government. In the nineteenth century, reformers called for legislative action to ameliorate the worst abuses of industrialization and urbanization. Reformers ranged from British industrialists who wanted to improve the quality of the labor force to French Social Catholics who sought to base solutions to societal problems on Christian principles to Prussia's "Iron Chancellor" Otto von Bismarck, who schemed to reduce the threat of socialist revolution. Whether impelled by religious, philanthropic, political, or economic motives, they shared the recognition that such innovations increased governmental powers over persons' lives. They also found that they could succeed, against strongly held liberal tenets favoring laissez-faire

practice, by exposing the physical, and allegedly moral, dangers to female (and young) persons posed by the new working and living conditions. Working women rarely spoke for themselves in these debates, and even feminist voices, largely from the middle class, were little heeded.

Beginning in the 1840s with the first laws limiting women's night work, every policy of the interventionist states, acting in lieu of a patriarchal family to regulate female behavior, extended the premise that women needed special consideration and that men must provide them with protection, even against themselves. The nineteenth-century debate over short hours and the twentieth-century controversy over state regulation of reproduction share the assumption that adult women, as individual citizens, cannot or should not be empowered to make decisions affecting their own persons. Whether arguing against a woman's working outside the home at night, on behalf of keeping her husband home from the cabaret, or championing limits on abortion, advocates of restrictive legislation link women's rights with those of others: husband, child, family, state.

Similar arguments may be employed on occasion in support of male-specific measures such as military conscription, which subordinates individual freedom to national security. Such denial of personal autonomy, however, remains the exception for men and, moreover, often brings with it rights of citizenship. Women, on the other hand, are assumed to serve the interests of others at all times, and rarely gain comparable advantage. Historically, legislation concerning women has not distinguished among them by race, ethnicity, or class, by marital status, age, preference, or capacity, assuming marriage and motherhood to be the overriding obligation and destiny of all women, and conflating childbearing with child rearing. As historians have highlighted in recent books, the interests of women and their calls for "freedom" may even be seen as at odds with those of the family. This, of course, is true especially of the type of family associated primarily with the white, Western world (Bell and Offen, 1983; Degler, 1980); studies of the African-American family in the United States, and of extended families in other cultures, stress their function as sources of strength as well (Jones, 1985).

The history of women in the twentieth century reveals the centrality of the "woman question" to the social, economic, and political concerns of many nations. During wars and revolutions, traditional notions of "women's place" and struggles over woman suffrage have been eclipsed by calls for female labor and patriotic support. Apparent feminist advances, however, have frequently led to the reinstitution of traditional norms. Following both world wars, women were summarily discharged from good-paying jobs or offered less skilled and less rewarding employment. However, structural changes in commerce and industry have escalated demand for female workers, especially in clerical, teaching, and other service occupations dominated by women; expansion of educational opportunities has augmented female literacy and professional expertise; advances in public health, nutrition, and medicine have continued to increase female life expectancy and decrease infant mortality; and new technologies have reduced the need for labor-intensive household chores. All of these changes tend to free many women for long periods of productive activity outside the family. As more and more countries have been swept into the global economy and information network, women's movements, often linked (and sometimes subordinated) to nationalism, have appeared around the world. Along with efforts to improve women's health and education, Third World feminists are challenging double standards in law and culture as well as such practices as clitoridectomy, marriage by capture, and sati (Johnson-Odim and Strobel, 1992).

Unlike earlier waves of feminist protest, the mid-twentieth-century rebirth of feminism called into action sufficient numbers of educated and strategically placed women and their male supporters to successfully challenge many social priorities and institutional structures. Though feminists are sometimes wrongly perceived as a "special interest" group reflecting only the needs and desires of middle-class white women in developed nations, their pressure, especially since the 1970s, has achieved significant change in legal status, medical treatment, and workplace conditions of benefit to all women. It has opened to women professions long monopolized by men, including medicine, law, the ministry, and the professoriate, whose collective powers of definition long buttressed gender biases. In some cases, most notably medicine, this represents a restoration to women of roles they held prior to the institution of professional schools and licensure, from which they were excluded. As health-care providers, women today often challenge the gender distinction between male doctors who "cure" and female nurses who "care." Women's health centers tend to stress women's need to question conventional medical procedures and to encourage women to assume an active role in determining their own treatment (Jaggar, 1983).

## Women challenging epistemology

Modeled on the "self-help" agencies for women's health that first developed in the late 1960s and influenced medical practice, this new women's liberation movement has flourished in the academy, especially in the United States but increasingly in Europe and in some instances in Africa, Asia, and Latin America. The field of women's studies, which began as a search for feminist foremothers and a female past lost to history, has expanded across the disciplines to question old methodologies, ask new questions, identify new sources, reinterpret received wisdom, develop new female perspectives, and challenge the very construction of knowledge—not only about the "nature" of women but also about all the constructs in the natural and social sciences based on androcentric experience. Grounded in advocacy for the rights of women to equality in education, culture, and society, it is a form of moral as well as scientific inquiry.

Among the earliest paradigms developed from the new scholarship in women's studies was the "social construction of feminity." Whether psychologists rereading Sigmund Freud, sociologists reinterpreting Erik Erikson, or historians rediscovering Heinrich Kramer and James Sprenger's notorious late-fifteenth-century handbook on witchcraft, these scholars found in the sciences as well as the humanities a pervasive confusion of description with prescription. Proceeding from male-imposed definitions of female nature and proscriptions limiting female behavior as old as written records of humankind, men as philosophers, preachers, physicians, politicians, patriarchs, and professors had labeled unconventional women abnormal, criminal, ill, even pathological—or, alternatively, not "real women." The "eternal feminine" of Western mythology falsely universalized descriptions of an idealized (implicitly) white woman (Spelman, 1988; Chaudhuri and Strobel, 1992).

Historical and cross-cultural studies that belie many such interpretations have now been done. The new women's history, increasingly inclusive of women of color and international perspectives (Offen et al., 1991; Johnson-Odim and Strobel, 1992), lays bare the many consequences of the absence of female voices and agency, and the fundamental ways in which justice has been denied to half the human species. Women's history tells a tale of misconceptions, biases, and injustices that have oppressed women and limited their freedom of choice—and, hence, their moral responsibility. It also reveals the many and differing contributions, perceptions, and struggles that constitute the female past. Although this historical perspective faces challenges, sometimes by groups of women who remain dependent on traditional sex roles for economic support and social recognition, it nevertheless offers the potential for transformation of benefit to all (Jaggar, 1983). It rests, moreover, on the principles of justice.

To the extent that ethical considerations require attribution of personhood and personal agency to every human being, ethical behavior toward women calls for disclosure and discussion of the full record of women in history. It demands that women be defined by their particular positions within specific and changing contexts and allowed choices reflecting the full range of their human attributes. It calls for major societal change. Inspired by new knowledge and the new feminisms, women have begun as never before to speak in their own voices and to claim equality despite their differences—envisioning difference without hierarchy. The "woman question," as posed by women today, can no longer be answered in terms of expediency. The ground has shifted: in the new world, women stand along with men as individuals endowed equally, if perhaps differently, with moral rights and moral responsibilities.

MARILYN J. BOXER

*Directly related to this article are the other articles in this entry:* HEALTH-CARE ISSUES, RESEARCH ISSUES, *and* WOMEN AS HEALTH PROFESSIONALS. *Also directly related are the entries* FEMINISM; JUSTICE; *and* MARRIAGE AND OTHER DOMESTIC PARTNERSHIPS. *For a further discussion of topics mentioned in this article, see the entries* AUTONOMY; CARE; RIGHTS; SEXISM; *and* UTILITY. *Other relevant material may be found under the entries* BIOLOGY, PHILOSOPHY OF; CIRCUMCISION, *article on* FEMALE CIRCUMCISION; ETHICS, *articles on* SOCIAL AND POLITICAL THEORIES, *and* RELIGION AND MORALITY; PATERNALISM; PROSTITUTION; *and* SEXUALITY IN SOCIETY, *article on* SOCIAL CONTROL OF SEXUAL BEHAVIOR.

## Bibliography

ANDERSON, BONNIE S., and ZINSSER, JUDITH P. 1988. *A History of Their Own: Women in Europe from Prehistory to the Present.* 2 vols. New York: Harper & Row.

BEAUVOIR, SIMONE DE. 1952. *The Second Sex.* Translated and edited by Howard Madison Parshley. New York: Alfred A. Knopf.

BELL, SUSAN GROAG, and OFFEN, KAREN M., eds. 1983. *Women, the Family, and Freedom: The Debate in Documents.* 2 vols. Stanford, Calif.: Stanford University Press.

BOXER, MARILYN J., and QUATAERT, JEAN H., eds. 1987. *Connecting Spheres: Women in the Western World, 1500 to the Present.* New York: Oxford University Press.

BRIDENTHAL, RENATE; KOONZ, CLAUDIA; and STUARD, SUSAN M., eds. 1987. *Becoming Visible: Women in European History.* 2d ed. Boston: Houghton Mifflin.

CHAUDHURI, NUPUR, and STROBEL, MARGARET, eds. 1992. *Western Women and Imperialism: Complicity and Resistance.* Bloomington: Indiana University Press.

COTT, NANCY F. 1977. *The Bonds of Womanhood: "Woman's Sphere" in New England, 1780–1835.* New Haven, Conn.: Yale University Press.

DEGLER, CARL N. 1980. *At Odds: Women and the Family in America from the Revolution to the Present.* Oxford: Oxford University Press.

EVANS, SARA M. 1989. *Born for Liberty: A History of Women in America.* New York: Free Press.

FOX-GENOVESE, ELIZABETH. 1991. *Feminism Without Illusions: A Critique of Individualism.* Chapel Hill: University of North Carolina Press.

GILLIGAN, CAROL. 1982. *In a Different Voice: Psychological Theory and Women's Development.* Cambridge, Mass.: Harvard University Press.

JAGGAR, ALISON M. 1983. *Feminist Politics and Human Nature.* Totowa, N.J.: Rowan Allanheld.

JOHNSON-ODIM, CHERYL, and STROBEL, MARGARET, eds. 1992. *Expanding the Boundaries of Women's History: Essays on Women in the Third World.* Bloomington: Indiana University Press.

JONES, JACQUELINE. 1985. *Labor of Love, Labor of Sorrow: Black Women, Work, and the Family from Slavery to the Present.* New York: Basic Books.

KERBER, LINDA K. 1980. *Women of the Republic: Intellect and Ideology in Revolutionary America.* Chapel Hill: University of North Carolina Press.

KRADITOR, AILEEN S. 1965. *The Ideas of the Woman Suffrage Movement, 1890–1920.* New York: Columbia University Press.

LARNER, CHRISTINA. 1981. *Enemies of God: The Witch-hunt in Scotland.* Baltimore: Johns Hopkins University Press.

OFFEN, KAREN M. 1988. "Defining Feminism: A Comparative Historical Approach." *Signs* 14, no. 1:119–157.

OFFEN, KAREN; PIERSON, RUTH ROACH; and RENDALL, JANE, eds. 1991. *Writing Women's History: International Perspectives.* Bloomington: Indiana University Press.

OKIN, SUSAN MOLLER. 1979. *Women in Western Political Thought.* Princeton, N.J.: Princeton University Press.

PATEMAN, CAROLE. 1987. "Feminist Critiques of the Public/Private Dichotomy." In *Feminism and Equality,* pp. 103–126. Edited by Anne Phillips. New York: New York University Press.

SANDAY, PEGGY REEVES. 1981. *Female Power and Male Dominance: On the Origins of Sexual Inequality.* Cambridge: At the University Press.

SCOTT, JOAN WALLACH. 1988. *Gender and the Politics of History.* New York: Columbia University Press.

SPELMAN, ELIZABETH V. 1988. *Inessential Woman: Problems of Exclusion in Feminist Thought.* Boston: Beacon Press.

TILLY, LOUISE A., and SCOTT, JOAN WALLACH. 1978. *Women, Work, and Family.* New York: Holt, Rinehart & Winston.

WAITHE, MARY ELLEN, ed. 1987. *A History of Women Philosophers.* 3 vols. Dordrecht, Netherlands: Kluwer.

WALKER, MARGARET URBAN. 1992. "Feminism, Ethics, and the Question of Theory." *Hypatia* 7, no. 3:23–38.

## II. HEALTH-CARE ISSUES

Most ethical issues in patient care and biomedical research affect men and women in the same ways, but there are some important differences related to biological factors, psychosocial experiences, and cultural background, as well as to differences in life experiences. These are exemplified in emerging health-care areas, such as the new reproductive technologies; in medical research; and in the data indicating that different treatment options are often made available to women and men (National Institutes of Health, 1990). This article will explore some of the ethical issues that arise in the health care of women. It will examine situations that characterize North American and European health-care settings, which therefore may not be relevant to other cultures or even to all segments of Western cultures. Areas of focus will be (1) aspects of the relationship between physicians, the health-care system, and female patients; and (2) specific aspects of the health care of women, including mental-health care.

## General aspects of the therapeutic relationship

The relationship between health-care providers and their patients has been described as paternalistic (Notman and Nadelson, 1978). Women have generally been subordinate in the relationship between the sexes in health care as well as in other areas of their lives (Baker Miller and Mothner, 1971; West, 1984). A large body of literature documents that norms of behavior and social roles for women have supported stereotypic expectations of greater compliance, dependence, and passivity, especially in relationships with men. Although many of these stereotyped roles of men and women have changed, aspects persist and are still reflected in the expectations and responses of women as patients (Nadelson and Notman, 1991). These stereotypes also influence the expectations of physicians and other health-care providers in caring for women.

Although research, consumerism, and the erosion of the authoritarian role of the physician have influenced understandings of and attitudes about men's and women's characteristics and social roles, vestiges of these old stereotypes persist. Women patients continue to be approached with advice, commands, directions, or decisions about their illness or treatment more often than they are included as partners or collaborators in plans for their care (Nadelson and Notman, 1977). The relationship between physician or researcher and patient can assume the quality of a parent–child interaction rather than a partnership.

Men also experience a kind of paternalism in their relationships with physicians and the health-care system, but there are differences in the ways that men and women are treated, based on beliefs about men's and women's capabilities and roles. Women's complaints, for example, are often pejoratively labeled "psychogenic," implying that they are not to be taken seriously (Lennane and Lennane, 1973). This labeling may, in part, explain some of the gender differences in the treatment of certain diseases, such as cardiac disease, which is often not recognized in women. As a result, when women have procedures like a coronary bypass, they are typically sicker and require emergency surgery. Women are also referred later for revascularization procedures, and fewer women are referred for exercise rehabilitation (Wenger et al., 1993).

Women also often perceive themselves in ways that are consistent with the view that they are passive or compliant. This parent–child model, in which the patient accepts that she will relinquish an active role in her treatment, can result in diminished communication and compromised care. At times of crisis and in gratitude for being helped, the patient may overlook the depreciation implicit in the paternalistic model. The dependent, compliant response of the woman patient can interfere with active efforts to recuperate, an important part of the process of recovery from trauma and illness (Notman and Nadelson, 1978). All people can regress, to some extent, in the face of illness and pain. The tension between active participation and the wish to be taken care of is a particular problem for women because of their socialization to be more passive, and because of the authority and power dynamics that have characterized their relationships with men.

**Professional–patient sexual relationships.**    Another problem in the relationship between the female patient and the male physician is the potential for sexualization of the relationship. The danger is reinforced in this relationship by the intimate nature of the interaction, which exposes private information as well as body parts.

Sexual relationships between patient and physician have received a great deal of attention, from the public as well as from the profession. Although the incidence of sexual contact between physicians and patients is difficult to document accurately, reports suggest that it is a significant problem (Council, 1990). In the past, sexual activity with patients was defended by some physicians as not necessarily harmful, and possibly therapeutic, but the profession has judged it to be categorically exploitative and unethical, and studies have determined that it is damaging (Bouhoutsos et al., 1983; Burgess, 1981; Feldman-Summers and Jones, 1984; Gabbard, 1989; Herman et al., 1987; Kluft, 1989; Pope and Bouhoutsos, 1986).

Efforts to enforce ethical guidelines forbidding sexual activity between doctor and patient have been hampered by concerns about confidentiality and public exposure that have made it difficult for patients to register formal complaints (Marmor, 1970). Substantial progress, however, has been made since the mid-1980s. Civil actions have been brought in the courts, and several states have adopted criminal, civil, and licensing regulations that specifically proscribe sexual behavior on the part of psychotherapists, physicians, other health-care providers, and others in positions of authority, such as teachers and employers (Jorgenson et al., 1991).

Many factors can lead to exploitative behavior by physicians and other health-care providers. Some behave unethically because of character flaws; others are vulnerable to sexual involvement because they are depressed, lonely, disappointed, or stressed. Their personal problems may lead them to respond sexually to a patient who enhances their feelings of importance and effectiveness, or who is physically appealing. Other physicians who become involved in exploitative behavior are compromised by alcoholism or substance abuse. Some women patients behave in ways that they do not consciously intend to be seductive, but can be interpreted to be, in response to the anxiety induced by their feelings about their illness. The physician can misinterpret this behavior and take advantage of the situation.

**Transference.**    Understanding the concept of transference can clarify aspects of the doctor–patient relationship that may otherwise be difficult to comprehend. It refers to the attitudes and feelings brought to a relationship from past experiences with important figures, such as parents. Thus the need to please, or to gain love—through acquiescence or seductive behavior—can be brought into the doctor–patient relationship as if it were a response by the patient to the physician. Because of the transference that is inevitable in the doctor–patient relationship, questions have been raised about whether the patient is able to give truly informed consent to a sexual relationship (Herman et al., 1987; Kluft, 1989). Sexual interaction with a patient or client has been considered analogous to rape or incest because of the exploitative nature of the act and the problem of consent in the context of a relationship where the power and influence of the physician is so disproportionate (Gabbard, 1989; Nadelson, 1989a; Council, 1990).

Almost any doctor–patient relationship can become sexual, regardless of the age of the patient and of the doctor, or of the appropriateness of the sexual activity. It is always incumbent on the doctor to maintain appropriate therapeutic boundaries.

## Specific problems in the health care of women

**Reproductive decisions.**    An important sphere of ethical consideration arises from the characteristics of women's bodies and their reproductive roles. Decisions about childbearing, the availability of contraception or sterilization, the performance of surgery involving reproductive organs, and the use of in utero fetal surgery to cure a fetal defect have profound consequences because they affect the family, the society, and future generations. Thus, how much autonomy a woman does or should have in deciding these questions has been a matter of intense debate.

> Social response to women's reproductive abilities typically has made their bodies part of the public domain in a way that men's are not. . . . And as wombs have become increasingly public spaces medically, they have also become increasingly public politically; women's choices, not only about how they manage their preg-

nancies, but also about how they will manage their work, their leisure, their use of both legal and illegal drugs, and their sexuality, are further subject to society's scrutiny and to the law's constraints. (Nelson, 1992, p. 13)

Historically and economically, women generally have not been in a position to set or achieve their own reproductive goals; such goals have not been considered by families or by society to be distinct from *their* goals and values. Decisions about medical or surgical procedures that have an impact on female sexuality and childbearing have often been made by the members of a family or community rather than by the woman affected. Such decisions have often been based on uninformed assumptions about the patient's best interest, or without consideration of the patient's desires. They have been based on societal or family considerations, such as the desire for more or fewer children.

These decisions also may reflect the views or values of the physician, although they may be presented as medically indicated. For example, a gynecologist may assume, without discussing the options with a woman, that she would not want additional children after she reaches the age of forty, because she would not want to run the potential risk of having a defective child. A hysterectomy may be recommended even though other options are available in her situation. Thus, the choice has been made for her, without her informed consent.

Decisions about abortion, the rights of the fetus as opposed to those of the pregnant woman, and other reproductive issues, such as surrogate motherhood and the prohibition of contraception in some countries, have brought attention to the role of the woman as an individual who is expected to fulfill societal responsibilities via her fertility, rather than making autonomous decisions.

*Hysterectomy.*    Hysterectomy remains the most frequently performed major surgery in the United States, and its incidence in younger women is increasing (Muller, 1990). There has been considerable debate, among gynecologists and others, about the appropriate indications for this procedure, often in disregard of the meaning of the uterus and bodily intactness for the self-image of many women. The uterus has been considered a "useless" and potentially disease-causing organ after the childbearing years.

The difficulty of establishing uniform indications for performing hysterectomies has been a long-standing problem. That the decision can be made arbitrarily and without specifically agreed-on criteria is suggested by the variation in the numbers of procedures performed in different communities with similar population bases, as well as by the differences in rates of hysterectomies performed by male and female gynecologists (Roos, 1984; Domenighetti et al., 1985).

Hysterectomies have been performed on women who are ambivalent about contraception or for whom contraception presents a problem because of religious beliefs or cultural practices. Thus a medical procedure, with its inherent risks, may be performed when there are safer alternatives available, in order to achieve contraception. Among the ethical questions raised by this practice are the use of medical procedures for nonmedical indications, especially when the risks may be greater, and the problem of whether a woman can make an informed choice in these circumstances.

*Contraception.* The development of new contraceptive methods over the past few decades has had a profound impact on women's lives by providing effective control of reproduction. Most research on contraceptives has been on techniques for women, and most widely available new contraceptives have been for women. Although this potentially offers reproductive control to women, who are most vulnerable to the hazards of pregnancy, women are also exposed to the risks and side effects of drugs and other potential long-term consequences of contraception that will not be determined for many years. The development of effective contraceptives for women has proceeded more quickly than for men, possibly reflecting the attitude that women should bear responsibility for contraception. It also may result from the pressure brought by women to gain more control of reproduction (Bremmer and de Kretzer, 1976).

The history of contraceptive research has been marred by ethical violations. In an early study, conducted on Mexican-American women, of the side effects of contraceptive pills, one group of women was given active contraceptive pills; another group was given placebos and a vaginal cream known to be a less effective contraceptive (Katz, 1972). The women were not clearly informed that some of them were not protected against pregnancy, and some became pregnant. Abortion was not made available to them, and even if it had been, many would have had moral and religious objections to it. The investigators deceived the women and misused the trust of their subjects by failing to obtain informed consent from those who participated in the study.

The case of the Dalkon Shield, an intrauterine device that was marketed for several years, also exemplifies problems in obtaining informed consent and not adequately testing contraceptive devices. After it had been used extensively, evidence was compiled indicating that uterine infections and deaths could result. The device was then withdrawn from the market (Mintz, 1985).

One consequence of the extensive litigation involving contraception has been a decrease in the development of new techniques and products. Many companies are unwilling to risk this litigation, or to assume the cost of more ethically and clinically responsible research.

This outcome illustrates the problems arising when research is dependent on an industry that is also at risk of litigation.

For many years, diethylstilbestrol (DES) was given to pregnant women to prevent spontaneous abortions, without adequate investigation of the other potential consequences of its use. Daughters of women who took DES were later found to be at risk for precancerous changes of the vaginal lining, and in some cases for carcinoma and infertility as well (Apfel and Fisher, 1984). Here, too, the greater vulnerability of women to unpredictable long-term hazards of medication arises from their reproductive roles; too little attention had been paid to the rigorous investigations necessary to establish the safety of medications (Chalmers, 1974).

*Sterilization.* In some situations, laws have permitted sterilization of women considered to be socially undesirable, psychologically deviant, or retarded. This practice has been justified in two ways: (1) the protection of the individual (e.g., a mentally retarded woman who is sexually active and may be exploited); and (2) the protection of society against reproduction by "unfit" individuals. Sterilization statutes may, however, be punitive and discriminatory rather than based on science. In many instances, the conditions considered to be indications for sterilization, such as psychosis, criminality, and retardation, have not been clearly evaluated or linked to genetic determinants. The children of psychotic or retarded people were expected to create social problems; society, then, was seen as justified in preventing the conception of such children. Permission for sterilization procedures has often not been obtained, or was obtained from parents or guardians under pressure and without the patient's full awareness of the implications of the procedure. For minors, the decisions have been made by social agencies or physicians. Many patients have been black, poor, and uneducated, and thus especially vulnerable (*Relf v. Weinberger*, 1974).

Sterilization raises another ethical issue that is not unique to the procedure, but serves to exemplify the problem of informed and autonomous consent in making irrevocable decisions, when there is a possibility that the procedure might be regretted in the future. A woman may not be informed that sterilization procedures such as tubal ligation are generally irreversible. But even if she is, it has been common practice for health professionals to raise questions about a woman's motivation for sterilization, and even to require psychiatric consultation. Thus, the right of an adult woman to make this choice, when she is appropriately informed, is questioned and this may even result in refusal of the procedure. A restriction based on suppositions about her motivation can be viewed as excessively paternalistic.

A small study of women in their early twenties who were seeking voluntary tubal ligation, and who had never been pregnant, found that they based their wish for childlessness on their own negative feelings toward children, on their judgment that they had limited capacity to be mothers, and on their desires to be independent. They had made reasoned decisions based on their beliefs and experiences. The researcher suggested that it is important to assess the character of the decision-making process, in order to determine that there has been no outside pressure and there are no major internal psychological conflicts (Lindenmayer, 1976).

Another study, of women under age thirty who had decided never to have children, reported a strong psychological motivation in these women to make their own decision to elect a tubal ligation (Kaltreider and Margolis, 1977). A history of family disruption, fear of motherhood, and dislike of children characterized this group. The authors suggested that for these women "the choice to be barren was multidetermined, persistent over time," and in agreement with other aspects of their psychological functioning. While there is clearly a need for longitudinal data about the long-term outcome of sterilization and subsequent requests for reversal of the procedure, the ethical consideration remains: that the competent woman be able to make her own informed decision, regardless of whether others believe that it is wrong or that she may change her mind.

Another ethical—as well as social, economic, and political—question involves the need to obtain the agreement of both marital partners for a married woman seeking sterilization or for any procedure that affects reproduction, since presumably both have an interest. For a woman this need has an immediate effect, since it directly affects her body; for a man it involves control of the woman as well as of his reproductive possibilities.

*New reproductive technologies.* For couples who are infertile due to organ or functional problems, new reproductive technologies have extended the possibility of pregnancy in ways that had previously been only the subject of science fiction. In addition to expanding reproductive options, potentially redirecting the use of health-care expertise and resources, and creating new clinical problems for women who may, for example, be using drugs or techniques that can result in complications or side effects, these techniques have created unusual ethical dilemmas.

Surrogate pregnancy, for example, involves the insemination of a woman who agrees to carry a pregnancy and surrender the baby after delivery. This arrangement has raised many legal and ethical questions, including who the "real" parents are, whether it is justified to offer financial incentives or rewards in such a case, who is responsible if the outcome is "undesirable," and what is the nature of the surrogate mother's consent. There has been controversy about whether a contract made with a surrogate can or should be binding, since the woman may have been under duress or not able to know how

she would feel after becoming pregnant and after the baby is born.

The issues were dramatically brought to public attention by the Baby M case, in which the birth mother changed her mind and refused to surrender the baby to the biological father and his wife (Harrison, 1990). Among the many problems raised are visitation rights, the nature of the relationship between the birth mother and the adoptive parents, and the rights of grandparents and siblings. These dilemmas acknowledge the special experience of pregnancy and the tie between the birth mother and the baby.

New reproductive techniques also include early prenatal diagnosis to detect fetal abnormalities. Since these techniques can also be used for sex selection, ethical dilemmas attendant on decisions about abortion, whether for fetal abnormality or for characteristics such as fetal sex, also arise.

Artificial insemination of a woman with sperm from her husband or from another man has been performed for centuries. It has been widely used in cases of male infertility and genetic abnormalities carried by the male, and to enable single women to conceive.

In recent years it has become technically possible to use donor ova as well as sperm, raising ethical questions about who the "real" parent is, and about ownership and responsibility for the fetus and baby. The technique of in vitro fertilization involves retrieving multiple ripe oocytes from a woman whose ovaries have been hormonally primed, mixing ova and sperm in the laboratory, and transferring fertilized ova or gametes into the uterus or fallopian tubes. The least complex situation involves retrieving oocytes from the same woman into whom the fertilized ova are implanted, and fertilization by sperm from a known donor, usually her husband. Ova and sperm can come from other donors, however, resulting in complicated legal and emotional issues of parenthood. Freezing techniques make it possible to keep the fertilized ovum or embryo alive almost indefinitely, thus creating a problem about future ownership and use, particularly if the genetic parents are divorced or if one, or both, dies.

Multiple ova are usually stimulated by the initial hormonal treatment of the woman, and multiple fertilized ova are usually implanted to ensure a greater likelihood of successful pregnancy. In most instances when there are multiple gametes, not all are allowed to continue to term because of the greater risks in multiple pregnancy. The parents and doctors then must select which to maintain and which to terminate.

In all of these situations, the woman bears the greater burden of the procedure and its outcome because of her physical connection to the pregnancy and delivery. Along with the risks of the pregnancy, the emotional consequences of potentially bearing a defective child are also greater for her, since in all societies women assume the major responsibilities for child rearing.

*Pregnancy.* Technological advances such as fetal monitoring have brought new ethical issues in the care of women during pregnancy and childbirth. These issues have focused on the responsibilities of a woman for the well-being of her fetus and the treatment of women without their consent when they are pregnant. In the past, because of the high morbidity and mortality rates during pregnancy and childbirth, physicians and parents viewed the fetus as a potential threat to the mother's life and health. As pregnancy and childbirth have become safer, attention has shifted to the well-being of the fetus, and prenatal diagnosis and treatment have become possible. This has caused a shift in perspective, so that women who do not agree to diagnostic and therapeutic procedures on their fetuses can be seen as not acting in the best interests of their unborn offspring (Nadelson, 1991).

Legal action and even prison sentences have resulted for women who are considered to be endangering their fetuses, such as pregnant alcoholics and drug addicts. The argument made in this situation is that the social costs of the effects of substance abuse on the fetus justify intervention. The autonomy of the woman, and the fact that she may not have willingly chosen to be pregnant, complicate the problem. Thus, in these situations the interests of the mother are pitted against those of the fetus to the degree that the fetus is considered to be a separate and equal person (Nadelson, 1993). These examples only begin to touch on the complexity of the issues raised by the changes in morbidity and mortality rates and the development of reproductive technologies. They do not, for example, address whether the stage of fetal development is an important consideration.

Discrimination because of socioeconomic or ethnic factors also appears to be an issue in some situations, for example, where cesarean section or other medical treatment is recommended in the interests of the fetus, and the mother refuses. One British author noted that the issue of forced cesarean section most often had arisen in cases involving poor or foreign women, or those with religious beliefs different from the physician's. This finding suggests that the cultural or socioeconomic dissimilarity between doctor and patient may have been a factor in the recommendation. In most cases, courts had ruled that the cesarean section be performed, but this position began to shift in the early 1990s. Arguments have supported the rights of the mother to the integrity and control of her body, even where refusing intervention may result in the death of the fetus. The reasoning, in one case, stemmed from a decision that a man did not have to take the risk required to donate a kidney to his child, who would otherwise die without the transplant (Shenkin, 1991).

A related issue involves consent for treatment of a fetus in utero, and whether failure to consent constitutes fetal abuse. Conceptualizing the problem in this way implies that the fetus and mother are separate individuals, and that the mother who refuses treatment has committed a crime against another person, a fetus. Thus the court can intervene. However, "Coercing the mother to protect the not-yet-born child poses serious threats to women's privacy and bodily autonomy" (Steinbock, 1992, p. 19). The American Medical Association and other medical groups have made a distinction between mother and fetus, holding that a pregnant woman cannot be coerced to accept a treatment to benefit her fetus. They also emphasize that it is the physician's ethical duty to be noncoercive and to accept the informed decision of the patient (Council, 1990).

The dilemma of whether the fetus and pregnant woman can be considered as a single or a dual unit can be further elucidated. "When the maternal–fetal dyad is regarded as an organic whole, what matters is that combined maternal–fetal benefits outweigh combined maternal–fetal burdens," but when "fetus and pregnant woman are conceptualized as two individual patients . . . it is no longer appropriate to consider effects of treatment on the two combined" (Mattingly, 1992, p. 14). Thus, in the latter view, the benefit and burden to each are separate. When fetal abnormalities pose no threat to maternal health, the risk of treatment is greater for the maternal patient, and she should not be obliged to undergo it. Physicians should not benefit one patient by forcing another to take unwarranted risks.

The arguments regarding endangerment of another person could mean that almost every act of a pregnant woman, even failing to follow a doctor's orders, could affect her fetus and make her vulnerable to legal action (Steinbock, 1992). Here we approach a logically and pragmatically impossible slippery slope.

*Abortion.* In 1973 the U.S. Supreme Court made abortion a legal procedure in the United States within limits of time and specific circumstances (*Roe v. Wade,* 1973). The decision then became the responsibility of the pregnant woman and her physician. Physicians and hospitals, however, may refuse to perform abortions or the grounds of moral convictions and limitation of funds (Nadelson and Notman, 1977). Although it may not be the intent, this policy effectively discriminates against women with limited mobility and finances, since they may have no way of obtaining abortion services if they are not available in their community. They may then be faced with the choice of illegal abortion or continuing an unwanted pregnancy, while women with more financial resources will be able to seek abortion elsewhere. Extralegal procedures increase in frequency in the face of restrictive laws (Callahan, 1970). In addition, illegal abortion is more hazardous to a woman's health, so that the risks for poorer women, who may perceive no alternative, are greater.

In the abortion issue there are differing ethical philosophies, perhaps in unresolvable conflict. Although some argue that, from the moment of conception, the right to life is absolute, others disagree and emphasize that the right to life is the right not to be killed unjustly (Thomson, 1971). Attempts to resolve these conflicting points of view have sometimes medicalized the decision, using physical- and mental-health criteria to justify terminating a pregnancy. Early abortion currently involves less risk than continuing a pregnancy to term. Since physical problems rarely make pregnancy hazardous, emotional indications, including the development of a "post-abortion syndrome" and threats of suicide, have been sought to justify restrictions on the availability of abortion. Emotional repercussions of abortion are rare. In order to emphasize that abortion could have deleterious consequences and therefore should be denied, some abortion opponents have proposed that a post-abortion syndrome exists, and that it has serious emotional sequelae. There are no data supporting the existence of such a syndrome. Invoking a post-abortion syndrome also pathologizes normal reactions to life experiences.

Legal and policy issues focus on the right to privacy, including control of one's body, the freedom of individual choice, and equality. It is clear that women, because they can become pregnant, face a risk and burden that men do not.

**Menstruation.**    Many myths persist about menstruation. The existence of behavioral and mood fluctuations with phases of the menstrual cycle and their possible physiological basis have been debated for years. On the grounds that they are too strongly affected by cyclic changes, women have been considered unsuitable for important positions. Although many women experience no changes premenstrually, for others the days before each menstrual period are characterized by irritability, mood lability, and other symptoms that disappear with the onset of the menstrual period.

Premenstrual syndrome (PMS), a nonspecific term, was said to be responsible for various types of social behavior and psychological phenomena. Crimes committed (Morton et al., 1953; Dalton, 1964), suicide attempts, misbehavior of schoolgirls, psychiatric admissions to emergency rooms, and visits to clinics (Sommer, 1973; Koeske, 1976) have been related to the premenstrual period. A number of studies of suicide attempts (Mandell and Mandell, 1967; MacKinnon et al., 1959) have indicated that a majority occurred in the bleeding phase of the cycle. Most of the early data on PMS consist of self-reports of functioning during the menstrual cycle; they indicate that a small percentage of women feel that their judgment and mental faculties are im-

paired to some extent, particularly in the premenstrual phase of the cycle.

Reviews of studies of cognitive and perceptual-motor behavior in relation to menstruation have pointed out methodological problems in much of the research (Sommer, 1973). The problem of determining the hormonal status of the subjects, the selection bias toward women with regular cycles, the use of self-reports, and the combination of objective with subjective data complicate evaluation of results. Many studies were not replicated, and correlational studies did not determine causality. A majority of studies using objective performance measures have failed to demonstrate significant cyclic fluctuation in performance.

Barbara Sommer concluded that cyclic effects are seen where the demands of the social milieu and the woman's own expectations predict them, and she suggested that altering these social-psychological expectations of menstrual debility results in the disappearance of the effect (1973). Menstrual variations may reflect responses of the individual to personal and social expectations, identification with important women in her life, or somatic expressions of a wide variety of feelings about herself, her femininity, and her body.

Although there are data suggesting cyclic effects in some women, the use of diagnoses like PMS and the assumption that menstrual fluctuations are pathologic are inappropriate bases for stereotyping women's behavior. The term PMS has been replaced in the *DSM-IV* (American Psychiatric Association, 1994) by the term Premenstrual Dysphoric Disorder (PMDD), which specifically delineates psychiatric symptoms. Including this term in any form in the official psychiatric nomenclature (*DSM-IV*) evoked considerable controversy about the stigmatizing effects of its use and the tendency to pathologize reactions to normal fluctuations of mood with variations in life experiences.

Although more research is continuing in this area, many studies still suffer from methodological problems, including the use of nonuniform criteria for the diagnosis, the lack of daily records of mood fluctuations, the failure to accurately correlate menstrual cycle phase with biological data, and the inaccuracies of data based on short periods of observation. Current research using the narrower and more specific criteria to define PMDD suggests that prevalence rates may be much lower than had been estimated for PMS. Using the criteria for Late Luteal Phase Dysphoric Disorder (LLPDD), from the *DSM-III-R* (American Psychiatric Association, 1987), the rates are as low as 4.6 percent in one study (Rivera-Tovar and Frank, 1990) and 6.8 percent in another (Stout and Steege, 1990). The problem of differentiating other disorders from PMDD remains.

The reappraisal undertaken for the *DSM-IV* was based on careful reviews of emerging research, so that the syndrome could validly apply to a very small percentage of women who are seriously incapacitated. The proponents of the PMDD diagnosis feel that it would be unethical to deny those women appropriate treatment, based on solid scientific evidence.

The stigmatizing effect of the diagnosis, however, as is true for many diagnoses, must be considered in the context of the cultural meaning of a body experience. In this case, menstruation and the taboos, beliefs, and expectations associated with it bring a complex set of responses. The diagnosis, even if legitimate, supports and is supported by popular expectations of menstrually related responses and pathology. This attribution can color research and confuse the results. The persistence of the use of the diagnosis of PMS illustrates the problems of addressing a behavior that is embedded in a complex context by questioning only one component of the behavior, raising questions about the diagnosis without considering cultural attitudes toward menstruation.

**Menopause.** Endocrinological and social-psychological data (McKinlay, 1989; Parlee, 1990) indicate that many misconceptions have existed about the nature and extent of the symptoms that can be directly ascribed to menopause. Multiple disorders said to be caused by the changing hormonal balance and equated with menopause may, in fact, not be due to these imbalances (Notman, 1990).

Research on menopause also suffers from serious methodological problems, such as relying on case histories, clinical impressions, or analyses of data from selected samples of women under the care of gynecologists or psychiatrists. More reliable studies show that psychological symptoms were not reported more frequently by so-called menopausal women than by younger women (McKinlay and Jeffreys, 1974).

Vasomotor instability, manifested as hot flashes, flushes, and excess perspiration, has been one of the consistent symptoms accompanying menopause. Such phenomena are present in a large number of menopausal women; up to 75 percent report some symptoms (Kronenberg, 1990). The other symptoms investigated—headaches, dizzy spells, palpitations, sleeplessness, depression, and weight increase—do not appear to show a direct relationship to menopause (McKinlay and Jeffreys, 1974).

Not only are many symptoms attributed to menopause not necessarily biological, but menopause itself may not be as central to the midlife crisis for women as had previously been thought (Neugarten et al., 1968; Parlee, 1990; Notman, 1990). The cessation of menses and the accompanying endocrine changes may be less critical than the reaction to menopause as a signal of aging and the awareness that a phase of life has ended. For many women there are concomitant changes in their social role at that time, including the loss of their status

as mothers and the disruption of a network of important social relationships.

The stereotyping of menopause as the determining diagnostic entity for midlife depression or midlife stress has led to inappropriate treatment decisions, with insufficient attention paid to social, family, or psychiatric conditions. A wide variety of treatments have been used, as for PMS, with insufficient investigation of the causes of the symptoms.

**Mastectomy.** The increase in incidence of breast cancer in the 1980s, and the sparse resources devoted to research on and treatment of it at that time, suggest either that it was not taken seriously enough, or that it is difficult to stimulate areas of research that do not have special meaning to investigators. Among the questions that need be addressed is the optimal treatment for an individual patient, including indications for a particular type and extent of surgery, for chemotherapy, or for radiation. Understanding of the risks and alternatives is critical. For some women, the knowledge that a disfiguring operation is not inevitable has made it easier for them to seek medical attention for a breast mass.

The controversy about the safety of silicone implants for postmastectomy patients complicates the problem enormously. If evidence regarding complications was indeed withheld from those making the decisions about the safety of silicone implants ("Patients and Surgeons," 1992), then patients were deceived into believing they were taking less risk than they actually did. This case raises questions similar to those regarding contraceptives.

It also raises important questions about patient autonomy. To what extent does the patient have the right to choose to accept a risk, and at what level of safety should a procedure be forbidden? Unavailability of silicone breast implants can have profound consequences for women who risk losing a breast with no recourse to a reconstructive procedure. The threat of disfiguring surgery causes many women to delay treatment. Not only is the possibility of reconstruction important in helping a woman confront and deal with her illness, but it also has implications for her self-image and relationships.

**Rape.** Women who have been raped are often blamed, disbelieved, and criticized. As a result, they may be reluctant to seek medical care or to report the rape. This often results in their receiving poor medical care, creating a disparity between them and victims of other aggressions or disasters (Notman and Nadelson, 1976).

Rape is a violent crime that is often misperceived as a sexual experience. The possibility of serious harm or death exists, and the victim's prime concern is to protect herself from injury. Since the absence of consent is crucial to the definition of rape, the victim often has had to demonstrate signs of struggle or to provide witnesses, in order to prove the absence of consent—a requirement that does not occur with other violent crimes.

Health-care personnel may be in dual and conflicting roles with rape victims. Those who first see the victim have to collect evidence for possible prosecution of the rapist, yet they are also obligated to attend to the best interests of their patient, who may not wish to report the crime. Sensitivity to the patient's condition may be in conflict with the need for complete information. The victim's need to gain control can conflict with the requirements for thoroughness in the evaluation.

## Mental health

Although women have generally been considered more vulnerable than men to a variety of emotional symptoms and mental illnesses, the actual incidence of mental illness is difficult to determine because descriptions of symptoms and definitions of mental illness vary widely. In an early study documenting variations in the way that men and women were evaluated and in recommendations for treatment, the researchers reported that clinicians' concepts of a mentally healthy, mature man were similar to their concepts of a mentally healthy adult; their concepts of a mentally healthy, mature woman were more like those for a child (Broverman et al., 1970). For instance, healthy women were seen as being more submissive, less independent, less adventurous, more sensitive to being hurt, less aggressive, and less competitive than were healthy men.

Although some controversy surrounds the data analysis from the original study and its current validity, there is still evidence that social stereotypes operate and influence patient care (Widiger and Settle, 1987; Hansen and Reekie, 1990). The differentiation between psychopathology and deviance from culturally accepted norms is particularly relevant for women, who often feel that the help they are offered, especially when they are suffering from psychological distress, supports traditional views about women's roles and behavior, rather than being responsive to their individual needs (Nadelson and Notman, 1991).

Since 1980 specific criteria have been formulated for the diagnosis of psychiatric disorders, enabling researchers to collect epidemiologic data to permit estimates of the incidence and prevalence of various mental disorders. There is increasing evidence that although there are no differences in the overall incidence of mental illness in the population at large, there are gender-related differences in the incidence, diagnosis, treatment, and outcome for mental illnesses (Regier et al., 1984; Weissman, 1991). Woman have been reported to have higher rates of depression, as well as somatization, anxiety, and eating and panic disorders (using *DSM-III-R* [American Psychiatric Association, 1987] criteria).

Men are more likely to be diagnosed with alcoholism, substance abuse, early-onset schizophrenia, and impulse and antisocial personality disorders.

There are also gender differences in symptom expression, such as suicide. Although more men commit suicide, more women attempt it (Farberow and Schneidman, 1965). Norman Farberow and Edwin Schneidman found that 69 percent of attempted suicides in the United States were women and 70 percent of completed suicides were men.

One difference in rates of mental illness between men and women involves marital status. Married men and single women have been reported to have the lowest rates of mental illness (Weissman and Klerman, 1985; Gove and Tudor, 1973). Contrary to popular expectations, marriage would seem to offer men some protection against mental illness and to make women more vulnerable. One hypothesis to explain these data suggests that wives provide care for their husbands, and that the marital relationship often imposes more constraints on women and provides less care for them. Additional data indicate that the women most vulnerable to symptoms are young married women with small children (Brown and Harris, 1978).

Another hypothesis suggests that women are labeled mentally ill when they cannot perform the service and maintenance functions of wife and mother, or other socially accepted roles for women (Chesler, 1972). An alternative explanation of the differences is that women are responding to the stresses of social isolation, particularly from other adults; the physical and emotional fatigue of dealing with small children (and often elderly relatives); and the tensions of confronting the impulses and feelings stirred up in parents by their young children. It has been suggested that women experience greater life stress because of their multiple roles, and because of the greater likelihood that they will live in poverty and be alone as they age (McBride, 1990; Belle, 1990; Rodeheaver and Datan, 1988).

Women experience more sexual and physical abuse than men, and this may be an important factor in the greater incidence of disorders such as depression, posttraumatic stress disorder, and anxiety (Koss, 1990). Depression, for example, has been linked with socialization toward compliance in women. The reasons for most gender differences in mental illness, however, remain unclear, although it appears that complex interactions between biological and psychosocial factors are responsible.

Differences between men and women in the incidence of mental illness are most apparent when they are related to biological and, in particular, reproductive functions. Women, not men, may suffer from reproductively and menstrually related disorders such as postpartum syndromes or symptoms related to menopause, hysterectomy, infertility, abortion, and miscarriage. With the exception of some forms of postpartum disorders and symptoms related to physiologic concomitants during the menstrual cycle and menopause, the psychological specificity of these other syndromes has not been demonstrated.

The readiness with which symptoms and behaviors are attributed to physical events experienced by women, such as menopause, a hysterectomy, or an abortion, attests to the power of societal expectations of women's weakness and vulnerability. These beliefs and values can affect investigators' care in examining data or researching these areas. It is also possible to objectify symptoms and impart causality without looking carefully at individual experience and variability.

Alcoholism and substance abuse are generally grouped with mental disorders. The data indicate that there is a substantial preponderance of men with these disorders. This discrepancy has resulted in a minimization of the incidence or impact of these disorders in women. There has been little research, and thus data on women's specific treatment needs and responses are sparse. Resources for the treatment of women are scarce. An Institute of Medicine report suggested that public concern about male behavior, especially violence, related to alcohol abuse may lead to the development of treatment methods that are less effective for women. Thus, differential access to care is a substantial ethical problem. It is also not clear what percentage of women actually receive treatment, in part because definitions of severe alcohol use vary and also because other variables related to differential access to treatment are not taken into account—such as the availability of child care, so that mothers with dependent children can seek treatment. There is a general tendency to deny the seriousness of alcoholism and substance abuse in women, and this leads to delays in treatment (Reed, 1991; Weisner, 1991).

## Conclusion

Social, economic, and technological changes have brought about alterations in relationships between men and women and patients and providers and in the delivery of health care. Although the paternalism that has existed in the health-care system has gradually changed, in part as a result of the changes that have taken place in women's roles since the 1970s, there continue to be inequities in research and clinical care between men and women. Some of this, as we have suggested, derives from the special aspects of women's reproductive roles and the potential consequences for society of allowing women to be autonomous in decisions about their care.

CAROL C. NADELSON
MALKAH T. NOTMAN

*Directly related to this article are the other articles in this entry, especially* HISTORICAL AND CROSS-CULTURAL PERSPECTIVES, *and* RESEARCH ISSUES. *Also directly related are the entries* FEMINISM; SEXISM; FREEDOM AND COERCION; PATERNALISM; REPRODUCTIVE TECHNOLOGIES, *article on* ETHICAL ISSUES; FERTILITY CONTROL, *article on* ETHICAL ISSUES; POPULATION POLICIES, *article on* HEALTH STANDARDS IN FERTILITY CONTROL; CIRCUMCISION, *article on* FEMALE CIRCUMCISION; *and* MENTAL ILLNESS, *article on* CONCEPTIONS OF MENTAL ILLNESS. *For a further discussion of topics mentioned in this article, see the entries* ABUSE, INTERPERSONAL, *articles on* ABUSE BETWEEN DOMESTIC PARTNERS, *and* ELDER ABUSE; AGING AND THE AGED, *article on* OLD AGE; AUTONOMY; COMPETENCY; INFORMED CONSENT, *articles on* CLINICAL ASPECTS OF CONSENT IN HEALTH CARE, *and* LEGAL AND ETHICAL ISSUES OF CONSENT IN HEALTH CARE (*with its* POSTSCRIPT); PROFESSIONAL–PATIENT RELATIONSHIP; SEXUAL ETHICS AND PROFESSIONAL STANDARDS; SUBSTANCE ABUSE, *article on* ALCOHOLISM; *and* SURGERY. *For a further discussion of fertility control and related ideas, see the entries* ABORTION, *section on* CONTEMPORARY ETHICAL AND LEGAL PERSPECTIVES; EUGENICS, *article on* ETHICAL ISSUES; FERTILITY CONTROL, *articles on* SOCIAL ISSUES, *and* LEGAL AND REGULATORY ISSUES; MATERNAL–FETAL RELATIONSHIP, *article on* ETHICAL ISSUES; *and* POPULATION POLICIES, *section on* STRATEGIES OF FERTILITY CONTROL. *For a further discussion of women and mental illness, see the entries* MENTAL-HEALTH SERVICES, *article on* ETHICAL ISSUES; MENTAL ILLNESS, *article on* ISSUES IN DIAGNOSIS; MENTALLY DISABLED AND MENTALLY ILL PERSONS, *article on* HEALTH-CARE ISSUES; *and* SUICIDE. *See also the* APPENDIX (CODES, OATHS, AND DIRECTIVES RELATED TO BIOETHICS), SECTION II: ETHICAL DIRECTIVES FOR THE PRACTICE OF MEDICINE, OATH OF HIPPOCRATES.

## Bibliography

AMERICAN PSYCHIATRIC ASSOCIATION. 1987. *Diagnostic and Statistical Manual of Mental Disorders: DSM-III-R.* 3d ed., rev. Washington, D.C.: Author.

———. 1994. *Diagnostic and Statistical Manual of Mental Disorders: DSM-IV.* 4th ed. Washington, D.C.: Author.

APFEL, ROBERTA J., and FISHER, SUSAN M. 1984. *To Do No Harm: DES and the Dilemmas of Modern Medicine.* New Haven, Conn.: Yale University Press.

BAKER MILLER, JEAN, and MOTHNER, ÌRA. 1971. "Psychological Consequences of Sexual Inequality." *American Journal of Orthopsychiatry* 41, no. 5:767–775.

BELLE, DEBORAH. 1990. "Poverty and Women's Mental Health." *American Psychologist* 45, no. 3:385–389.

BOK, SISSELA. 1974. "Ethical Problems of Abortion." *Hastings Center Studies* 2, no. 1:33–52. Reprinted in *Ethics in Medicine: Historical Perspectives and Contemporary Concerns.*

Edited by Stanley Joel Reiser, Arthur J. Dyck, and William J. Curran. Cambridge, Mass.: MIT Press, 1977.

BOUHOUTSOS, JACQUELINE; HOLROYD, JEAN; LERMAN, HANNAH; FORER, BERTRAM R; and GREENBERG, MIMI. 1983. "Sexual Intimacy Between Psychotherapists and Patients." *Professional Psychology: Research and Practice* 14, no. 2:185–196.

BREMMER, WILLIAM J., and DE KRETZER, DAVID M. 1976. "The Prospects for New, Reversible Male Contraceptives." *New England Journal of Medicine* 295, no. 20:1111–1117.

BROVERMAN, INGE K; BROVERMAN, DONALD M.; CLARKSON, FRANK E.; ROSENKRANTZ, PAUL S.; and VOGEL, SUSAN R. 1970. "Sex-Role Stereotypes and Clinical Judgments of Mental Health." *Journal of Consulting and Clinical Psychology* 34, no. 1:1–7.

BROWN, GEORGE W., and HARRIS, TIRRIL. 1978. *Social Origins of Depression: A Study of Psychiatric Disorders in Women.* New York: Free Press.

BURGESS, A. 1981. "Physician Sexual Misconduct and Patients' Responses." *American Journal of Psychiatry* 138, no. 10:1335–1342.

CALLAHAN, DANIEL J. 1970. *Abortion: Law, Choice, and Morality.* New York: Macmillan.

CHALMERS, THOMAS C. 1974. "The Impact of Clinical Trials in Medical Practice." In vol. 1 of *Principles and Techniques of Human Research and Therapeutics*, pp. 193–203. Edited by F. Gilbert McMahon. Mt. Kisco, N.Y.: Futura.

CHESLER, PHYLLIS. 1972. *Women and Madness.* New York: Avon.

COUNCIL ON ETHICAL AND JUDICIAL AFFAIRS, AMERICAN MEDICAL ASSOCIATION. 1990. "Sexual Misconduct in the Practice of Medicine." Report of the council presented to and passed by the House of Delegates in Miami, Fla., December 19. Reprinted in *Journal of the American Medical Association* 266, no. 19:2741–2745.

DALTON, KATHARINA. 1964. *The Premenstrual Syndrome.* Springfield, Ill.: Charles C. Thomas.

DOMENIGHETTI, GIANFRANCO; LURASCHI, PIERANGELO; and MARAZZI, ALFIO. 1985. "Hysterectomy and Sex of the Gynecologist." *New England Journal of Medicine* 313, no. 23:1482.

FARBEROW, NORMAN L., and SCHNEIDMAN, EDWIN S. 1965. "Statistical Comparisons Between Attempted and Committed Suicides." In *The Cry for Help*, pp. 19–47. Edited by Norman L. Farberow and Edwin S. Schneidman. New York: McGraw-Hill.

FELDMAN-SUMMERS, S., and JONES, G. 1984. "Psychological Impacts on Sexual Contact Between Therapists or Other Health Care Practitioners and Their Clients." *Journal of Consulting and Clinical Psychology* 52, no. 6:1054–1061.

GABBARD, GLEN O., ed. 1989. *Sexual Exploitation in Professional Relationships.* Washington, D.C.: American Psychiatric Press.

GOVE, W. R., and TUDOR, JEANETTE F. 1973. "Adult Sex Roles and Mental Illness." In *Changing Women in a Changing Society*, pp. 50–73. Edited by Joan Huber. Chicago: University of Chicago Press.

HANSEN, FINY JOSEPHINE, and REEKIE, LILIAN-JEAN. 1990.

"Sex Differences in Clinical Judgements of Male and Female Therapists." *Sex Roles* 23, nos. 1–2:51–64.

HARRISON, MICHELLE. 1990. "Psychological Ramifications of 'Surrogate' Motherhood." In *Psychiatric Aspects of Reproductive Technology*, pp. 97–112. Edited by Nada L. Stotland. Washington, D.C.: American Psychiatric Press.

HERMAN, JUDITH L.; GARTRELL, NANETTE; OLARTE, SYLVIA; FELDSTEIN, MICHAEL; and LOCALIO, RUSSELL. 1987. "Psychiatrist-Patient Sexual Contact: Results of a National Survey, II: Psychiatrists' Attitudes." *American Journal of Psychiatry* 144, no. 2:164–169.

JORGENSON, LINDA; RANDLES, REBECCA; and STRASBURGER, LARRY. 1991. "The Furor over Psychotherapist-Patient Sexual Contact: New Solutions to an Old Problem." *William and Mary Law Review* 32, no. 3:645–732.

KALTREIDER, NANCY B., and MARGOLIS, ALAN G. 1977. "Childless by Choice: A Clinical Study." *American Journal of Psychiatry* 134, no. 2:179–182.

KATZ, JAY; CAPRON, ALEXANDER M.; and GLASS, ELEANOR SWIFT, eds. 1972. *Experimentation with Human Beings: The Authority of the Investigator, Subject, Professions, and State in the Human Experimentation Process.* New York: Russell Sage Foundation.

KLUFT, RICHARD P. 1989. "Treating the Patient Who Has Been Exploited by a Previous Therapist." *Psychiatric Clinics of North America* 12, no. 2:483–500.

KOESKE, RANDI DAIMON. 1976. "Premenstrual Emotionality: Is Biology Destiny?" *Women and Health* 1, no. 3:11–14.

KOSS, MARY P. 1990. "The Women's Mental Health Research Agenda: Violence Against Women." *American Psychologist* 45, no. 3:374–380.

KRONENBERG, FREDI. 1990. "Hot Flashes: Epidemiology and Physiology." In *Multidisciplinary Perspectives on Menopause*, pp. 52–86. Edited by Marcha Flint, Fredi Kronenberg, and Wulf Utian. Annals of the New York Academy of Sciences, no. 592. New York: New York Academy of Sciences.

LENNANE, K. JEAN, and LENNANE, R. JOHN. 1973. "Alleged Psychogenic Disorders in Women—A Possible Manifestation of Sexual Prejudice." *New England Journal of Medicine* 288, no. 6:288–292.

LINDENMAYER, JEAN-PIERRE. 1976. "More Young, Childless Women Seek Surgical Sterilization." *Roche Report: Frontiers of Psychiatry* 15 (June):5–6.

MACKINNON, E. L.; MACKINNON, P. C. B.; and THOMPSON, A. D. 1959. "Lethal Hazards of the Luteal Phase of the Menstrual Cycle." *British Medical Journal* 1, no. 2:1015–1017.

MANDELL, ARNOLD J., and MANDELL, MARY P. 1967. "Suicide and the Menstrual Cycle." *Journal of the American Medical Association* 200, no. 9:792–793.

MARMOR, JUDD. 1970. "The Seductive Psychotherapist." *Psychiatry Digest* 31, no. 10:10–16.

MATTINGLY, SUSAN S. 1992. "The Maternal-Fetal Dyad: Exploring the Two-Patient Obstetric Model." *Hastings Center Report* 22, no. 1:13–18.

McBRIDE, ANGELA B. 1990. "Mental Health Effects of Women's Multiple Roles." *American Psychologist* 45, no. 3:381–384.

McKINLAY, SONJA M., and JEFFREYS, MARGOT. 1974. "The

Menopausal Syndrome." *British Journal of Preventive and Social Medicine* 28, no. 2:108–115.

McKinlay, Sonja M., and McKinlay, John B. 1989. "The Impact of Menopause and Social Factors on Health." In *Menopause: Evaluation, Treatment and Health Concerns*, pp. 137–161. Edited by Charles B. Hammond, Florence P. Hazeltine, and Isaac Schiff. Progress in Clinical and Biological Research, vol. 320. New York: Alan R. Liss.

Mintz, Morton. 1985. *At Any Cost: Corporate Greed, Women and the Dalkon Shield*. New York: Pantheon.

Morton, J. H.; Additon, J.; Addison, R. G.; Hunt, L.; and Sullivan, J. J. 1953. "A Clinical Study of Premenstrual Tension." *American Journal of Obstetrics and Gynecology* 65, no. 6:1182–1191.

Muller, Charlotte F. 1990. *Health Care and Gender*. New York: Russell Sage Foundation.

Nadelson, Carol C. 1989. "Afterword." In *Sexual Exploitation in Professional Relationships*. Edited by Glen Gabbard. Washington, D.C.: American Psychiatric Press.

———. 1991. "Emerging Issues in Medical Ethics." *British Journal of Psychiatry* 158 (suppl. 10):9–16.

———. 1993. "Ethics, Empathy and Gender in Health Care." *American Journal of Psychiatry* 150, no. 9:1309–1314.

Nadelson, Carol C., and Notman, Malkah T. 1977. "Emotional Aspects of the Symptoms, Functions and Disorders of Women." In *Psychiatric Medicine*, pp. 334–397. Edited by Gene L. Usdin. New York: Brunner/Mazel.

———. 1991. "The Impact of the New Psychology of Men and Women on Psychotherapy." *American Psychiatric Press Review of Psychiatry* 10:608–612.

National Institutes of Health (U.S.). 1990. "Report." Washington, D.C.: Author.

Nelson, James L. 1992. Introduction to papers presented by Susan S. Mattingly and Bonnie Steinbock. *Hastings Center Report* 22, no. 1:13.

Neugarten, Bernice L.; Wood, Vivian; Kraines, Ruth; and Loomis, Barbara. 1968. "Women's Attitudes Toward the Menopause." In *Middle Age and Aging: A Reader in Social Psychology*, pp. 195–200. Edited by Bernice Levin Neugarten. Chicago: University of Chicago Press.

Notman, Malkah T. 1990. "Menopause and Adult Development." In *Multidisciplinary Perspectives on Menopause*, pp. 149–155. Edited by Marcha Flint, Fredi Kronenberg, and Wulf Utian. Annals of the New York Academy of Sciences, no. 592. New York: New York Academy of Sciences.

Notman, Malkah T., and Nadelson, Carol C. 1976. "The Rape Victim: Psychodynamic Considerations." *American Journal of Psychiatry* 133, no. 4:408–413.

———. 1978. "Women as Patients and Experimental Subjects." In vol. 4 of *Encyclopedia of Bioethics*, pp. 1704–1713. Edited by Warren T. Reich. New York: Macmillan.

Parlee, Mary B. 1990. "Integrating Biological and Social Scientific Research on Menopause." In *Multidisciplinary Perspectives on Menopause*, pp. 379–389. Edited by Marcha Flint, Fredi Kronenberg, and Wulf Utian. Annals of the New York Academy of Sciences, no. 592. New York: New York Academy of Sciences.

"Patients and Surgeons Backing Implants Sue." 1992. *New York Times*, February 9, 1992, p. C1.

Pope, Kenneth S., and Bouhoutsos, Jacqueline C. 1986. *Sexual Intimacy Between Therapists and Patients*. New York: Praeger.

Reed, Beth G. 1991. "Services Research and Drug-Involved Women: Concepts, Questions, and Options." In *Assessing Future Research Needs: Mental and Addictive Disorders in Women*, pp. 91–97. Summary of an Institute of Medicine Conference, October. Washington, D.C.: Institute of Medicine.

Regier, Darrel A.; Myers, Jerome K.; Kramer, Morton; Robins, Lee N.; Blazer, Dan G.; Hough, Richard L.; Eaton, William W.; and Locke, Ben Z. 1984. "The NIMH Epidemiologic Catchment Area Program: Historical Context, Major Objectives, and Study Population Characteristics." *Archives of General Psychiatry* 41, no. 10:934–941.

*Relf v. Weinberger and National Welfare Rights Org*. 1974. 372 F. Supp. 1196 (D.C.D.).

Rivera-Tovar, Ana D., and Frank, Ellen. 1990. "Late Luteal Phase Dysphoric Disorder in Young Women." *American Journal of Psychiatry* 147, no. 12:1634–1636.

Rodeheaver, Dean, and Datan, Nancy. 1988. "The Challenge of Double Jeopardy: Toward a Mental Health Agenda for Aging Women." *American Psychologist* 43, no. 8:648–654.

*Roe v. Wade*. 1973. 410 U.S. 113.

Roos, Noralou P. 1984. "Hysterectomies in One Canadian Province: A New Look at Risks and Benefits." *American Journal of Public Health* 74, no. 1:39–46.

"Selective Reduction in Multifetal Pregnancy." 1990. *European Journal of Obstetrics & Gynecology and Reproductive Biology* 38, no. 3:181–182.

Shenkin, Henry A. 1991. *Medical Ethics: Evolution, Rights and the Physician*. Dordrecht, Netherlands: Kluwer.

Sommer, Barbara. 1973. "The Effect of Menstruation on Cognitive and Perceptual-Motor Behavior: A Review." *Psychosomatic Medicine* 35, no. 6:515–534.

Steinbock, Bonnie. 1992. "The Relevance of Illegality." *Hastings Center Report* 22, no. 1:19–22.

Stout, Anna L., and Steege, John F. 1990. Paper presented at the annual meeting of the American Society of Psychosomatic Obstetrics and Gynecology.

Thomson, Judith J. 1971. "A Defense of Abortion." *Philosophy and Public Affairs* 1, no. 1:45–66.

Weisner, Constance. 1991. "Treatment Services Research and Alcohol Problems: Treatment Entry, Access, and Effectiveness." In *Assessing Future Research Needs: Mental and Addictive Disorders in Women*, pp. 85–90. Summary of an Institute of Medicine Conference, October. Washington, D.C.: Institute of Medicine.

Weissman, Myrna M. 1991. "Gender Differences in the Rates of Mental Disorders." In *Assessing Future Research Needs: Mental and Addictive Disorders in Women*, pp. 8–13. Summary of an Institute of Medicine Conference, October. Washington, D.C.: Institute of Medicine.

Weissman, Myrna M., and Klerman, Gerald L. 1985. "Gender and Depression." *Trends in Neurosciences* 8: 416–420.

Wenger, Nanette K.; Speroff, Leon; and Packard, Barbara. 1993. "Cardiovascular Health and Disease in

Women." *New England Journal of Medicine* 329, no. 34:247–256.

WEST, CANDICE. 1984. "When the Doctor Is a 'Lady': Power, Status, and Gender in Physician-Patient Encounters." *Symbolic Interaction* 7, no. 1:87–106.

WIDIGER, THOMAS A., and SETTLE, SHIRLEY A. 1987. "Broverman et al. Revisited: An Artifactual Sex Bias." *Journal of Personality and Social Psychology* 53, no. 3:463–469.

## III. RESEARCH ISSUES

The early 1990s brought considerable attention to the response of biomedical research to women's health. Recognition emerged that to a large extent, women's only health concern had been primarily perceived to be related to the reproductive functions and that although research in these areas had been inadequate, research that promoted other important aspects of women's health had been practically nonexistent. Moreover, it was recognized that research findings had been generalized to apply to women when women had not served as subjects in studies. This article reviews the recent controversy that has brought these concerns to public attention, describes the injustices that are present in the way research has involved women, and discusses current attempts to redress the problems of the past.

### Controversy regarding women as research subjects

The early 1990s represented a time of intensifying interest in women's health and shifting perceptions of how women should be involved in biomedical research. This surge of interest originated from many sources but may be most concretely traced to the work of a U.S. Public Health Service Task Force on Women's Health Issues that was created in response to pressure from women researchers within the largest publicly funded U.S. research agency, the National Institutes of Health (NIH). Following a two-year study, this task force issued a report in 1985, concluding that

> Many methodological problems, as well as a lack of data, limit our understanding of the status of women's health, women's particular needs, and the services women require. The need for data that are relevant to health and are sex- and age-specific by race and ethnicity is crucial. (U.S. Public Health Service Task Force on Women's Health Issues, 1985, p. 81)

The NIH subsequently established an Advisory Committee on Women's Health Issues and in 1986, with the Alcohol, Drug Abuse and Mental Health Administration, published a joint policy statement that "urged" grant applicants to include more women in research efforts and also to evaluate any gender differences that were found.

The language of and commitment to this new policy were insufficient. In late 1989, members of the U.S. Congress requested that the U.S. General Government Accounting Office (GAO) investigate how the NIH was implementing its new policy (Nadel, 1990). Contention was mounting in response to a growing perception that too little research was being undertaken on diseases and conditions affecting women, such as breast cancer, menopause, and acquired immunodeficiency syndrome (AIDS). In addition, there was increased sensitivity regarding the effects of exclusionary practices represented by NIH-supported studies. Specifically, the Multiple Risk Factor Intervention Trial (MRFIT) examined the prevention of cardiac events with a sample of nearly 13,000 men (Multiple Risk Factor Intervention Trial Research Group, 1982); the Physician Health Study began in 1981 and involved over 22,000 male doctors and examined the benefits of prophylactic aspirin in decreasing the risk of myocardial infarction (Steering Committee of the Physicians' Health Study Research Group, 1989); and the Baltimore Longitudinal Study of Aging (National Institute Advisory Council, 1991) in its initial stages in the late 1950s included only men, despite the fact that women comprise nearly two-thirds of the elderly population in the United States.

When the GAO reported the results of its investigation to Congress indicating that the NIH had made "little progress" in implementing its 1986 policy on the inclusion of women in research (Nadel, 1990), immediate change began to occur within this research agency. Though it took until 1993 for it to be statutorily authorized, within months of the GAO report, the NIH established an Office of Research on Women's Health. Language regarding the inclusion of women in research was also strengthened with revisions specifying that applications "should employ a study design with gender representation appropriate to the known incidence/prevalence of the disease or condition being studied" (National Institutes of Health/Alcohol, Drug Abuse, and Mental Health Administration, 1990, p. 18). The NIH also initiated large-scale research studies that specifically address women's health concerns.

Bernadine Healy, the first woman to serve as director of the NIH, was appointed in 1991 and in this role began to advocate a strengthened research agenda on health concerns facing women. She also voiced her observation that the women's movement of the 1960s emphasized equality of rights for women but was accompanied by an unfortunate side effect in that the ways in which women differ from men have not received the attention they deserve from the medical community (Healy, 1991a; 1991b). She observed that this had particularly been true with coronary artery disease. Sex-exclusive research has created the myth that heart disease is primarily a male affliction, and male-generated findings have been extrapolated to women, leading to biased standards of care for women. Recognizing this reality and similar gender disparities in the treatment of other diseases, the Council on Ethical and Judicial Affairs of the American Medical Association recommended in 1991 that "results of medical testing done solely on men should not be generalized to women without evidence that results can be applied safely and effectively to both sexes" (Council on Ethical and Judicial Affairs, American Medical Association, 1991, p. 562).

The U.S. Congress included in the NIH Revitalization Act of 1993 several provisions to strengthen research as it relates to women and minority groups. One of these provisions requires that all NIH studies include representative samples of subpopulations, particularly women and ethnic and racial minorities (U.S. Department of Health and Human Services, 1994). In addition, in 1993, the Food and Drug Administration (FDA), which also was the subject of a GAO investigation in 1992, lifted its 1977 guideline that had restricted, with few exceptions, women "with childbearing potential" from early phases of drug development research. The FDA now expects research on new drugs to include the study of gender differences (Merkatz et al., 1993).

Why has it been that males and not females have been the primary subjects and recipients of the benefits of research, and why has it taken so long for concern about this practice to be expressed? Responses to these questions highlight the injustice apparent in how biomedical research has been conceptualized and the complacency regarding the need for research to better respond to the health concerns of women. Specifically, a variety of factors play a role in how these injustices have evolved. They include protectionistic policies, disparities in attention to women's as opposed to men's health problems, the conceptualization of the white male as the norm for society and women as "special," and the perception that development of adequate sample sizes for findings that are generalizable to women would be too difficult or too expensive to achieve. These injustices will be reviewed.

## Protectionism

The very policies and attitudes that have provoked controversy regarding the exclusion of women from research are to a considerable degree the outcome of attempts to protect women and fetuses from risks that are inherent in participation in research. There is a long and unfortunate history of the way in which populations of women and men have been abused by research; this has been redressed with clear ethical standards such as those presented in the Belmont Report published by the U.S. National Commission for the Protection of Human Sub-

jects of Biomedical and Behavioral Research in 1978. This report articulates the importance of the researcher's adherence to the ethical principles of respect for persons, beneficence, and justice; it represented opposition to the paternalistic practices of the past. Nonetheless, current concerns about women and research are focused on the way in which protective policies have prevented women from making autonomous decisions regarding their participation in research.

At approximately the same time that the Belmont Report was published, the FDA issued a guideline in 1977 barring women of childbearing potential from early phases of drug trials regardless of their or their mate's fertility status, use of contraceptives, or sexual behavior (FDA, 1977). Though exceptions were made for circumstances where an experimental drug could be lifesaving or life-prolonging, the 1977 guideline essentially disallowed premenopausal women from having the opportunity to participate in drug-related research.

The recognition of the tragic malformations caused during fetal development when pregnant women in the late 1950s and early 1960s took the drug thalidomide as a mild sedative, prompted such exclusionary practices and little opposition was expressed initially regarding them. The philosophy represented by the limitations placed on women's participation in research was reinforced in the late 1970s with the recognition that the drug diethylstilbestrol (DES), taken by pregnant women in the 1940s and 1950s to prevent miscarriage, is a carcinogen for their daughters.

The fear of fatal damage clearly overpowered concerns that were raised regarding how failure to evaluate the effects of drugs on menstruating women could outweigh risks to a potential pregnancy (Kinney et al., 1981). Recognition of protectionistic policies was slow in coming. These policies assume that an adult woman is not competent to decide whether to participate in a study or to decide whether to use contraception or, if contraceptive efforts fail, to terminate pregnancy (Chavkin and Fox, 1990). In addition, little attention has been given to how such a policy violated the basic premise of equal protection, because fertile men were not excluded from studies—the potential risk of participation in research to their reproductive functions has essentially been ignored (Institute of Medicine, 1994b).

The exclusion of women from drug research is also prompted by concerns regarding legal liability for potential fetal injury. Reviews, however, show that drug manufacturers have not faced substantial litigation by those who have participated in clinical trials. Alternatively, litigation occurs when an approved drug has been used in a population in whom it had not been well researched (Merkatz et al., 1993). Furthermore, it is suggested that women participating in a clinical trial who consent to the risk of harm to potential offspring and who decide against contraception or terminating a pregnancy resulting from a contraceptive failure would be unlikely to recover damages if fetal damage occurs (Dresser, 1992). Nonetheless, legislative immunity may be needed to protect researchers from possible claims brought by injured children (Dresser, 1992).

Protectionistic policies represent greater concern for the well-being of the fetus than for women and their future children. In addition, concerns about litigation as a rationale for excluding potentially pregnant women from research trials essentially place more value on the prevention of potential lawsuits than on promoting women's health with research. Overall, these policies fail to provide women with the opportunity to make autonomous, informed decisions regarding their involvement in research.

### Gender disparities in research

Much of the impetus that has led to policy changes regarding women's involvement in research has come from the perception that women's health-care needs have been inadequately recognized by the research community. Specifically, examples abound of inadequate attention to women in the studies of coronary heart disease in the 1960s and 1970s. The formulation of these specific studies and the biomedical research agenda in general, however, may reflect ageism as much as sexism (Angell, 1993).

The studies conducted by the NIH that initially excluded women were based on findings from the massive epidemiological data base from the Framingham Heart study that began in 1948 and included both women and men (Higgins, 1990). Twelve-year follow-up data from this study showed that for those subjects under sixty-five years of age there was a threefold difference in mortality rates between men and women. Interpretations of these findings created the impression that coronary heart disease was a male problem although it was the leading cause of death for women over sixty-five years of age. The fact that women live longer than men and experience cardiac and other problems later in life contributes to a perception that women are healthier. In actuality, many conditions affecting women significantly affect the quality of their lives but have been perceived as a part of "normal aging" and, until recently, have not been essential topics for biomedical research. Indeed, research agendas often reflect the interests, power, and privilege of those who set them (Sherwin, 1994). The absence of women in science has been a contributing factor in the exclusion of women from clinical studies and the failure of research to address adequately conditions affecting women (LaRosa and Pinn, 1993).

Research pertaining to women is also often conceived in a manner that fails to address fairly women's health concerns. For example, AIDS research initially explored the disease process in women with a focus on the way in which they transmit the human immunodeficiency virus to the fetus or to the newborn (Institute of Medicine, 1994c). Less attention was paid to how women themselves respond to the virus, regardless of the fact that data show that women with AIDS do not live as long as men live, which may be related to the medical treatment they receive (Lemp et al., 1992).

While data are clear in documenting the underrepresentation of women in cardiac- and AIDS-related research and gaps in knowledge are recognized in research related to aging and women, there is less empirical evidence to support the claim that women have not been fairly represented in the whole of clinical research. The Committee on the Ethical and Legal Issues Related to the Inclusion of Women in Clinical Studies of the Institute of Medicine attempted to address this concern and reported that it was "frustrated by the lack of any systematic, centralized collection of data on the gender composition of study populations" (Institute of Medicine, 1994a, p. 3). A variety of studies, however, have made observations similar to a review of articles that appeared in the *Journal of the American Medical Association* between 1991 and 1992. This review shows that women are more often underrepresented in research samples than are men (Bird, 1994). Nonetheless, the Committee recognized the need for a systematized collection of these data in order to draw firm conclusions about the relative participation of men and women in research.

Former perceptions of involvement in research primarily recognized it in terms of its altruistic contributions to society. Increasingly, instead, it has come to be viewed as a potential personal benefit for participants who gain access to investigational drugs and treatments and who cooperate with protocols. With this changing view of the meaning of serving as a research subject, biases affecting the design of research are recognized for how they affect personal health care. Protests regarding these biases emphasize how the benefits of research (that is primarily publicly funded) should be justly enjoyed by both the male and female citizens who provide its financial support.

### Perception of men as the norm and women as "special"

The style of discussion used in the consideration of research affects its conceptualization and contributes to the creation of biases. Traditionally society has had a tendency to use the male gender to express universal statements regarding humanity, thus creating the notion that males represent the norm for society. As issues regarding women and research are considered, queries arise regarding "when women need to be included in studies" rather than posing questions in a manner that would reflect gender equity such as, "When is it possible to exclude men or women from research?" (National Academy of Sciences, 1991). Discussion regarding women as a "special population" (a term used by the Pharmaceutical Manufacturers Association) also implies the traditional assumption that men represent the norm for society and similarly for research.

Though women essentially have gained this "special" status by virtue of not being men, the fact that they menstruate, may become pregnant, and experience menopause is highlighted as a reason why researchers need to show special consideration if women are to be involved in studies. Alternatively, men could be, but are not, considered special because they do not menstruate, gestate, or experience menopause.

The biases inherent in how language has been used foster the impression that women's involvement in research is often not essential and thus unnecessarily costly and time-consuming. Attributing special status to women also prevents researchers from paying closer attention to concerns such as the vulnerability of male fertility to the unknown effects of research protocols.

## Methodological issues

A variety of methodological rationales for women's exclusion from research are offered by investigators. For example, critiques of the Physician Health Study's (Steering Committee, 1989) failure to include women in its protocol are countered with the typical justifications of gender exclusion of women. These include the lower incidence of heart attacks among women in the age groups studied and anticipated disinterest among women in following the protocol (Cotton, 1990).

For research findings to be meaningful, sample sizes must not only be sufficiently large, but also must be representative of the group to whom findings are to be generalized. However, a basic premise for the development of an experimental design is that it use a sample that excludes subjects whose characteristics may interfere with a clear explanation of differences between an experimental and a control group. Thus, the more homogeneous the research sample, the more secure the conclusions drawn from it. Alternatively, the more homogeneous the subjects that comprise a research sample are, the less generalizable the findings of a study are. Extremely large samples may be needed to detect significant differences among subgroups representing gender, age, or racial differences.

Consequently, in concert with the prevailing perception that women are special (because of their variable hormonal makeup related to the menstrual cycle, menopause, and use of oral contraceptives or estrogen-replacement therapy), they have been excluded from studies because controlling for these variables would demand larger and more expensive sample sizes. In such cases, simplifying research has taken precedence over the value of understanding women's concerns (e.g., how hormonal variation affects response to drugs or other forms of medical treatment). As a consequence, women's health care is frequently based on findings from male subjects, whose hormonal makeup is different from that of females. The shortsightedness of this approach is evidenced in findings published in 1994 showing that survival among premenopausal women with breast cancer is related significantly to the timing of surgery in relation to the menstrual cycle (Saad et al., 1994). Though other investigations have not made similar observations (Wobbes et al., 1994), it has taken until the end of the twentieth century to consider the role played by such a basic variable of female physiology, highlighting the biases that have guided research activities. It also represents a failure to recognize the possible untoward expenses of not including in a study's methodology an examination of variables that are unique to women.

The involvement of women in research may require that consideration be given to their needs for time away from hourly employment, transplantation, and child-care services (Stoy, 1994). Though such considerations may also be needed for male subjects, women's responsibilities and life circumstances may require different provisions to enable their involvement in research.

## Conclusions

Between 1990 and 1994 there were major policy and legal shifts related to research on women. The Congress, major federal research and service agencies, women's advocacy groups, professionals, the lay press, and the public have been among those involved in activities that have led to these changes.

The NIH Revitalization Act of 1993 was a mandate that women "must be included in all NIH-supported biomedical and behavioral research projects unless a clear and compelling rationale and justification is established" (U.S. Department of Health and Human Services, 1994, p. 14509). Furthermore, the guidelines state that "cost is not an acceptable reason for exclusion" and that "women of childbearing potential should not be routinely excluded from participation in clinical research" (U.S. Department of Health and Human Services, 1994, p. 14509). Each of these statements represents a major shift from previous policies and perspectives on women as research subjects.

The challenge becomes one of interpreting these guidelines so that a balance can be achieved between developing sufficient diversity in samples for findings to be optimally generalizable yet maintaining feasible methodologies. It must be recognized that more than gender representation is necessary for data to be generalizable to women. The new guidelines demand that minorities must also be represented. Attention also needs to be given to the importance of the age of subjects as research designs are constructed.

The early 1990s represented an awakening to the need to be sensitive to the importance of gender in research as it is pursued. However, what must not be sacrificed is mindfulness of how rigid adherence to guidelines for inclusiveness may blind awareness to knowledge that comes with reasoned judgment and the creative probing of questions. A broad and keen perspective is necessary as research continues to improve the health of women and society.

ANN L. WILSON

*Directly related to this article are the other articles in this entry, especially* HISTORICAL AND CROSS-CULTURAL PERSPECTIVES, *and* HEALTH-CARE ISSUES. *Also directly related are the entries* RESEARCH POLICY, *articles on* SUBJECT SELECTION, *and* RISK AND VULNERABLE GROUPS; RESEARCH BIAS; MULTINATIONAL RESEARCH; JUSTICE; *and* COMPETENCY. *For a further discussion of topics mentioned in this article, see the entries* AGING AND THE AGED, *article on* HEALTH-CARE AND RESEARCH ISSUES; INFORMED CONSENT, *article on* CONSENT ISSUES IN HUMAN RESEARCH; OCCUPATIONAL SAFETY AND HEALTH, *article on* ETHICAL ISSUES; *and* RESEARCH METHODOLOGY, *article on* CONCEPTUAL ISSUES. *For a discussion of related ideas, see the entry* SEXISM.

## Bibliography

ANGELL, MARCIA. 1993. "Caring for Women's Health—What Is the Problem?" *New England Journal of Medicine* 329, no. 4:271–272.

BIRD, CHLOE E. 1994. "Women's Representation as Subjects in Clinical Studies: A Pilot Study of Research Published in JAMA in 1990 and 1992." In vol. 2 of *Women and Health Research: Ethical and Legal Issues of Including Women in Clinical Studies*, pp. 151–173. Edited by Anna C. Mastroianni, Ruth Faden, and Daniel Federman. Washington, D.C.: National Academy Press.

CHAVKIN, WENDY and FOX, HAROLD. 1990. "Ethical Implications of Rejecting Patients for Clinical Trials." *Journal of the American Medical Association* 264, no. 8:973–974.

COTTON, PAUL. 1990. "Examples Abound of Gaps in Medical Knowledge Because of Groups Excluded from Scientific Study." *Journal of the American Medical Association* 263, no. 8:1051 and 1055.

COUNCIL ON ETHICAL AND JUDICIAL AFFAIRS, AMERICAN MEDICAL ASSOCIATION. 1991. "Gender Disparities in Clinical Decision Making." *Journal of the American Medical Association* 266, no. 4:559–562.

DRESSER, REBECCA. 1992. "Wanted: Single, White Male for Medical Research." *Hastings Center Report* 22, no. 1: 24–29.

HEALY, BERNADINE. 1991a. Statement before the U.S. Senate Labor and Human Resources Aging Subcommittee, April 19.

———. 1991b. "The Yentl Syndrome." *New England Journal of Medicine* 325, no. 4:274–276.

HIGGINS, MILLICENT. 1990. "Women and Coronary Heart Disease: Then and Now." In *Women's Health Issues*, pp. 5–11. Presentation at the 159th meeting of the National Heart, Lung, and Blood Advisory Council, National Institutes of Health, U.S. Department of Health and Human Services.

INSTITUTE OF MEDICINE. 1994a. "Executive Summary." In vol. 1 of *Women and Health Research: Ethical and Legal Issues of Including Women in Clinical Studies*, pp. 1–25. Edited by Anna C. Mastroianni, Ruth Faden, and Daniel Federman. Washington, D.C.: National Academy Press.

———. 1994b. "Legal Considerations." In vol. 1 of *Women and Health Research: Ethical and Legal Issues of Including Women in Clinical Studies*, pp. 128–174. Edited by Anna C. Mastroianni, Ruth Faden, and Daniel Federman. Washington, D.C.: National Academy Press.

———. 1994c. "Women's Participation in Clinical Studies." In vol. 1 of *Women and Health Research: Ethical and Legal Issues of Including Women in Clinical Studies*, pp. 36–74. Edited by Anna C. Mastroianni, Ruth Faden, and Daniel Federman. Washington, D.C.: National Academy Press.

KINNEY, ELVIN L.; TRAUTMANN, JOANNE; GOLD, JAY A.; VESELL, ELLIOTT S.; and ZELIS, ROBERT. 1981. "Underrepresentation of Women in New Drug Trials." *Annals of Internal Medicine* 95, no. 4:495–499.

LaROSA, JUDITH H., and PINN, VIVIAN W. 1993. "Gender Bias in Biomedical Research." *Journal of the American Medical Women's Association* 48, no. 5:145–151.

LEMP, GEORGE F.; HIROZAWA, ANNE M.; COHEN, JUDITH B.; DERISH, PAMELA A.; McKINNEY, KEVIN C.; and HERNANDEZ, SANDRA R. 1992. "Survival for Women and Men with AIDS." *Journal of Infectious Diseases* 166, no. 1:74–79.

MERKATZ, RUTH B.; TEMPLE, ROBERT; SUBEL, SOLOMON; FEIDEN, KARYN; and KESSLER, DAVID A. 1993. "Women in Clinical Trials of New Drugs: A Change in the Food and Drug Administration Policy." *New England Journal of Medicine* 329, no. 4:292–296.

MULTIPLE RISK FACTOR INTERVENTION TRIAL RESEARCH GROUP. 1982. "Multiple Risk Factor Intervention Trial: Risk Factor Changes and Mortality Results." *Journal of the American Medical Association* 248, no. 12:1465–1477.

NADEL, MARK V. 1990. *National Institutes of Health: Problems in Implementing Policy on Women in Study Populations.* Statement Before the Subcommittee on Health and the Environment, Committee on Energy and Commerce, House of Representatives. Washington, D.C.: General Accounting Office

NATIONAL ACADEMY OF SCIENCES. 1991. "Issues in the Inclusion of Women in Clinical Trials." Report of a Planning Panel of the Institute of Medicine, Division of Health Sciences Policy, Washington, D.C.

NATIONAL INSTITUTE ADVISORY COUNCIL ON AGING. 1991. *Research on Older Women: Highlights from the Baltimore Longitudinal Study of Aging.* Washington, D.C.: National Institute on Aging, National Institutes of Health, Public Health Service, Department of Health and Human Services.

NATIONAL INSTITUTES OF HEALTH/ALCOHOL, DRUG ABUSE, AND MENTAL HEALTH ADMINISTRATION. 1990. "NIH/ADAMHA Policy Concerning Inclusion of Women in Study Populations." *NIH Guide for Grants and Contracts* 19:18–19.

SAAD, Z.; BRAMWELL, V.; DUFF, J.; GIROTTI, M.; JORY, T.; HEATHCOTE, G.; TURNBULL, I.; GARCIA, B.; and STITT, L. 1994. "Timing of Surgery in Relation to the Menstrual Cycle in Premenopausal Women with Operable Breast Cancer." *British Journal of Surgery* 81, no. 2:217–220.

SHERWIN, SUSAN. 1994. "Women in Clinical Studies: A Feminist View." In vol. 2 of *Women and Health Research: Ethical and Legal Issues of Including Women in Clinical Studies,* pp. 11–17. Edited by Anna C. Mastroianni, Ruth Faden, and Daniel Federman. Washington, D.C.: National Academy Press.

STEERING COMMITTEE OF THE PHYSICIANS' HEALTH STUDY RESEARCH GROUP. 1989. "Final Report on the Aspirin Component of the Ongoing Physicians' Health Study." *New England Journal of Medicine* 321, no. 3:129–135.

STOY, DIANE B. 1994. "Recruitment and Retention of Women in Clinical Studies: Theoretical Perspectives and Methodological Considerations." In vol. 2 of *Women and Health Research: Ethical and Legal Issues of Including Women in Clinical Studies,* pp. 41–45. Edited by Anna C. Mastroianni, Ruth Faden, and Daniel Federman. Washington, D.C.: National Academy Press.

U.S. DEPARTMENT OF HEALTH AND HUMAN SERVICES. NATIONAL INSTITUTES OF HEALTH. 1994. "NIH Guidelines on the Inclusion of Women and Minorities as Subjects in Clinical Research; Notice." *Federal Register* 59, no. 59 (March 28):14508–14513.

U.S. FOOD AND DRUG ADMINISTRATION (FDA). 1977. *General Considerations for the Clinical Evaluation of Drugs.* Publication no. (FDA) 77–3040. Washington, D.C.: U.S. Government Printing Office.

U.S. GOVERNMENT ACCOUNTING OFFICE. 1990. "National Institutes of Health: Problems in Implementing Policy on Women in Study Populations." Testimony before the Subcommittee on Housing and Consumer Interest and Select Committee on Aging, U.S. House of Representatives, July 24.

U.S. NATIONAL COMMISSION FOR THE PROTECTION OF HUMAN SUBJECTS OF BIOMEDICAL AND BEHAVIORAL RESEARCH. 1978. *The Belmont Report: Ethical Principles and Guidelines for the Protection of Human Subjects of Research.* Washington, D.C.: U.S. Government Printing Office.

U.S. PUBLIC HEALTH SERVICE TASK FORCE ON WOMEN'S HEALTH ISSUES. 1985. "Women's Health: Report of the Public Health Service Task Force on Women's Health Issues." *Public Health Reports* 100, no. 1:73–105.

WOBBES, THOMAS; THOMAS, C. M. G.; SEGERS, M. F. G.; PEER, P. G. M.; BRUGGINK, E. D. M.; and BEEX, L. V. 1994. "The Phase of the Menstrual Cycle Has No Influence on the Disease-Free Survival of Patients with Mammary Carcinoma." *British Journal of Cancer* 69, no. 3:599–600.

## IV. WOMEN AS HEALTH PROFESSIONALS
### A. HISTORY

Historically, women in health care have primarily been caretakers and nurturers in their roles as wives, mothers, and nurses and in their responsibilities for the care of the sick, the aged, and the disabled. When healing roles became more organized, formally structured, and financially lucrative, women met resistance to being included. This was often based on fear, suspicion, and mistrust of their capacities and their departure from more traditional roles, as well as the possibility that they would compete with men.

### Early history of women in health care

Women have always been healers as well as caretakers; they have acted as pharmacists, physicians, nurses, herbalists, abortionists, counselors, midwives, and "sagae" or "wise women." They have also been called witches. In the physician role, however, society rarely permitted them to perform in the same capacities and positions as men.

Early Egyptian stele refer to a Chief Woman Physician, Peseshet; and in 1500 B.C.E., women studied in the Egyptian medical school in Heliopolis. The Chinese record, in 1000 B.C.E., female physicians in positions that encompassed activities other than traditional midwifery and herb gathering. Medical roles also existed for women in the Greek and Roman civilizations. In Rome physicians were often slaves or freed slaves; it is likely that many were women. Women who entered medicine were frequently members of medical families and practiced together with family members. The physician husband of a second-century woman physician wrote for his wife's epitaph, "You guided straight the rudder of life in our home and raised high our common fame in healing—though you were a woman you were not behind me in skill" (Anderson and Zinsser, 1988, p. 61).

Throughout history women have been special attendants to other women, assisting with labor and delivery, advising them on the functions and disorders of their bodies, and tending newborns. Since childbirth was considered to be a normal, not a pathological process, it was not thought to be part of medicine. Soranus of Ephesus, a first-century C.E. physician practicing in Rome, believed that women were divinely appointed to care for sick women and children. Among the criteria he included for those practicing were literacy, anatomic understanding, a sense of patient responsibility, and ethical concerns, particularly about confidentiality.

During the first few centuries of the spread of Christianity, women ordained as deaconesses by bishops with the consent of the congregation appear to have played a significant role in health care. Although little is known about their actual work, many of these deaconesses became the first parish workers and district nurses (Shryock, 1959). Among these women were Saint Monica, the mother of Saint Augustine, and Fabiola, who founded a hospital at Ostia in Italy in 398 c.e.

After the fall of the Roman Empire, medicine continued along two paths: Monastic medicine, which lost touch with older traditions, and Arabic medicine, which developed in Persia and transmitted the heritage of Greek medicine back into Europe. Arabic medicine produced notable practitioners and established hospitals run by male and female "nurses." During the Crusades women staffed infirmaries and clinics in Jerusalem and along the European routes to the Holy Land.

Medical scholarship flourished in the ninth century at the University of Salerno in Italy and continued to do so throughout the tenth and eleventh centuries (Corner, 1937). At that time women apparently studied medicine at the university. Although little is known about most of those early women physicians, eleventh-century records reveal the existence of Trotula, a woman faculty member at Salerno, who is said to have written important texts on obstetrics and gynecology, and also headed a department of women's diseases. Her major work, *De passionibus mulierum*, remained the major reference on the subject for several centuries. Its authorship was attributed to her husband or to other male colleagues. She suggested that infertility could be attributed to the male as well as the female. In cooperation with the "Ladies of Salerno," a group of women physicians, Trotula established the first center of medicine that was not under church control.

The M.D. degree was first awarded in 1180, apparently only to men. One of the notable figures of the twelfth century was Hildegard of Bingen, a scientific scholar, abbess, writer, composer, and political adviser to kings and to the pope. She wrote two medical textbooks, *Liber Simplicis Medicinae* and *Liber Compositae Medicinae*, presumably for use by the nurses in charge of the infirmaries of Benedictine monasteries. The books described a number of diseases, including their courses, symptoms, and treatment, as well as scientific data on the pulsation of blood and the regulation of vital activities by the nervous system. Hildegard's writings also demonstrated an understanding of normal and abnormal psychology.

In the medieval period affluent women were active in medicine, particularly in Italy, where the universities were accessible to them. In 1390 Dorotea Bocchi earned a degree in medicine from the University of Bologna and followed her father as a lecturer in medicine at that university. In 1423 Constanza Calenda, the daughter of the dean of the medical faculty at Salerno, lectured on medicine at the university in Naples. Women also qualified and were permitted to practice in France, England, and Germany. They generally had to practice in specifically defined and limited roles, including bleeding, administration of herbs and medicines, and reducing fractures, as well as in midwifery. As early as 1292, however, women in Paris were "barber surgeons," practicing what was known of surgery. Until 1694 widows were automatically allowed to continue practicing as such if it had been their husbands' field.

From the thirteenth to the seventeenth centuries, the number of physicians was small, and the role of women healers was particularly important in meeting the health-care needs of the population. During this period women practiced as physicians, surgeons, bone setters, eye healers, and midwives. It was generally believed that women were better suited for the treatment of women's diseases.

During the fifteenth century women were obtaining higher degrees by presenting medical theses, and during the fifteenth and early part of the sixteenth centuries women began to excel in innovative techniques and make important contributions in medicine. They served kings, royal families, and even armies in Europe.

Although we assume that the number of women in medicine was small, their presence did seem to cause enough concern that by 1220, the University of Paris succeeded in preventing them from gaining admission to medical school. In 1485 Charles VIII of France decreed that women could not work as surgeons.

By the fourteenth century the licensing of physicians was well established, although women were rarely allowed to sit for licensing examinations. In 1322 university-trained male physicians brought a suit against Jacoba Felicie de Almania in France; they claimed that in practicing without appropriate training and licensing, she endangered patients. Patients testified to her skill; she herself argued that she was both physician and nurse to her patients. She also emphasized that many women would not seek treatment for their illnesses if they had to see a male physician. Because she did not have the correct university degree, she was not only barred from medicine; she was also excommunicated from the church. Women who practiced outside their licensed specialty—for example, midwives who functioned as physicians—were also condemned.

By the end of the fifteenth century, as medicine became an academic discipline and a more established profession in various centers in Europe, the movement to exclude women from the formal practice of medicine gained momentum. This movement coincided with the ideology of misogyny as it was articulated by Heinrich Kraemer and James Sprenger in *The Malleus Maleficarum*

(1486), a treatise on how to identify and what to do with witches. Witch-hunting capitalized on the widespread belief in the spiritual and mental inferiority of women, a belief that was fueled by the church. Even when active witch-hunts subsided, their effects remained. Women were effectively eliminated from performing in medical roles other than traditional caretaking and midwifery.

Before the sixteenth century, it was not possible for a male to be a midwife; in fact, it was a capital offense in some places. As medicine and surgery differentiated from each other in the fifteenth and sixteenth centuries, some of the male barber surgeons began to practice midwifery. By the late fifteenth century, licensing examinations were given, generally by a doctor and a midwife. Increasingly, concern was expressed by physicians and the laity about whether midwives were knowledgeable enough to recognize when it was appropriate to call for consultation from male physicians and surgeons.

The sixteenth to eighteenth centuries produced several outstanding female midwives, including Louyse Bourgeois, who in 1609 was the first midwife to publish a work on obstetrics. It became the basic text for midwifery in Europe. Nonetheless, with the invention of the obstetrical forceps in the seventeenth century by the Chamberlens, a family of male midwives and barber surgeons, obstetrics was pushed closer to the realm of the male practitioner. In 1634 Peter Chamberlen III attempted to establish a corporation of midwives in England with himself as governor—a move that was resented by female midwives. Increasingly, men began to participate and compete in this profession, particularly in serving the upper classes. By the eighteenth century men controlled all medical areas except midwifery and nursing, and even in these areas, women were increasingly required to practice only under male supervision.

By the beginning of the seventeenth century women were denied access to medical training and then prohibited from belonging to professional associations. University training was required, and women were not admitted to universities. Despite exclusion from formal training and practice, women continued to provide for the health-care needs of family members and others in the community, especially the poor, who had no other access to health care.

## Women in early American medicine

In colonial North America the healing role of women was critical to survival; many women assumed medical roles. Ann Hutchinson, the early seventeenth-century dissident religious leader, functioned as a general practitioner and midwife. Since there were relatively few university-trained physicians and no medical schools in the colonies, medicine was practiced by those who appeared to be particularly talented, and an apprenticeship system began to evolve. Two women listed as physicians in Boston in the seventeenth century were later denounced as witches, and no other woman practiced medicine in Boston until Harriot Hunt, after apprenticeship training, opened her office in 1835.

Eighteenth-century American medicine had no unified concept of medical care; a variety of views of practice and training offered various programs of study and concepts of healing. In this setting, the role of women was extensive and complex, since the medical care of families was frequently the responsibility of the women.

Most women practitioners were midwives. Many went to Europe to train, since the first school for midwives in the English colonies was not started until 1762. The early training of midwives was based on the assumption that most obstetrical practice would remain in the hands of women. This did not occur in colonial North America, although it did in many parts of Europe.

In 1765 John Morgan founded the first university-connected, so-called regular American medical school at the University of Pennsylvania. Its formal, scientifically based curriculum departed from the almost exclusive apprenticeship training that existed in the colonies and was more reflective of European standards of the time. By excluding women, it began a tradition of barring them from formal medical training and forcing them into "irregular" training. Many women without diplomas, however, did set up flourishing practices. They were trained in the homeopathic, eclectic, or "irregular" traditions, which tended to be less prestigious.

## Women in nineteenth-century medicine

In 1847 Elizabeth Blackwell became the first woman to be admitted to a "regular" medical school in the United States. She graduated first in her class from Geneva (New York) Medical School in 1849. The New York State Medical Association promptly censured the school, and when her sister, Emily Blackwell, applied a few years later, she was rejected. Emily subsequently received her M.D. from Western Reserve Medical College in Cleveland, Ohio, after her acceptance to Rush Medical College in Chicago, Illinois, had been rescinded in response to pressure from the state medical society.

Ann Preston began her medical studies in 1847 as an apprentice to a Quaker physician. After two years she applied to and was rejected by four medical schools. In 1850, she established the first regular women's medical college in the world, the Women's Medical College of Pennsylvania. She and her students recalled their experiences at the Pennsylvania Hospital: "We entered in a body, amidst jeerings, groaning, whistlings, and stamping of feet by the men students. . . . On leaving the hospital, we were actually stoned by those so-called gentlemen" (Alsop, 1950, pp. 54–55). This account was corroborated by the Philadelphia *Evening Bulletin*.

In 1847, Harriot K. Hunt, who had earlier established herself in an irregular practice in Boston without an M.D., applied to Harvard Medical School. Although supported by the dean, Oliver Wendell Holmes, she was rejected for admission. After hearing about Elizabeth Blackwell's acceptance, she again applied for admission and was accepted. However, she was denied her seat when the all-male class threatened to leave if women or blacks were admitted. Not until almost one hundred years later, in 1946, did Harvard Medical School begin to admit women.

By 1850 two additional all-female medical colleges were founded, one in Boston and one in Cincinnati. Both were irregular schools. The Boston Female Medical College was designed primarily to prevent male midwifery, which its founder, Dr. Samuel Gregory, felt trespassed on female delicacy. The school was founded in 1848 and offered a medical degree by 1853, but it was always financially troubled and did not enjoy a good reputation. In 1856 it changed its name to the New England Female Medical College and began to recruit good faculty, including Marie Zakrzewska, who was able to help develop a pioneering clinical training program. In 1873 the school merged with Boston University.

In 1855 the National Eclectic Medical Association formally approved the education of women in medicine, and in 1870 it became the first medical society to accept them for membership. Traditional medical societies, however, continued to be closed to women. In his 1871 American Medical Association (AMA) presidential address, Alfred Stille criticized female physicians for being women who seek to rival men, who "aim toward a higher type than their own" (Ehrenreich and English, 1967, p. 26). Negative attitudes toward the presence of women in medicine appeared to be supported by accumulating "scientific" evidence that supposedly supported the inferior status of women on biological grounds, including that their brain capacity was less than men's. A book published in 1873 by Edward Hammond Clarke fueled the controversy: in *Sex in Education: or, A Fair Chance for the Girls* he stated, "Higher education for women produces monstrous brains and puny bodies" (Clarke, 1873). It echoed Charles Meigs's 1847 statement, "She [woman] has a head almost too small for the intellect but just big enough for love" (Meigs, 1847).

The debate about women's intellectual capacity induced Harvard Medical School to offer the Boylston Medical Prize in 1874 for the best paper on the topic, "Do women require mental and bodily rest during menstruation and to what extent?" The winning research was submitted by Mary Putnam Jacobi; when the judges discovered who the author was, they hesitated about awarding the prize, but finally did so (Walsh, 1977). Putnam Jacobi had found, contrary to prevailing views, that the majority of her sample did not suffer incapacity. Her study was followed by several others, all with similar findings. Despite such work and evidence, the barriers to women did not fall.

Even those women who managed to obtain medical training were refused admittance to medical societies, and hospitals denied them appointments. Female physicians in the United States began to open their own hospitals and clinics. In 1857 Elizabeth and Emily Blackwell founded the New York Infirmary for Women, where they cared largely for indigent women, and in 1865 the Women's Medical College of the New York Infirmary was opened. Paternalistic attitudes coupled with the difficulty women had in obtaining hospital privileges also led Marie Zakrzewska, in 1862, to found the New England Hospital for Women, owned and operated entirely by women.

The role of women in medicine, including the productivity and lifestyle of female physicians, continued to be hotly debated. In 1881 Rachel Bodley, dean of the Women's Medical College of Pennsylvania, surveyed the 244 living graduates of the school and found that, despite the persistent mythology to the contrary, the overwhelming majority were in active practice. Those who had married reported that their profession had had no adverse effect on their marriages, nor had marriage interfered with their work.

By the end of the nineteenth century, 75 percent of women medical students were being trained in regular medical schools, and women physicians were being accepted into many medical societies. The Massachusetts Medical Society admitted women in 1884, and the AMA seated a woman delegate in 1876 but did not formally accept women until 1915 (Morantz-Sanchez, 1985). Women physicians began to form their own associations. There were several attempts to build a national organization of women physicians, beginning in 1867. The *Women's Medical Journal* was started in 1872. In 1915, the National Women's Medical Association was founded. It was renamed the American Medical Women's Association (AMWA) in 1919 and was condemned by many male physicians. In order to alleviate fears, AMWA required that its members also join the AMA, and it held its meetings together with theirs.

Female separatism was a double-edged sword. While it gave women a special place in the care of women and children, it was also used to exclude women from more extensive roles in medical education and from the increasing influence and prestige of the profession.

Financial contributions of women philanthropists forced the Johns Hopkins Medical School, in 1889, to accept women on the same terms as it accepted men. However, this did not result in large numbers of women being admitted, nor did it appear to increase the number of appointments of women to faculty and leadership positions (Walsh, 1977).

Following Johns Hopkins's lead, however, 75 percent of other, already existing medical schools also began to accept women as students. By 1894, over 66 percent of women medical students were enrolled in regular medical schools (Walsh, 1977). Tufts Medical School had 42 percent women. Women also received a disproportionate number of the academic honors in their graduating classes.

This direction was quickly reversed. At Johns Hopkins the percentage of women students dropped from 33 percent in 1896 to 10 percent in 1916. At the University of Michigan, the percentage of women students dropped from 25 percent in 1890 to 3 percent in 1910 (Walsh, 1977).

## Women physicians in Europe and Canada

In 1859 America's Elizabeth Blackwell was placed on the British Medical Register; the following year, the British Medical Association ruled that those with foreign medical degrees could not practice in England. Elizabeth Garrett Anderson, in 1865, was the first woman who qualified to practice medicine in England. She did this by passing the apothecaries' examination; their guild regulations did not exclude women. The rules were changed shortly thereafter. In France, although women were allowed to study at the Faculty of Medicine in Paris, they could not become interns and thus could not complete their training.

The Royal College of Physicians in Edinburgh attempted to exclude Sophia Jex-Blake from medical school in 1869 by stating that a single woman could not attend. She organized a group of seven women and together they completed the first year. Attacks on female students from peers, however, prompted some public support from people who were outraged that these "indelicate and ungentlemanly" men would be seeing female patients. Four years later the university won a lawsuit allowing it to refuse to grant degrees to women.

Women in other European countries also experienced hostile and even violent attacks by their male peers. Many of the women who graduated from medical schools in those countries were from middle-class or upper-class backgrounds. Often they had fathers or other family members in medicine; they entered the profession to join the family practice.

The first continental European university to accept women was the University of Zurich, in 1865. By the 1870s other Swiss universities followed. In Russia, women were allowed to attend medical schools in 1872, partly because a number of Russian women had already studied medicine at Zurich. Negative attitudes toward women were fueled by the assassination of Czar Alexander II by a woman. Following this event, from 1881 through 1905, universities in Russia were closed to women.

The first woman doctor to practice medicine in Canada, James Barry, a graduate of the University of Edinburgh, was a British army medical officer who became Inspector General of hospitals in Canada in 1857. She was able to practice because she was thought to be a man; after her death, Dr. Barry was discovered to have been a woman (Hacker, 1974).

## Nineteenth-century midwifery

There was considerable opposition to the practice of midwifery by women in the mid-nineteenth century, particularly in the United States. In 1820 John Ware, a Boston physician, is said to have written *Remarks on the Employment of Females as Practitioners of Midwifery*, in which he raised objections based on his view of women's moral qualities. He stated: "Where the responsibility in scenes of distress and danger does not fall upon them when there is someone on whom they can lean, in whose skill and judgement they have entire confidence, they retain their collection and presence of mind; but where they become the principal agents, the feelings of sympathy are too powerful for the cool exercise of judgment" (Ware, 1820, p. 7).

Economic and class issues also played a part in women's exclusion from medicine. Midwives came primarily from working-class, rural, and poor backgrounds. They charged less than physicians for their services and were more likely to care for the poor. With the beginning of obstetrics as a medical discipline, physicians feared economic competition from midwives.

Some physicians objected to midwives on grounds of the allegedly lower quality of health care they provided. In fact, in the 1840s, two physicians, Oliver Wendell Holmes and Ignaz Semmelweiss, reported on the spread of puerperal sepsis (childbirth infection); Semmelweiss found that there was actually a lower incidence of it in women delivered by midwives. He deduced that, because medical students and physicians did not wash their hands when they moved from autopsy to delivery room, they spread disease. The warnings of both doctors were ignored by most of the medical profession at that time, and controversy continued about the adequacy of midwives.

By the turn of the twentieth century, about 50 percent of all babies in the United States were delivered by midwives. Midwives were held responsible for childbirth illness or puerperal sepsis, as well as neonatal ophthalmia (inflammation of the eyes generally related to maternal gonorrhea), because it was widely believed, especially by the medical profession, that they were not sufficiently trained to prevent these illnesses. Under mounting pressure, many states began to pass laws forbidding midwifery, many of which remain in effect today.

## Evolution of nursing in the nineteenth century

The practice of nursing was sponsored primarily by the Church until the mid-eighteenth century, when the London Infirmary appointed a lay nurse. Nursing was seen as a low-status occupation; records show long working hours and low pay. Dickens's novel *Martin Chuzzlewit* (1844) focused attention on the quality of the nursing care given by pardoned criminals, aging prostitutes, and other women of questionable morality and interest who functioned as nurses.

At the time of the Crimean War, Florence Nightingale responded to the need for nursing reform and established military and then civilian nursing. In 1860 she founded a school for nurses in London with a rigorous curriculum and specific guidelines for nursing as a profession. She met opposition from the medical profession, many of whose members felt that "nurses are in much the same position as housemaids and need little teaching beyond poultice-making and the enforcement of cleanliness and attention to the patient's wants" (Dolan, 1916, p. 230).

The first nursing schools recruited upper-class women who were "refugees from the enforced leisure of Victorian ladyhood" (Ehrenreich and English, 1967, p. 34). Despite their aristocratic image, nursing schools began to change and to attract more women from working-class and lower-middle-class homes. Those advocating the nursing profession saw the nurse as the embodiment of Victorian femininity and nursing as a natural vocation for women, second only to motherhood. Nightingale viewed women as instinctive nurses, not physicians: "They have only tried to be men, and they have succeeded only in being third-rate men" (Ehrenreich and English, 1967, p. 36).

## Women in twentieth-century medicine

By the beginning of the twentieth century, women were seeking admission to medical schools in increasing numbers. Because of an oversupply of physicians, however, both salaries and prestige were diminishing. Some blamed the situation on the "feminization" of the profession, and many schools began to decrease their acceptances of women. Women also had more difficulty obtaining internships and residencies. Since all but one of the female institutions (the Women's Medical College of Pennsylvania) had consolidated or closed, many women had nowhere to train.

The conviction that women were not able to perform effectively as physicians, and the belief that women would be damaged by pursuing a difficult career, intensified. Women physicians seemed unable to develop a consolidated and effective strategy to resist the negativism. In 1905, Dr. F. W. Van Dyke, the president of the Oregon State Medical Society, stated, "Hard study killed sexual desire in women, took away their beauty, brought on hysteria, neurasthenia, dyspepsia, astigmatism and dysmenorrhea. . . . Educated women could not bear children with ease because study arrested the development of the pelvis at the same time it increased the size of the child's brain and therefore its head. This caused extensive suffering in childbirth" (Bullough and Voght, 1973, pp. 74–75).

At this time, academic medical schools were evolving formal medical curricula. Proprietary medical schools were also increasing in numbers. Their education was primarily focused on an apprenticeship model, and there was little monitoring of the quality of the education they provided. Because of the oversupply of doctors produced by these two systems, with consequent competition for patients as well as the lack of mechanisms to assess quality and monitor performance, the AMA asked the Carnegie Foundation to investigate the condition of medicine and make appropriate recommendations. The Foundation commissioned Abraham Flexner, a schoolteacher with no medical expertise, to do this. In his 1910 report, Flexner stated: "Medical education is now, in the United States and Canada, open to women upon practically the same terms as men. If all institutions do not receive women, so many do, that no woman desiring an education in medicine is under any disability in finding a school to which she may gain admittance. . . . Now that women are freely admitted to the medical profession, it is clear that they show a decreasing inclination to enter it" (Flexner, 1910, pp. 178–179, 296).

Flexner's report concluded that medical education required higher standards for training, and it was an important impetus in establishing medicine as an academic discipline. It resulted in the closing of many medical schools, especially the proprietary ones; unfortunately, since women continued to have difficulty gaining admission to many of the university-affiliated and more prestigious medical schools, those schools that were closed were the ones that had admitted substantial numbers of women and minorities.

Women physicians gained some status for their patriotism during World War I, when the AMWA campaigned to have women physicians commissioned on the same basis as men. Although this effort was rejected by the government, the AMWA did urge women physicians to contribute to the war effort. Fifty-five women physicians did practice by signing specific contracts with the military. They received neither military status nor benefits.

By this time the number of female physicians in the United States dropped precipitously and continued to be exceedingly low until the 1970s. Other countries did not experience this abrupt drop and continued to report greater percentages of female physicians. In 1965, for example, women comprised 7 percent of all U.S. physicians; the Soviet Union reported 65 percent female physicians, Poland 30 percent, the Philippines 25 percent, the German Federal Republic 20 percent, Italy 19 percent, the United Kingdom and Denmark 16 percent, and Japan 9 percent (Lopate, 1968).

Medicine has been viewed as a male profession in the United States more than in most other countries. Some hypothesize that this occurred because medicine has had higher prestige and income than many other professions, and thus interested men more. Others believe that the dominance of men adds prestige and that men demand better compensation. The reasons for gender stereotyping of professions, however, is complex and has cultural as well as political determinants. Many areas of work are sex-role stereotyped, which is often related to the perception that women are best at certain functions. For example, women are considered to be more suited to caretaking roles and men to be better in more instrumental activities. Medicine presents a melding of these stereotypes. The caretaking functions of physicians do not inherently contradict "traditional" views of women and women's roles, whereas the technological and instrumental aspects do. Even in a revolutionary society like Cuba, where these stereotypes are disparaged, there is a persistence of traditional roles for women in health care; 30 to 40 percent of Cuban physicians are women and virtually all nurses and midwives are women.

The choice of specialty as well as the specific positions held by women within their fields of expertise reveal a pattern that has held since women were admitted to medical schools in the United States. Women have characteristically entered pediatrics, internal medicine, psychiatry, family practice, and, increasingly, obstetrics and gynecology. There is more diversification in the choice of medical specialty for women in other countries.

Within each specialty there are also some important differentiations in status and role. In the United States and other countries, academic and administrative appointments as well as other decision-making positions are almost exclusively held by men, whereas women tend to be involved in direct patient care; 90 percent of U.S. female physicians are involved directly in patient care. In the 1970s, the fact that women assumed this role was used as an argument for increasing their numbers in medical school. It was presumed that they could be counted on to meet the needs of the health-care system in delivering primary care.

In countries where women have made significant progress in their influence on the health fields, changes have occurred most often in times of war, physician shortages, or major cultural reorganization. In Russia, midwives proved themselves effective as doctors in the Russo-Turkish War of 1870, thus beginning the influx of women into medical schools. After the 1917 revolution, as the prestige of medicine declined, women were admitted in great numbers to medical school. By 1940, 62 percent of Soviet physicians were women, and by 1970, 72 percent. As in the United States and other countries, however, Russian women held a disproportionately small number of senior positions. The *Feldschers* (semiprofessional health workers officially known as physician assistants) in the Soviet Union were often women, and this situation presumably continues in Russia and the other former Soviet republics. The large number of women in medicine, especially in lower-prestige positions, serves to reduce the differentiation between doctors and paramedical workers.

The rise of female health professionals in China occurred along with the reorganization of the medical-care system and of Chinese society under the People's Republic. About half of Chinese physicians are women. In 1950, 50,000 midwives were reeducated as local health workers. Since then the Chinese have emphasized hospital deliveries by fully trained obstetricians. In the countryside, "barefoot doctors" (peasants who have had basic medical training and provide medical care without leaving their regular productive labor) meet the needs of fellow workers. Women primarily fill this role (Sidel and Sidel, 1973).

### Changes for women in health care

The blurring of roles and overlapping of areas of function in a number of fields have caused considerable confusion. What are the similarities and differences among the functions of a psychologist, psychiatrist, psychiatric social worker, and psychiatric nurse? Among those of a primary-care physician, a physician assistant, and a nurse practitioner? In these situations, similar functions may be performed by people who have somewhat different training and skills. It is often difficult to differentiate what are appropriate functions and responsibilities.

Economic factors, rather than expertise or experience, have become important determinants of decisions about which practitioners will provide certain types of care, rather than the expertise and skill of caregivers. Less skilled practitioners may be favored by insurance or managed-care companies because their services are less costly. Objective guidelines have not been developed that provide guidance for assessing scope of practice or expertise. For example, in psychotherapy, sexual therapy, routine physical exams, obstetrical care, anesthesia, and minor medical and surgical procedures, professionals of varied backgrounds and training may provide similar services, and there are currently no adequate means of assessing outcome.

In many of these areas women have functioned as the less highly trained professionals and paraprofessionals. Since skills are less easily identifiable than training and credentials and since the accountability of certain professions is increasingly important, women may find themselves again in the position of nineteenth-century midwives—they have the experience and expertise, but not the credentials. They may thus find themselves displaced and superseded unless training and recognition validate their skills. Since women have always been important providers of care, future planning calls for ways of utilizing women creatively and widely in the healing professions.

CAROL C. NADELSON
MALKAH T. NOTMAN

*Directly related to this article are the companion article on* WOMEN AS HEALTH PROFESSIONALS: B. CONTEMPORARY ISSUES, *and the other articles in this entry:* HISTORICAL AND CROSS-CULTURAL PERSPECTIVES, HEALTH-CARE ISSUES, *and* RESEARCH ISSUES. *For a further discussion of topics mentioned in this article, see the entries* ALTERNATIVE THERAPIES, *article on* SOCIAL HISTORY; CARE; FEMINISM; MEDICAL EDUCATION; NURSING AS A PROFESSION; PATERNALISM; *and* SEXISM. *Other relevant material may be found under the entries* ALLIED HEALTH PROFESSIONS; JUSTICE; LICENSING, DISCIPLINE, AND REGULATION IN THE HEALTH PROFESSIONS; MEDICINE AS A PROFESSION; *and* SEXUAL ETHICS AND PROFESSIONAL STANDARDS.

## Bibliography

ABRAM, RUTH J., ed. 1985. *"Send Us a Lady Physician": Women Doctors in America, 1835–1920.* New York: W. W. Norton.

ACHTERBERG, JEANNE. 1990. *Woman as Healer.* Boston: Shambhala.

ALSOP, GULIELMA FELL. 1950. *History of the Woman's Medical College, Philadelphia, Pennsylvania, 1850–1950.* Philadelphia: J.B. Lippincott.

ANDERSON, BONNIE S., and ZINSSER, JUDITH P. 1988. *A History of Their Own: Women in Europe from Prehistory to the Present.* 2 vols. New York: Harper & Row.

APPLE, RIMA D., ed. 1990. *Women, Health, and Medicine in America: A Historical Handbook.* New York: Garland.

BONNER, THOMAS N. 1992. *To the Ends of the Earth: Women's Search for Education in Medicine.* Cambridge, Mass.: Harvard University Press.

BULLOUGH, VERN, and VOGHT, MARTHA. 1973. "Women, Menstruation and Nineteenth-Century Medicine." *Bulletin of the History of Medicine* 47, no. 1:66–82.

CALDER, JEAN MCKINLAY. 1963. *The Story of Nursing.* 4th rev. ed. London: Methuen.

CLARKE, EDWARD HAMMOND. 1873. *Sex in Education: or, A Fair Chance for the Girls.* Boston: J. R. Osgood.

CORNER, GEORGE W. 1937. "The Rise of Medicine at Salerno in the Twelfth Century." In *Lectures on the History of Medicine: A Series of Lectures at the Mayo Foundation and the Universities of Minnesota, Wisconsin, Iowa, Northwestern and the Des Moines Academy of Medicine, 1926–1932,* pp. 371–399. Philadelphia: W. B. Saunders.

CUTTER, IRVING S., and VIETS, HENRY R. 1964. [1933]. *A Short History of Midwifery.* Philadelphia: W. B. Saunders.

DALLY, ANN G. 1991. *Women Under the Knife: A History of Surgery.* New York: Routledge.

DOLAN, JOSEPHINE A. 1963. *Goodnow's History of Nursing.* 11th ed. Philadelphia: W. B. Saunders.

DRACHMAN, VIRGINIA G. 1984. *Hospital with a Heart: Women Doctors and the Paradox of Separatism at the New England Hospital, 1862–1969.* Ithaca, N.Y.: Cornell University Press.

EHRENREICH, BARBARA, and ENGLISH, DEIRDRE. 1967. *Witches, Midwives, and Nurses: A History of Women Healers.* 2d ed. Glass Mountain Pamphlet, no. 1. Old Westbury, N.Y.: Feminist Press.

FLEXNER, ABRAHAM. 1972 [1910]. *Medical Education in the United States and Canada: A Report to the Carnegie Foundation for the Advancement of Teaching.* Bulletin of the Carnegie Foundation for the Advancement of Teaching, no. 4. New York: Arno.

HACKER, CARLOTTA. 1974. *The Indomitable Lady Doctors.* Toronto: Clarke, Irwin.

HUME, RUTH FOX. 1964. *Great Women of Medicine.* New York: Random House.

LEAVITT, JUDITH WALZER, ed. 1984. *Women and Health in America: Historical Readings.* Madison: University of Wisconsin Press.

LOPATE, CAROL. 1968. *Women in Medicine.* Baltimore: Johns Hopkins University Press.

LORBER, JUDITH. 1984. *Women Physicians: Careers, Status, and Power.* New York: Tavistock.

MARKS, GEOFFREY, and BEATTY, WILLIAM K. 1972. *Women in White.* New York: Charles Scribner.

MCPHERSON, MARY PATTERSON. 1981. "'On the Same Terms Precisely': The Women's Medical Fund and the Johns Hopkins School of Medicine." *Journal of the American Medical Women's Association* 36, no. 2:37–40.

MEAD, KATE CAMPBELL HURD. 1938. *A History of Women in Medicine: From the Earliest Times to the Beginning of the Nineteenth Century.* Haddam, Conn.: Haddam Press.

MORANTZ, REGINA M. 1982. "Introduction: From Art to Science: Women Physicians in American Medicine, 1600–1980." In *In Her Own Words: Oral Histories of Women Physicians,* pp. 3–44. Edited by Regina M. Morantz, Cynthia

S. Pomerleau, and Carol H. Fenichel. New Haven, Conn.: Yale University Press.

MORANTZ-SANCHEZ, REGINA M. 1985. *Sympathy and Science: Women Physicians in American Medicine.* New York: Oxford University Press.

NADELSON, CAROL C. 1983. "The Woman Physician: Past, Present, and Future." In *The Physician: A Professional Under Stress,* pp. 261–278. Edited by John P. Callan. Norwalk, Conn.: Appleton-Century-Crofts.

———. 1989. "Professional Issues for Women." *Psychiatric Clinics of North America* 3, no. 1:25–33.

NADELSON, CAROL C., and NOTMAN, MALKAH T. 1972. "The Woman Physician." *Journal of Medical Education* 47, no. 3:176–183.

NOTMAN, MALKAH T., and NADELSON, CAROL C. 1973. "Medicine: A Career Conflict for Women." *American Journal of Psychiatry* 130, no. 10:1123–1127.

PIRADOVA, M. D. 1976. "USSR—Women Health Workers." *Women and Health* 1, no. 3:24–29.

ROSENBERG, CHARLES E. 1987. *The Care of Strangers: The Rise of America's Hospital System.* New York: Basic Books.

SCHULMAN, SAM. 1958. "Basic Functional Roles in Nursing: Mother Surrogate and Healer." In *Patients, Physicians and Illness: A Sourcebook in Behavioral Science and Medicine,* pp. 528–537. Edited by E. Gartly Jaco. New York: Free Press.

SHRYOCK, RICHARD H. 1959. *The History of Nursing: An Interpretation of the Social and Medical Factors Involved.* Philadelphia: W. B. Saunders.

———. 1966. "Women in American Medicine." In his *Medicine in America: Historical Essays,* pp. 177–200. Baltimore: Johns Hopkins University Press.

SIDEL, VICTOR W., and SIDEL, RUTH. 1973. *Serve the People: Observations on Medicine in the People's Republic of China.* New York: Josiah Macy, Jr., Foundation.

WALSH, MARY ROTH. 1977. *"Doctors Wanted: No Women Need Apply": Sexual Barriers in the Medical Profession, 1835–1975.* New Haven, Conn.: Yale University Press.

WARE, JOHN. 1820. *Remarks on the Employment of Females as Practitioners in Midwifery.* American Imprints, no. 4171. Boston: Cummings & Hilliard. This work has also been ascribed to Walter Channing.

## B. CONTEMPORARY ISSUES

Although they fill many roles in the health professions, women face a number of challenges, with gender stereotyping topping the list. No matter how complex the technical requirements of a woman's occupation, Western culture expects her to be more nurturing and emotionally accessible than a man. At the same time, it places a low value on roles traditionally assigned to women, particularly caretaking roles, in terms of both prestige and financial remuneration (Reverby, 1987). In the professions, women earn less than men in equivalent positions. Women's struggle to achieve parity with men continues on other fronts as well, particularly in acquiring the best possible education and in terms of career options. These struggles exact costly tolls in energy, self-confidence, and relationships with others. Moreover, because medicine is such a powerful social institution, the stereotyping of women health professionals reinforces social constructs that hamper the opportunity for women to achieve equality in all fields of endeavor.

### Gender bias

Health-care professions reflect their culture, and most cultures evidence gender bias; that is, they ascribe stereotypical characteristics to groups or individuals on the basis of gender. For example, U.S. society associates courage, rationality, and ambition with men, and gentleness, empathy, and nurturance with women (Tong, 1993). Such patterning serves the purpose of allowing individuals to make generalizations about each new situation. Busy and powerful people use stereotypes as shortcuts when many people are competing for their attention (Fiske, 1993). Stereotypes can be harmful, however, for they deny individuals, both men and women, the opportunity to be appraised positively on the basis of their unique traits. Indeed, men or women who act "against type" tend to be dismissed or marginalized. The "feminine" man who displays more sensitivity or emotion than is culturally normative for his gender risks derision; the woman who is more assertive in pursuit of career goals is perceived as "unfeminine."

Gender-specific roles for health professionals have a long history. Elizabeth Blackwell, a mid-nineteenth-century leader in women's medical education, and Rebecca Lee, who in 1864 was the first African-American woman to obtain a medical degree in the United States, accepted the prevalent Victorian view that women—and, by extension, women physicians—were by nature responsible for domestic hygiene and maternal and child welfare. Florence Nightingale, founder of the first formal school of nursing at St. Thomas' Hospital in London following the Crimean War, not only accepted the "natural division of labor" between men and women, but felt that the "special nature" of women uniquely suited them for the nursing profession.

Gender stereotypes may create wedges between individuals who actually share the burden of a stereotype. For example, the gender identification of women with nursing continues to create challenges for both women physicians and nurses. Women medical students complain among themselves about patients mistaking them for nurses and assigning them nursing tasks. Some nurses evidence mixed reactions to and confusion about the role of women physicians, expecting more of female medical students than of males in such tasks as emptying bedpans and doing routine paperwork. The woman physician is faced with a dilemma: to reinforce her legitimacy as a physician, she may need to reject assignment to nursing roles; yet in doing so, she risks implying denigration of the nurse.

The social allocation of gender roles can also unnecessarily and unfairly constrain individual choice. Although men may take on many parenting responsibilities, social emphasis remains on the woman as the primary parent. One result is that women's careers in health care tend to be much more frequently disrupted by parenting responsibilities than are men's. However, stereotyping cuts both ways; allowing women to take paid leave related to childbirth excludes men who might desire a more active role in their infants' care.

Gender stereotyping may also discourage men and women from learning effective behaviors from each other, especially if one sex is perceived to be less adequate in some dimensions, such as moral development, than the other. Carol Gilligan's *In a Different Voice* (1982) challenged the prevailing assumptions that women are not as morally developed as men. Such assumptions stemmed from Lawrence Kohlberg's work in moral development, which was conducted largely on male subjects; Kohlberg concluded that decisions based on an impersonal principle of justice reflected the highest form of moral development. Gilligan's studies led her to describe women's ethical decision making not as a disengaged, principle-based, rule-governed endeavor but rather as a commitment to caring governed by a responsiveness to others (Gilligan, 1982). Feminist philosophers have in turn developed a variety of theoretical arguments for an ethic of "caring," drawing heavily on experiences and preferences traditionally ascribed to women (Tong, 1993).

The emergence of this new train of moral analysis is highly relevant to the experience and future success of women in health care. The distanced, impersonal judgments of Kohlberg's schema are embodied to some extent in the medical model, which insists that doctors remain detached from patients. Furthermore, lack of expressed emotional response to the patient's experience was until very recently deemed the mark of the effective, psychologically well-balanced physician. As a result, many women who completed medical training in the 1960s, 1970s, and 1980s (with the possible exception of those entering psychiatry) were criticized or ignored when they focused on a patient's emotional well-being. Expressions of grief over a patient's death (especially in the form of tears) were met with frank rejection. Discussion about emotions and relationships, often important to women physicians and their patients, remained outside the parlance of much of medicine.

Feminist philosophy, far from rejecting such behavior, offers philosophical support for the approach of many women physicians to their patient relationships. Emphasis on the quality of physician–patient communication and relationships certainly finds justification in traditional medical ethics but can be even more robustly grounded in an ethic of caring. However, these arguments risk perpetuating the stereotyping of women as more suited and committed to caring than men are. In fact, these arguments ignore men's actual and potential affections and attachments. Feminine moral theories should not be misconstrued to equate with moral capacities unique to women, any more than abstract ideals of justice should be construed as intellectual constructs especially accessible to men. Stereotyping by gender, as opposed to approaches valuing characteristics of women's culturally or otherwise determined characteristics, would have the effect of inhibiting dialogue between the sexes as well as progress toward the goals of facilitating "caring" and "leading" on the part of both women and men.

Fortunately, since the late 1980s there has been increasing emphasis on the need for formal education in and evaluation of the humane behavior of physicians (American Board of Internal Medicine, 1985). And what women doctors often emphasize, perhaps as a result of their acculturation outside of medicine, is acquiring greater value within medical practice generally. In fact, the pressing need to improve and humanize health care demands that all providers become better at caring. For instance, researchers found that male medical students were less willing to work with the underserved in their final year of medical school than in their first year, whereas female students' willingness remained constant. This finding should stimulate exploration of why women medical students have a more robust concern for such populations (Crandall et al., 1993).

Critical comparison of the codes of ethics of nurses and physicians seems to suggest that professional identities may well emanate from gender-specific attributes and concerns; nurses' codes emphasize patient empowerment while those of physicians typically focus on the rights and duties of the profession. The codes embody the relative responsibilities of physicians (historically men) and nurses (historically women) in the medical hierarchy. The mutual reinforcement of gender stereotyping embodied by these codes and the gender association of these two health professions potentially limits rather than encourages the exploration of how both professions and sexes can respond more effectively to patients' needs.

Also to be considered is how sexism—gender bias that systematically places women at a disadvantage—limits women's options in medicine. Susan Fiske (1993) observes that stereotypes reinforce one group's power over another by limiting the other's options. Those who are more powerful will predetermine how the less powerful are expected to behave. Should members of the less powerful group behave differently than expected, such behavior is likely to be ignored or actively discouraged. Both sexes must operate in medical institutions that are typically hierarchical and competitive. Typically, women are taught the attributes of followers in such organizations, while men learn how to be leaders.

Though discrimination on the basis of gender is now illegal in education and the workplace, men have been the "normal" frame of reference for so long that bias continues to interject itself. A common example is the tendency of physicians to refer to a patient as "he," unless the disease is of psychogenic origin, when the pronoun becomes "she." Other examples, as apparent in the health-care context as in any other, are sexual humor disparaging women in general; a woman's having her suggestions attributed to a man; and the focus on a woman's appearance while her professional attributes are downplayed (Lenhart and Evans, 1991). Sometimes deliberately, sometimes unconsciously, men may undermine women by treating them with condescending chivalry, friendly harassment, benevolent exploitation, considerate domination, and collegial exclusion (Lorber, 1991). Under such conditions, women cannot realize their full potential, nor can they care for their patients with maximum effectiveness. These behaviors also maintain an asymmetrical relationship in which men dominate (Epstein, 1988).

Sexism contributes to other inequities as well. Susan Sherwin (1992) notes that the institution of medicine not only reflects social values, but is in fact so powerful that its characteristics affect society as a whole. Thus, she argues, the inequitable treatment of women within the medical hierarchy reinforces and even validates gender bias throughout the social system. For instance, the relative paucity of women who are principal investigators and leaders in the medical science community helps to explain the relative lack of research into conditions affecting women and of women in clinical trials, which results in large gaps in knowledge regarding the appropriate treatment of women patients.

Finally, it is worth noting that women of color face even greater difficulties in finding their way to leadership and policymaking positions within the medical profession. For instance, whereas African-Americans make up 12 percent of the U.S. population, they comprise only 3 percent of M.D.s (Sherwin, 1992). In 1993, U.S. medical schools had a total of 1,097 African-American men on the faculty (less than 2 percent of all male faculty) and 651 African-American women (less than 4 percent of all female faculty) (Association of American Medical Colleges, 1993).

In summary, gender stereotyping in the health-care context limits the options of women, thereby reducing their effectiveness. Sexism not only reflects an unjust distribution of power based on irrelevant considerations, but also perpetuates stereotypes insofar as they serve to enforce the dominance of men over women. As Sherwin notes: "When predominantly white female nurses accept the authority of mostly male doctors and follow their directions, they convey gender messages to patients and health care workers alike" (1992, p. 235).

The moral imperative to treat men and women patients equitably demands that such a system be critically examined. The remainder of this article explores in more detail several key issues that continue to shape women's experience as health professionals—access to education, professional opportunities and status, role conflicts, and leadership.

## Access to education

Three virtually simultaneous phenomena largely solved the problem of women's access to medical education in the United States: (a) the enactment in 1972 of Title IX of the Higher Education Amendments prohibiting institutions receiving federal funds from practicing discrimination based on sex; (b) a sizable expansion of medical school places; and (c) cultural changes that raised the sights of young women. Between 1970 and 1980 alone, the number of women applying to medical schools rose from 3,390 to 16,141, while the number of men rose from 22,166 to 25,436 (Bickel and Quinnie, 1993). In 1993, women comprised 42 percent of new entrants, compared to 9 percent in 1970. Between 1970 and 1990 the number of women physicians more than quadrupled, from 25,401 to 104,194 (17 percent of the total) (Women in Medicine Services, 1991).

Informal barriers to full gender parity in medical education, however, have remained. One large-scale study of young physicians found that, as medical students, white women and African-Americans and Latinos of both sexes had greater reservations than white men about asking questions and volunteering for assignments (Hadley et al., 1992); as a result, these women and minorities had less positive experiences during their clinical years of medical school. This study's additional finding that as young physicians these groups were more likely to have second thoughts about a medical career is therefore not surprising. Likewise, a study of medical students in a surgery clerkship found that, even though the women's performances were evaluated as favorably as the men's, only half as many of the women as of the men entered surgery as a field of specialty training. Moreover, the women rated twelve of fifteen aspects of the clerkship experience less positively than the men did. These findings suggest that more women might select surgery if they were offered as many satisfying and relevant work and skill development opportunities as men receive (Calkins et al., 1992). Studies such as these suggest an interaction between gender and educational opportunity that discourages women from affiliating with particular specialties and reinforces gender-associated distinctions within the profession.

Overt sexism also affects the relative quality of the educational experience. In response to the question on the Association of American Medical Colleges' Graduation Questionnaire, "Have you ever been subjected to sexual harassment or discrimination while in medical school?" 60 percent of women and 14 percent of men said yes. When asked what form the discrimination took, men most commonly noted favoritism, hostility, and denied opportunity. Although many women also noted these, three times more women than men reported sexist slurs, sexist teaching materials, and sexual advances. Although they are difficult to measure, such environmental features as sexual harassment can damage self-confidence and career aspirations (Lenhart and Evans, 1991).

Both sexes' preparation for treating women patients is another educational access concern. Increasing evidence of disparities related to women's health is surfacing with regard to many diagnostic and therapeutic interventions, and the results of research on men are too often generalized to women without sufficient evidence of applicability (Council on Ethical and Judicial Affairs, 1991). Another concern is that women students may not be as well-trained in the examination of the prostate as men are of the female pelvis; some women still report difficulties in gaining training in urology.

Women who select other health careers have also faced inequities. Not until 1931, when the New York Maternity Center Association opened its Midwifery School, could women pursue advanced training in the profession they had held almost by birthright. In nursing, there were no formal educational barriers. However, individuals of low socioeconomic status have been less likely to complete hospital-based programs leading to careers as registered nurses and to collegiate curricula resulting in bachelor's of science degrees in nursing. Until the late 1930s, few nurses of any socioeconomic background had the opportunity to advance within nursing if they wished to continue doing clinical work. Women's routes to clinical autonomy were very few indeed. The development of nurse practitioner programs since the 1970s has afforded nurses a gateway to greater independence and autonomy (Koch et al., 1992; Safriet, 1992).

## Professional opportunities and status

Women deserve access to as wide a range of career choices as men enjoy, but this range is not represented by the career choices of men and women in medicine. Looking first at physicians in the United States, it is no surprise to find that both historically and currently, a higher proportion of women physicians than men specialize in pediatrics, general internal medicine, and family practice. Men are more evenly distributed across specialties and are much more likely than women to be surgeons or subspecialists. Thus, the more prestigious (and better paid) "curing" specialties continue to be male dominated (Bickel, 1988). One concern women physicians have about their concentration in what might be termed the "caring" specialties is that listening and counseling skills are sometimes viewed as qualities inherent in women rather than acknowledged as technical proficiencies.

In 1989, 73 percent of men compared to 49 percent of women physicians were self-employed; women are more likely than men to be employees of a hospital, an HMO, or other physician groups (Women in Medicine Services, 1991). This tendency toward salaried positions may reflect women's desire for regular hours because of family responsibilities. The willingness to work within larger organized groups may also reflect social stereotyping that encourages interdependence and collaboration in women, and independence and entrepreneurship in men.

Another reflection of unequal access to opportunity and status for women in the health professions is seen in their experience as nurses. Imbalances in power between physicians and nurses detract from nurses' identity as colleagues and professionals. Hospitals continue to exercise power over nurses' wages, which are not billed separately as "professional services." The nurse-practitioner is an exception. An outgrowth of the shortage of primary-care physicians, the nurse-practitioner developed in a context very different from that of the Victorian nurse. Nurse-practitioners envision themselves collaborating with, more than depending on physicians. In fact, in an ever-increasing number of states, nurse-practitioners have sought and been granted legal licensure for independent practice. Many of the ensuing battles with the medical profession have reprised the turf, gender, and class issues all nurses face. Physicians and institutions continue to be the largest "buyers" of nurse-practitioner services; as a result, many nurse-practitioners experience dissonance between the autonomy they seek and the dependence they encounter (Pearson, 1994). Despite some evidence of progress in geriatrics and family practice, the nurse-practitioner's struggle to be recognized as an autonomous clinician will likely continue. Whether as physicians, as nurses, or as other health professionals, women continue to experience the impact of gender stereotyping.

## Role conflicts: Professional parents

Most women health professionals are also mothers. In the United States in 1988, 75 percent of female and 89 percent of male physicians were married with the spouse present; 85 percent of the women and 93 percent of men reported having children (Women in Medicine Services, 1991). The process of accruing credentials, however, conflicts with women's biological clocks. Becoming a doctor typically takes eight years of education after college graduation, with no time out and with periods of virtually around-the-clock patient care. The subsequent years of building a practice and, for faculty, meeting tenure and promotion deadlines and attaining standards requiring excellence in research and teaching achievements, may be even more demanding than the years of clinical training.

In 1991, only 34 percent of U.S. medical schools had specific maternity-leave policies for their faculty and only 10 percent had written provisions for paternity leave (Grisso et al., 1991). The personnel policies of many hospitals and medical schools may be responsible for undermining residents' health in general, through sleep deprivation at the very least. Such policies may be especially deleterious to childbearing residents (Merritt, 1993). Even when workable policies exist, those doctors who take advantage of the leave may be labeled "uncommitted." Family-related decisions can escalate into genuine moral dilemmas. The traditional obligation of physicians to set patients' needs above their own confronts physician-parents (and especially couples who are both in practice) with difficult choices between the needs of patients and those of their own children. How are they to decide when a patient must take priority over their children? What seems to be needed is an account of the ethics of child rearing as related to the ethics of medicine, as well as systems that promote attention to both.

Except for the higher earnings that make more paid child care and other help possible, women physicians may be at a disadvantage relative to, say, nurses or physical therapists with respect to role expectations and support as parents and family members. A physician's commitment to medicine may be called into question when, however infrequently, she puts her family first. Other women health professionals have somewhat greater leeway in balancing their personal and professional responsibilities. However, nursing education has also remained inflexible, possibly because of nurse educators' ongoing concern to be taken seriously by their physician counterparts.

### Leadership positions

In 1992, women comprised 22 percent of full-time U.S. medical school faculty; however, only 8 percent of full professors and about 4 percent of academic department chairs were women. Two medical schools out of a total 126 were headed by women deans. The continuing paucity of women in top positions, especially in academia, remains a complex challenge. For one thing, women faculty do not progress to the rank of full professor at the same rate as men. Of all faculty who had their first full-time medical-school appointment in 1976, 22 percent of men but only 10 percent of women had gained the rank of professor by 1991 (Bickel and Whiting, 1991). Likewise, women physicians are more likely than men to be on nontenured clinical faculty tracks (Bickel and Whiting, 1991). Another study explored the status and productivity of women and men in academic internal medicine. Women had similar job descriptions and allocations of work among research, clinical, and teaching activity; in the number of grants funded as principal investigator, abstracts accepted, and papers published in refereed journals, the statistics were also comparable. However, women had lower academic rank and received less compensation (Carr et al., 1993). In considering the many variables contributing to career development, it is helpful to think in terms of "accumulated" advantages and disadvantages, or negative and positive "kicks," as shaping one's opportunity structure (Zuckerman et al., 1991). A prestigious fellowship is likely to pay off in a variety of ways over the course of a career, for instance, by increasing the total number of articles published. Similarly, having a child during residency—and, in so doing, losing the support of one's mentor—is likely to have negative career consequences. The interaction of such variables as subtle and overt sexist behavior, inflexible personnel policies, and inadequate mentoring suggests the necessity of continuing efforts to assist women's professional development.

With respect to professional advancement, gender bias is at work within nursing as well as within medicine. On the one hand, there have been relatively few men in nursing, probably because of gender bias among men and within nursing. Yet although men make up fewer than 4 percent of nurses, they advance more quickly than women nurses; this faster rate cannot be explained by education, work experience, or such variables as having children or marital status. Women may advance less rapidly because, relative to male nurses, they may focus more on family roles; men may also receive more encouragement both within and outside the nursing profession to seek out leadership roles. It might even be suggested that men more often than women pursue paths affording social recognition because they do not have the social option afforded most women of substituting child rearing as a socially approved alternative to career success.

### Future directions

This article aims to provide an understanding of the powerful role that gender bias has played in medicine. But changes, probably mirroring shifts in the larger social context, are taking place. Developments in the organization of health care and in medical education are mitigating the impact of some gender stereotypes and breaking down others altogether. For example:

1. Since women are likelier to enter primary-care fields than men, the rising status of primary care may lift the status of women physicians along with it. Competition is increasing among health-care enterprises to sign up primary-care physicians with excellent communication and networking skills. Kaiser Permanente and other large HMOs are now paying such physicians more than those with greater technical skills. Health-care reform is also likely to expand career opportunities for nurse-practitioners and physician assistants.

2. The traditional "transactional," hierarchical management style (that is, viewing performance as a series of transactions with subordinates and using the power that comes from formal authority) is becoming outmoded (Senge, 1990). Studies of managers have shown that women are more likely to use "transformational" methods, getting subordinates to see their own self-interest more in terms of the interest of the group through a common concern for a broader goal (Rosener, 1990). As teamwork becomes ever more necessary in the delivery of patient care, transformational management styles become more desirable. This shift not only draws on many women's strengths, but is also likely to foster environments where women will be able to achieve leadership without having to copy the styles of men they do not admire. Furthermore, the trend away from hierarchical organizations and top-down decision making should enhance the value of "feminine" styles of interaction, making them more desirable and economically rewarded attributes for both women and men.

3. More young physicians and medical trainees are seeking a better balance between work and family than did most of their predecessors. Increasing opportunities for physicians in managed-care settings will abet this trend because in such settings schedules are more predictable and less onerous than in private practice. Even in residencies, the proportion of programs offering paternity leave is increasing (Bickel, 1991).

4. While only 15 percent of all surgical residents are women (numbering almost 1,200 in 1991), this proportion continues to increase each year. Some of these women, even those who bear a child during residency, are becoming chief residents. Perhaps the most radical shift has occurred over the last two decades in obstetrics and gynecology, almost exclusively a male specialty in the United States since the early 1800s. As of 1993, 48 percent of the residents are women (Bickel and Quinnie, 1993).

5. The National Institutes of Health Office for Research on Women's Health was created in 1990 to ensure that women are appropriately represented in clinical trials, to increase the numbers of women principal in-

vestigators, and to support efforts of medical schools to enhance their focus on women's health issues. The *Journal of Women's Health,* established in 1992, publishes many articles that add significantly to both biomedical and psychosocial knowledge about women. This is especially timely, since more patients and professionals of both sexes are calling for a definition of health that includes both spiritual and social dimensions missing from the strictly biomedical model.

Reducing the power of gender stereotypes in medicine is a moral imperative because health-care professionals have a duty to ensure that perceptual bias does not interfere either with the best possible patient care or with clinicians' responsibilities as role models for and teachers of students of both genders. Health-care professionals' effectiveness depends in large part on their sensitivities to others, that is, their ability to "hear" and "see" individual patients. These abilities are best nurtured in a gender-neutral educational environment that is free of harassment. In such an environment those with power will attend equally to the strengths and needs of both men and women, and all trainees, staff, and patients will benefit.

JANET BICKEL
GAIL J. POVAR

*Directly related to this article are the preceding article on* WOMEN AS HEALTH PROFESSIONALS: A. HISTORY, *and the other articles in this entry:* HISTORICAL AND CROSS-CULTURAL PERSPECTIVES, HEALTH-CARE ISSUES, *and* RESEARCH ISSUES. *Also directly related are the entries* FEMINISM; SEXISM; *and* SEXUAL ETHICS AND PROFESSIONAL STANDARDS. *For a further discussion of topics mentioned in this article, see the entries* ALLIED HEALTH PROFESSIONS; CARE; MEDICAL EDUCATION; MEDICINE, SOCIOLOGY OF; MEDICINE AS A PROFESSION; NURSING AS A PROFESSION; *and* RESEARCH BIAS. *Other relevant material may be found under the entry* ALTERNATIVE THERAPIES, *article on* SOCIAL HISTORY.

## Bibliography

AMERICAN BOARD OF INTERNAL MEDICINE. 1985. *A Guide to Awareness and Evaluation of Humanistic Qualities in the Internist.* Portland, Oreg.: Author.

ASSOCIATION OF AMERICAN MEDICAL COLLEGES. 1993. *U.S. Medical School Faculty, 1993.* Washington, D.C.: Author.

BICKEL, JANET W. 1988. "Women in Medical Education: A Status Report." *New England Journal of Medicine* 319, no. 24:1579–1584.

———. 1991. *Medicine and Parenting: A Resource for Medical Students, Residents, Faculty and Program Directors.* Washington, D.C.: Association of American Medical Colleges.

BICKEL, JANET W., and QUINNIE, RENÉE. 1993. *Women in Academic Medicine: Statistics.* Rev. ed. Washington, D.C.: Association of American Medical Colleges.

BICKEL, JANET W., and WHITING, BROOKE E. 1991. "Comparing the Representation and Promotion of Men and Women Faculty at U.S. Medical Schools." *Academic Medicine* 66, no. 8:497.

BONNER, THOMAS N. 1992. *To the Ends of the Earth: Women's Search for Education in Medicine.* Cambridge, Mass.: Harvard University Press.

BOWMAN, MARJORIE A., and ALLEN, DEBORAH I. 1991. "The Experience of Women as Physicians." *Journal of Medical Practice Management* 6, no. 4:235–239.

BUTTER, IRENE H.; CARPENTER, EUGENIA; KAY, BONNIE; and SIMMONS, RUTH. 1985. *Sex and Status: Hierarchies in the Health Workforce.* Washington, D.C.: American Public Health Association.

CALKINS, E. VIRGINIA; WILLOUGHLY, T. LEE; and ARNOLD, LOUISE M. 1992. "Women Medical Students' Ratings of the Required Surgery Clerkship: Implications for Career Choice." *Journal of the American Medical Women's Association* 47, no. 2:58–60.

CARR, PHYLLIS L.; FRIEDMAN, ROBERT H.; MOSKOWITZ, MARK A.; and KAZIS, LEWIS E. 1993. "Comparing the Status of Women and Men in Academic Medicine." *Annals of Internal Medicine* 119, no. 9:908–913.

COUNCIL ON ETHICAL AND JUDICIAL AFFAIRS. AMERICAN MEDICAL ASSOCIATION. 1991. "Gender Disparities in Clinical Decision Making." *Journal of the American Medical Association* 266, no. 4:559–562.

CRANDALL, SONIA J. S.; VOLK, ROBERT J.; and LOEMKER, VICKI. 1993. "Medical Students' Attitudes Toward Providing Care for the Underserved: Are We Training Socially Responsible Physicians?" *Journal of the American Medical Association* 269, no. 19:2519–2523.

EPSTEIN, CYNTHIA FUCHS. 1988. *Deceptive Distinctions: Sex, Gender and Social Order.* New Haven, Conn.: Yale University Press.

FISKE, SUSAN T. 1993. "Controlling Other People: The Impact of Power on Stereotyping." *American Psychologist* 48, no. 6:621–628.

FLOGE, LILIANE, and MERRILL, DEBORAH H. 1986. "Tokenism Reconsidered: Male Nurses and Female Physicians in a Hospital Setting." *Social Forces* 64, no. 4:925–947.

GILLIGAN, CAROL. 1982. *In a Different Voice: Psychological Theory and Women's Development.* Cambridge, Mass.: Harvard University Press.

GRISSO, JEAN ANN; HANSEN, LESLIE; ZELLING, INGE; BICKEL, JANET; and EISENBERG, JOHN. 1991. "Parental Leave Policies for Faculty in U.S. Medical Schools." *Annals of Internal Medicine* 114, no. 1:43–45.

HADLEY, JACK; CANTOR, JOEL C.; WILLKE, RICHARD J.; FEDER, JUDITH; and COHEN, ALAN B. 1992. "Young Physicians Most and Least Likely to Have Second Thoughts About a Career in Medicine." *Academic Medicine* 67, no. 3: 180–189.

KOCH, LARRY W.; PAZAKI, S. H.; and CAMPBELL, JAMES D. 1992. "The First 20 Years of Nurse Practitioner Literature: An Evolution of Joint Practice Issues." *Nurse Practitioner* 17, no. 2:62–71.

LENHART, SHARYN A., and EVANS, CLYDE H. 1991. "Sexual Harassment and Gender Discrimination: A Primer for Women Physicians." *Journal of the American Medical Women's Association* 46, no. 3:77–82.

LORBER, JUDITH. 1991. "Can Women Physicians Ever Be True Equals in the American Medical Profession?" *Current Research on Occupations and Professions* 6:25–37.

MARIESKIND, HELEN I. 1980. *Women in the Health System: Patients, Providers and Programs.* St. Louis: Mosby.

MELOSH, BARBARA. 1982. *The Physician's Hand: Work, Culture, and Conflict in American Nursing.* Philadelphia: Temple University Press.

MERRIT, ELI F. 1993. "Family and the Medical Profession: Conflicting Claims." *Journal of the American Medical Association* 270, no. 13:1606–1607.

PEARSON, LINDA J. 1994. "Annual Update on How Each State Stands on Legislative Issues Affecting Advanced Nursing Practice." *Nurse Practitioner* 19, no. 1:11–13, 17–18, 21.

REVERBY, SUSAN M. 1987. *Ordered to Care.* New York: Cambridge University Press.

RISKA, ELIANNE, and WEGAR, KATARINA. 1993. "Women Physicians: A New Force in Medicine?" In *Gender, Work and Medicine.* Edited by Elianne Riska and Katarina Wegar. London: Sage.

ROSENER, JUDY B. 1990. "Ways Women Lead." *Harvard Business Review,* November-December, pp. 119–125.

SAFRIET, BARBARA J. 1992. "Health Care Dollars and Regulatory Sense: The Role of Advanced Nursing Practice." *Yale Journal on Regulation* 9, no. 2:417–488.

SANDAY, PEGGY REEVES. 1981. *Female Power and Male Dominance: On the Origins of Sexual Inequality.* New York: Cambridge University Press.

SHERWIN, SUSAN. 1992. *No Longer Patient: Feminist Ethics and Health Care.* Philadelphia: Temple University Press.

TONG, ROSEMARIE. 1993. *Feminine and Feminist Ethics.* Belmont, Calif.: Wadsworth.

WARREN, VIRGINIA L. 1992. "Feminist Directions in Medical Ethics." In *Feminist Perspectives in Medical Ethics,* pp. 32–45. Edited by Helen B. Holmes and Laura M. Purdy. Bloomington: Indiana University Press.

WOMEN IN MEDICINE SERVICES. AMERICAN MEDICAL ASSOCIATION. 1992. *In the Mainstream: Women in Medicine in America.* Chicago: Author.

ZUCKERMAN, HARRIET; COLE, JONATHAN; and BRUER, JOHN T., eds. 1991. *The Outer Circle: Women in the Scientific Community.* New York: W. W. Norton.

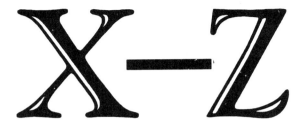

# XENOGRAFTS

Humankind's fascination with transplantation dates back to early mythology. Legendary creatures such as the centaur and the chimera, formed by combinations of actual animals, are described in the myths of various ancient cultures. Today, the transplantation of human organs has become commonplace and is recognized as the treatment of choice for conditions such as end-stage heart failure.

The great shortcoming of transplantation in the twentieth century is the shortage of human donor organs. The Registry of the International Society for Heart and Lung Transplantation lists fewer than 2,500 people as having received heart transplants during 1991 (Kaye, 1992). In addition, approximately 30 percent of patients on heart transplant waiting lists die before a suitable donor can be located (United Network for Organ Sharing [UNOS], 1990). There are an estimated 14,000 potential organ donors each year in the United States, but only a fraction of these are utilized (Evans, 1991). Neither educational programs nor "required request" legislation designed to increase the supply of donor organs has had a significant impact on donation rates. In addition, laws requiring the use of seat belts and motorcycle helmets preserve life but also reduce the size of the potential donor pool.

The immense disparity between organ supply and demand has led transplant physicians to reconsider the ancient notion of the centaur and the chimera. Cross-species transplantation, or xenotransplantation, has several appealing characteristics. Xenografts are biological transplants and therefore are totally implantable, do not require an external power source, and do not present the high risk of blood clot formation seen with many mechanical devices. Xenografts have been investigated as bridges to eventual human-to-human transplantation (allotransplantation). In other words, the heart of an animal would be implanted in a human recipient until a suitable human organ could be found, at which time the animal heart would be removed and a human one implanted. Although potentially lifesaving, this procedure would not alleviate the donor shortage and would likely increase the competition for suitable organs because it would keep alive more people on waiting lists. Therefore, investigators argue that xenografts must be viewed as a permanent alternative to allografts for transplantation. Though early results using nonhuman primate organs have been judged promising by some investigators, a number of ethical concerns have been expressed regarding the experimental and clinical use of these primates.

## Historical perspective

The earliest recorded attempts at clinical xenotransplantation occurred in the early 1900s and involved kidney grafts from the rabbit, pig, goat, nonhuman primate, and lamb. In some cases, organ function was noted, but none of the patients survived more than several days (Reemtsma, 1991). Following these early studies, the scientific literature was devoid of reports of xenotransplantation for nearly forty years. However, following Sir Peter Medawar's work detailing the immunologic nature of the rejection response (Billingham et al., 1956) and the development of more potent immunosuppressive drugs, Keith Reemtsma and his colleagues at Tulane University transplanted a chimpanzee kidney into a uremic human patient on November 5, 1963. Six people received kidney xenografts in the Tulane study, with one patient surviving for more than nine months after the transplant (Reemtsma, 1991).

The first heart xenotransplant was performed on January 23, 1964, by James Hardy and his colleagues at the University of Mississippi. This operation predated the world's first heart allotransplant by nearly four years. The chimpanzee xenograft functioned for approximately two hours before it failed, presumably because it was too small to support the recipient's circulation (Hardy et al., 1964). In 1985, the heart of a baboon was transplanted into a newborn infant with hypoplastic left heart syndrome at Loma Linda Medical Center (Bailey et al., 1985). "Baby Fae" survived for twenty days. Her short life sparked a lively controversy regarding the ethics of human experimentation in general and xenografts in particular. More recently, Jeremi Czaplicki and his colleagues in Poland performed heart xenotransplantation using a pig as the donor in 1992 (Czaplicki et al., 1992). The patient survived for twenty-four hours. As in Hardy's original case, the cause of death was attributed to the donor pig's small size and the heart's inability to support the recipient's circulation.

In June 1992, Thomas Starzl and his colleagues at the University of Pittsburgh transplanted a baboon liver into a thirty-five-year-old HIV-positive man suffering hepatic damage as a result of hepatitis B infection. Because of this dual viral infection, he was not a candidate for human liver allotransplantation (patients with HIV are routinely excluded from waiting lists). Function of the organ was noted following transplantation, but the patient died within seventy days due to damage of the baboon liver ducts and an acute bacterial infection (Starzl et al., 1993).

## The barrier to success

The surgical technique of xenotransplantation is no different from the transplantation of human organs. The primary barrier to successful cross-species transplantation is the immunologic disparity between donor and recipient. To a lesser degree, this can be a problem in human-to-human transplantation. When a person receives an organ from a human donor, the recipient's immune system recognizes the foreign tissue and attempts to destroy it. For this reason, a transplant recipient must take immunosuppressive drugs for the rest of his or her life. These drugs (such as cyclosporine) inhibit the func-

tion of the immune system, thus thwarting the rejection response. Of course, the immune system serves other functions as well, such as protection of the body from infection. Thus, the transplant recipient must be carefully monitored so as to maintain a balance between rejection and infection, thereby ensuring function of the transplanted organ as well as general health.

As mentioned above, the immunologic reaction is even more pronounced in cross-species transplantation. It is the degree of genetic disparity between different species that dictates the severity of the rejection reaction. For example, the human immune system will attack the heart of a pig more quickly and intensely than it will the heart of a chimpanzee (and that heart more quickly and intensely than a human heart). Thus, even within the realm of xenotransplantation, the degree of genetic disparity between species results in significant differences in transplantation immune responses.

From the time of birth, animals have natural antibodies (protective molecules of the immune system) circulating in their bodies that are prepared to attack the tissue of a distantly related species. The presence of these antibodies accounts for the rapid and vigorous "hyperacute rejection" of organs between certain species combinations (such as pig-to-human). Hyperacute rejection is a rapid and aggressive rejection reaction that occurs within minutes to hours of implantation; it is mediated by circulating antibodies. However, more closely related species combinations (such as chimpanzee-to-human) do not involve these natural antibodies and, therefore, rarely exhibit hyperacute rejection. A species pair that has these natural antibodies is known as a discordant pair, while one without them is referred to as concordant (Calne, 1970). This is relevant to current research and practice because humans have natural antibodies to some farm animals, such as pigs, but not to more closely related nonhuman primates, such as chimpanzees. For this reason, successful discordant xenotransplantation must take into account the control of this antibody response as well as the cellular rejection response seen in concordant xenotransplantation and allotransplantation.

Current research efforts in xenotransplantation are aimed at a better understanding of the rejection response and eventual clinical application of cross-species transplantation. In studies of concordant xenotransplantation, it has been noted that combinations of drugs and techniques that act on the immune system often work better than any single therapy alone. Robert Michler and his colleagues at Columbia University achieved tenfold prolongation of heart graft survival from cynomolgus monkeys to baboons by employing the immunosuppressive drug cyclosporine along with other agents (Michler et al., 1985). Since that time, many studies have illustrated the importance of using a variety of techniques to act on the immune system in order to prevent rejection.

Discordant xenotransplantation has proved to be a more difficult area of research. Not only must methods like the ones used in concordant xenotransplantation be employed, but the natural antibody response must also be controlled. Various techniques to remove these antibodies and to prevent their resynthesis have been investigated, but results to date have been limited in their clinical utility. Hyperacute rejection remains a major problem.

In order for xenotransplantation to be clinically applicable, an appropriate donor species must be identified and the immune system controlled. The ideal donor animal would be available in large numbers and free of transmissible diseases, and it must have organs that are available in all sizes. Nonhuman primates are an attractive choice because of their genetic similarity to humans. Both baboon and chimpanzee organs were used in the early human xenograft studies mentioned above. The similarity between nonhuman primates and humans also leads to the fact that many of the ethical arguments against xenotransplantation focus on these animals. Discordant xenograft research has increasingly focused on farm animals such as the pig, which may prove to be a more ethically appropriate alternative to the use of nonhuman primates, despite the greater immunologic barrier.

## Ethical issues

The motivation for using animals as a source of organs for human transplantation is the scarcity of suitable human organs and the thousands of people dying each year who might have benefited from transplantation. This situation shows no sign of resolution in the near future. Indeed, it has been referred to as an "insurmountable obstacle" (Caplan, 1992). Transplantation is the treatment of choice for end-stage organ failure, yet many fewer people actually receive transplants than could benefit from them. Even educational initiatives and large organ-sharing networks have not appreciably enlarged the donor pool. One alternative that has shown promise in Europe is "presumed consent" legislation. This legislation identifies all brain-dead individuals as having consented to organ donation unless they have previously indicated otherwise. In addition, the question of whether transplants are fiscally responsible procedures at a time when many people lack even the most basic health care is widely debated. Some analysts view expensive lifesaving therapies such as transplantation as secondary to disease prevention for resource allocation; however, even if effective prevention measures were to be instituted immediately, the number of patients who could benefit from transplantation would still outstrip

the number of potential human donors for many years. Thus, it has seemed reasonable for physicians and researchers to look outside of the normal pool of human organs for possible sources for transplantation. Naturally, the use of animals in both experimental and clinical settings raises considerable ethical concerns. Is it appropriate for human beings to use animals in this way, both to determine the feasibility of cross-species transplantation through experimental studies and, if these are successful, to serve as a source of supply of organs for humans?

As Thomasine Kushner and Raymond Belliotti point out in their examination of the Baby Fae case (1985), in order for unequal treatment of two groups to be moral, it must be justified. That is, the unequal treatment of two beings X and Y must be justified by a morally relevant difference between X and Y. In this context we find justification for relieving children of many of the social responsibilities held by adults, and it is also in this context that we can begin to examine whether the use of animals (especially nonhuman primates) can be justified in xenograft research and clinical application. Clearly, in order for this research to be justifiable, there must be a morally relevant distinction between humans and nonhuman primates. It is not enough to state, though some may believe it to be true, that primates can be used for any purpose humans deem fit simply because they are members of a different species. This arbitrary distinction cannot be morally justified, for to allow that argument would be to engage in "speciesism," the favoring of the members of a species simply by virtue of their being members of that species. Peter Singer argues against this sort of prejudicial logic. "When you think about it, it is not difficult to see that there is no morally important feature which *all* human beings possess, and *no* nonhuman animals have" (Singer, 1992, p. 729).

Singer is presumably referring to the fact that there are humans with diminished mental capacities (such as severely retarded individuals and anencephalic infants) who could never approach the cognitive and emotional level that some primates exhibit. How, then, can the use of animals for experimentation be justified? Is there a morally relevant difference between the species that can be pointed to as a rationale for continuing xenograft experimentation? If not, the procedures could not be justified because the act of doing good for the human (beneficence) would not outweigh the absence of regard (denial of nonmaleficence) for the animal. Kushner and Belliotti (1985) point to the human ability to carry out complex cognitions as the morally significant difference between species, while Arthur Caplan (1992) identifies the capacity for complex emotional relationships between human beings.

Even if one accepts the above distinctions as morally valid, what should be said about human beings with diminished mental capacities? Are they less than human? Should they be used as experimental subjects or as organ donors? Proponents of research involving primates who oppose the use of anencephalic or cortically dead humans focus the arguments on the effect that the use of these individuals would have on other human beings, most notably the subject's family. Caplan states, "It is in the relationships with others, both family and strangers, that the moral worth and standing of these children are grounded" (1992, p. 726). If one accepts that the morally reasonable distinction between humans and nonhuman primates has something to do with the complex emotional relationships that humans share and nonhumans do not, then Caplan's argument appears valid. That is, because these humans may be part of a familial or social structure that is weighted emotionally with regard to other people, they should be given moral preference over nonhuman primates. In some instances, families have taken great comfort at the donation of the organs of their anencephalic child. If this is the case, then donation for transplantation or research is certainly acceptable. However, if this is not the case, Caplan's rationale for the use of primates rather than severely impaired humans seems to hold.

If we do accept that there is a valid moral distinction between humans and nonhuman primates, we should next ask, "Is it necessary to use primates in this manner?" Ethical justification does not make an action a moral imperative. Do we need to use primates in order to determine whether xenotransplantation is clinically feasible? Efforts have been made to use more in vitro techniques and smaller animal species, such as rats, to study the immunologic properties of xenograft rejection. However, significant physiological and immunological differences between rodents and primates (including humans) make complete evaluation of xenotransplantation therapies impossible in small animal models. For example, certain therapeutic regimens that show great promise in rodents do not work in primates.

If xenotransplantation technology progresses to the point where it becomes a feasible clinical option, it will then be necessary to address a host of new issues regarding the use of these animals. That a technology can be employed does not necessarily mean that it ought to be or that it is appropriate in all situations. We must keep in mind that the use of primates depends on the need to supplement the available pool of donor organs from human cadavers. Clearly, in a situation where there is a choice between using an organ from a human cadaver and one from a living animal, the human organ ought to be used. To kill an animal in that case would be excessive and unnecessary. Xenotransplantation cannot be seen as a quick fix for the problem of organ scarcity. Efforts to expand the human donor pool and advances in areas of alternative therapies, such as mechanical

hearts and improved medical management of organ failure, should still be aggressively pursued. Progress has been made in the area of mechanical assist devices as bridges to heart transplants, but the development of permanently implantable devices is necessary to make an impact on the donor shortage (Chen and Michler, 1993).

Other issues regarding the clinical application of xenografts include the eventual development of large-scale breeding colonies to meet the immense demand for organs. Care must be taken in allowing these "organ farms" to come into existence. That is, the use of these animals must always be regarded as a necessary consequence of a widespread problem rather than as an obvious right of the human race. The use of farm animals such as pigs would be a more ethically palatable alternative to the use of primates. Pigs are already bred in vast numbers for food, and problems regarding the physical condition of the colonies and the well-being of the animals would be greatly reduced.

Attention must be given to the recipients of xenografts as well. Informed consent must always be obtained for procedures such as transplantation, but the medical profession must be prepared to deal with a host of potential psychosocial problems brought about by the implantation of an organ from a member of another species into a human. Issues of autonomy and of proper consent procedures must be given high priority.

## Conclusion

Transplantation of human organs is the treatment of choice for end-stage organ failure. However, there is a critical shortage of human organs for transplantation. For that reason, physicians and scientists have turned to the idea of cross-species transplantation as a means of alleviating the disparity between organ supply and demand. Xenotransplantation is currently an area of active research and may, in the near future, become a clinical reality. Meanwhile, great steps are being made to overcome the immunologic barriers to cross-species transplantation. It is also a subject rich with ethical dilemmas that must be articulated and fully explored before widespread research in and application of these technologies can be permitted.

ADAM J. RATNER
ROBERT E. MICHLER
ERIC A. ROSE

*Directly related to this entry are the entries* ORGAN AND TISSUE PROCUREMENT; ORGAN AND TISSUE TRANSPLANTS, *article on* ETHICAL AND LEGAL ISSUES; *and* ANIMAL RESEARCH, *article on* PHILOSOPHICAL ISSUES. *For a further discussion of topics mentioned in this entry, see the entries*

Health-Care Resources, Allocation of, *article on* microallocation; Informed Consent, *article on* consent issues in human research; *and* Research Policy, *article on* risk and vulnerable groups. *For a discussion of related ideas, see the entry* Body, *article on* social theories. *See also the* Appendix (Codes, Oaths, and Directives Related to Bioethics), *section* v: ethical directives pertaining to the welfare and use of animals.

## Bibliography

Bailey, Leonard L.; Nehlsen-Cannarella, Sandra L.; Concepcion, Waldo; and Jolley, Weldon B. 1985. "Baboon-to-Human Cardiac Xenotransplantation in a Neonate." *Journal of the American Medical Association* 254, no. 23:3321–3329.

Billingham, R. E.; Brent, L.; and Medawar, Peter B. 1956. "Quantitative Studies on Tissue Transplantation Immunity: III. Actively Acquired Tolerance." *Philosophical Transactions of the Royal Society of London: Series B* 239:357–412.

Calne, Roy Y. 1970. "Organ Transplantation Between Widely Disparate Species." *Transplantation Proceedings* 2, no. 4:550–553.

Caplan, Arthur L. 1992. "Is Xenografting Morally Wrong?" *Transplantation Proceedings* 24, no. 2:722–727.

Chen, Jonathan M., and Michler, Robert E. 1993. "Heart Xenotransplantation: Lessons Learned and Future Prospects." *Journal of Heart and Lung Transplantation* 12, no. 5:869–875.

Czaplicki, Jeremi; Blonska, Barbara; and Religa, Zbigniew. 1992. "The Lack of Hyperacute Xenogenic Heart Transplant Rejection in a Human." *Journal of Heart and Lung Transplantation* 11, no. 2, pt. 1:393–397.

Evans, Roger W. 1991. "The Actual and Potential Supply of Organ Donors in the United States." In *Clinical Transplants 1990*, pp. 329–341. Edited by Paul I. Terasaki. Los Angeles: UCLA Tissue Typing Laboratory.

Hardy, James D.; Chavez, Carlos M.; Kurrus, Fred D.; Neely, William A.; Eraslan, Sadan; Turner, M. Don; Fabian, Leonard W.; and Labecki, Thaddeus D. 1964. "Heart Transplantation in Man: Developmental Studies and Report of a Case." *Journal of the American Medical Association* 188, no. 13:1132–1140.

Kaye, Michael P. 1992. "The Registry of the International Society for Heart and Lung Transplantation Ninth Official Report—1992." *Journal of Heart and Lung Transplantation* 11, no. 4:599–606.

Kushner, Thomasine, and Belliotti, Raymond. 1985. "Baby Fae: A Beastly Business." *Journal of Medical Ethics* 11, no. 4:178–183.

Michler, Robert E.; McManus, Robert P.; Sadeghi, Ali M.; Smith, Craig R.; Marboe, Charles C.; Thomas, William; Hardy, Mark A.; Reemtsma, Keith; and Rose, Eric A. 1985. "Prolonged Primate Cardiac Xenograft Survival with Cyclosporine." *Surgical Forum* 36:359–365.

Reemtsma, Keith. 1991. "Xenotransplantation—A Brief History of Clinical Experiences: 1900–1965." In *Xenotransplantation: The Transplantation of Organs and Tissues Between Species*, pp. 9–22. Edited by David K. C. Cooper, Ejvind Kemp, Keith Reemtsma, and David J. G. White. New York: Springer-Verlag.

Singer, Peter. 1992. "Xenotransplantation and Speciesism." *Transplantation Proceedings* 24, no. 2:728–732.

Starzl, Thomas E.; Fung, J.; Tzakis, A.; Todo, S.; Demetris, A. J.; Marino, I. R.; Doyle, H.; Zeevi, A.; Warty, V.; Michaels, M.; Kusne, S.; Rudert, W. A.; and Trucco, M. 1993. "Baboon-to-Human Liver Transplantation." *Lancet* 341, no. 8837:65–71.

United Network for Organ Sharing (UNOS). 1990. *Annual Report of the U.S. Scientific Registry of Transplant Recipients and the Organ Procurement and Transplantation Network 1990*. Bethesda, Md.: U.S. Department of Health and Human Services, Public Health Service, Bureau of Health Resources and Development, Division of Organ Transplantation.

# YUGOSLAVIA

*See* Medical Ethics, History of, *section on* europe, *subsection on* contemporary period, *article on* central and eastern europe.

# ZOOS AND ZOOLOGICAL PARKS

*See* Animal Welfare and Rights, *article on* zoos and zoological parks.

# APPENDIX

## Codes, Oaths, and Directives Related to Bioethics

*Appendix Editor:*

Carol Mason Spicer

*Appendix Advisory Group:*

Glenn C. Graber, Chair

Patricio Figueroa
Doris Goldstein
Rihito Kimura
Charles R. McCarthy
Ruth B. Purtilo
Holmes Rolston, III
Robert M. Veatch
LeRoy Walters

# Contents

**Nature and Role of Codes and Other Ethics Directives**
*Carol Mason Spicer*

**Introduction to the Codes, Oaths, and Directives**

**Section I. Directives on Health-Related Rights and Patient Responsibilities**

**Section II: Ethical Directives for the Practice of Medicine**

1. *Fourth century* B.C.E.–*Early twentieth century* C.E.

2. *Mid-twentieth century–1994*

### Section III. Ethical Directives for Other Health-Care Professions

Occupational Therapy Code of Ethics, American Occupational Therapy Association [1988]

Code of Ethics of the Physician Assistant Profession, American Academy of Physician Assistants [1983, amended 1985, reaffirmed 1990]

Ethical Principles of Psychologists and Code of Conduct, American Psychological Association [1992]

Code of Ethics, National Association of Social Workers [1979, revised 1990]

Code of Ethics, American College of Healthcare Executives [amended 1990]

Ethical Conduct for Health Care Institutions, American Hospital Association [1992]

## Section IV. Ethical Directives for Human Research

German Guidelines on Human Experimentation [1931]

Nuremberg Code [1947]

Principles for Those in Research and Experimentation, World Medical Association [1954]

Article Seven, International Covenant on Civil and Political Rights, General Assembly of the United Nations [1958]

Declaration of Helsinki, World Medical Association [1964, revised 1975, 1983, 1989]

The Belmont Report: Ethical Principles and Guidelines for the Protection of Human Subjects of Research, National Commission for the Protection of Human Subjects of Biomedical and Behavioral Research [1979]

DHHS Regulations for the Protection of Human Subjects (45 CFR 46) [June 18, 1991]

Summary Report of the International Summit Conference on Bioethics [1987]

Recommendation No. R (90) 3 of the Committee of Ministers to Member States Concerning Medical Research on Human Beings, Council of Europe [1990]

International Ethical Guidelines for Biomedical Research Involving Human Subjects, Council for International Organizations of Medical Sciences (CIOMS) in collaboration with the World Health Organization [1993]

## Section V. Ethical Directives Pertaining to the Welfare and Use of Animals

1. *Veterinary Medicine*

Veterinarian's Oath, American Veterinary Medical Association (AVMA) [1954, revised 1969]

Principles of Veterinary Medical Ethics, American Veterinary Medical Association (AVMA) [revised 1993]

2. *Research Involving Animals*

International Guiding Principles for Biomedical Research Involving Animals, Council for International Organizations of Medical Sciences (CIOMS), World Health Organization [1984]

Principles for the Utilization and Care of Vertebrate Animals Used in Testing, Research, and Education, U.S. Interagency Research Animal Committee [1985]

Ethics of Animal Investigation, Canadian Council on Animal Care [revised 1989]

Australian Code of Practice for the Care and Use of Animals for Scientific Purposes, National Health and Medical Research Council, Commonwealth Scientific and Industrial Research Organization, and Australian Agricultural Council [revised 1989]

World Medical Association Statement on Animal Use in Biomedical Research, World Medical Association [1989]

Guidelines for Ethical Conduct in the Care and Use of Animals, American Psychological Association [1985, revised 1992]

Principles and Guidelines for the Use of Animals in Precollege Education, Institute of Laboratory Animal Resources, National Research Council [1989]

### Section VI. Ethical Directives Pertaining to the Environment

World Charter for Nature, General Assembly of the United Nations [1982]

Rio Declaration on Environment and Development, United Nations Conference on Environment and Development [1992]

Conservation Policies of the Wildlife Society, The Wildlife Society [1988]

Code of Ethics for Members of the Society of American Foresters, Society of American Foresters [1976, amended 1986, 1992]

Code of Ethics and Standards of Practice for Environmental Professionals, National Association of Environmental Professionals [1979, revised 1994]

Code of Ethics, National Environmental Health Association [revised 1992]

### Bibliography

### Credits

# Nature and Role of Codes and Other Ethics Directives

The earliest extant documents regulating the practice of medicine are records of Egyptian laws from the sixteenth century B.C.E. and the Babylonian Code of Hammurabi, dated about 2000 B.C.E. These legal documents included guidance on what fees could be charged, what constituted competent medical care, the conditions under which a physician could be held accountable for malpractice, and what sanctions would apply. The first significant statement on medical *morality*, however, is the Hippocratic Oath (fourth century B.C.E.). Although all cultures have their historical equivalents, the Oath is the cornerstone of traditional Western medical ethics.

With the notable exception of religious precepts being brought to bear on the conduct of physicians, most medical ethics documents written prior to World War II were professionally generated, that is, they were developed by physicians for physicians. Given the general deference paid to professionals at the time, it is not surprising that ethics directives pertaining to them were authored by the profession. Since the mid-1900s, however, a complex set of factors has challenged the traditional authority of the medical profession.

The atrocities committed by Nazi physician-researchers, which led to the Nuremberg Code (Germany, 1949), and infamous cases of abuse of research subjects in the United States, such as the Tuskegee syphilis study, began to undermine trust in the profession. The various rights movements of the 1960s and 1970s and the anti–Vietnam War movement emphasized individual liberty and contributed to a general willingness to challenge authoritative traditions. At the same time, the dramatic increase in scientific knowledge and the development and use of medical technology powerfully increased the ability of health-care professionals to affect the course of people's lives and deaths. These factors, among others, contributed to an increased emphasis on respect for the autonomy and self-determination of individuals seeking health care.

With these changes came a proliferation of bioethics documents pertaining to research on human subjects, to health professionals other than physicians, and to health-care institutions. Furthermore, growing concerns over the alleged mistreatment of research animals and claims that the use of animals for any research purpose is immoral, coupled with concerns for the protection of the environment, resulted in bioethics directives that extend well beyond human medical practice. Concurrent with the increased diversity in the focus of bioethics documents, the authorship of such documents has diversified as well. Professional organizations no longer monopolize the formulation of directives governing professional behavior; religious organizations, institutions, and government agencies, for example, also set moral or legal standards for clinicians and researchers.

The resulting array of bioethics documents may be divided into three fundamental types: (1) professionally generated documents that govern behavior within the profession; (2) documents that set standards of behavior for professionals but are generated outside the profession; and (3) documents that specify values and standards of behavior for persons who are not members of a profession.

## Documents generated by and for a profession

Although controversy exists over precisely what constitutes a profession, professions may be distinguished from occupations on several grounds (see, e.g., Barber, 1963; Greenwood, 1982; Kultgen, 1988). Professions involve a specialized body of knowledge and skill that requires lengthy education and training to acquire and provides a service to clients and to society. Once a field has achieved professional status, a trained practitioner is considered a professional regardless of employment status. Another characteristic of professions is their claim to be autonomous and self-regulating; however, with the freedom and power of self-regulation comes a concurrent obligation to establish and enforce standards of ethical behavior. Indeed, some have argued that the existence of a professional ethic is the hallmark of a profession (see, e.g., Barber, 1963; Newton, 1988; Campbell, 1982).

Professionally generated ethics documents may take the form of prayers, oaths, or codes. Prayers, such as that once attributed to the Jewish physician-philosopher Moses Maimonides, express gratitude to a deity and ask for divine assistance in developing one's skills and meeting one's responsibilities. Oaths are vows taken by individuals entering a profession to uphold specified obligations. They were frequently employed in ancient times; more recent examples include the Declaration of Geneva (World Medical Association, 1983) and the Solemn Oath of a Physician of Russia (1993), among others. In contrast to the personal, interactive nature of prayers and oaths, codes, which are often accompanied by more detailed "interpretive statements," are collective summaries of the moral ideals and conduct that are expected of the professional.

**Roles of professional ethics directives.** The importance to an emerging profession of producing its own ethics directives indicates a primary role of such documents. They help to define and legitimate a profession as well as to maintain, promote, and protect its prestige. Simultaneously, the documents function as a promise to society that the profession will maintain specified standards of practice in return for the power and autonomy that society is being asked to grant the profession.

Protection of the unity, integrity, and power of the profession, which appears to be a primary goal of the rules of etiquette governing the relationship between professionals, is a "quasi-moral" role of professional ethics documents. Although maintenance of a profession has a limited moral component in that its existence promotes the well-being of society, it especially serves the interests of those within the profession who stand to lose the monopoly on their practice should society lose faith in them. In contrast, the explicitly moral role of professional ethics documents lies in the articulation of both ideal and minimal standards of character and conduct for the professional. Both the moral and some of the "quasi-moral" guidelines form the content of the profession's promise to society and serve as a guide for determining when sanctions should be brought to bear against a member of the profession.

**The nature of professional codes.**   In professionally generated codes, the same guideline may simultaneously help to fulfill both categories of function.

*"Quasi-moral" guidelines.*   In addition to having an ethic, professions are characterized by the possession and practice of a specialized body of knowledge. Consequently, frequently articulated requirements include: competency to practice; restriction of professional status to those who have undergone specific educational and training programs; keeping one's knowledge current; and working to advance the existing knowledge in one's field through research (see, e.g., American Nurses' Association, 1985; Canadian Nurses Association, 1991; American Dental Association, 1994; American Psychological Association, 1992; and American Chiropractic Association, 1992).

Such requirements serve a dual purpose—to maintain the profession and to serve society's well-being. By maintaining a specialized body of knowledge, the profession ensures a monopoly in providing its services. At the same time, restricting the practice of a profession to those who are qualified and requiring that they keep their skills and knowledge current are essential elements in fulfilling society's mandate to the profession: to provide a specialized service competently and safely.

Rules of professional etiquette, such as prohibitions on criticizing colleagues in the presence of clients, the proper procedures for consultation, and the process for the adjudication of disputes, constitute another characteristic of professional ethics documents. Thomas Percival's *Medical Ethics* (1803), originally commissioned to address conflicts among physicians, surgeons, and apothecaries at Manchester Infirmary, epitomizes this characteristic. Like the competency requirements,

rules governing intraprofessional behavior serve the dual purpose of maintaining the profession and serving the well-being of society. Regarding the former, public criticism of colleagues could, as Percival noted, undermine the credibility of the professional and might ultimately damage the reputation of the profession. Professionally generated documents require that questions one practitioner has about another's competence or conduct be brought to the attention of the appropriate authorities, but none to my knowledge explicitly states that the client be advised of the concern. The presumption seems to be that this arrangement, at least in most cases, will protect the client from incompetent practice at the same time as it safeguards the reputation of the professional.

In addition, rules that foster harmony between members of a profession presumably promote not only the self-interest of the profession(als) but also the well-being of society. Rules of etiquette help to maintain the unity of the profession and promote teamwork, two factors that are widely perceived to optimize the quality of patient care (see, e.g., American Chiropractic Association, 1992).

Similarly, rules governing professionals' association with practitioners outside of the profession serve multiple functions. The American Medical Association, for example, proscribes the association of its physicians with "nonscientific practitioners" but permits its physicians to refer patients to nonphysician practitioners provided the referrals are believed to benefit the patients and the services "will be performed competently and in accordance with accepted scientific standards and legal requirements." In part, such rules protect the standing of a profession by not allowing a competing practice to infringe upon its professional monopoly. But if the competing practice truly is "quackery," the rules may also protect the professional's clients from harm.

Many codes include guidelines on the setting of fees as well as prohibitions of fee-splitting, deceptive advertising, and misrepresenting one's professional qualifications (see, e.g., American Dental Association, 1994; American Psychological Association, 1992). Once again, the dual purpose of protecting the profession and safeguarding its clients is evident. With regard to deceptive practices, the prohibition benefits both the consumer and the profession. Over time, deceptive practices undermine the credibility of the profession, resulting in diminished status and externally imposed sanctions. The setting of fees promotes the interests of professionals by allowing them the discretion to set fees in return for the expertise over which they hold a monopoly. However, professional codes also may admonish the professional to take into account the client's ability to pay when setting the fee in a particular case (see, e.g.,

Canadian Medical Association, 1990a, 1990b; International Chiropractors Association, 1990).

A common component of the "quasi-moral" elements of professional ethics codes is a description of the procedures for reviewing, adjudicating, and, if necessary, sanctioning alleged violations of professional conduct (see, e.g., American Chiropractic Association, 1992; American Psychiatric Association, 1989). There are several reasons for this often lengthy discussion. Allegations of moral impropriety can harm the reputation of the accused as well as the profession. Consequently, every effort must be made to ensure due process and the fair treatment of all parties. In addition, the potentially explosive nature of such allegations and the serious consequences if they are proved true set the stage for vehement denial and rebuttal by the professional accused. It is not unreasonable for the professional organization to protect itself, the process, and any victims, by making the rules clear in advance.

*Moral guidelines.* Professional ethics is best understood as a subset of ethics in general, although this might be disputed by some. The moral dictates of professional ethics documents ought to relate general moral values, duties, and virtues to the unique situations encountered in professional practice. A professional ethic cannot make a practitioner ethical; it can only hope to inform and guide a previously existing moral conscience. Lisa Newton (1988) has distinguished between the internal and external aspects of ethics in professional practice. The internal aspect is ontologically prior to the external; it is the personal conscience that each professional brings to the professional enterprise. The external aspect consists of the publicly specified moral requirements of the profession, that is, those elements of professional morality that are addressed in the profession's ethics documents. Despite the potential conflict between the internal and external aspects, both of them are important.

The external aspect may prompt professionals to reflect critically on their personal moral beliefs and values, a process that helps practitioners refine their internal ethic. The internal ethic then guides professionals when they encounter the myriad situations and conflicts of duty to which ethics documents can only allude. However, since only the external aspect is accessible to public scrutiny, the remainder of this section will explore that aspect in more detail.

The moral guidelines of ethics documents generally involve three elements: (1) values; (2) duties; and (3) virtues.

1. At the center of the professional ethic lies the value that the profession perceives to be the primary good, or its objective. Professional ethics documents often identify this value explicitly and include a pledge to promote it as their means of serving the public interest. Some professional organizations focus on general values, citing the benefit, well-being, or greatest good of their clients as the fundamental value to be pursued (see, e.g., National Federation of Societies for Clinical Social Work, 1987; American Chiropractic Association, 1992). Although including values in ethics documents helps provide a touchstone for guiding conduct when duties that are specified conflict, a problem can arise when it is the profession that articulates the value central to the client–provider relationship. An individual's well-being generally involves all aspects of his or her life, and practitioners, who might be qualified to assess and advance more specific goods, such as health, can claim no particular expertise in judging what constitutes a client's total well-being (Veatch, 1991).

Even the professional organizations that cite the health of clients as the central value encounter difficulties (see, e.g., International Council of Nurses, 1973; American Pharmaceutical Association, 1981; World Medical Association, 1983). In this case, the problem arises because a client's real goal is usually total well-being. Even if the practitioner can claim expertise in "health," it is still only one factor in the client's overall welfare. The Canadian Nurses Association (1991) takes particular care to avoid this difficulty by admonishing nurses to respect the "individual needs and values" of their clients; this injunction appears to recognize the client as the expert in judging what is in his or her own best interests.

2. The moral duties articulated in professional ethics documents may be broad (such as respecting the dignity and self-determination of one's clients) or specific (such as maintaining client confidentiality or not engaging in sexual relations with a client). The more general duties permit a certain amount of interpretation in their implementation by the individual practitioner, whereas the more specific ones establish particular minimum standards for professional behavior.

There are, of course, gray areas, such as the duty of confidentiality. The duty to keep professional confidences secret is found in almost every professional ethic since the Hippocratic Oath. Yet exceptions to the general rule can be found. Until 1980, for example, the American Medical Association's "Principles of Medical Ethics" included an exception clause that permitted the disclosure of confidential information not only when required by law but also when "necessary in order to protect the welfare of the individual or of the community." Although most professional ethics documents allow for at least limited disclosure to ensure the safety of third parties, disclosure without consent for the benefit of the patient is suspect and subsequently has been dropped from the AMA "Principles of Medical Ethics." Also, although it is generally acceptable to disclose patient information when consulting with colleagues, there are rules governing such disclosure.

The presence of guidelines on safeguarding and disposing of written and computerized patient records emphasizes how seriously the duty to keep confidences is viewed by professions (see, e.g., British Medical Association, 1988; International Chiropractors Association, 1990). Although some discretion is permitted, the rules governing confidentiality still have the force of minimum requisite standards rather than ideals.

Some professional documents are organized around the distinction between ideal and minimalist standards (see, e.g., American Psychological Association, 1992, American College of Radiology, 1991). They begin with a set of general guidelines that are admittedly broad and explicitly not subject to sanction by the professional organization. These ideals are followed by the minimal rules of professional conduct, violations of which may be punishable by the organization.

3. Traditionally, philosophers have argued that moral behavior is governed primarily in one of two ways. Moral obligations, ideal or minimalist, may be specified, as in the documents just discussed. Alternatively, moral guidelines may focus on the character of the individual, with the assumption that moral behavior will flow naturally from a moral person.

Although the Prayer of Moses Maimonides is concerned primarily with specifying the virtues of a moral physician (Purtilo, 1977), many other professional ethics documents incorporate both basic standards of conduct and specific character traits, such as honesty, compassion, and integrity.

Even though a good or virtuous character may help a professional respond morally to a complex dilemma (in which, for example, specific duties conflict), the possession of a good character does not ensure morally right conduct. The moral character of an individual does, however, affect the way others perceive him or her. One is apt to have more regard for persons who act morally from good motives than for those who act morally simply because the rules require them to do so. Arguably a professional of good character is more trustworthy than one of poor character, and trust is an extremely important element in the relationship between client and professional.

**Difficulties with professional codes.** Professionally generated ethics documents are subject to a number of criticisms.

*Monopoly and self-regulation.* The most serious problems stem from the profession's power as an autonomous and self-regulating entity. The profession's monopoly on both setting and enforcing rules of conduct raises charges of elitism and opens the door to abuse of power. The presumption is that only professionals can know what constitutes ethical conduct for professionals and thus that they are the only ones who can evaluate the technical and moral quality of the services rendered.

It is true that professionals have been trained in a specialized body of knowledge that is not generally available to the layperson. That knowledge and professional judgment is part of the reason that society grants power and respect to a profession. However, professionals are neither uniquely nor the best equipped to make moral decisions (Veatch, 1973). Even if professionals were able to determine a client's best interest, they would have no special expertise in determining whether, for example, the client's interest, the client's rights, or the interests of society should take moral precedence in a given case.

*Competing ethics.* Historically, prayers, oaths, and certain codes have incorporated appeals to deities and/or the precepts of a broader religious or philosophical ethic into the professional mandate. Ludwig Edelstein (1943), for example, has argued that the Hippocratic Oath involves an application of Pythagorean principles to medicine. Some modern professional documents, such as the *Health Care Ethics Guide* of the Catholic Health Association of Canada (1991) and the *Islamic Code of Medical Ethics* (Islamic Organization of Medical Sciences, 1981), also explicitly place professional practice in the context of a larger ethic.

The generation of a professional ethic by modern secular professional organizations makes those organizations the functional equivalent of a religious or philosophical system and places them in direct competition with those systems, at least in their claim to know what is morally right in professional practice. In short, what the profession determines to be ethical is so, regardless of whether clients or other individuals in society agree. Of course, as illustrated by the variations between the codes authored by, for example, the medical associations of different countries (see Appendix, Section II), even secular professional ethics are influenced by the underlying values of the societies in which they are written. Furthermore, professional ethics are evolutionary and specific changes can be brought to bear from outside the profession. The significant moderation, if not obliteration, of traditional medical paternalism by societal demands for information and "informed consent" in decision making is one example of this point.

*Self-policing.* The self-policing of professionals raises a similar problem. If the profession does not find a practitioner to be at fault in an alleged ethics violation, there is no recourse to a general moral standard. Despite the requirement of many codes that unethical behavior by a colleague be reported, professionals may have a vested interest in not reporting or condemning violations by colleagues for fear of reprisal. They also may be deterred by the recognition that "everyone makes mistakes" and that they might be in a similar position in the future. An example of the closing of professional ranks appears in the American Academy of Orthopaedic Surgeons' *Guide to the Ethical Practice of Orthopaedic Surgery* (A.A.O.S., 1992, pp. 4–5, 9). Allegations raised by a professional against a colleague are investigated confidentially, and allegations brought by a patient, which admittedly are explicitly outside the auspices of the academy, are forwarded directly to the practitioner with a letter "urging him or her to contact the patient about the concern."

Although abuses of power can and do occur, mechanisms exist to limit them. International professional organizations, such as the World Medical Association, have arisen in part in an effort to forestall idiosyncratic, immoral practices of the sort that occurred in Nazi medicine. In addition, requiring that professionals report suspected violations, as well as maintaining, to the extent possible, the confidentiality of individuals who report them, and protecting such individuals from reprisal, helps to ensure that professionals will not be absolved of their responsibilities.

*Business interests.*    Another criticism of professional codes is their excessive concern with nonmoral "business" interests, such as etiquette, fees, advertising, and the like, and the use of such measures to enhance professional prestige and prosperity. However, although such concerns are not specifically moral, they do have a moral component and their presence in an ethics document can thereby be justified. Furthermore, although the potential for abuse exists, the same type of safeguards outlined above apply here as well.

*Generality.*    The remaining concerns with professional ethics documents are directed at the vagueness, conflicts, and idealism found in them. Many of the guidelines found in professional codes are intentionally vague. No document can or should pretend to foresee all eventualities and eliminate the need for individual discretion. In addition, ethics statements are "consensus documents." They reflect the general values and obligations held by most of the profession's members. The more specific such statements become, the more likely it is that there will be disagreement and loss of support for the moral authority of the document. For this reason, professional organizations address the more controversial topics in bioethics in separate documents that do not require ratification by the entire membership (Gass, 1978).

Similarly, resolutions to all conflicts of duty cannot be specified. The professional must rely on the values underlying the ethic, as well as his or her own conscience as informed by virtue, to determine the correct action when multiple duties conflict. Ethics codes may idealize the profession by suggesting that all professionals consistently possess all the virtues, uphold all the ideals, and reason through conflicts flawlessly. Holding professionals to such standards is, of course, unreasonable and may even be detrimental by undermining the motivation of those professionals who cannot, but feel they must, satisfy such expectations. Nevertheless, ideals serve as guides, as something to aspire to; if one aims high, one may land close to the goal.

As long as the difficulties with professionally generated ethics documents are recognized and accounted for both within and outside the profession, it seems that the documents do provide a standard by which questionable professional behavior can be judged. In addition, they are useful tools for generating professional awareness of the need for ethical discourse, which in turn helps to inform the internal ethic of individual practitioners.

## Documents directed toward a profession, but generated outside it

This category encompasses all bioethics documents that have direct implications for professional behavior, yet are authored by an "extraprofessional" group. The term "extraprofessional" refers to individuals who, in a specified setting, are not engaged in professional practice. Most commonly such documents are authored by an entity representing the public at large, such as a state licensing agency or other government body; a group within a field such as health care but outside of the profession(s) addressed; or a group representing a religious or philosophical ethic.

**The nature and roles of "extraprofessional" ethics directives.**    Typically, documents generated outside of a profession serve two main functions, either independently or concurrently. The first purpose is to regulate professional practice, thereby helping to limit the professional authority discussed in the previous section and addressing some of its potential abuses. Laws, regulations, and judicial decisions governing informed consent, advance directives, and research practices are examples of outside controls placed on professional practice.

Directives from outside professional organizations, such as the American Hospital Association's Patient's Bill of Rights (1973, 1992) serve a similar purpose. Rights documents are complex because they pertain not only to the individuals whose rights are being enumerated but also to the persons who are obliged to respect those rights. The American Hospital Association is, in effect, issuing guidelines governing ethical behavior for all individuals working at the facility, although in several instances the duties of physicians are singled out.

Extraprofessional documents that seek to regulate professional behavior tend to be minimalistic. Whereas professionally generated statements frequently articulate the ideals of character and behavior to which professionals should aspire, externally imposed standards are often generated in response to professional indiscretion and are designed to specify the limits to the range of acceptable professional conduct.

The second principal function of extraprofessional ethics statements is to focus attention on a broader ethic of which professional ethics is perceived by the authoring group to be a subset. Such documents derive norms for ethical practice from the values underlying a whole ethic or world view, rather than from the values underlying a specific profession. Whereas secular associations of health care professionals generally derive their ethical principles from the values of the profession, such as the health and well-being of clients, bioethics directives generated by religious bodies derive standards of practice from the values of the religion.

For example, the *Ethical and Religious Directives for Catholic Health Facilities* (United States Catholic Conference, 1975) outlines the practices that may and may not take place in Catholic facilities. Although many of the directives correspond directly to precepts already adhered to by health-care practitioners, other directives, such as those concerning abortion and sterilization, reflect distinctly Catholic values and teaching. Although the directives are addressed to institutions, their force applies to the institutions' employees, including the professionals.

Other examples of religious or philosophical ethics being brought to bear on professional practice include the application of Jewish law to medical practice, for instance, to ascertain the moral licitness of neurological criteria for determining death, and the admonition of the old Oath of Soviet Physicians (1971) to follow the principles of communist morality in all of one's actions.

Documents that explicitly locate professional ethics within a religious or philosophical ethic tend to be idealistic in the same way that many professionally generated documents are. The goal is to provide a moral framework for professional practice. In contrast to the policing function of other extraprofessional documents, these documents attempt to define an ideal standard at which to aim.

Although some of the obligations articulated in extraprofessional documents—for example, those emphasizing duties to clients or to society—parallel those articulated in professionally generated statements, others specify the duties of professionals to an organization, institution, government, or other authority. In such cases, conflicts between the values and duties perceived by a profession and those articulated by the extraprofessional group are likely to arise.

Researchers, for example, might perceive their professional mandate to be the expansion of scientific knowledge, either generally or with the goal of aiding a specific population, such as persons with Alzheimer's disease, that might potentially benefit from the information acquired. They might further believe that the best means of advancing those goals is to violate an externally imposed ban on human fetal tissue transplantation research. Or nurses might believe that their professional mandate to care for the well-being of their client requires the violation of an institutional policy. In such cases, professionals face potential legal, monetary, or moral sanctions, on the one hand, or the loss of personal and/or professional integrity, on the other.

Such conflicts illustrate the more global problem of reconciling competing values in a pluralistic society (cf. Veatch and Mason, 1987). Professionals who simultaneously subscribe to a general religious or philosophical ethic—such as Catholicism, Islam, or libertarianism—and are members of a professional organization, or employees of an institution, that does not explicitly reflect that ethic are apt to find themselves in an untenable situation if personal values and professional duties conflict.

Some professionally generated documents attempt to address such conflicts by proscribing practices forbidden by law and by allowing, within certain confines, practitioners to withdraw from practices they find morally objectionable. The American Nurses' Association (1985) cautions its members that "neither physicians' orders nor the employing agency's policies relieve the nurse of accountability for actions taken and judgments made," implying that the precepts of the profession may outweigh the requirements of an institutional obligation. The Canadian Nurses Association (1991) advises that "prospective employers be informed of the provisions of [its] Code so that realistic and ethical expectations may be established at the beginning of the nurse–employer relationship."

Although such provisions may be of some assistance, their value may be limited by other provisions of the code. For example, a professional's right to withdraw from practices he or she deems morally offensive is conditional upon ensuring that the client is not abandoned, that is, the fundamental professional duty to care for the client ultimately takes precedence over one's personal ethic. Furthermore, even if a professional's personal morality were compatible with those of the professional association and the employing institution, the professional may still encounter conflict when a client with different values and beliefs requests a service deemed morally offensive by the professional.

## Documents directed toward "nonprofessionals"

The term "nonprofessional" here refers to two groups: (1) clients, for instance, patients or research subjects, and (2) persons engaged in nonprofessional work, such as orderlies, hospital volunteers, or laboratory assistants. Since these groups do not have a self-imposed ethic other than a broad, societal one, bioethics directives pertaining to them usually are generated outside of the group by the same sources that apply to professionals. The implications, however, are rather different.

**Directives pertaining to clients.** Rights statements are directed at two distinct groups, those who hold rights and those who must respect them. Most of the rights documents in bioethics are not generated by individuals specifically representing the holders of the rights. For example, although groups advocating for health-care consumers helped to precipitate its establishment, the American Hospital Association's Patient's Bill of Rights (1973, 1992) was written by individuals representing member hospitals. Although the intention of protecting the interests of patients is admirable, it is not clear that the authoring group has any special expertise in determining what the rights of hospital patients actually are or should be. Similarly, the American Medical Association's Fundamental Elements of the Physician–Patient Relationship is a professionally generated document that outlines patients' rights to information, confidentiality, continuity of care, and so forth. Again, in one sense, this document sets forth the obligation of physicians to advance these rights (as such it is subject to the discussion in the first section), but in another sense, it claims authority for knowing what rights patients have, a task for which physicians are not necessarily the best suited.

In addition, rights documents, which presumably are intended to protect the rights-bearer, increasingly are accompanied by statements of the responsibilities of the rights-bearer. The American Medical Association, for example, includes among the responsibilities of patients the provision of accurate and complete information and compliance with the treatment plan and instructions of those responsible for the patient's care. It is not clear in any of the documents that issue joint statements of rights and responsibilities whether respect for the rights identified is contingent upon fulfillment of the specified responsibilities. Also not clear is why the authoring body has the moral authority to specify the responsibilities of those not members of the group.

Other bioethics documents affecting patients or research subjects are regulatory and/or governmental. Judicial and legislative actions as well as regulatory agencies and advisory bodies that represent the general populace are the closest the recipients of professional services come to a self-generated ethic. Even here, however, controversy arises over the extent to which patients and research subjects should be protected from others (and themselves). In the United States, the debates over access to experimental drugs by seriously ill patients and silicone implants by women seeking breast augmentation exemplify the dilemma.

Religious and broad philosophical ethics also affect individuals in this category. Usually individuals have elected to follow the precepts of a particular ethic in their overall existence and bring that ethic into whatever situation they encounter. As noted earlier, difficulties arise when one encounters a competing ethic. A traditional example is the difficulty faced by a Jehovah's Witness who refuses a potentially life-saving blood transfusion. On a larger scale, the imposition of one culture's beliefs upon another—for example, through regulations attached to financial assistance—poses the same problem.

**Directives pertaining to nonprofessional workers.** The final documents to be discussed are those that articulate standards for nonprofessional workers. Rights documents and other statements directed at institutions set minimal standards for all personnel, insofar as they apply, not just for professionals. Ethics directives that pertain to nonprofessionals tend to be minimalistic. They set guidelines protecting basic concerns such as respect, privacy, and competence, but unlike their professional counterparts, the job descriptions of nonprofessionals do not include a unique ethical mandate.

Nonprofessionals, like their professional counterparts, may be subject to certain duties to the institution or organization employing them. Similarly, nonprofessional workers are subject to moral standards articulated by legal and governmental bodies, as well as those stemming from religious or philosophical worldviews. The problem of conflicting duties arising from multiple moral authorities affects nonprofessionals, but not to the same degree as it plagues professionals. The conflicts faced by the nonprofessional are more analogous to those faced by any human being when the demands of law or one's employer conflict with a broader ethic that is perceived to be more fundamental. This is not to imply that these conflicts are any less difficult to resolve, only that their nature is different.

## Conclusion

The number and diversity of bioethics documents reflect the pluralism of our world. When the ideologies expressed in these documents clash, controversy and conflicts may arise. In such cases, it is to be hoped that the documents will provide a basis for dialogue between the disagreeing parties. Ethical dialogue can promote understanding and a resolution to the conflict, as well as an ongoing assessment of the precepts in question relative to their underlying ideologies.

CAROL MASON SPICER

## Bibliography

AMERICAN ACADEMY OF ORTHOPAEDIC SURGEONS. 1992. *Guide to the Ethical Practice of Orthopaedic Surgery.* 2d ed. Park Ridge, Ill.: Author.

AMERICAN CHIROPRACTIC ASSOCIATION. 1992. "Code of Ethics 1992–1993." In *1992–93 Membership Directory*, pp. B1–B11. Arlington, Va.: Author.

AMERICAN COLLEGE OF RADIOLOGY. 1991. *ACR 1991 Bylaws*. Reston, Va.: Author.

AMERICAN DENTAL ASSOCIATION. 1994. *ADA Principles of Ethics and Code of Professional Conduct*. Chicago: Author.

AMERICAN HOSPITAL ASSOCIATION. 1973, revised 1992. *A Patient's Bill of Rights*. Chicago: Author.

———. 1992. *A Patient's Bill of Rights Handbook*. Chicago: Author.

AMERICAN NURSES' ASSOCIATION. 1985. *Code for Nurses with Interpretive Statements*. Kansas City, Mo.: Author.

AMERICAN PHARMACEUTICAL ASSOCIATION. 1981. *Code of Ethics*. Washington, D.C.: Author.

AMERICAN PSYCHIATRIC ASSOCIATION. 1989. *The Principles of Medical Ethics with Annotations Especially Applicable to Psychiatry*. Washington, D.C.: Author.

AMERICAN PSYCHOLOGICAL ASSOCIATION. 1992. "Ethical Principles of Psychologists and Code of Conduct." *American Psychologist* 47, no. 12:1597–1611.

BARBER, BERNARD. 1963. "Some Problems in the Sociology of the Professions." *Daedalus* 92, no. 4:669–688.

BRITISH MEDICAL ASSOCIATION. 1988. *Philosophy and Practice of Medical Ethics*. London: Author.

CAMPBELL, DENNIS M. 1982. *Doctors, Lawyers, Ministers: Christian Ethics in Professional Practice*. Nashville, Tenn.: Abingdon Press.

CANADIAN MEDICAL ASSOCIATION. 1990a. *Code of Ethics*. Ottawa: Author.

——— 1990b. *Guide to the Ethical Behaviour of Physicians*. Ottawa: Author.

CANADIAN NURSES ASSOCIATION. 1991. *Code of Ethics for Nursing*. Ottawa: Author.

CATHOLIC HEALTH ASSOCIATION OF CANADA. 1991. *Health Care Ethics Guide*. Ottawa: Author.

EDELSTEIN, LUDWIG. 1943. "The Hippocratic Oath: Text, Translation, and Interpretation." *Bulletin of the History of Medicine*. Suppl. no. 1:1–64.

FREEDMAN, BENJAMIN. 1989. "Bringing Codes to Newcastle: Ethics for Clinical Ethicists." In *Clinical Ethics: Theory and Practice*, pp. 125–139. Edited by Barry Hoffmaster, Benjamin Freedman, and Gwen Fraser. Clifton, N.J.: Humana.

GASS, RONALD S. 1978. "Codes of the Health-Care Professions." In *Encyclopedia of Bioethics*, vol. 4, pp. 1725–1730. Edited by Warren T. Reich. New York: Macmillan and Free Press.

GERMANY (TERRITORY UNDER ALLIED OCCUPATION, 1945–1955: U.S. ZONE). MILITARY TRIBUNALS. 1949. "Permissible Medical Experiments." In vol. 2 of *Trials of War Criminals Before the Nuremberg Military Tribunals Under Control Council Law No. 10, Nuremberg, October 1946–April 1949*, pp. 181–183. Washington D.C.: U.S. Government Printing Office.

GREENWOOD, ERNEST. 1982. "Attributes of a Profession." In *Moral Responsibility and the Professions*, pp. 20–33. Edited by Benjamin Freedman and Bernard H. Baumrin. New York: Haven.

INTERNATIONAL CHIROPRACTORS ASSOCIATION. 1990. "ICA Code of Professional Ethics [1987]." In *ICA Policy Handbook and Code of Ethics*. 2d. ed., pp. 153–169. Arlington, Va.: Author.

INTERNATIONAL COUNCIL OF NURSES. 1973. *Code for Nurses: Ethical Concepts Applied to Nursing*. Geneva: Author.

INTERNATIONAL ORGANIZATION OF ISLAMIC MEDICINE. 1981. *Islamic Code of Medical Ethics: Kuwait Document*. Kuwait: Author.

JOINT COMMISSION ON ACCREDITATION OF HEALTHCARE ORGANIZATIONS. 1989. "Rights and Responsibilities of Patients." In *Accreditation Manual for Hospitals, 1990*, pp. xiii–xvii. Chicago: Author.

KULTGEN, JOHN H. 1988. *Ethics and Professionalism*. Philadelphia: University of Pennsylvania Press.

MAHOWALD, MARY A. 1984. "Are Codes of Professional Ethics Ethical?" *Health Matrix* 8, no. 2:37–42.

NATIONAL FEDERATION OF SOCIETIES FOR CLINICAL SOCIAL WORK. COMMITTEE ON PROFESSIONAL STANDARDS. 1987. "National Federation of Societies for Clinical Social Work—Code of Ethics." *Clinical Social Work Journal* 15, no. 1:81–91.

NEWTON, LISA H. 1988. "Lawgiving for Professional Life: Reflections of the Place of the Professional Code." In *Professional Ideals*, pp. 47–55. Edited by Albert Flores. Belmont, Calif.: Wadsworth.

"Oath of Soviet Physicians." 1971. *Journal of the American Medical Association* 217, no. 6:834.

PERCIVAL, THOMAS. 1927. [1803]. *Percival's Medical Ethics, 1803*. Reprint. Edited by Chauncey D. Leake. Baltimore, Md.: Williams and Wilkins.

PETERSON, SUSAN R. 1987. "Professional Codes and Ethical Decision Making." In *Health Care Ethics: A Guide for Decision Makers*, pp. 321–329. Edited by Gary R. Anderson and Valerie A. Glesnes-Anderson. Rockville, Md.: Aspen Publishers.

PURTILO, RUTH B. 1977. "The American Physical Therapy Association's Code of Ethics." *Physical Therapy* 57, no. 9:1001–1006.

"Solemn Oath of the Physician of Russia [1992]." 1993. *Kennedy Institute of Ethics Journal* 3, no. 4:419.

UNITED STATES CATHOLIC CONFERENCE. 1975. *Ethical and Religious Directives for Catholic Health Facilities*. Washington, D.C.: Author.

VEATCH, ROBERT M. 1973. "Generalization of Expertise: Scientific Expertise and Value Judgments." *Hastings Center Studies* 1, no. 2:29–40.

———. 1991. "Is Trust of Professionals a Coherent Concept?" In *Ethics, Trust, and the Professions*, pp. 159–173. Edited by Edmund D. Pellegrino, Robert M. Veatch, and John P. Langan. Washington, D.C.: Georgetown University Press.

VEATCH, ROBERT M., and MASON, CAROL G. 1987. "Hippocratic vs. Judeo-Christian Medical Ethics: Principles in Conflict." *Journal of Religious Ethics* 15, no. 1:86–105.

WORLD MEDICAL ASSOCIATION. 1983. "Declaration of Geneva." Ferney-Voltaire, France: Author.

# INTRODUCTION
## TO THE
## CODES, OATHS, AND DIRECTIVES

The bioethics documents included in this Appendix are divided into six sections as listed in the table of contents. The first section contains documents that outline the health-related rights of individuals or address topics that are designed to implement such rights. The remaining sections contain directives that address the responsibilities of professionals, many of which can be understood as correlates of the rights of the individuals under their care or supervision. The Appendix concludes with a bibliography that references more than 150 additional bioethics directives and several anthologies of documents.

The number of directives related to bioethics has increased exponentially since the publication of the first edition of the *Encyclopedia of Bioethics* in 1978. The process of revising the Appendix began with a search of the BIOETHICS-LINE database, accessed through the National Library of Medicine's MEDLARS system, and a review of several hundred pertinent documents in the collection of the National Reference Center for Bioethics Literature at Georgetown University. The staff of the National Reference Center played an essential role in this search and document-retrieval process. In addition, we reviewed approximately 3,000 listings in the *Encyclopedia of Associations*, the *Encyclopedia of Medical Organizations and Agencies*, and the *Yearbook of International Organizations* and selected approximately 120 organizations, primarily on the basis of the size of their membership and the duration of their existence, to whom we sent letters soliciting "codes of ethics and other ethics statements/guidelines" that they had issued. We also contacted experts from all parts of the world for assistance in compiling and screening documents for inclusion, and in several instances we engaged translators to prepare English transcripts of documents. The Appendix Advisory Group provided indispensable assistance both in selecting the 84 documents that appear in the Appendix from the approximately 125 that remained following the first cut and in excerpting documents that could not be included *in toto*.

Credits for the documents that appear in the Appendix can be found at the end of the Appendix, following the bibliography.

# SECTION I

## Directives on Health-Related Rights and Patient Responsibilities

Constitution of the World Health Organization [1948]

Universal Declaration of Human Rights, General Assembly of the United Nations [1948]

Declaration of the Rights of the Child, General Assembly of the United Nations [1959]

Declaration on the Rights of Mentally Retarded Persons, General Assembly of the United Nations [1971]

A Patient's Bill of Rights, American Hospital Association [1973, revised 1992]

Declaration of Lisbon on the Rights of the Patient, World Medical Association [1981]

Declaration on Physician Independence and Professional Freedom, World Medical Association [1986]

Fundamental Elements of the Patient–Physician Relationship, American Medical Association [1990, updated 1993]

Patient Responsibilities, American Medical Association [1993]

Patient Rights, Joint Commission on Accreditation of Healthcare Organizations [1994]

*The use of rights language has emerged in recent decades as a strong feature of contemporary bioethics documents. Although the language of rights cannot embrace all that must be said in bioethics, this collection of directives on health-related rights and patient responsibilities heads the Appendix both because it reinforces the common doctrine that all health care is patient-centered and because rights language has become typical of the period on which this edition is reporting.*

*Most of the documents in this section outline the health-related rights of specific groups of individuals, such as children, mentally retarded persons, and patients. Two documents, however, address topics that are designed to implement these rights. The World Medical Association's Declaration on Physician Independence and Professional Freedom addresses the importance of physicians' professional freedom to support patient rights. The American Medical Association (AMA) perceives patient rights and the corresponding patient responsibilities to be two elements of a mutually respectful alliance between patients and physicians. The AMA's directive on patient responsibilities elaborates upon the view expressed in the AMA's patient rights document, Fundamental Elements of the Patient–Physician Relationship, that "patients share with physicians the responsibility for their own health care."*

# CONSTITUTION OF THE WORLD HEALTH ORGANIZATION
## 1948

*Originally adopted by the International Health Conference held in New York in June–July 1946 and signed by the representatives of sixty-one nations, the following statement is found in the Preamble to the Constitution of the World Health Organization, established in 1948. Especially significant elements are the controversial definition of health as "a state of complete physical, mental and social well-being and not merely the absence of disease or infirmity" and the recognition of health as a fundamental human right.*

The States Parties to this Constitution declare, in conformity with the Charter of the United Nations, that the following principles are basic to the happiness, harmonious relations and security of all peoples:

Health is a state of complete physical, mental and social well-being and not merely the absence of disease or infirmity.

The enjoyment of the highest attainable standard of health is one of the fundamental rights of every human being without distinction of race, religion, political belief, economic or social condition.

The health of all peoples is fundamental to the attainment of peace and security and is dependent upon the fullest co-operation of individuals and States.

The achievement of any State in the promotion and protection of health is of value to all. Unequal development in different countries in the promotion of health and control of disease, especially communicable disease, is a common danger.

Healthy development of the child is of basic importance; the ability to live harmoniously in a changing total environment is essential to such development.

The extension to all peoples of the benefits of medical, psychological and related knowledge is essential to the fullest attainment of health.

Informed opinion and active co-operation on the part of the public are of the utmost importance in the improvement of the health of the people.

Governments have a responsibility for the health of their peoples which can be fulfilled only by the provision of adequate health and social measures.

Accepting these principles, and for the purpose of co-operation among themselves and with others to promote and protect the health of all peoples, the Contracting parties agree to the present Constitution and hereby establish the World Health Organization as a specialized agency within the terms of Article 57 of the Charter of the United Nations.

# UNIVERSAL DECLARATION OF HUMAN RIGHTS
## General Assembly of the United Nations
## 1948

*Adopted in 1948 by the General Assembly of the United Nations, the Universal Declaration of Human Rights is, as stated in its preamble, "a common standard of achievement for all peoples in all nations, to the end that every individual and every organ of society . . . shall strive by teaching and education to promote respect for these rights and freedoms and by progressive mea-*

*sures, national and international, to secure their universal and effective recognition and obser-
vance. . . ."*

*Article five should be compared to article seven of the International Covenant on Civil and
Political Rights (Section IV). Article 25 directly pertains to health and health care.*

### Article 1

All human beings are born free and equal in dignity and rights. They are endowed
with reason and conscience and should act towards one another in a spirit of brotherhood.

• • •

### Article 3

Everyone has the right to life, liberty and the security of person.

• • •

### Article 5

No one shall be subjected to torture or to cruel, inhuman or degrading treatment or
punishment.

• • •

### Article 16

1. Men and women of full age, without any limitation due to race, nationality or
religion, have the right to marry and to found a family. They are entitled to equal rights
as to marriage, during marriage and at its dissolution.

2. Marriage shall be entered into only with the free and full consent of the intending
spouses.

3. The family is the natural and fundamental group unit of society and is entitled to
protection by society and the State.

• • •

### Article 25

1. Everyone has the right to a standard of living adequate for the health and well-
being of himself and of his family, including food, clothing, housing and medical care
and necessary social services, and the right to security in the event of unemployment,
sickness, disability, widowhood, old age or other lack of livelihood in circumstances
beyond his control.

2. Motherhood and childhood are entitled to special care and assistance. All children,
whether born in or out of wedlock, shall enjoy the same social protection.

# DECLARATION OF THE RIGHTS OF THE CHILD
## General Assembly of the United Nations
1959

*Adopted unanimously by the General Assembly of the United Nations on November 20, 1959,
the Declaration of the Rights of the Child emphasizes the physical, mental, and moral health and
development of children.*

• • •

"*Whereas* the child by reason of his physical and mental immaturity, needs special
safeguards and care, including appropriate legal protection, before as well as after birth,

• • •

"*The General Assembly*
"*Proclaims* this Declaration of the Rights of the Child to the end that he may have a
happy childhood and enjoy for his own good and for the good of society the rights and
freedoms herein set forth, and calls upon parents, upon men and women as individuals,
and upon voluntary organizations, local authorities and national Governments to recognize these rights and strive for their observance by legislative and other measures progressively taken in accordance with the following principles:

#### PRINCIPLE 1

"The child shall enjoy all the rights set forth in this Declaration. Every child, without
any exception whatsoever, shall be entitled to these rights, without distinction or discrimination on account of race, colour, sex, language, religion, political or other opin-

ion, national or social origin, property, birth or other status, whether of himself or of his family.

### PRINCIPLE 2

"The child shall enjoy special protection, and shall be given opportunities and facilities, by law and by other means, to enable him to develop physically, mentally, morally, spiritually and socially in a healthy and normal manner and in conditions of freedom and dignity. In the enactment of laws for this purpose, the best interests of the child shall be the paramount considerations.

### PRINCIPLE 3

"The child shall be entitled from his birth to a name and a nationality.

### PRINCIPLE 4

"The child shall enjoy the benefits of social security. He shall be entitled to grow and develop in health; to this end, special care and protection shall be provided both to him and to his mother, including adequate pre-natal and post-natal care. The child shall have the right to adequate nutrition, housing, recreation and medical services.

### PRINCIPLE 5

"The child who is physically, mentally or socially handicapped shall be given the special treatment, education and care required by his particular condition.

### PRINCIPLE 6

"The child, for the full and harmonious development of his personality, needs love and understanding. He shall, wherever possible, grow up in the care and under the responsibility of his parents, and, in any case, in an atmosphere of affection and of moral and material security; a child of tender years shall not, save in exceptional circumstances, be separated from his mother. Society and the public authorities shall have the duty to extend particular care to children without a family and to those without adequate means of support. Payment of State and other assistance towards the maintenance of children of large families is desirable.

### PRINCIPLE 7

"The child is entitled to receive education, which shall be free and compulsory, at least in the elementary stages. He shall be given an education which will promote his general culture, and enable him, on a basis of equal opportunity, to develop his abilities, his individual judgement, and his sense of moral and social responsibility, and to become a useful member of society.

"The best interests of the child shall be the guiding principle of those responsible for his education and guidance; that responsibility lies in the first place with his parents.

"The child shall have full opportunity for play and recreation, which should be directed to the same purposes as education; society and the public authorities shall endeavour to promote the enjoyment of this right.

### PRINCIPLE 8

"The child shall in all circumstances be among the first to receive protection and relief.

### PRINCIPLE 9

"The child shall be protected against all forms of neglect, cruelty and exploitation. He shall not be the subject of traffic, in any form.

"The child shall not be admitted to employment before an appropriate minimum age; he shall in no case be caused or permitted to engage in any occupation or employment which would prejudice his health or education, or interfere with his physical, mental or moral development.

### PRINCIPLE 10

"The child shall be protected from practices which may foster racial, religious and any other form of discrimination. He shall be brought up in a spirit of understanding, tolerance, friendship among peoples, peace and universal brotherhood, and in full consciousness that his energy and talents should be devoted to the service of his fellow men."

# DECLARATION ON THE RIGHTS OF MENTALLY RETARDED PERSONS
## General Assembly of the United Nations
### 1971

*The following Declaration on the Rights of Mentally Retarded Persons was adopted by the General Assembly of the United Nations on December 20, 1971. It is a revised and amended version of the Declaration of General and Special Rights of the Mentally Retarded that was adopted in 1968 by the International League of Societies for the Mentally Handicapped.*

• • •

1. The mentally retarded person has, to the maximum degree of feasibility, the same rights as other human beings.

2. The mentally retarded person has a right to proper medical care and physical therapy and to such education, training, rehabilitation and guidance as will enable him to develop his ability and maximum potential.

3. The mentally retarded person has a right to economic security and to a decent standard of living. He has a right to perform productive work or to engage in any other meaningful occupation to the fullest possible extent of his capabilities.

4. Whenever possible, the mentally retarded person should live with his own family or with foster parents and participate in different forms of community life. The family with which he lives should receive assistance. If care in an institution becomes necessary, it should be provided in surroundings and other circumstances as close as possible to those of normal life.

5. The mentally retarded person has a right to a qualified guardian when this is required to protect his personal well-being and interests.

6. The mentally retarded person has a right to protection from exploitation, abuse and degrading treatment. If prosecuted for any offence, he shall have a right to due process of law with full recognition being given to his degree of mental responsibility.

7. Whenever mentally retarded persons are unable, because of the severity of their handicap, to exercise all their rights in a meaningful way or it should become necessary to restrict or deny some or all of these rights, the procedure used for that restriction or denial of rights must contain proper legal safeguards against every form of abuse. This procedure must be based on an evaluation of the social capability of the mentally retarded person by qualified experts and must be subject to periodic review and to the right of appeal to higher authorities.

# A PATIENT'S BILL OF RIGHTS
## American Hospital Association
### 1973, revised 1992

*In 1973, the American Hospital Association's House of Delegates adopted A Patient's Bill of Rights, which was influential in the development of similar documents in other parts of the world. The first revision of the document, and the only one to date, was approved in 1992. Some of the most notable changes from the 1973 document include: (1) deletion of the "therapeutic privilege" clause that permitted information regarding a patient's condition to be disclosed to family, rather than to the patient, when it was "not medically advisable to give such information to the patient"; (2) addition of the right to execute advance directives; (3) addition of a clause indicating that otherwise confidential information may be released when permitted or required by law for the benefit of third parties; (4) addition of the patients' right to review their medical records; (5) addition of the clarification that a patient's right to expect a hospital to reasonably respond to requests for care and services is limited to those that are "appropriate and medically indicated"; and (6) addition of a list of patient responsibilities.*

## Introduction

Effective health care requires collaboration between patients and physicians and other health care professionals. Open and honest communication, respect for personal and professional values, and sensitivity to differences are integral to optimal patient care. As the setting for the provision of health services, hospitals must provide a foundation for understanding and respecting the rights and responsibilities of patients, their families, physicians, and other caregivers. Hospitals must ensure a health care ethic that respects the role of patients in decision making about treatment choices and other aspects of their care. Hospitals must be sensitive to cultural, racial, linguistic, religious, age, gender, and other differences as well as the needs of persons with disabilities.

The American Hospital Association presents A Patient's Bill of Rights with the expectation that it will contribute to more effective patient care and be supported by the hospital on behalf of the institution, its medical staff, employees, and patients. The American Hospital Association encourages health care institutions to tailor this bill of rights to their patient community by translating and/or simplifying the language of this bill of rights as may be necessary to ensure that patients and their families understand their rights and responsibilities.

## Bill of Rights*

1. The patient has the right to considerate and respectful care.

2. The patient has the right to and is encouraged to obtain from physicians and other direct caregivers relevant, current, and understandable information concerning diagnosis, treatment, and prognosis.

Except in emergencies when the patient lacks decision-making capacity and the need for treatment is urgent, the patient is entitled to the opportunity to discuss and request information related to the specific procedures and/or treatments, the risks involved, the possible length of recuperation, and the medically reasonable alternatives and their accompanying risks and benefits.

Patients have the right to know the identity of physicians, nurses, and others involved in their care, as well as when those involved are students, residents, or other trainees. The patient also has the right to know the immediate and long-term financial implications of treatment choices, insofar as they are known.

3. The patient has the right to make decisions about the plan of care prior to and during the course of treatment and to refuse a recommended treatment or plan of care to the extent permitted by law and hospital policy and to be informed of the medical consequences of this action. In case of such refusal, the patient is entitled to other appropriate care and services that the hospital provides or transfer to another hospital. The hospital should notify patients of any policy that might affect patient choice within the institution.

4. The patient has the right to have an advance directive (such as a living will, health care proxy, or durable power of attorney for health care) concerning treatment or designating a surrogate decision maker with the expectation that the hospital will honor the intent of that directive to the extent permitted by law and hospital policy.

Health care institutions must advise patients of their rights under state law and hospital policy to make informed medical choices, ask if the patient has an advance directive, and include that information in patient records. The patient has the right to timely information about hospital policy that may limit its ability to implement fully a legally valid advance directive.

5. The patient has the right to every consideration of privacy. Case discussion, consultation, examination, and treatment should be conducted so as to protect each patient's privacy.

6. The patient has the right to expect that all communications and records pertaining to his/her care will be treated as confidential by the hospital, except in cases such as suspected abuse and public health hazards when reporting is permitted or required by law. The patient has the right to expect that the hospital will emphasize the confidentiality of this information when it releases it to any other parties entitled to review information in these records.

7. The patient has the right to review the records pertaining to his/her medical care and to have the information explained or interpreted as necessary, except when restricted by law.

8. The patient has the right to expect that, within its capacity and policies, a hospital will make reasonable response to the request of a patient for appropriate and medically indicated care and services. The hospital must provide evaluation, service, and/or referral as indicated by the urgency of the case. When medically appropriate and legally permissible, or when a patient has so requested, a patient may be transferred to another facility. The institution to which the patient is to be transferred must first have accepted the patient for transfer. The patient must also have the benefit of complete information and explanation concerning the need for, risks, benefits, and alternatives to such a transfer.

*These rights can be exercised on the patient's behalf by a designated surrogate or proxy decision maker if the patient lacks decision-making capacity, is legally incompetent, or is a minor.

9. The patient has the right to ask and to be informed of the existence of business relationships among the hospital, educational institutions, other health care providers, or payers that may influence the patient's treatment and care.

10. The patient has the right to consent to or decline to participate in proposed research studies or human experimentation affecting care and treatment or requiring direct patient involvement, and to have those studies fully explained prior to consent. A patient who declines to participate in research or experimentation is entitled to the most effective care that the hospital can otherwise provide.

11. The patient has the right to expect reasonable continuity of care when appropriate and to be informed by physicians and other caregivers of available and realistic patient care options when hospital care is no longer appropriate.

12. The patient has the right to be informed of hospital policies and practices that relate to patient care, treatment, and responsibilities. The patient has the right to be informed of available resources for resolving disputes, grievances, and conflicts, such as ethics committees, patient representatives, or other mechanisms available in the institution. The patient has the right to be informed of the hospital's charges for services and available payment methods.

The collaborative nature of health care requires that patients, or their families/surrogates, participate in their care. The effectiveness of care and patient satisfaction with the course of treatment depend, in part, on the patient fulfilling certain responsibilities. Patients are responsible for providing information about past illnesses, hospitalizations, medications, and other matters related to health status. To participate effectively in decision making, patients must be encouraged to take responsibility for requesting additional information or clarification about their health status or treatment when they do not fully understand information and instructions. Patients are also responsible for ensuring that the health care institution has a copy of their written advance directive if they have one. Patients are responsible for informing their physicians and other caregivers if they anticipate problems in following prescribed treatment.

Patients should also be aware of the hospital's obligation to be reasonably efficient and equitable in providing care to other patients and the community. The hospital's rules and regulations are designed to help the hospital meet this obligation. Patients and their families are responsible for making reasonable accommodations to the needs of the hospital, other patients, medical staff, and hospital employees. Patients are responsible for providing necessary information for insurance claims and for working with the hospital to make payment arrangements, when necessary.

A person's health depends on much more than health care services. Patients are responsible for recognizing the impact of their life-style on their personal health.

## Conclusion

Hospitals have many functions to perform, including the enhancement of health status, health promotion, and the prevention and treatment of injury and disease; the immediate and ongoing care and rehabilitation of patients; the education of health professionals, patients, and the community; and research. All these activities must be conducted with an overriding concern for the values and dignity of patients.

## DECLARATION OF LISBON ON THE RIGHTS OF THE PATIENT
### World Medical Association
### 1981

*Whereas most of the early documents on patients' rights, such as the American Hospital Association's A Patient's Bill of Rights, focus on the rights of individuals within health care facilities (hospitals, nursing homes), the Declaration of Lisbon, adopted in 1981 by the 34th World Medical Assembly at Lisbon, is an international statement of the rights of patients in general. In conjunction with the International Code of Medical Ethics (Section II), it illustrates the relatively recent emphasis placed on "the rights of patients" in addition to the traditional "duties of physicians." Physicians not only "ought" to behave in certain ways, but patients also are entitled to have them do so.*

Recognizing that there may be practical, ethical or legal difficulties, a physician should always act according to his/her conscience and always in the best interest of the patient. The following Declaration represents some of the principal rights which the medical profession seeks to provide to patients. Whenever legislation or government action denies these rights of the patient, physicians should seek by appropriate means to assure or to restore them.

a) The patient has the right to choose his physician freely.
b) The patient has the right to be cared for by a physician who is free to make clinical and ethical judgements without any outside interference.
c) The patient has the right to accept or to refuse treatment after receiving adequate information.
d) The patient has the right to expect that his physician will respect the confidential nature of all his medical and personal details.
e) The patient has the right to die in dignity.
f) The patient has the right to receive or to decline spiritual and moral comfort including the help of a minister of an appropriate religion.

## DECLARATION ON PHYSICIAN INDEPENDENCE AND PROFESSIONAL FREEDOM
### World Medical Association
### 1986

*Adopted in 1986 by the 38th World Medical Assembly at Rancho Mirage, California, this declaration elaborates on section (b) of the 1981 Declaration of Lisbon. Of interest is the declaration's assertion of the need for professional independence in order to ensure the rights of patients and to fulfill professional obligations to them. The document emphasizes concern over conflicts of interest in the area of cost containment and asserts that physicians must advocate for their individual patients.*

The World Medical Association, Inc., recognizing the importance of the physician's independence and professional freedom, hereby adopts the following declaration of principles:

Physicians must recognize and support the rights of their patients, particularly as set forth in the World Medical Association Declaration of Lisbon (1981).

Physicians must have the professional freedom to care for their patients without interference. The exercise of the physician's professional judgement and discretion in making clinical and ethical decisions in the care and treatment of patients must be preserved and protected.

Physicians must have the professional independence to represent and defend the health needs of patients against all who would deny or restrict needed care for those who are sick or injured.

Within the context of their medical practice and the care of their patients, physicians should not be expected to administer governmental or social priorities in the allocation of scarce health resources. To do so would be to create a conflict of interest with the physician's obligation to his patients, and would effectively destroy the physician's professional independence, upon which the patient relies.

While physicians must be conscious of the cost of medical treatment and actively participate in cost containment efforts within medicine, it is the physician's primary obligation to represent the interests of the sick and injured against demands by society for cost containment that would endanger patients' health and perhaps patients' life.

By providing independence and professional freedom for physicians to practice medicine, a community assures the best possible health care for its citizens, which in turn contributes to a strong and secure society.

## FUNDAMENTAL ELEMENTS OF THE PATIENT–PHYSICIAN RELATIONSHIP
### American Medical Association
### 1990, updated 1993

*This document, which constitutes one part of the American Medical Association's complete code of ethics, extends the rights language introduced in the 1980 Principles of Medical Ethics (Section II) to a separate statement listing the specific rights of patients. The opening paragraph of the Fundamental Elements also mentions the responsibilities of patients. Points of particular interest include: (1) Right #4 on confidentiality, which contains the therapeutic privilege exception dropped from the Principles of Medical Ethics in 1980 and still not restored to the principles themselves; (2) Right #5 on continuity of care, which implies that treatment may be discontin-ued, without making alternative arrangements for care, when further treatment is not "medically indicated"; and (3) Right #6, which establishes a basic right to adequate health care, but ex-plicitly does not guarantee the fulfillment of such a right.*

From ancient times, physicians have recognized that the health and well-being of patients depends upon a collaborative effort between physician and patient. Patients share with physicians the responsibility for their own health care. The patient-physician relationship is of greatest benefit to patients when they bring medical problems to the attention of their physicians in a timely fashion, provide information about their medical condition to the best of their ability, and work with their physicians in a mutually respectful alliance. Physicians can best contribute to this alliance by serving as their patients' advocate and by fostering these rights:

1. The patient has the right to receive information from physicians and to discuss the benefits, risks, and costs of appropriate treatment alternatives. Patients should receive guidance from their physicians as to the optimal course of action. Patients are also entitled to obtain copies or summaries of their medical records, to have their questions answered, to be advised of potential conflicts of interest that their physicians might have, and to receive independent professional opinions.

2. The patient has the right to make decisions regarding the health care that is recommended by his or her physician. Accordingly, patients may accept or refuse any recommended medical treatment.

3. The patient has the right to courtesy, respect, dignity, responsiveness, and timely attention to his or her needs.

4. The patient has the right to confidentiality. The physician should not reveal confidential communications or information without the consent of the patient, unless provided for by law or by the need to protect the welfare of the individual or the public interest.

5. The patient has the right to continuity of health care. The physician has an obligation to cooperate in the coordination of medically indicated care with other health care providers treating the patient. The physician may not discontinue treatment of a patient as long as further treatment is medically indicated, without giving the patient reasonable assistance and sufficient opportunity to make alternative arrangements for care.

6. The patient has a basic right to have available adequate health care. Physicians, along with the rest of society, should continue to work toward this goal. Fulfillment of this right is dependent on society providing resources so that no patient is deprived of necessary care because of an inability to pay for the care. Physicians should continue their traditional assumption of a part of the responsibility for the medical care of those who cannot afford essential health care. Physicians should advocate for patients in dealing with third parties when appropriate.

# PATIENT RESPONSIBILITIES
## American Medical Association
### 1993

*The American Medical Association's (AMA) Patient Responsibilities draws upon the recognition, articulated in the preceding Fundamental Elements of the Patient–Physician Relationship, that successful medical care depends upon a collaborative effort between physicians and patients. Originally published in July 1993 as Report 52 in the AMA Code of Medical Ethics: Reports of the Council on Ethical and Judicial Affairs, Patient Responsibilities expands upon the Fundamental Elements document by specifying the responsibilities of patients for their own health care.*

*The background section of the original report states: "Like patients' rights, patients' responsibilities are derived from the principle of autonomy. . . . With that exercise of self-governance and free choice comes a number of responsibilities." The list of those patient responsibilities, which also appears in the 1994 AMA Current Opinions, follows.*

1. Good communication is essential to a successful physician-patient relationship. To the extent possible, patients have a responsibility to be truthful and to express their concerns clearly to their physicians.

2. Patients have a responsibility to provide a complete medical history, to the extent possible, including information about past illnesses, medications, hospitalizations, family history of illness and other matters relating to present health.

3. Patients have a responsibility to request information or clarification about their health status or treatment when they do not fully understand what has been described.

4. Once patients and physicians agree upon the goals of therapy, patients have a responsibility to cooperate with the treatment plan. Compliance with physician instructions is often essential to public and individual safety. Patients also have a responsibility to disclose whether previously agreed upon treatments are being followed and to indicate when they would like to reconsider the treatment plan.

5. Patients generally have a responsibility to meet their financial obligations with regard to medical care or to discuss financial hardships with their physicians. Patients should be cognizant of the costs associated with using a limited resource like health care and try to use medical resources judiciously.

6. Patients should discuss end of life decisions with their physicians and make their wishes known. Such a discussion might also include writing an advance directive.

7. Patients should be committed to health maintenance through health-enhancing behavior. Illness can often be prevented by a healthy lifestyle, and patients must take personal responsibility when they are able to avert the development of disease.

8. Patients should also have an active interest in the effects of their conduct on others and refrain from behavior that unreasonably places the health of others at risk. Patients should inquire as to the means and likelihood of infectious disease transmission and act upon that information which can best prevent further transmission.

9. Patients should discuss organ donation with their physicians and make applicable provisions. Patients who are part of an organ allocation system and await needed treatment or transplant should not try to go outside of or manipulate the system. A fair system of allocation should be answered with public trust and an awareness of limited resources.

10. Patients should not initiate or participate in fraudulent health care and should report illegal or unethical behavior by providers to the appropriate medical societies, licensing boards, or law enforcement authorities.

## PATIENT RIGHTS
### Joint Commission on Accreditation of Healthcare Organizations
### 1994

*Patient Rights is a section of the Joint Commission on Accreditation of Healthcare Organizations' (JCAHO) Accreditation Manual for Hospitals, 1994. Although many health-care organizations demonstrate their recognition and support of patient/client rights by issuing lists of those rights, no list can assure that the rights are respected. The standards on patient rights included in JCAHO's Accreditation Manual are designed to reflect the implementation, as well as the existence, of institutional policies and procedures for the exercise and protection of a specified set of patient rights.*

The scoring of the standards in this chapter will reflect evidence of the implementation of policies and procedures as well as the existence of such policies and procedures.

*RI.1    The organization supports the rights of each patient.*

*RI.1.1    Organizational policies and procedures describe the mechanisms by which the following rights are protected and exercised:*

### Intent of RI.1 and RI.1.1

The policies and procedures that guide the organization's interaction with and care of the patient demonstrate its recognition and support of patient rights.

No listing of patient rights can assure the respect of those rights. It is the intent of these standards that the organization's interaction with and care of the patient reflect concern and respect for the rights of the patient.

The organization's policies and procedures describe the mechanisms or processes established to support the following patient rights:
- Reasonable access to care;
- Considerate (and respectful) care that respects the patient's personal value and belief systems;
- Informed participation in decisions regarding his/her care;
- Participation in the consideration of ethical issues that arise in the provision of his/her care;
- Personal privacy and confidentiality of information; and

- Designation of a representative decision maker in the event that the patient is incapable of understanding a proposed treatment or procedure or is unable to communicate his/her wishes regarding care.

• • •

*RI.1.1.1* [*Organizational policies and procedures describe the mechanisms by which the following rights are protected and exercised:*] *The right of the patient to the hospital's reasonable response to his/her requests and needs for treatment or service, within the hospital's capacity, its stated mission, and applicable law and regulation;*

## Intent of RI.1.1.1

In response to the patient's request and need, the organization provides care that is within its capacity, its stated mission and philosophy, and applicable law and regulation. When the organization cannot meet the request or need for care because of a conflict with its mission or philosophy or incapacity to meet the patient's needs or requests, the patient may be transferred to another facility when medically permissible. Such a transfer is made only after the patient has received complete information and explanation concerning the need for and alternatives to such a transfer. The transfer must be acceptable to the receiving organization.

• • •

*RI.1.1.2* [*Organizational policies and procedures describe the mechanisms by which the following rights are protected and exercised:*] *The right of the patient to considerate and respectful care;*

*RI1.1.2.1* *The care of the patient includes consideration of the psychosocial, spiritual, and cultural variables that influence the perceptions of illness.*

## Intent of RI.1.1.2 and RI.1.1.2.1

The provision of patient care reflects consideration of the patient as an individual with personal values and a belief system that impact his/her attitude toward and response to the care provided by the organization. The organizational policies and procedures that guide patient care include recognition of the psychosocial, spiritual, and cultural values that affect the patient's response to the care given. Organizational policies and procedures allow the patient to express spiritual beliefs and cultural practices that do not harm others or interfere with the planned course of medical therapy for the patient.

• • •

*RI.1.1.2.2* *The care of the dying patient optimizes the comfort and dignity of the patient through*

*RI.1.1.2.2.1* *treating primary and secondary symptoms that respond to treatment as desired by the patient or surrogate decision maker;*

*RI.1.1.2.2.2* *effectively managing pain; and*

*RI.1.1.2.2.3* *acknowledging the psychosocial and spiritual concerns of the patient and the family regarding dying and the expression of grief by the patient and family.*

**Note:** *The term dying is used to refer to an incurable and irreversible condition such that death is imminent. Imminent is seen as impending or about to happen.*

## Intent of RI.1.1.2.2 Through RI.1.1.2.2.3

All hospital staff are sensitized to the needs of the dying patient in an acute care hospital. Support for the psychological, social, emotional, and spiritual needs of the patient and family demonstrates respect for the patient's values, religion, and philosophy. The goal of respectful, responsive care of the dying patient is to optimize the patient's comfort and dignity by providing appropriate treatment for primary and secondary symptoms as desired by the patient or surrogate decision maker, responding to the psychosocial, emotional, and spiritual concerns of the patient and family, and managing pain aggressively. (The management of pain is appropriate for all patients, not just dying patients. Guidelines such as those published by the Agency for Health Care Policy and Research for Acute Pain Management reflect the state of knowledge on effective and appropriate care for all patients experiencing acute pain.)

• • •

*RI.1.1.3    [Organizational policies and procedures describe the mechanisms by which the following rights are protected and exercised:]The right of the patient, in collaboration with his/her physician, to make decisions involving his/her health care, including*

*RI.1.1.3.1    the right of the patient to accept medical care or to refuse treatment to the extent permitted by law and to be informed of the medical consequences of such refusal, and*

*RI.1.1.3.2    the right of the patient to formulate advance directives and appoint a surrogate to make health care decisions on his/her behalf to the extent permitted by law.*

*RI.1.1.3.2.1    The organization has in place a mechanism to ascertain the existence of and assist in the development of advance directives at the time of the patient's admission.*

*RI.1.1.3.2.2    The provision of care is not conditioned on the existence of an advance directive.*

*RI.1.1.3.2.3    Any advance directive(s) is in the patient's medical record and is reviewed periodically with the patient or surrogate decision maker.*

### Intent of RI.1.1.3 Through RI.1.1.3.2.3

The quality of patient care is enhanced when the patient's preferences are incorporated into plans for care. The process by which care and treatment decisions are made elicit respect and incorporate the patient's preferences. Sound medical judgment is provided to the patient or the patient's surrogate decision maker for informed decision making.

In hospitals providing services to neonate, child, and adolescent patients, a mechanisms exists that is designed to coordinate and facilitate the family's and/or guardian's involvement in decision making throughout the course of treatment. The patient is responsible for providing, to the best of his/her knowledge, accurate and complete information about present complaints, past illnesses, hospitalizations, medications, advance directives, and other matters relevant to his/her health or care. The patient is also responsible for reporting whether he/she clearly comprehends a contemplated course of action and what is expected of him/her.

The hospital ascertains the existence of advance directives, and health care professionals and surrogate decision makers honor them within the limits of the law and the organization's mission and philosophy. An advance directive is a document a person uses to give directions about future medical care or to designate another person to give directions about medical care should he/she lose decision-making capacity. Advance directives may include living wills, durable powers of attorney, or similar documents and contain the patient's preferences.

• • •

*RI.1.1.4    [Organizational policies and procedures describe the mechanisms by which the following rights are protected and exercised:] The right of the patient to the information necessary to enable him/her to make treatment decisions that reflect his/her wishes;*

*RI.1.1.4.1    A policy on informed decision making is developed by the medical staff and governing body and is consistent with any legal requirements.*

### Intent of RI.1.1.4 and RI.1.1.4.1

The patient is given clear, concise explanation of his/her condition and of any proposed treatment(s) or procedure(s), the potential benefit(s) and the potential drawback(s) of the proposed treatment(s) or procedure(s), problems related to recuperation, and the likelihood of success. Information is also provided regarding any significant alternative treatment(s) or procedure(s).

This information includes the identity of the physician or other practitioner who has primary responsibility for the patient's care and the identity and professional status of individuals responsible for authorizing and performing procedures or treatments. The information also includes the existence of any professional relationship among individuals treating the patient, as well as the relationship to any other health care or educational institutions involved in his/her care.

• • •

*RI.1.1.5    [Organizational policies and procedures describe the mechanisms by which the following rights are protected and exercised:] The right of the patient to information, at the time of admission, about the hospital's*

*RI.1.1.5.1    patient rights policy(ies), and*

*RI.1.1.5.2   mechanism designed for the initiation, review, and, when possible, resolution of patient complaints concerning the quality of care;*

## Intent of RI.1.1.5 Through RI.1.1.5.2

The organization assists the patient in exercising his/her rights by informing the patient of those rights during the admission process. The information is given to the patient or his/her representative in a form that is understandable to the patient (for example, in a language that is understood by the patient).

The patient has the right, without recrimination, to voice complaints regarding the care received, and to have those complaints reviewed and, when possible, resolved. This right, and the mechanism(s) established by the organization to assist the patient in exercising this right, are explained to the patient during the admission process.

• • •

*RI.1.1.6   [Organizational policies and procedures describe the mechanisms by which the following rights are protected and exercised:] The right of the patient or the patient's designated representative to participate in the consideration of ethical issues that arise in the care of the patient;*

*RI.1.1.6.1   The organization has in place a mechanism(s) for the consideration of ethical issues arising in the care of patients and to provide education to caregivers and patients on ethical issues in health care.*

## Intent of RI.1.1.6 and RI.1.1.6.1

Health care professionals provide patient care within an ethical framework established by their profession, the hospital, and the law. The health care professional has an obligation to respect the views of the patient or the patient's designated representative when ethical issues arise during the patient's care. Moreover, the hospital has an obligation to involve the patient or the patient's representative in the organizational mechanism for considering such issues. Such mechanisms may include community programs, education programs for patients or their representatives, and education programs for staff members. The hospital also has an obligation to provide education on important ethical issues in health care to caregivers, care recipients, and the community.

• • •

*RI.1.1.7   [Organizational policies and procedures describe the mechanisms by which the following rights are protected and exercised:] The right of the patient to be informed of any human experimentation or other research/educational projects affecting his/her care or treatment;*

## Intent of RI.1.1.7

The patient has the right to know of any experimental, research, or educational activities involved in his/her treatment: the patient also has the right to refuse to participate in any such activity.

• • •

*RI.1.1.8   [Organizational policies and procedures describe the mechanisms by which the following rights are protected and exercised:] The right of the patient, within the limits of law, to personal privacy and confidentiality of information; and*

*RI.1.1.8.1   The patient and/or the patient's legally designated representative has access to the information contained in the patient's medical record, within the limits of the law.*

## Intent of RI.1.1.8 and RI.1.1.8.1

The patient has the following rights:
- To be interviewed, examined, and treated in surroundings designed to give reasonable visual and auditory privacy;
- To have access to his/her medical record and to have his/her medical record read only by individuals directly involved in his/her care, or by individuals monitoring the quality of the patient's care, or by individuals authorized by law or regulation (other individuals may read the medical record only with the patient's written consent or that of a legally authorized or designated representative); and

- To request a transfer to a different room if another patient or a visitor in the room is unreasonably disturbing him/her and if another room equally suitable for his/her care needs is available.

• • •

*RI.1.1.9    [Organizational policies and procedures describe the mechanisms by which the following rights are protected and exercised:] The right of the patient's guardian, next of kin, or a legally authorized responsible person to exercise, to the extent permitted by law, the rights delineated on behalf of the patient if the patient has been adjudicated incompetent in accordance with the law, is found by his/her physician to be medically incapable of understanding the proposed treatment or procedure, is unable to communicate his/her wishes regarding treatment, or is a minor.*

### Intent of RI.1.1.9

Although the patient is recognized as having the right to participate in his/her care and treatment to the fullest extent possible, there are circumstances under which the patient may be unable to do so. In these situations, the patient's rights are to be exercised by the patient's designated representative or other legally authorized person.

• • •

*RI.2    There are hospitalwide policies on the withholding of resuscitative services from patients and the forgoing or withdrawing of life-sustaining treatment.*

### Intent of RI.2

No single set of policies can anticipate the varied situations in which the difficult decisions about withholding resuscitative services or forgoing or withdrawing life-sustaining treatment will need to be made. However, organizations can develop the framework for a decision-making process. Such a framework would include policies designed to assist the organization in identifying its position on the initiation of resuscitative services and the use and removal of life-sustaining treatment. Policies of this nature need to conform to the legal requirements of the organization's jurisdiction.

• • •

*RI.2.1    The policies are developed in consultation with the medical staff, nursing staff, and other appropriate bodies and are adopted by the medical staff and approved by the governing body.*

### Intent of RI.2.1

Organizational policies that provide a framework for the decision-making process for withholding resuscitative services or forgoing or withdrawing life-sustaining treatment offer guidance to health professionals on the ethical and legal issues involved in such decisions and decrease the uncertainty about the practices permitted by the organization. It is vital that the policies guiding such decisions be formally adopted by the organization's medical staff and approved by the governing body in order to assure that the process is consistent and that there is accountability for the decisions made.

• • •

*RI.2.2    The policies describe*

*RI.2.2.1    the mechanism(s) for reaching decisions about the withholding of resuscitative services from individual patients or forgoing or withdrawing of life-sustaining treatment;*

*RI.2.2.2    the mechanism(s) for resolving conflicts in decision making, should they arise; and*

*RI.2.2.3    the roles of physicians and, when applicable, of nursing personnel, other appropriate staff, and family members in decisions to withhold resuscitative services or forgo or withdraw life-sustaining treatment.*

### Intent of RI.2.2 Through RI.2.2.3

Organizational policies regarding the withholding of resuscitative services or the forgoing or withdrawing of life-sustaining treatment outline a process for reaching such decisions. This process protects the decision-making rights of the patient or his/her designated representative; decreases staff uncertainty about practices permitted by the organization; clarifies the roles and duties, and therefore the accountability, of health professionals; and reduces arbitrary decision-making procedures.

• • •

*RI.2.3    The policies include provisions designed to assure that the rights of patients are respected.*

## Intent of RI.2.3

Organizational policies regarding the withholding of resuscitative services or the forgoing or withdrawing of life-sustaining treatment empower the patient or designated representative to make such decisions and assure that such decisions made by a patient or designated representative explicitly affirm the patient's responsibility for such decision making.

• • •

*RI.2.4    The policies include the requirement that appropriate orders be written by the physician primarily responsible for the patient and that documentation be made in the patient's medical record if life-sustaining treatment is to be withdrawn or resuscitative services are to be withheld.*

## Intent of RI.2.4

Decisions regarding the withholding of resuscitative services or the withdrawal of life-sustaining treatment are communicated to all health professionals involved in the patient's treatment to assure that the decision is implemented.

**Note:** *This does not mean that for all deaths in which resuscitative services were not utilized there must be an order to withhold resuscitative services.*

• • •

*RI.2.5    The policies address the use of advance directives in patient care to the extent permitted by law.*

## Intent of RI.2.5

The organization is expected to use any advance directives prepared by the patient and known to the organization in the decision-making process surrounding the consideration of the withholding of resuscitative services or the initiation or withdrawal of life-sustaining treatment, to the extent permitted by law and supported by the organization's mission and philosophy.

• • •

# SECTION II
## Ethical Directives for the Practice of Medicine

### 1. Fourth century B.C.E.–Early twentieth century C.E.

Oath of Hippocrates [Fourth Century B.C.E.]

Oath of Initiation (Caraka Samhita) [First Century C.E.?]

Oath of Asaph [Third Century–Seventh Century C.E.?]

Advice to a Physician, Advice of Haly Abbas (Ahwazi) [Tenth Century C.E.]

The 17 Rules of Enjuin (For Disciples of Our School) [Sixteenth Century C.E.]

Five Commandments and Ten Requirements [1617]

A Physician's Ethical Duties from *Kholasah al Hekmah* [1770]

Daily Prayer of a Physician ("Prayer of Moses Maimonides") [1793?]

Code of Ethics, American Medical Association [1847]

Venezuelan Code of Medical Ethics, National Academy of Medicine [1918]

### 2. Mid-twentieth century–1994

Declaration of Geneva, World Medical Association [1948, amended 1968, 1983]

International Code of Medical Ethics, World Medical Association [1949, amended 1968, 1983]

Principles of Medical Ethics (1957), American Medical Association [1957]

Principles of Medical Ethics (1980), American Medical Association [1980]

Current Opinions of the Council on Ethical and Judicial Affairs, American Medical Association [1994]

The Moral and Technical Competence of the Ophthalmologist, American Academy of Ophthalmology [1991]

Code of Ethics, American Osteopathic Association [revised 1985]

Code of Ethics and Guide to the Ethical Behaviour of Physicians, Canadian Medical Association [revised 1990]

Code of Ethics and Guide to the Ethical Behaviour of Physicians, New Zealand Medical Association [1989, last amended 1992]

Code of Ethics of the Chilean Medical Association, Chilean Medical Association [1983]

Code of Medical Ethics, Brazil, Federal Council of Medicine [1988]

European Code of Medical Ethics, Conférence Internationale des Ordres et des Organismes d' Attributions Similaires [1987]

Code of Ethics for Doctors, Norwegian Medical Association [amended 1992]

Final Report Concerning Brain Death and Organ Transplantation, Japan Medical Association [1988]

*The ethical directives for the practice of medicine included in this section are organized in two primary groups: (1) codes, oaths, prayers, and other directives from the fourth century B.C.E. through the early twentieth century; and (2) directives from the mid-twentieth century through 1994. Documents in the first group are arranged in chronological order; those in the second group are arranged chronologically within thematic clusters, for example, by issuing body, area of the world, and philosophical or religious tradition.*

*Some of the documents in this section address not only physicians but also health-care institutions and the health professions in general; they are included in this section because many medical ethics codes historically have applied not only to physicians but also to the practice of health care more generally. Ethical directives for medical specialties generally have not been included in this Appendix, due to space constraints; references for a selection of specialty documents appear in the bibliography to the Appendix.*

# OATH OF HIPPOCRATES
## Fourth Century B.C.E.

*Attributed to Hippocrates, the oath, which exemplifies the Pythagorean school rather than Greek thought in general, differs from other, more scientific, writings in the Hippocratic corpus. Written later than some of the other treatises in the corpus, the Oath of Hippocrates is one of the earliest and most important statements on medical ethics. Not only has the oath provided the foundation for many succeeding medical oaths, such as the Declaration of Geneva, but it is still administered to the graduating students of many medical schools, either in its original form or in an altered version.*

I swear by Apollo Physician and Asclepius and Hygieia and Panaceia and all the gods and goddesses, making them my witnesses, that I will fulfil according to my ability and judgment this oath and this covenant:

To hold him who has taught me this art as equal to my parents and to live my life in partnership with him, and if he is in need of money to give him a share of mine, and to regard his offspring as equal to my brothers in male lineage and to teach them this art—if they desire to learn it—without fee and covenant; to give a share of precepts and oral instruction and all the other learning to my sons and to the sons of him who has instructed me and to pupils who have signed the covenant and have taken an oath according to the medical law, but to no one else.

I will apply dietetic measures for the benefit of the sick according to my ability and judgment; I will keep them from harm and injustice.

I will neither give a deadly drug to anybody if asked for it, nor will I make a suggestion to this effect. Similarly I will not give to a woman an abortive remedy. In purity and holiness I will guard my life and my art.

I will not use the knife, not even on sufferers from stone, but will withdraw in favor of such men as are engaged in this work.

Whatever houses I may visit, I will come for the benefit of the sick, remaining free of all intentional injustice, of all mischief and in particular of sexual relations with both female and male persons, be they free or slaves.

What I may see or hear in the course of the treatment or even outside of the treatment in regard to the life of men, which on no account one must spread abroad, I will keep to myself holding such things shameful to be spoken about.

If I fulfil this oath and do not violate it, may it be granted to me to enjoy life and art, being honored with fame among all men for all time to come; if I transgress it and swear falsely, may the opposite of all this be my lot.

# OATH OF INITIATION (CARAKA SAMHITA)
## First Century C.E.?

*This ancient Indian oath for medical students appears in the Caraka Samhita (or, Charaka Samhita), a medical text written around the first century C.E. by the Indian physician Caraka. Unlike the Hippocratic Oath, which exemplifies only one, minority, school of ancient Greek thought, the Oath of the Caraka Samhita reflects concepts and beliefs found throughout ancient nonmedical Indian literature. The oath contains several uniquely Hindu elements, including the requirements to lead the life of a celibate, eat no meat, and carry no arms.*

1. The teacher then should instruct the disciple in the presence of the sacred fire, Brāhmanas [Brahmins] and physicians.

2. [saying] "Thou shalt lead the life of a celibate, grow thy hair and beard, speak only the truth, eat no meat, eat only pure articles of food, be free from envy and carry no arms.

3. There shall be nothing that thou should not do at my behest except hating the king, causing another's death, or committing an act of great unrighteousness or acts leading to calamity.

4. Thou shalt dedicate thyself to me and regard me as thy chief. Thou shalt be subject to me and conduct thyself for ever for my welfare and pleasure. Thou shalt serve and dwell with me like a son or a slave or a supplicant. Thou shalt behave and act without arrogance, with care and attention and with undistracted mind, humility, constant reflection and ungrudging obedience. Acting either at my behest or otherwise, thou shalt conduct thyself for the achievement of thy teacher's purposes alone, to the best of thy abilities.

5. If thou desirest success, wealth and fame as a physician and heaven after death, thou shalt pray for the welfare of all creatures beginning with the cows and Brāhmanas.

6. Day and night, however thou mayest be engaged, thou shalt endeavour for the relief of patients with all thy heart and soul. Thou shalt not desert or injure thy patient for the sake of thy life or thy living. Thou shalt not commit adultery even in thought. Even so, thou shalt not covet others' possessions. Thou shalt be modest in thy attire and appearance. Thou shouldst not be a drunkard or a sinful man nor shouldst thou associate with the abettors of crimes. Thou shouldst speak words that are gentle, pure and righteous, pleasing, worthy, true, wholesome, and moderate. Thy behaviour must be in consideration of time and place and heedful of past experience. Thou shalt act always with a view to the acquisition of knowledge and fullness of equipment.

7. No persons, who are hated by the king or who are haters of the king or who are hated by the public or who are haters of the public, shall receive treatment. Similarly, those who are extremely abnormal, wicked, and of miserable character and conduct, those who have not vindicated their honour, those who are on the point of death, and similarly women who are unattended by their husbands or guardians shall not receive treatment.

8. No offering of presents by a woman without the behest of her husband or guardian shall be accepted by thee. While entering the patient's house, thou shalt be accompanied by a man who is known to the patient and who has his permission to enter; and thou shalt be well-clad, bent of head, self-possessed, and conduct thyself only after repeated consideration. Thou shalt thus properly make thy entry. Having entered, thy speech, mind, intellect and senses shall be entirely devoted to no other thought than that of being helpful to the patient and of things concerning only him. The peculiar customs of the patient's household shall not be made public. Even knowing that the patient's span of life has come to its close, it shall not be mentioned by thee there, where if so done, it would cause shock to the patient or to others.

Though possessed of knowledge one should not boast very much of one's knowledge. Most people are offended by the boastfulness of even those who are otherwise good and authoritative.

9. There is no limit at all to the Science of Life, Medicine. So thou shouldst apply thyself to it with diligence. This is how thou shouldst act. Also thou shouldst learn the skill of practice from another without carping. The entire world is the teacher to the intelligent and the foe to the unintelligent. Hence, knowing this well, thou shouldst listen and act according to the words of instruction of even an unfriendly person, when his words are worthy and of a kind as to bring to you fame, long life, strength and prosperity."

10. Thereafter the teacher should say this—"Thou shouldst conduct thyself properly with the gods, sacred fire, Brāhmanas, the guru, the aged, the scholars and the preceptors. If thou has conducted thyself well with them, the precious stones, the grains and the gods become well disposed towards thee. If thou shouldst conduct thyself otherwise, they become unfavorable to thee." To the teacher that has spoken thus, the disciple should say, "Amen."

# OATH OF ASAPH
## Third Century–Seventh Century C.E.?

*The Oath of Asaph appears at the end of the* Book of Asaph the Physician *(Sefer Asaph ha-Rofe), which is the oldest Hebrew medical text. It was written by Asaph Judaeus, also known as Asaph ben Berachyahu, a Hebrew physician from Syria or Mesopotamia, who lived sometime between the third and seventh centuries* C.E., *probably in the sixth century. The oath, which in part resembles the Oath of Hippocrates, was taken by medical students when they received their diplomas.*

And this is the oath adminstered by Asaph, the son of Berachyahu, and by Jochanan, the son of Zabda, to their disciples; and they adjured them in these words: Take heed that ye kill not any man with the sap of a root; and ye shall not dispense a potion to a woman with child by adultery to cause her to miscarry; and ye shall not lust after beautiful women to commit adultery with them; and ye shall not disclose secrets confided unto you; and ye shall take no bribes to cause injury and to kill; and ye shall not harden your hearts against the poor and the needy, but heal them; and ye shall not call good evil or evil good; and ye shall not walk in the way of sorcerers to cast spells, to enchant and to bewitch with intent to separate a man from the wife of his bosom or woman from the husband of her youth.

And ye shall not covet wealth or bribes to abet depraved sexual commerce.

And ye shall not make use of any manner of idol-worship to heal thereby, nor trust in the healing powers of any form of their worship. But rather must ye abhor and detest and hate all their worshippers and those that trust in them and cause others to trust in them, for all of them are but vanity and of no avail, for they are naught; and they are demons. Their own carcasses they cannot save; how, then, shall they save the living?

And now, put your trust in the Lord your God, the God of truth, the living God, for He doth kill and make alive, smite and heal. He doth teach man understanding and also to do good. He smiteth in righteousness and justice and healeth in mercy and loving-kindness. No crafty device can be concealed from Him, for naught is hidden from His sight.

He causeth healing plants to grow and doth implant in the hearts of sages skill to heal by His manifold mercies and to declare marvels to the multitude, that all that live may know that He made them, and that beside Him there is none to save. For the peoples trust in their idols to succour them from their afflictions, but they will not save them in their distress, for their hope and their trust are in the Dead. Therefore it is fitting that ye keep apart from them and hold aloof from all the abominations of their idols and cleave unto the name of the Lord God of all flesh. And every living creature is in His hand to kill and to make alive; and there is none to deliver from His hand.

Be ye mindful of Him at all times and seek Him in truth uprightness and rectitude that ye may prosper in all that ye do; then He will cause you to prosper and ye shall be praised by all men. And the peoples will leave their gods and their idols and will yearn to serve the Lord even as ye do, for they will perceive that they have put their trust in a thing of naught and that their labour is in vain; (otherwise) when they cry unto the Lord, He will not save them.

As for you, be strong and let not your hands slacken, for there is a reward for your labours. God is with you when ye are with Him. If ye will keep His covenant and walk in His statutes to cleave unto them, ye shall be as saints in the sight of all men, and they shall say: "Happy is the people that is in such a case; happy is that people whose God is the Lord."

And their disciples answered them and said: All that ye have instructed us and commanded us, that will we do, for it is a commandment of the Torah, and it behooves us to perform it with all our heart and all our soul and all our might: to do and to obey and to turn neither to the right nor to the left. And they blessed them in the name of the Highest God, the Lord of Heaven and earth.

And they admonished them yet again and said unto them: Behold, the Lord God and His saints and His Torah be witness unto you that ye shall fear Him, turning not aside from His commandments, but walking uprightly in His statutes. Incline not to covetousness and aid not the evildoers to shed innocent blood. Neither shall ye mix poisons for a man or a woman to slay his friend therewith; nor shall ye reveal which roots be poisonous or give them into the hand of any man, or be persuaded to do evil. Ye shall not cause the shedding of blood by any manner of medical treatment. Take heed that ye do not cause a malady to any man; and ye shall not cause any man injury by hastening to cut through flesh and blood with an iron instrument or by branding, but shall first observe twice and thrice and only then shall ye give your counsel.

Let not a spirit of haughtiness cause you to lift up your eyes and your hearts in pride. Wreak not the vengeance of hatred on a sick man; and alter not your prescriptions for them that do hate the Lord our God, but keep his ordinances and commandments and walk in all His ways that ye may find favour in His sight. Be ye pure and faithful and upright.

Thus did Asaph and Jochanan instruct and adjure their disciples.

# ADVICE TO A PHYSICIAN
## Advice of Haly Abbas (Ahwazi)
### Tenth Century C.E.

*A leading Persian figure in medicine and medical ethics, Haly Abbas (Ahwazi), who died in 994 C.E., devoted the first chapter of his work* Liber Regius (Kamel Al Sanaah al Tibbia) *to the ethics of medicine. An excerpt of his ethical admonition follows.*

The first advice is to worship God and obey his commands; then be humble toward your teacher and endeavor to hold him in esteem, to serve and show gratitude to him, to hold him equally dear as you do your parents, and to share your possessions with him as with your parents.

Be kind to the children of your teachers and if one of them wants to study medicine you are to teach him without any remuneration.

You are to prohibit the unsuited and undeserving from studying medicine.

A physician is to prudently treat his patients with food and medicine out of good and spiritual motives, not for the sake of gain. He should never prescribe or use a harmful drug or abortifacient.

A physician should be chaste, pious, religious, well-spoken, and graceful, and must avoid any kind of sinfulness or impurity. He should not look upon women with lust and never go to their home except to visit a patient.

A physician should respect confidences and protect the patient's secrets. In protecting a patient's secrets, he must be more insistent than the patient himself. A physician should follow the Hippocratic counsels. He must be kind, compassionate, merciful and benevolent, and give himself unstintingly to the treatment of patients, especially the poor. He must never expect remuneration from the poor but rather provide them free medicine. If it is not impossible, he must visit them graciously whenever it is necessary, day or night, especially when they suffer from an acute disease, because the patient's condition changes very quickly with this kind of disease.

It is not proper for a physician to live luxuriously and become involved in pleasure-seeking. He must not drink alcohol because it injures the brain. He must study medical books constantly and never grow tired of research. He has to learn what he is studying and repeat and memorize what is necessary. He has to study in his youth because it is easier to memorize the subject at this age than in old age, which is the mother of oblivion.

A medical student should be constantly present in the hospital so as to study disease processes and complications under the learned professor and proficient physicians.

To be a learned and skillful physician, he has to follow this advice, develop an upright character and never hesitate to put this advice into practice so as to make his work effective, to win the patient's trust, and to receive the benefit of the patient's friendship and gratitude.

The Almighty God knows better than all. . . .

# THE 17 RULES OF ENJUIN
# (FOR DISCIPLES OF OUR SCHOOL)
### Sixteenth Century C.E.

*The 17 Rules of Enjuin were developed for students by practitioners of the Ri-shu school, an approach to disease that was practiced in sixteenth-century Japan. The text reflects the priestly role of the physician and emphasizes the idea, also found in the Hippocratic Oath, that medical knowledge should not be disclosed outside of the school.*

1. Each person should follow the path designated by Heaven (Buddha, the Gods).

2. You should always be kind to people. You should always be devoted to loving people.

3. The teaching of Medicine should be restricted to selected persons.

4. You should not tell others what you are taught, regarding treatments without permission.

5. You should not establish association with doctors who do not belong to this school.

6. All the successors and descendants of the disciples of this school shall follow the teachers' ways.

7. If any disciples cease the practice of Medicine, or, if successors are not found at

the death of the disciple, all the medical books of this school should be returned to the SCHOOL OF ENJUIN.

8. You should not kill living creatures, nor should you admire hunting or fishing.

9. In our school, teaching about poisons is prohibited, nor should you receive instructions about poisons from other physicians. Moreover, you should not give abortives to the people.

10. You should rescue even such patients as you dislike or hate. You should do virtuous acts, but in such a way that they do not become known to people. To do good deeds secretly is a mark of virtue.

11. You should not exhibit avarice and you must not strain to become famous. You should not rebuke or reprove a patient, even if he does not present you with money or goods in gratitude.

12. You should be delighted if, after treating a patient without success, the patient receives medicine from another physician, and is cured.

13. You should not speak ill of other physicians.

14. You should not tell what you have learned from the time you enter a woman's room, and, moreover, you should not have obscene or immoral feelings when examining a woman.

15. Proper or not, you should not tell others what you have learned in lectures, or what you have learned about prescribing medicine.

16. You should not like undue extravagance. If you like such living, your avarice will increase, and you will lose the ability to be kind to others.

17. If you do not keep the rules and regulations of this school, then you will be cancelled as a disciple. In more severe cases, the punishment will be greater.

# FIVE COMMANDMENTS AND TEN REQUIREMENTS
## 1617

*The Five Commandments and Ten Requirements of physicians constitute the most comprehensive statement on medical ethics in China. They were written by Chen Shih-kung, an early-seventeenth-century Chinese physician, and appear in his work* An Orthodox Manual of Surgery.

## Five Commandments

1. Physicians should be ever ready to respond to any calls of patients, high or low, rich or poor. They should treat them equally and care not for financial reward. Thus their profession will become prosperous naturally day by day and conscience will remain intact.

2. Physicians may visit a lady, widow or nun only in the presence of an attendant but not alone. The secret diseases of female patients should be examined with a right attitude, and should not be revealed to anybody, not even to the physician's own wife.

3. Physicians should not ask patients to send pearl, amber or other valuable substances to their home for preparing medicament. If necessary, patients should be instructed how to mix the prescriptions themselves in order to avoid suspicion. It is also not proper to admire things which patients possess.

4. Physicians should not leave the office for excursion and drinking. Patients should be examined punctually and personally. Prescriptions should be made according to the medical formulary, otherwise a dispute may arise.

5. Prostitutes should be treated just like patients from a good family and gratuitous services should not be given to the poor ones. Mocking should not be indulged for this brings loss of dignity. After examination physicians should leave the house immediately. If the case improves, drugs may be sent but physicians should not visit them again for lewd reward.

## Ten Requirements

1. A physician or surgeon must first know the principles of the learned. He must study all the ancient standard medical books ceaselessly day and night, and understand them thoroughly so that the principles enlighten his eyes and are impressed on his heart. Then he will not make any mistake in the clinic.

2. Drugs must be carefully selected and prepared according to the refining process of Lei Kung. Remedies should be prepared according to the pharmaceutical formulae but may be altered to suit the patient's condition. Decoctions and powders should be freely made. Pills and distilled medicine should be prepared in advance. The older the plaster is the more effective it will be. Tampons become more effective on standing. Don't spare valuable drugs; their use is eventually advantageous.

3. A physician should not be arrogant and insult other physicians in the same district. He should be modest and careful towards his colleagues; respect his seniors, help his juniors, learn from his superiors and yield to the arrogant. Thus there will be no slander and hatred. Harmony will be esteemed by all.

4. The managing of a family is just like the curing of a disease. If the constitution of a man is not well cared for and becomes over-exhausted, diseases will attack him. Mild ones will weaken his physique, while serious ones may result in death. Similarly, if the foundation of the family is not firmly established and extravagance be indulged in, reserves will gradually drain away and poverty will come.

5. Man receives his fate from Heaven. He should not be ungrateful to the Heavenly decree. Professional gains should be approved by the conscience and conform to the Heavenly will. If the gain is made according to the Heavenly will, natural affinity takes place. If not, offspring will be condemned. Is it not better to make light of professional gain in order to avoid the evil retribution?

6. Gifts, except in the case of weddings, funerals and for the consolation of the sick, should be simple. One dish of fish and one of vegetable will suffice for a meal. This is not only to reduce expenses but also to save provisions. The virtue of a man lies not in grasping but rather in economy.

7. Medicine should be given free to the poor. Extra financial help should be extended to the destitute patients, if possible. Without food, medicine alone can not relieve the distress of a patient.

8. Savings should be invested in real estate but not in curios and unnecessary luxuries. The physician should also not join the drinking club and the gambling house which would hinder his practice. Hatred and slander can thus be avoided.

9. Office and dispensary should be fully equipped with necessary apparatus. The physician should improve his knowledge by studying medical books, old and new, and reading current publications. This really is the fundamental duty of a physician.

10. A physician should be ready to respond to the call of government officials with respect and sincerity. He should inform them of the cause of the disease and prescribe accordingly. After healing he should not seek for a complimentary tablet [a wooden board inscribed with complimentary words, hung in the physician's office for propaganda] or plead excuse for another's difficulty. A person who respects the law should not associate with officials.

# A PHYSICIAN'S ETHICAL DUTIES
### From *Kholasah al Hekmah*
#### 1770

*In 1770* C.E., *during Persia's Islamic era, Mohamad Hosin Aghili of Shiraz wrote the work* Kholasah al Hekmah. *The first chapter of that work contains a list of ethical duties for the physician, which are printed here in condensed form.*

1. A physician must not be conceited; he should know that the actual healer is God.

2. He should praise his teachers and professor and return thanks to them for their kindnesses.

3. He should never slander another physician. The fault of others should occasion the recognition of his own fault, not be the occasion for pride and conceit.

4. He must speak to patients with civility and good humor and never get angry at the misbehavior and insults of patients.

5. He must protect the patients' secrets and not betray them, especially to those the patients do not want to know.

6. In the case of the transmission of disease, the physician must not turn the second patient against the first.

7. He must be energetic in studying diseases and drugs and earnest in the diagnosis and treatment of a patient or disease.

8. He must never be tenacious in his opinion, and continue in his fault or mistake but, if it is possible, he is to consult with proficient physicians and ascertain the facts.

9. If someone mentions a useless or wrong idea, he must not turn it down definitely

but say politely, "Maybe it is true in some cases but, in my opinion, in this case it is more probably such and such."

10. If a prior physician has a better knowledge of a patient or disease, he has to encourage the patient to return to the first physician.

11. If he is not successful in the treatment of a case or if he has found the patient did not have confidence in his work or that the patient would like to refer to another physician, it is better to offer an excuse and ask him to consult another physician.

12. He must not be prejudiced against any method of treatment and never continue any wrong practice.

13. In the treatment of disease, he must begin with simple medicine and not recommend any drug as long as the nature of the disease is resistant to it and it would not be effective.

14. If a patient has several diseases, first of all he has to cure the main disease which may be the cause of complications.

15. He should never recommend any kind of fatal, harmful or enfeebling drugs; he has to know that as a physician he has to do what is conducive to the patient's temperament, and temperament itself is an efficient corrector and protector of the body, not fatal or destructive.

16. He must not be proud of his class or his family and must not regard others with contempt.

17. He must not withhold medical knowledge; he should teach it to everyone in medicine without any discrimination between poor or rich, noble or slave.

18. He must not hold his students or his patients under his obligation.

19. He must be content, grateful, generous and magnanimous, and never be covetous, greedy, ravenous or jealous.

20. He must never covet another's property. If someone offers him a present while he himself is in need of it, he must not accept it.

21. He must never claim that he can cure an impoverished patient who has gone to many physicians, and should not jeopardize his own reputation.

22. He should never be gluttonous and become involved in pleasure-seeking, buffoonery, drinking, and other sins.

23. He must not look upon women with lust but must look at them as he looks at his daughter, sister, or mother.


## DAILY PRAYER OF A PHYSICIAN
## ("PRAYER OF MOSES MAIMONIDES")
### 1793?

*Although there is considerable debate about this prayer's true authorship, it was first attributed to Moses Maimonides, a twelfth-century Jewish physician in Egypt. Many now believe it was in fact authored by Marcus Herz, a German physician, pupil of Immanuel Kant, and physician to Moses Mendelssohn. The prayer first appeared in print in 1793 as "Tägliches Gebet eines Arztes bevor er seine Kranken besucht—Aus der hebräischen Handschrift eines berühmten jüdischen Arztes in Egypten aus dem zwölften Jahrhundert" ("Daily prayer of a physician before he visits his patients—From the Hebrew manuscript of a renowned Jewish physician in Egypt from the twelfth century"). The Prayer of Moses Maimonides and the Oath of Hippocrates are probably the best known of the older statements on medical ethics.*

Almighty God, Thou has created the human body with infinite wisdom. Ten thousand times ten thousand organs hast Thou combined in it that act unceasingly and harmoniously to preserve the whole in all its beauty—the body which is the envelope of the immortal soul. They are ever acting in perfect order, agreement and accord. Yet, when the frailty of matter or the unbridling of passions deranges this order or interrupts this accord, then forces clash and the body crumbles into the primal dust from which it came. Thou sendest to man diseases as beneficent messengers to foretell approaching danger and to urge him to avert it.

Thou has blest Thine earth, Thy rivers and Thy mountains with healing substances; they enable Thy creatures to alleviate their sufferings and to heal their illnesses. Thou hast endowed man with the wisdom to relieve the suffering of his brother, to recognize his disorders, to extract the healing substances, to discover their powers and to prepare and to apply them to suit every ill. In Thine Eternal Providence Thou hast chosen me to watch over the life and health of Thy creatures. I am now about to apply myself to the duties of my profession. Support me, Almighty God, in these great labors that they may benefit mankind, for without Thy help not even the least thing will succeed.

Inspire me with love for my art and for Thy creatures. Do not allow thirst for profit, ambition for renown and admiration, to interfere with my profession, for these are the enemies of truth and of love for mankind and they can lead astray in the great task of attending to the welfare of Thy creatures. Preserve the strength of my body and of my soul that they ever be ready to cheerfully help and support rich and poor, good and bad, enemy as well as friend. In the sufferer let me see only the human being. Illumine my mind that it recognize what presents itself and that it may comprehend what is absent or hidden. Let it not fail to see what is visible, but do not permit it to arrogate to itself the power to see what cannot be seen, for delicate and indefinite are the bounds of the great art of caring for the lives and health of Thy creatures. Let me never be absent-minded. May no strange thoughts divert my attention at the bedside of the sick, or disturb my mind in its silent labors, for great and sacred are the thoughtful deliberations required to preserve the lives and health of Thy creatures.

Grant that my patients have confidence in me and my art and follow my directions and my counsel. Remove from their midst all charlatans and the whole host of officious relatives and know-all nurses, cruel people who arrogantly frustrate the wisest purposes of our art and often lead Thy creatures to their death.

Should those who are wiser than I wish to improve and instruct me, let my soul gratefully follow their guidance; for vast is the extent of our art. Should conceited fools, however, censure me, then let love for my profession steel me against them, so that I remain steadfast without regard for age, for reputation, or for honor, because surrender would bring to Thy creatures sickness and death.

Imbue my soul with gentleness and calmness when older colleagues, proud of their age, wish to displace me or to scorn me or disdainfully to teach me. May even this be of advantage to me, for they know many things of which I am ignorant, but let not their arrogance give me pain. For they are old and old age is not master of the passions. I also hope to attain old age upon this earth, before Thee, Almighty God!

Let me be contented in everything except in the great science of my profession. Never allow the thought to arise in me that I have attained to sufficient knowledge, but vouchsafe to me the strength, the leisure and the ambition ever to extend my knowledge. For art is great, but the mind of man is ever expanding.

Almighty God! Thou has chosen me in Thy mercy to watch over the life and death of Thy creatures. I now apply myself to my profession. Support me in this great task so that it may benefit mankind, for without Thy help not even the least thing will succeed.

# CODE OF ETHICS
## American Medical Association
### 1847

*The American Medical Association's (AMA) first code of ethics can be understood only in light of the work in medical ethics done by Thomas Percival, an eighteenth-century English physician. Percival wrote the first comprehensive modern statement of medical ethics in response to a request from the trustees of the Manchester Infirmary to draw up a "scheme of professional conduct relative to hospitals and other medical charities" that would resolve conflicts among infirmary physicians and prevent future conflicts. In 1794, after three years of writing and revising, Percival privately distributed a book titled Medical Ethics. Finally published in 1803, Percival's Medical Ethics served for many years as a model for the ethics codes of medical societies in both England and the United States.*

*When the AMA was founded in 1847, its first tasks were to establish standards for medical education and to formulate a code of ethics. Because most of the existing American codes of medical ethics relied heavily on Thomas Percival's work, the AMA followed suit, frequently preserving Percival's wording. The code of 1847, adopted by both the AMA and the New York Academy of Medicine, is excerpted below.*

Chapter I. OF THE DUTIES OF PHYSICIANS TO THEIR PATIENTS, AND OF THE OBLIGATIONS OF PATIENTS TO THEIR PHYSICIANS

ART. I—*Duties of Physicians to their Patients*

1. A physician should not only be ever ready to obey the calls of the sick, but his mind ought also to be imbued with the greatness of his mission, and of the responsibility he habitually incurs in its discharge. Those obligations are the more deep and enduring, because there is no tribunal other than his own conscience, to adjudge penalties for carelessness or neglect. Physicians should, therefore, minister to the sick with due impressions of the importance of their office; reflecting that the ease, the health, and the lives

of those committed to their charge, depend on their skill, attention and fidelity. They should study, also, in their deportment, so to unite *tenderness* with *firmness*, and *condescension* with *authority*, as to inspire the minds of their patients with gratitude, respect and confidence.

2. Every case committed to the charge of a physician should be treated with attention, steadiness and humanity. Reasonable indulgence should be granted to the mental imbecility and caprices of the sick. Secrecy and delicacy, when required by peculiar circumstances, should be strictly observed; and the familiar and confidential intercourse to which physicians are admitted in their professional visits, should be used with discretion, and with the most scrupulous regard to fidelity and honor. The obligation of secrecy extends beyond the period of professional services;—none of the privacies of personal and domestic life, no infirmity of disposition or flaw of character observed during professional attendance, should ever be divulged by him except when he is imperatively required to do so. The force and necessity of this obligation are indeed so great, that professional men have, under certain circumstances, been protected in their observance of secrecy by courts of justice.

3. Frequent visits to the sick are in general requisite, since they enable the physician to arrive at a more perfect knowledge of the disease,—to meet promptly every change which may occur, and also tend to preserve the confidence of the patient. But unnecessary visits are to be avoided, as they give useless anxiety to the patient, tend to diminish the authority of the physician, and render him liable to be suspected of interested motives.

4. A physician should not be forward to make gloomy prognostications, because they savor of empiricism, by magnifying the importance of his services in the treatment or cure of the disease. But he should not fail, on proper occasions, to give to the friends of the patient timely notice of danger, when it really occurs; and even to the patient himself, if absolutely necessary. This office, however, is so peculiarly alarming when executed by him, that it ought to be declined whenever it can be assigned to any other person of sufficient judgment and delicacy. For, the physician should be the minister of hope and comfort to the sick; that, by such cordials to the drooping spirit, he may smooth the bed of death, revive expiring life, and counteract the depressing influence of those maladies which often disturb the tranquility of the most resigned, in their last moments. The life of a sick person can be shortened not only by the acts, but also by the words or the manner of a physician. It is, therefore, a sacred duty to guard himself carefully in this respect, and to avoid all things which have a tendency to discourage the patient and to depress his spirits.

5. A physician ought not to abandon a patient because the case is deemed incurable; for his attendance may continue to be highly useful to the patient, and comforting to the relatives around him, even to the last period of a fatal malady, by alleviating pain and other symptoms, and by soothing mental anguish. To decline attendance, under such circumstances, would be sacrificing to fanciful delicacy and mistaken liberality, that moral duty, which is independent of, and far superior to all pecuniary consideration.

6. Consultations should be promoted in difficult or protracted cases, as they give rise to confidence, energy, and more enlarged views in practice.

7. The opportunity which a physician not unfrequently enjoys of promoting and strengthening the good resolutions of his patients, suffering under the consequences of vicious conduct, ought never to be neglected. His counsels, or even remonstrances, will give satisfaction, not offence, if they be proffered with politeness, and evince a genuine love of virtue, accompanied by a sincere interest in the welfare of the person to whom they are addressed.

Art. II—*Obligations of Patients to their Physicians*

1. The members of the medical profession, upon whom are enjoined the performance of so many important and arduous duties towards the community, and who are required to make so many sacrifices of comfort, ease, and health, for the welfare of those who avail themselves of their services, certainly have a right to expect and require, that their patients should entertain a just sense of the duties which they owe to their medical attendants.

2. The first duty of a patient is, to select as his medical adviser one who has received a regular professional education. In no trade or occupation do mankind rely on the skill of an untaught artist; and in medicine, confessedly the most difficult and intricate of the sciences, the world ought not to suppose that knowledge is intuitive.

3. Patients should prefer a physician whose habits of life are regular, and who is not devoted to company, pleasure, or to any pursuit incompatible with his professional obligations. A patient should also confide the care of himself and family, as much as possible, to one physician, for a medical man who has become acquainted with the

peculiarities of constitution, habits, and predispositions, of those he attends, is more likely to be successful in his treatment than one who does not possess that knowledge.

A patient who has thus selected his physician, should always apply for advice in whatever may appear to him trivial cases, for the most fatal results often supervene on the slightest accidents. It is of still more importance that he should apply for assistance in the forming stage of violent diseases; it is to a neglect of this precept that medicine owes much of the uncertainty and imperfection with which it has been reproached.

4. Patients should faithfully and unreservedly communicate to their physician the supposed cause of their disease. This is the more important, as many diseases of a mental origin simulate those depending on external causes, and yet are only to be cured by ministering to the mind diseased. A patient should never be afraid of thus making his physician his friend and adviser; he should always bear in mind that a medical man is under the strongest obligations of secrecy. Even the female sex should never allow feelings of shame and delicacy to prevent their disclosing the seat, symptoms and causes of complaints peculiar to them. However commendable a modest reserve may be in the common occurrences of life, its strict observance in medicine is often attended with the most serious consequences, and a patient may sink under a painful and loathsome disease, which might have been readily prevented had timely intimation been given to the physician.

5. A patient should never weary his physician with a tedious detail of events or matters not appertaining to his disease. Even as relates to his actual symptoms, he will convey much more real information by giving clear answers to interrogatories, than by the most minute account of his own framing. Neither should he obtrude the details of his business nor the history of his family concerns.

6. The obedience of a patient to the prescriptions of his physician should be prompt and implicit. He should never permit his own crude opinions as to their fitness, to influence his attention to them. A failure in one particular may render an otherwise judicious treatment dangerous, and even fatal. This remark is equally applicable to diet, drink, and exercise. As patients become convalescent, they are very apt to suppose that the rules prescribed for them may be disregarded, and the consequence, but too often, is a relapse. Patients should never allow themselves to be persuaded to take any medicine whatever, that may be recommended to them by the self-constituted doctors and doctoresses, who are so frequently met with, and who pretend to possess infallible remedies for the cure of every disease. However simple some of their prescriptions may appear to be, it often happens that they are productive of much mischief, and in all cases they are injurious, by contravening the plan of treatment adopted by the physician.

7. A patient should, if possible, avoid even the *friendly visits of a physician* who is not attending him—and when he does receive them, he should never converse on the subject of his disease, as an observation may be made, without any intention of interference, which may destroy his confidence in the course he is pursuing, and induce him to neglect the directions prescribed to him. A patient should never send for a consulting physician without the express consent of his own medical attendant. It is of great importance that physicians should act in concert; for, although their modes of treatment may be attended with equal success when employed singly, yet conjointly they are very likely to be productive of disastrous results.

8. When a patient wishes to dismiss his physician, justice and common courtesy require that he should declare his reasons for so doing.

9. Patients should always, when practicable, send for their physician in the morning, before his usual hour of going out; for, by being early aware of the visits he has to pay during the day, the physician is able to apportion his time in such a manner as to prevent an interference of engagements. Patients should also avoid calling on their medical adviser unnecessarily during the hours devoted to meals or sleep. They should always be in readiness to receive the visits of their physician, as the detention of a few minutes is often of serious inconvenience to him.

10. A patient should, after his recovery, entertain a just and enduring sense of the value of the services rendered him by his physician; for these are of such a character, that no mere pecuniary acknowledgment can repay or cancel them.

Chapter II. OF THE DUTIES OF PHYSICIANS TO EACH OTHER AND TO THE PROFESSION AT LARGE

ART. 1—*Duties for the support of professional character*

1. Every individual, on entering the profession, as he becomes thereby entitled to all its privileges and immunities, incurs an obligation to exert his best abilities to maintain its dignity and honor, to exalt its standing, and to extend the bounds of its usefulness. He should therefore observe strictly, such laws as are instituted for the government of its

members;—should avoid all contumelious and sarcastic remarks relative to the faculty, as a body; and while, by unwearied diligence, he resorts to every honorable means of enriching the science, he should entertain a due respect for his seniors, who have, by their labors, brought it to the elevated condition in which he finds it.

2. There is no profession, from the members of which greater purity of character and a higher standard of moral excellence are required, than the medical; and to attain such eminence, is a duty every physician owes alike to his profession, and to his patients. It is due to the latter, as without it he cannot command their respect and confidence; and to both, because no scientific attainments can compensate for the want of correct moral principles. It is also incumbent upon the faculty to be temperate in all things, for the practice of physic requires the unremitting exercise of a clear and vigorous understanding; and, on emergencies for which no professional man should be unprepared, a steady hand, an acute eye, and an unclouded head, may be essential to the well-being, and even life, of a fellow creature.

3. It is derogatory to the dignity of the profession, to resort to public advertisements or private cards or handbills, inviting the attention of individuals affected with particular diseases—publicly offering advice and medicine to the poor gratis, or promising radical cures; or to publish cases and operations in the daily prints, or suffer such publications to be made;—to invite laymen to be present at operations—to boast of cures and remedies—to adduce certificates of skill and success, or to perform any other similar acts. These are the ordinary practices of empirics, and are highly reprehensible in a regular physician.

4. Equally derogatory to professional character is it, for a physician to hold a patent for any surgical instrument, or medicine; or to dispense a secret *nostrum,* whether it be the composition or exclusive property of himself or of others. For, if such nostrum be of real efficacy, any concealment regarding it is inconsistent with beneficence and professional liberality; and, if mystery alone give it value and importance, such craft implies either disgraceful ignorance, or fraudulent avarice. It is also reprehensible for physicians to give certificates attesting the efficacy of patent or secret medicines, or in any way to promote the use of them.

ART. II—*Professional services of Physicians to each other*

1. All practitioners of medicine, their wives, and their children while under the paternal care, are entitled to the gratuitous services of any one or more of the faculty residing near them, whose assistance may be desired. A physician afflicted with disease is usually an incompetent judge of his own case; and the natural anxiety and solicitude which he experiences at the sickness of a wife, a child, or any one who by the ties of consanguinity is rendered peculiarly dear to him, tend to obscure his judgment, and produce timidity and irresolution in his practice. Under such circumstances, medical men are peculiarly dependent upon each other, and kind offices and professional aid should always be cheerfully and gratuitously afforded. Visits ought not, however, to be obtruded officiously; as such unasked civility may give rise to embarrassment, or interfere with that choice on which confidence depends. But, if a distant member of the faculty, whose circumstances are affluent, request attendance, and an honorarium be offered, it should not be declined; for no pecuniary obligation ought to be imposed, which the party receiving it would wish not to incur.

• • •

ART. IV—*Of the duties of Physicians in regard to consultations*

1. A regular medical education furnishes the only presumptive evidence of professional abilities and acquirements, and ought to be the only acknowledged right of an individual to the exercise and honors of his profession. Nevertheless, as in consultations, the good of the patient is the sole object in view, and this is often dependent on personal confidence, no intelligent regular practitioner, who has a license to practise from some medical board of known and acknowledged respectability, recognised by this association, and who is in good moral and professional standing in the place in which he resides, should be fastidiously excluded from fellowship, or his aid refused in consultation when it is requested by the patient. But no one can be considered as a regular practitioner, or fit associate in consultation, whose practice is based on an exclusive dogma, to the rejection of the accumulated experience of the profession, and of the aids actually furnished by anatomy, physiology, pathology, and organic chemistry.

2. In consultations, no rivalship or jealousy should be indulged; candor, probity, and all due respect, should be exercised towards the physician having charge of the case.

3. In consultations, the attending physician should be the first to propose the necessary questions to the sick; after which the consulting physician should have the opportunity to make such farther inquiries of the patient as may be necessary to satisfy him of the true character of the case. Both physicians should then retire to a private place for

deliberation; and the one first in attendance should communicate the directions agreed upon to the patient or his friends, as well as any opinions which it may be thought proper to express. But no statement or discussion of it should take place before the patient or his friends, except in the presence of all the faculty attending, and by their common consent; and no *opinions* or *prognostications* should be delivered, which are not the result of previous deliberation and concurrence.

4. In consultations, the physician in attendance should deliver his opinion first; and when there are several consulting, they should deliver their opinions in the order in which they have been called in. No decision, however, should restrain the attending physician from making such variations in the mode of treatment, as any subsequent unexpected change in the character of the case may demand. But such variation and the reasons for it ought to be carefully detailed at the next meeting in consultation. The same privilege belongs also to the consulting physician if he is sent for in an emergency, when the regular attendant is out of the way, and similar explanations must be made by him, at the next consultation.

• • •

7. All discussions in consultation should be held as secret and confidential. Neither by words nor manner should any of the parties to a consultation assert or insinuate, that any part of the treatment pursued did not receive his assent. The responsibility must be equally divided between the medical attendants—they must equally share the credit of success as well as the blame of failure.

8. Should an irreconcilable diversity of opinion occur when several physicians are called upon to consult together, the opinion of the majority should be considered as decisive; but if the numbers be equal on each side, then the decision should rest with the attending physician. It may, moreover, sometimes happen, that two physicians cannot agree in their views of the nature of a case, and the treatment to be pursued. This is a circumstance much to be deplored, and should always be avoided, if possible, by mutual concessions, as far as they can be justified by a conscientious regard for the dictates of judgment. But in the event of its occurrence, a third physician should, if practicable, be called to act as umpire; and if circumstances prevent the adoption of this course, it must be left to the patient to select the physician in whom he is most willing to confide. But as every physician relies upon the rectitude of his judgment, he should, when left in the minority, politely and consistently retire from any further deliberation in the consultation, or participation in the management of the case.

• • •

10. A physician who is called upon to consult, should observe the most honorable and scrupulous regard for the character and standing of the practitioner in attendance: the practice of the latter, if necessary, should be justified as far as it can be, consistently with a conscientious regard for truth, and no hint or insinuation should be thrown out, which could impair the confidence reposed in him, or affect his reputation. The consulting physician should also carefully refrain from any of those extraordinary attentions or assiduities, which are too often practiced by the dishonest for the base purpose of gaining applause, or ingratiating themselves into the favor of families and individuals.

Art. V—*Duties of Physicians in cases of interference*
1. Medicine is a liberal profession, and those admitted into its ranks should found their expectations of practice upon the extent of their qualifications, not on intrigue or artifice.

2. A physician in his intercourse with a patient under the care of another practitioner, should observe the strictest caution and reserve. No meddling inquiries should be made; no disingenuous hints given relative to the nature and treatment of his disorder; nor any course of conduct pursued that may directly or indirectly tend to diminish the trust reposed in the physician employed.

3. The same circumspection and reserve should be observed, when, from motives of business or friendship, a physician is prompted to visit an individual who is under the direction of another practitioner. Indeed, such visits should be avoided, except under peculiar circumstances; and when they are made, no particular inquiries should be instituted relative to the nature of the disease, or the remedies employed, but the topics of conversation should be as foreign to the case as circumstances will admit.

• • •

Art. VI—*Of differences between Physicians*
1. Diversity of opinion, and opposition of interest, may, in the medical, as in other professions, sometimes occasion controversy and even contention. Whenever such cases

unfortunately occur, and cannot be immediately terminated, they should be referred to the arbitration of a sufficient number of physicians, or a *court-medical.*

As peculiar reserve must be maintained by physicians towards the public, in regard to professional matters, and as there exist numerous points in medical ethics and etiquette through which the feelings of medical men may be painfully assailed in their intercourse with each other, and which cannot be understood or appreciated by general society, neither the subject-matter of such differences nor the adjudication of the arbitrators should be made public, as publicity in a case of this nature may be personally injurious to the individuals concerned, and can hardly fail to bring discredit on the faculty.

• • •

Chapter III. OF THE DUTIES OF THE PROFESSION TO THE PUBLIC, AND OF THE OBLIGATIONS OF THE PUBLIC TO THE PROFESSION

ART. I—*Duties of the profession to the public*

1. As good citizens, it is the duty of physicians to be ever vigilant for the welfare of the community, and to bear their part in sustaining its institutions and burdens: they should also be ever ready to give counsel to the public in relation to matters especially appertaining to their profession, as on subjects of medical police, public hygiene, and legal medicine. It is their province to enlighten the public in regard to quarantine regulations,—the location, arrangement, and dietaries of hospitals, asylums, schools, prisons, and similar institutions,—in relation to the medical police of towns, as drainage, ventilation, &c.,—and in regard to measures for the prevention of epidemic and contagious diseases; and when pestilence prevails, it is their duty to face the danger, and to continue their labors for the alleviation of the suffering, even at the jeopardy of their own lives.

2. Medical men should also be always ready, when called on by the legally constituted authorities, to enlighten coroners' inquests and courts of justice, on subjects strictly medical,—such as involve questions relating to sanity, legitimacy, murder by poisons or other violent means, and in regard to the various other subjects embraced in the science of Medical Jurisprudence. But in these cases, and especially where they are required to make a post-mortem examination, it is just, in consequence of the time, labor and skill required, and the responsibility and risk they incur, that the public should award them a proper honorarium.

3. There is no profession, by the members of which, eleemosynary services are more liberally dispensed, than the medical; but justice requires that some limits should be placed to the performance of such good offices. Poverty, professional brotherhood, and certain public duties referred to in section 1 of this chapter, should always be recognised as presenting valid claims for gratuitous services; but neither institutions endowed by the public or by rich individuals, societies for mutual benefit, for the insurance of lives or for analogous purposes, nor any profession or occupation, can be admitted to possess such privilege. Nor can it be justly expected of physicians to furnish certificates of inability to serve on juries, to perform militia duty, or to testify to the state of health of persons wishing to insure their lives, obtain pensions, or the like, without a pecuniary acknowledgment. But to individuals in indigent circumstances, such professional services should always be cheerfully and freely accorded.

4. It is the duty of physicians, who are frequent witnesses of the enormities committed by quackery, and the injury to health and even destruction of life caused by the use of quack medicines, to enlighten the public on these subjects, to expose the injuries sustained by the unwary from the devices and pretensions of artful empirics and impostors. Physicians ought to use all the influence which they may possess, as professors in Colleges of Pharmacy, and by exercising their option in regard to the shops to which their prescriptions shall be sent, to discourage druggists and apothecaries from vending quack or secret medicines, or from being in any way engaged in their manufacture and sale.

ART. II—*Obligations of the public to Physicians*

1. The benefits accruing to the public directly and indirectly from the active and unwearied beneficence of the profession, are so numerous and important, that physicians are justly entitled to the utmost consideration and respect from the community. The public ought likewise to entertain a just appreciation of medical qualifications;—to make a proper discrimination between true science and the assumption of ignorance and empiricism,—to afford every encouragement and facility for the acquisition of medical education,—and no longer to allow the statute books to exhibit the anomaly of exacting knowledge from physicians, under liability to heavy penalties, and of making them obnoxious to punishment for resorting to the only means of obtaining it.

# VENEZUELAN CODE OF MEDICAL ETHICS
## National Academy of Medicine
### 1918

The Venezuelan Code, first promulgated by the National Academy of Medicine of Venezuela in 1918, was largely the work of Dr. Luis Razetti and for this reason is sometimes called the "Razetti Code." It served as a model for other Latin American codes of medical ethics (Colombia, 1919; Peru, 1922). The Sixth Latin American Medical Congress, meeting in Havana in 1922, recommended that the Venezuelan Code (slightly revised in 1922) serve to unify medical ethical concerns in Latin America. The First Brazilian Medical Congress, held in Rio de Janeiro in 1931, was similarly influenced by the Venezuelan Code.

The Venezuelan Code of 1918 includes many elements characteristic of the codes of its day, with heavy emphasis on the protection of the dignity of the profession, the maintenance of high standards of competence and training, duties toward patients (even regarding their health habits), the rendering of professional services to other doctors, obligations regarding substitute physicians and consultants, professional discipline, fees, and the like.

There are several interesting features in the Venezuelan Code that deserve comparison with other codes:

1. The code insists that there are "rules of medical deontology" that apply to the entire "medical guild"—physicians, surgeons, pharmacists, dentists, obstetricians, internes, and nurses.

2. It places emphasis on physicians' virtues and qualities of character—circumspection, honesty, honor, good faith, respect, and so forth—that serve as a basis for those practices of etiquette that support the honorable practice of medicine.

3. The code prohibits abortion and premature childbirth (morally and legally), except "for a therapeutic purpose in cases indicated by medical science"; but it permits embryotomy if the mother's life is in danger and no alternative medical skills are available.

4. The excerpt below contains an interesting and detailed set of instructions on "medical confidentiality." It combines a strong affirmation of the moral obligation of health professionals to observe confidentiality with many attenuations of that obligation in the interests of the public welfare.

## Chapter IX. On Medical Confidentiality

*Article 68.* Medical confidentiality is a duty inherent in the very nature of the medical profession; the public interest, the personal security of the ill, the honor of families, respect for the physician, and the dignity of the art require confidentiality. Doctors, surgeons, dentists, pharmacists, and midwives as well as interns and nurses are morally obligated to safeguard privacy of information in everything they see, hear, or discover in the practice of their profession or outside of their services and which should not be divulged.

*Article 69.* Confidential information may be of two forms: that which is explicitly confidential—formal, documentary information confided by the client—and that which is implicitly confidential, which is private due to the nature of things, which nobody imposes, and which governs the relations of clients with medical professionals. Both forms are inviolable, except for legally specified cases.

*Article 70.* Medical professionals are prohibited from revealing professionally privileged information except in those cases established by medical ethics. A revelation is an act which causes the disclosed fact to change from a private to a publicly known fact. It is not necessary to publish such a fact to make it a revealed one: it suffices to confide it to a single person.

*Article 71.* Professionally confidential information belongs to the client. Professionals do not incur any responsibility if they reveal the private information received by them when they are authorized to do so by the patient in complete freedom and with a knowledge of the consequences by the person or persons who have confided in them, provided always that such revelation causes no harm to a third party.

*Article 72.* A medical person incurs no responsibility when he reveals private information in the following cases:

1. When in his capacity as a medical expert he acts as a physician for an insurance company giving it information concerning the health of the applicant sent to him for examination; or when he is commissioned by a proper authority to identify the physical or mental health of a person; or when he has been designated to perform autopsies or give medico-legal expert knowledge of any kind, as in civil or criminal cases; or when he acts as a doctor of public health or for the city; and in general when he performs the functions of a medical expert.

2. When the treating physician declares certain diseases infectious and contagious before a health authority; and when he issues death certificates.

In any of the cases included in (1), the medical professional may be exempt from the charge of ignoring the right of privacy of a person who is the object of his examination if said person is his client at the time or if the declaration has to do with previous conditions for which the same doctor was privately consulted.

*Article 73.* The physician shall preserve utmost secrecy if he happens to detect a venereal disease in a married woman. Not only should he refrain from informing her of the nature of the disease but he should be very careful not to let suspicion fall on the husband as responsible for the contagion. Consequently, he shall not issue any certification or make any disclosure even if the husband gives his consent.

*Article 74.* If a physician knows that one of his patients in a contagious period of a venereal disease plans to be married, he shall take pains to dissuade his patient from doing so, availing himself of all possible means. If the patient ignores his advice and insists on going ahead with his plan to marry, the physician is authorized without incurring responsibility not only to give the information the bride's family asks for, but also to prevent the marriage without the bridegroom's prior consultation or authorization.

*Article 75.* The doctor who knows that a healthy wet-nurse is nursing a syphilitic child should warn the child's parents that they are obligated to inform the nurse. If they refuse to do so, the doctor without naming the disease will impose on the nurse the necessity of immediately ceasing to nurse the child, and he should arrange to have her remain in the house for the time needed to make sure that she has not caught the disease. If the parents do not give their consent and insist that the wet-nurse continue to nurse the child, the doctor shall offer the necessary arguments, and if they nevertheless persist he shall inform the nurse of the risk she runs of contracting a contagious disease if she continues to nurse the child.

*Article 76.* The doctor can without failing in his duty denounce crimes of which he may have knowledge in the exercise of his profession, in accord with article 470 of the [Venezuelan] Penal Code.

*Article 77.* When it is a matter of making an accusation in court in order to avoid a legal violation the doctor is permitted to disclose private information.

*Article 78.* When a doctor is brought before a court as a witness to testify to certain facts known to him, he may refuse to disclose professionally private facts about which he is being interrogated, but which he considers privileged.

*Article 79.* When a doctor finds himself obliged to claim his fees legally, he should limit himself to stating the number of visits and consultations, specifying the days and nights, the number of operations he has performed, specifying the major and minor ones, the number of trips made outside the city to attend the patient, indicating the distance and time involved in travel in each visit, etc., but in no case should he reveal the nature of the operations performed, nor the details of the care that was given to the patient. The explanation of these circumstances, if necessary, shall be referred by the doctor to the medical experts so designated by the court.

*Article 80.* The doctor should not answer questions concerning the nature of his patient's disease; however, he is authorized not only to tell the prognosis of the case to those closest to the patient but also the diagnosis if on occasion he considers it necessary, in view of his professional responsibility or the best treatment of his patient. . . .

# DECLARATION OF GENEVA
## World Medical Association
### 1948, amended 1968, 1983

*The Declaration of Geneva was adopted by the second General Assembly of the World Medical Association (WMA) at Geneva in 1948, and subsequently amended by the twenty-second World Medical Assembly at Sydney in 1968 and the thirty-fifth World Medical Assembly at Venice in 1983. The declaration, which was one of the first and most important actions of the WMA, is a declaration of physicians' dedication to the humanitarian goals of medicine, a pledge that was especially important in view of the medical crimes that had just been committed in Nazi Germany. The Declaration of Geneva was intended to update the Oath of Hippocrates, which was no longer suited to modern conditions. Of interest is the fact that the WMA considered this short declaration to be a more significant statement of medical ethics than the succeeding International Code of Medical Ethics.*

*Only two changes have been made in the declaration since 1948. In 1968, the phrase "even after the patient has died" was added to the confidentiality clause. In the 1983 version, which follows, the sentence regarding respect for human life was modified. Prior to 1983, it read, "I will maintain the utmost respect for human life from the time of conception. . . ."*

At the time of being admitted as a member of the medical profession:

I solemnly pledge myself to consecrate my life to the service of humanity;
I will give to my teachers the respect and gratitude which is their due;
I will practice my profession with conscience and dignity;
The health of my patient will be my first consideration;
I will respect the secrets which are confided in me, even after the patient has died;
I will maintain by all the means in my power, the honor and the noble traditions of the medical profession;
My colleagues will be my brothers;
I will not permit considerations of religion, nationality, race, party politics or social standing to intervene between my duty and my patient;
I will maintain the utmost respect for human life from its beginning even under threat and I will not use my medical knowledge contrary to the laws of humanity;

I make these promises solemnly, freely and upon my honor.

# INTERNATIONAL CODE OF MEDICAL ETHICS
**World Medical Association**
1949, amended 1968, 1983

*The International Code of Medical Ethics was adopted by the third General Assembly of the World Medical Association (WMA) at London in 1949, and amended in 1968 by the twenty-second World Medical Assembly at Sydney and in 1983 by the thirty-fifth World Medical Assembly at Venice. The code, which was modeled after the Declaration of Geneva and the medical ethics codes of most modern countries, states the most general principles of ethical medical practice.*

*The original draft of the code included the statement, "Therapeutic abortion may only be performed if the conscience of the doctors and the national laws permit," which was deleted from the adopted version because of its controversial nature. In addition, the words "from conception" were deleted from the statement regarding the doctor's obligation to preserve human life.*

*The 1983 version of the code, which is still current, reflects several changes from the version originally adopted. There are numerous changes in language, for example, the phrase "A physician shall . . ." replaces "A doctor must. . . ." Substantive changes include the addition of the paragraphs on providing competent medical service; on honesty and exposing physicians deficient in character; and on respecting rights and safeguarding confidences. Also, as in the Declaration of Geneva, the duty of confidentiality is extended to "even after the patient has died." Under practices deemed unethical, collaboration "in any form of medical service in which the doctor does not have professional independence" has been deleted, but the importance of professional independence is emphasized elsewhere in the text.*

## Duties of Physicians in General

A physician shall always maintain the highest standards of professional conduct.
A physician shall not permit motives of profit to influence the free and independent exercise of professional judgement on behalf of patients.
A physician shall, in all types of medical practice, be dedicated to providing competent medical service in full technical and moral independence, with compassion and respect for human dignity.
A physician shall deal honestly with patients and colleagues, and strive to expose those physicians deficient in character or competence, or who engage in fraud or deception.
The following practices are deemed to be unethical conduct:
a) Self-advertising by physicians, unless permitted by the laws of the country and the Code of Ethics of the National Medical Association.
b) Paying or receiving any fee or any other consideration solely to procure the referral of a patient or for prescribing or referring a patient to any source.
A physician shall respect the rights of patients, of colleagues, and of other health professionals, and shall safeguard patient confidences.
A physician shall act only in the patient's interest when providing medical care which might have the effect of weakening the physical and mental condition of the patient.
A physician shall use great caution in divulging discoveries or new techniques or treatment through non-professional channels.
A physician shall certify only that which he has personally verified.

### Duties of Physicians to the Sick

A physician shall always bear in mind the obligation of preserving human life.
A physician shall owe his patients complete loyalty and all the resources of his science. Whenever an examination or treatment is beyond the physician's capacity he should summon another physician who has the necessary ability.
A physician shall preserve absolute confidentiality on all he knows about his patient even after the patient has died.
A physician shall give emergency care as a humanitarian duty unless he is assured that others are willing and able to give such care.

### Duties of Physicians to Each Other

A physician shall behave towards his colleagues as he would have them behave towards him.
A physician shall not entice patients from his colleagues.
A physician shall observe the principles of the "Declaration of Geneva" approved by the World Medical Association.

## PRINCIPLES OF MEDICAL ETHICS (1957)
### American Medical Association
### 1957

*Until 1957, the American Medical Association's (AMA) Code of Ethics was basically that adopted in 1847, although there were revisions in 1903, 1912, and 1947. A major change in the code's format occurred in 1957 when the Principles of Medical Ethics printed here were adopted. The ten principles, which replaced the forty-eight sections of the older code, were intended as expressions of the fundamental concepts and requirements of the older code, unencumbered by easily outdated practical codifications. Of note are the therapeutic-privilege exception to the confidentiality clause in Section 9—confidences may be disclosed if "necessary in order to protect the welfare of the individual"—and Section 10, which highlights the tension between physicians' duties to patients and those to society.*

Preamble. These principles are intended to aid physicians individually and collectively in maintaining a high level of ethical conduct. They are not laws but standards by which a physician may determine the propriety of his conduct in his relationship with patients, with colleagues, with members of allied professions, and with the public.

Section 1. The principal objective of the medical profession is to render service to humanity with full respect for the dignity of man. Physicians should merit the confidence of patients entrusted to their care, rendering to each a full measure of service and devotion.

Section 2. Physicians should strive continually to improve medical knowledge and skill, and should make available to their patients and colleagues the benefits of their professional attainments.

Section 3. A physician should practice a method of healing founded on a scientific basis; and he should not voluntarily associate professionally with anyone who violates this principle.

Section 4. The medical profession should safeguard the public and itself against physicians deficient in moral character or professional competence. Physicians should observe all laws, uphold the dignity and honor of the profession and accept its self-imposed disciplines. They should expose, without hesitation, illegal or unethical conduct of fellow members of the profession.

Section 5. A physician may choose whom he will serve. In an emergency, however, he should render service to the best of his ability. Having undertaken the care of a patient, he may not neglect him; and unless he has been discharged he may discontinue his services only after giving adequate notice. He should not solicit patients.

Section 6. A physician should not dispose of his services under terms or conditions which tend to interfere with or impair the free and complete exercise of his medical judgment and skill or tend to cause a deterioration of the quality of medical care.

Section 7. In the practice of medicine a physician should limit the source of his professional income to medical services actually rendered by him, or under his supervision, to his patients. His fee should be commensurate with the services rendered and the patient's ability to pay. He should neither pay nor receive a commission for referral of patients. Drugs, remedies or appliances may be dispensed or supplied by the physician provided it is in the best interests of the patient.

Section 8. A physician should seek consultation upon request; in doubtful or difficult cases; or whenever it appears that the quality of medical service may be enhanced thereby.

Section 9. A physician may not reveal the confidences entrusted to him in the course of medical attendance, or the deficiencies he may observe in the character of patients, unless he is required to do so by law or unless it becomes necessary in order to protect the welfare of the individual or of the community.

Section 10. The honored ideals of the medical professional imply that the responsibilities of the physician extend not only to the individual, but also to society where these responsibilities deserve his interest and participation in activities which have the purpose of improving both the health and the well-being of the individual and the community.

# PRINCIPLES OF MEDICAL ETHICS (1980)
## American Medical Association
### 1980

*The American Medical Association's (AMA) complete code of ethics currently consists of four parts: (1) the Principles of Medical Ethics, which "broadly define the parameters of ethical conduct for physicians" and are the primary component of the Code; (2) the Current Opinions with Annotations of the Council on Ethical and Judicial Affairs, which is "a comprehensive set of concise statements addressing specific ethical issues in the practice of medicine" and includes extensive annotations of court opinions and pertinent medical, ethical, and legal literature; (3) the Fundamental Elements of the Patient–Physician Relationship, which "enunciates the basic rights to which patients are entitled from their physicians"; and (4) the Reports of the Council on Ethical and Judicial Affairs, which "discuss the rationale behind many of the Council's opinions, providing a detailed analysis of the relevant ethical considerations." The Principles of Medical Ethics are printed below, and selections from Current Opinions comprise the next entry in this section of the Appendix. The Fundamental Elements of the Patient–Physician Relationship appears above, in Section I.*

*The current Principles of Medical Ethics were adopted in 1980, when the earlier, 1957 principles were revised "to clarify and update the language, to eliminate reference to gender, and to seek a proper and reasonable balance between professional standards and contemporary legal standards. . . ." Among the changes, the 1980 principles, which were shortened to seven principles, introduced the language of rights to replace the traditional language of benefits and burdens and dispensed with the therapeutic-privilege exception to maintaining confidentiality.*

## Preamble

The medical profession has long subscribed to a body of ethical statements developed primarily for the benefit of the patient. As a member of this profession, a physician must recognize responsibility not only to patients, but also to society, to other health professionals, and to self. The following Principles adopted by the American Medical Association are not laws, but standards of conduct which define the essentials of honorable behavior for the physician.

I. A physician shall be dedicated to providing competent medical service with compassion and respect for human dignity.

II. A physician shall deal honestly with patients and colleagues, and strive to expose those physicians deficient in character or competence, or who engage in fraud or deception.

III. A physician shall respect the law and also recognize a responsibility to seek changes in those requirements which are contrary to the best interests of the patient.

IV. A physician shall respect the rights of patients, of colleagues, and of other health professionals, and shall safeguard patient confidences within the constraints of the law.

V. A physician shall continue to study, apply and advance scientific knowledge, make relevant information available to patients, colleagues, and the public, obtain consultation, and use the talents of other health professionals when indicated.

VI. A physician shall, in the provision of appropriate patient care, except in emergencies, be free to choose whom to serve, with whom to associate, and the environment in which to provide medical services.

VII. A physician shall recognize a responsibility to participate in activities contributing to an improved community.

# CURRENT OPINIONS OF THE COUNCIL ON ETHICAL AND JUDICIAL AFFAIRS

**American Medical Association**
1994

*The 1994 revision of the Current Opinions of the Council on Ethical and Judicial Affairs, which replaces the 1992 version, "reflects the application of the Principles of Medical Ethics to more than 125 specific ethical issues in medicine, including health care rationing, genetic testing, withdrawal of life-sustaining treatment, and family violence." A complete list of topics of the Current Opinions and the text of selected opinions follow; the annotations of court opinions and pertinent medical, ethical, and legal literature that follow many of the opinions are not included.*

• • •

## 2.00    Opinions on Social Policy Issues

**2.01    Abortion.** The Principles of Medical Ethics of the AMA do not prohibit a physician from performing an abortion in accordance with good medical practice and under circumstances that do not violate the law. (III, IV)

**2.015    Mandatory Parental Consent to Abortion.** Physicians should ascertain the law in their state on parental involvement to ensure that their procedures are consistent with their legal obligations.

Physicians should strongly encourage minors to discuss their pregnancy with their parents. Physicians should explain how parental involvement can be helpful and that parents are generally very understanding and supportive. If a minor expresses concerns about parental involvement, the physician should ensure that the minor's reluctance is not based on any misperceptions about the likely consequences of parental involvement.

Physicians should not feel or be compelled to require minors to involve their parents before deciding whether to undergo an abortion. The patient—even an adolescent—generally must decide whether, on balance, parental involvement is advisable. Accordingly, minors should ultimately be allowed to decide whether parental involvement is appropriate. Physicians should explain under what circumstances (e.g., life-threatening, emergency) the minor's confidentiality will need to be abrogated.

Physicians should try to ensure that minor patients have made an informed decision after giving careful consideration to the issues involved. They should encourage their minor patients to consult alternative sources if parents are not going to be involved in the abortion decision. Minors should be urged to seek the advice and counsel of those adults in whom they have confidence, including professional counselors, relatives, friends, teachers, or the clergy. (III, IV)

Issued June 1994 based on the report "Mandatory Parental Consent to Abortion," issued June 1992. (JAMA. 1993; 269: 82–86)

**2.02    Abuse of Children, Elderly Persons, and Others at Risk.** The following are guidelines for detecting and treating family violence:

Due to the prevalence and medical consequences of family violence, physicians should routinely inquire about abuse as part of the medical history. Physicians must also consider battering in the differential diagnosis for a number of medical complaints, particularly when treating women.

Physicians who are likely to have the opportunity to detect abuse in the course of their work have an obligation to familiarize themselves with protocols for diagnosing and treating abuse and with community resources for battered women, children and elderly persons.

Physicians also have a duty to be aware of societal misconceptions about abuse and prevent these from affecting the diagnosis and management of abuse. Such misconceptions include the belief that abuse is a rare occurrence; that abuse does not occur in "normal" families; that abuse is a private problem best resolved without outside interference; and that victims are responsible for the abuse.

In order to improve physician knowledge of family violence, physicians must be better trained to identify signs of abuse and to work cooperatively with the range of community services currently involved. Hospitals should require additional training for those physicians who are likely to see victims of abuse. Comprehensive training on family violence should be required in medical school curricula and in residency programs for specialties in which family violence is likely to be encountered.

The following are guidelines for the reporting of abuse:

Laws that require the reporting of cases of suspected abuse of children and elderly persons often create a difficult dilemma for the physician. The parties involved, both the suspected offenders and the victims, will often plead with the physician that the matter be kept confidential and not be disclosed or reported for investigation by public authorities.

Children who have been seriously injured, apparently by their parents, may nevertheless try to protect their parents by saying that the injuries were caused by an accident, such as a fall. The reason may stem from the natural parent-child relationship or fear of further punishment. Even institutionalized elderly patients who have been physically maltreated may be concerned that disclosure of what has occurred might lead to further and more drastic maltreatment by those responsible.

The physician who fails to comply with the laws requiring reporting of suspected cases of abuse to children and elderly persons and others at risk can expect that the victims could receive more severe abuse that may result in permanent bodily injury, emotional or psychological injury or even death.

Public officials concerned with the welfare of children and elderly persons have expressed the opinion that the incidence of physical violence to these persons is rapidly increasing and that a very substantial percentage of such cases is unreported by hospital personnel and physicians. A child or elderly person brought to a physician with a suspicious injury is the patient whose interests require the protection of law in a particular situation, even though the physician may also provide services from time to time to parents or other members of the family.

The obligation to comply with statutory requirements is clearly stated in the Principles of Medical Ethics. In addition, physicians have an ethical obligation to report abuse even when the law does not require it. However, for mentally competent adult victims of abuse, physicians must not disclose an abuse diagnosis to spouses or any other third party without the consent of the patient. Physicians must discuss the problem of family violence with adult patients in privacy and safety. (I, III)

Issued December 1982.

Updated June 1994 based on the report "Physicians and Family Violence: Ethical Considerations," issued December 1991. (JAMA. 1992; 267: 3190–3193)

2.03    **Allocation of Limited Medical Resources.** A physician has a duty to do all that he or she can for the benefit of the individual patient. Policies for allocating limited resources have the potential to limit the ability of physicians to fulfill this obligation to patients. Physicians have a responsibility to participate and to contribute their professional expertise in order to safeguard the interests of patients in decisions made at the societal level regarding the allocation or rationing of health resources.

Decisions regarding the allocation of limited medical resources among patients should consider only ethically appropriate criteria relating to medical need. These criteria include likelihood of benefit, urgency of need, change in quality of life, duration of benefit, and, in some cases, the amount of resources required for successful treatment. In general, only very substantial differences among patients are ethically relevant; the greater the disparities, the more justified the use of these criteria becomes. In making quality of life judgments, patients should first be prioritized so that death or extremely poor outcomes are avoided; then, patients should be prioritized according to change in quality of life, but only when there are very substantial differences among patients.

Nonmedical criteria, such as ability to pay, age, social worth, perceived obstacles to treatment, patient contribution to illness, or past use of resources should not be considered.

Allocation decisions should respect the individuality of patients and the particulars of individual cases as much as possible. When very substantial differences do not exist among potential recipients of treatment on the basis of the appropriate criteria defined above, a "first-come-first-served" approach or some other equal opportunity mechanism should be employed to make final allocation decisions. Though there are several ethically acceptable strategies for implementing these criteria, no single strategy is ethically mandated. Acceptable approaches include a three-tiered system, a minimal threshold approach, and a weighted formula. Decision-making mechanisms should be objective, flexible, and consistent to ensure that all patients are treated equally.

The treating physician must remain a patient advocate and therefore should not make allocation decisions. Patients denied access to resources have the right to be informed of the reasoning behind the decision. The allocation procedures of institutions controlling scarce resources should be disclosed to the public as well as subject to regular peer review from the medical profession. (I, VII)

Issued March 1981.

Updated June 1994 based on the report "Ethical Considerations in the Allocation of Organs and Other Scarce Medical Resources Among Patients," issued June 1993.

**2.035    Futile Care.** Physicians are not ethically obligated to deliver care that, in their best professional judgment, will not have a reasonable chance of benefitting their patients. Patients should not be given treatments simply because they demand them. Denial of treatment should be justified by reliance on openly stated ethical principles and acceptable standards of care, as defined in opinions 2.03 and 2.095, not on the concept of "futility," which cannot be meaningfully defined. (I, IV)

Issued June 1994.

• • •

**2.06    Capital Punishment.** An individual's opinion on capital punishment is the personal moral decision of the individual. A physician, as a member of a profession dedicated to preserving life when there is hope of doing so, should not be a participant in a legally authorized execution. Physician participation in execution is defined generally as actions which would fall into one or more of the following categories: (1) an action which would directly cause the death of the condemned; (2) an action which would assist, supervise, or contribute to the ability of another individual to directly cause the death of the condemned; (3) an action which could automatically cause an execution to be carried out on a condemned prisoner.

Physician participation in an execution includes, but is not limited to, the following actions: prescribing or administering tranquilizers and other psychotropic agents and medications that are part of the execution procedure; monitoring vital signs on site or remotely (including monitoring electrocardiograms); attending or observing an execution as a physician; and rendering of technical advice regarding execution.

In the case where the method of execution is lethal injection, the following actions by the physician would also constitute physician participation in execution: selecting injection sites; starting intravenous lines as a port for a lethal injection device; prescribing, preparing, administering, or supervising injection drugs or their doses or types; inspecting, testing, or maintaining lethal injection devices; and consulting with or supervising lethal injection personnel.

The following actions do not constitute physician participation in execution: (1) testifying as to competence to stand trial, testifying as to relevant medical evidence during trial, or testifying as to medical aspects of aggravating or mitigating circumstances during the penalty phase of a capital case; (2) certifying death, provided that the condemned has been declared dead by another person; (3) witnessing an execution in a totally nonprofessional capacity; (4) witnessing an execution at the specific voluntary request of the condemned person, provided that the physician observes the execution in a nonprofessional capacity; and (5) relieving the acute suffering of a condemned person while awaiting execution, including providing tranquilizers at the specific voluntary request of the condemned person to help relieve pain or anxiety in anticipation of the execution.

Organ donation by condemned prisoners is permissible only if (1) the decision to donate was made before the prisoner's conviction, (2) the donated tissue is harvested after the prisoner has been pronounced dead and the body removed from the death chamber, and (3) physicians do not provide advice on modifying the method of execution for any individual to facilitate donation. (I)

Issued July 1980.
Updated June 1994 based on the report "Physician Participation in Capital Punishment," issued December 1992. (JAMA. 1993; 270: 365–368)

• • •

2.09    **Costs.** While physicians should be conscious of costs and not provide or prescribe unnecessary services, concern for the quality of care the patient receives should be the physician's first consideration. This does not preclude the physician, individually, or through medical organizations, from participating in policy-making with respect to social issues affecting health care. (I, VII)

Issued March 1981.
Updated June 1994.

2.095    **The Provision of Adequate Health Care.** Because society has an obligation to make access to an adequate level of health care available to all of its members regardless of ability to pay, physicians should contribute their expertise at a policy-making level to help achieve this goal. In determining whether particular procedures or treatments should be included in the adequate level of health care, the following ethical principles should be considered: (1) degree of benefit (the difference in outcome between treatment and no treatment), (2) likelihood of benefit, (3) duration of benefit, (4) cost, and (5) number of people who will benefit (referring to the fact that a treatment may benefit the patient and others who come into contact with the patient, as with a vaccination or antimicrobial drug).

Ethical principles require that the ethical criteria be combined with a fair process to determine the adequate level of health care. Among the many possible alternative processes, the Council recommends the following two:

(1) Democratic decisionmaking with broad public input at both the developmental and final approval stages can be used to develop the package of benefits. With this approach, enforcement of anti-discrimination laws will be necessary to ensure that the interests of minorities and historically disadvantaged groups are protected.

(2) Equal opportunity mechanisms can also be used to determine the package of health care benefits. After applying the five ethical criteria listed above, it will be possible to designate some kinds of care as either clearly basic or clearly discretionary. However, for care that is not clearly basic or discretionary, a random selection or other equal consideration mechanism may be used to determine which kinds of care will be included in the basic benefits package.

The mechanism for providing an adequate level of health care should ensure that the health care benefits for the poor and disadvantaged will not be eroded over time. There should also be ongoing monitoring for variations in care that cannot be explained on medical grounds with special attention to evidence of discriminatory impact on historically disadvantaged groups. Finally, adjustment of the adequate level over time should be made to ensure continued and broad public acceptance.

Issued June 1994 based on the report "Ethical Issues in Health System Reform: The Provision of Adequate Health Care," issued December 1993. (JAMA. 1994; 272)

2.10    **Fetal Research Guidelines.** The following guidelines are offered as aids to physicians when they are engaged in fetal research:
(1) Physicians may participate in fetal research when their activities are part of a competently designed program, under accepted standards of scientific research, to produce data which are scientifically valid and significant.
(2) If appropriate, properly performed clinical studies on animals and nongravid humans should precede any particular fetal research project.

(3) In fetal research projects, the investigator should demonstrate the same care and concern for the fetus as a physician providing fetal care or treatment in a non-research setting.

(4) All valid federal or state legal requirements should be followed.

(5) There should be no monetary payment to obtain any fetal material for fetal research projects.

(6) Competent peer review committees, review boards, or advisory boards should be available, when appropriate, to protect against the possible abuses that could arise in such research.

(7) Research on the so called "dead fetus," macerated fetal material, fetal cells, fetal tissue, or fetal organs should be in accord with state laws on autopsy and state laws on organ transplantation or anatomical gifts.

(8) In fetal research primarily for treatment of the fetus:

   A. Voluntary and informed consent, in writing, should be given by the gravid woman, acting in the best interest of the fetus.

   B. Alternative treatment or methods of care, if any, should be carefully evaluated and fully explained. If simpler and safer treatment is available, it should be pursued.

(9) In research primarily for treatment of the gravid female:

   A. Voluntary and informed consent, in writing, should be given by the patient.

   B. Alternative treatment or methods of care should be carefully evaluated and fully explained to the patient. If simpler and safer treatment is available, it should be pursued.

   C. If possible, the risk to the fetus should be the least possible, consistent with the gravid female's need for treatment.

(10) In fetal research involving a fetus in utero, primarily for the accumulation of scientific knowledge:

   A. Voluntary and informed consent, in writing, should be given by the gravid woman under circumstances in which a prudent and informed adult would reasonably be expected to give such consent.

   B. The risk to the fetus imposed by the research should be the least possible.

   C. The purpose of research is the production of data and knowledge which are scientifically significant and which cannot otherwise be obtained.

   D. In this area of research, it is especially important to emphasize that care and concern for the fetus should be demonstrated. (I, III, V)

Issued March 1980.
Updated June 1994.

**2.11**   **Gene Therapy.** Gene therapy involves the replacement or modification of a genetic variant to restore or enhance cellular function.

Two types of gene therapy have been identified: (1) somatic cell therapy, in which human cells other than germ cells are genetically altered, and (2) germ line therapy, in which a replacement gene is integrated into the genome of human gametes or their precursors, resulting in expression of the new gene in the patient's offspring and subsequent generations. The fundamental difference between germ line therapy and somatic cell therapy is that germ line therapy affects the welfare of subsequent generations and may be associated with increased risk and the potential for unpredictable and irreversible results. Because of the far-reaching implications of germ line therapy, it is appropriate to limit genetic intervention to somatic cells only until all the short and long-term effects of germ line therapy are certain.

The goal of both somatic and germ line therapy is to alleviate human suffering and disease by remedying disorders for which available therapies are not satisfactory. This goal should be pursued only within the ethical tradition of medicine, which gives primacy to the welfare of the patient whose safety and well-being must be vigorously protected. To the extent possible, experience with animal studies must be sufficient to assure the effectiveness and safety of the techniques used, and the predictability of the results.

Moreover, genetic manipulation generally should be utilized only for therapeutic purposes. Efforts to enhance "desirable" characteristics through the insertion of a modified or additional gene, or efforts to "improve" complex human traits—the eugenic development of offspring—are contrary not only to the ethical tradition of medicine, but also to the egalitarian values of our society. Because of the potential for abuse, genetic manipulation to affect non-disease traits may never be acceptable and perhaps should never be pursued. If it is ever allowed, however, at least three conditions would have to be met before it could be deemed ethically acceptable: (1) there would have to be a clear and meaningful benefit to the child, (2) there would have to be no trade-off with other characteristics or traits, and (3) all citizens would have to have equal access to the genetic technology, irrespective of income or other socioeconomic characteristics. These criteria should be viewed as a minimal, not an exhaustive, test of the ethical propriety of non-disease-related genetic intervention. As genetic technology and knowledge of the human genome develop further, additional guidelines may be required.

All gene therapy should conform to the Council on Ethical and Judicial Affairs' guidelines on clinical investigation and genetic engineering and should adhere to stringent safety considerations. (I, V)

Issued December 1988.
Updated June 1994 based on the report "Prenatal Genetic Screening," issued December 1992. (Arch. Fam. Med. 1994; 3)

• • •

2.162    **Anencephalic Infants as Organ Donors.** Anencephaly is a congenital absence of a major portion of the brain, skull, and scalp. Infants born with this condition are born without a forebrain and without a cerebrum. While anencephalics are born with a rudimentary functional brain stem, their lack of functioning cerebrum permanently forecloses the possibility of consciousness.

It is ethically permissible to consider the anencephalic as a potential organ donor, although still alive under the current definition of death only if: (1) the diagnosis of anencephaly is certain and is confirmed by two physicians who are not part of the organ transplant team; (2) the parents of the infant desire to have the infant serve as an organ donor and indicate such in writing; and (3) there is compliance with the Council's Guidelines for the Transplantation of Organs (see Opinion 2.16: Organ Transplantation Guidelines).

In the alternative, a family wishing to donate the organs of their anencephalic infant may choose to provide the infant with ventilator assistance and other medical therapies that would sustain organ perfusion and viability until such time as a determination of death can be made in accordance with current medical standards and relevant law. In this situation, the family must be informed of the possibility that the organs might deteriorate in the process, rendering them unsuitable for transplantation.

It is normally required that the donor be legally dead before permitting the harvesting of the organs ("Dead Donor Rule"). The use of the anencephalic infant as a live donor is a limited exception to the general standard because of the fact that the infant has never experienced, and will never experience, consciousness. (I, III, V)

Issued March 1992 based on the report "Anencephalic Infants as Organ Donors," issued December 1988.
Updated June 1994.

• • •

2.17    **Quality of Life.** In the making of decisions for the treatment of seriously disabled newborns or of other persons who are severely disabled by injury or illness, the primary consideration should be what is best for the individual patient and not the avoidance of a burden to the family or to society. Quality of life, as defined by the patient's interests and values, is a factor to be considered in determining what is best for the individual. It is permissible to consider quality of life when deciding about life-sustaining treatment in accordance with opinions 2.20, 2.215, and 2.22 (I, III, IV)

Issued March 1981.
Updated June 1994.

• • •

2.19    **Unnecessary Services.** Physicians should not provide, prescribe, or seek compensation for services that are known to be unnecessary. (II, VII)

Updated June 1994.

2.20    **Withholding or Withdrawing Life-Sustaining Medical Treatment.** The social commitment of the physician is to sustain life and relieve suffering. Where the performance of one duty conflicts with the other, the preferences of the patient should prevail. The principle of patient autonomy requires that physicians respect the decision to forego life-sustaining treatment of a patient who possesses decisionmaking capacity. Life-sustaining treatment is any treatment that serves to prolong life without reversing the underlying medical condition. Life-sustaining treatment may include, but is not limited to, mechanical ventilation, renal dialysis, chemotherapy, antibiotics, and artificial nutrition and hydration.

There is no ethical distinction between withdrawing and withholding life-sustaining treatment.

A competent, adult patient may, in advance, formulate and provide a valid consent to the withholding or withdrawal of life-support systems in the event that injury or illness renders that individual incompetent to make such a decision.

If the patient receiving life-sustaining treatment is incompetent, a surrogate decisionmaker should be identified. Without an advance directive that designates a proxy, the patient's family should become the surrogate decisionmaker. Family includes persons with whom the patient is closely associated. In the case when there is no person closely associated with the patient, but there are persons who both care about the patient and have sufficient relevant knowledge of the patient, such persons may be appropriate surrogates. Physicians should provide all relevant medical information and explain to surrogate decisionmakers that decisions regarding withholding or withdrawing life-sustaining treatment should be based on substituted judgment (what the patient would have decided) when there is evidence of the patient's preferences and values. In making a substituted judgment, decisionmakers may consider the patient's advance directive (if any); the patient's values about life and the way it should be lived; and the patient's attitudes towards sickness, suffering, medical procedures, and death. If there is not adequate evidence of the incompetent patient's preferences and values, the decision should be based on the best interests of the patient (what outcome would most likely promote the patient's well-being).

Though the surrogate's decision for the incompetent patient should almost always be accepted by the physician, there are four situations that may require either institutional or judicial review and/or intervention in the decisionmaking process: (1) there is no available family member willing to be the patient's surrogate decisionmaker, (2) there is a dispute among family members and there is no decisionmaker designated in an advance directive, (3) a health care provider believes that the family's decision is clearly not what the patient would have decided if competent, and (4) a health care provider believes that the decision is not a decision that could reasonably be judged to be in the patient's best interests. When there are disputes among family members or between family and health care providers, the use of ethics committees specifically designed to facilitate sound decisionmaking is recommended before resorting to the courts.

When a permanently unconscious patient was never competent or had not left any evidence of previous preferences or values, since there is no objective way to ascertain the best interests of the patient, the surrogate's decision should not be challenged as long as the decision is based on the decisionmaker's true concern for what would be best for the patient.

Physicians have an obligation to relieve pain and suffering and to promote the dignity and autonomy of dying patients in their care. This includes providing effective palliative treatment even though it may foreseeably hasten death.

Even if the patient is not terminally ill or permanently unconscious, it is not unethical to discontinue all means of life-sustaining medical treatment in accordance with a proper substituted judgment or best interests analysis. (I, III, IV, V)

Issued March 1981 (Opinion 2.11: Terminal Illness) and December 1984 (Opinion 2.19: Withholding or Withdrawing Life-Prolonging Medical Treatment: Patient's Preferences, renumbered as Opinion 2.21 in August 1989).

In March 1986, the Council on Ethical and Judicial Affairs updated Opinion 2.11 by adopting its policy statement, "Withholding or Withdrawing Life-Prolonging Medical Treatment." This statement was identified as Opinion 2.18 (July 1986) [in August 1989, the Opinion number was changed to Opinion 2.20]. Numerous cases cited below simply note the March 1986 statement, without specific reference to the Opinions.

Updated June 1994 based on the reports "Decisions Near the End of Life" and "Decisions to Forgo Life-Sustaining Treatment for Incompetent Patients," both issued June 1991. ("Decisions Near the End of Life." JAMA. 1992; 267: 2229–2233)

2.21 **Euthanasia.** Euthanasia is the administration of a lethal agent by another person to a patient for the purpose of relieving the patient's intolerable and incurable suffering.

It is understandable, though tragic, that some patients in extreme duress—such as those suffering from a terminal, painful, debilitating illness—may come to decide that death is preferable to life. However, permitting physicians to engage in euthanasia would ultimately cause more harm than good. Euthanasia is fundamentally incompatible with the physician's role as healer, would be difficult or impossible to control, and would pose serious societal risks.

Instead of engaging in euthanasia, physicians must aggressively respond to the needs of patients at the end of life. Patients should not be abandoned once it is determined that cure is impossible. Patients near the end of life must continue to receive emotional support, comfort care, adequate pain control, respect for patient autonomy, and good communication. (I, IV)

Issued June 1994 based on the report "Decisions Near the End of Life," issued June 1991. (JAMA. 1992; 267: 2229–2233)

2.211 **Physician Assisted Suicide.** Physician assisted suicide occurs when a physician facilitates a patient's death by providing the necessary means and/or information to enable the patient to perform the life-ending act (e.g., the physician provides sleeping pills and information about the lethal dose, while aware that the patient may commit suicide).

It is understandable, though tragic, that some patients in extreme duress—such as those suffering from a terminal, painful, debilitating illness—may come to decide that death is preferable to life. However, allowing physicians to participate in assisted suicide would cause more harm than good. Physician assisted suicide is fundamentally incompatible with the physician's role as healer, would be difficult or impossible to control, and would pose serious societal risks.

Instead of participating in assisted suicide, physicians must aggressively respond to the needs of patients at the end of life. Patients should not be abandoned once it is determined that cure is impossible. Patients near the end of life must continue to receive emotional support, comfort care, adequate pain control, respect for patient autonomy, and good communication. (I, IV)

Issued 1994 based on the reports "Decisions Near the End of Life," issued June 1991, and "Physician-Assisted Suicide," issued December 1993. (JAMA. 1992; 267: 2229–2233)

2.215 **Treatment Decisions for Seriously Ill Newborns.** The primary consideration for decisions regarding life-sustaining treatment for seriously ill newborns should be what is best for the newborn. Factors that should be weighed are (1) the chance that therapy will succeed, (2) the risks involved with treatment and nontreatment, (3) the degree to which the therapy, if successful, will extend life, (4) the pain and discomfort associated with the therapy, and (5) the anticipated quality of life for the newborn with and without treatment.

Care must be taken to evaluate the newborn's expected quality of life from the child's perspective. Life-sustaining treatment may be withheld or withdrawn from a newborn when the pain and suffering expected to be endured by the child will overwhelm any potential for joy during his or her life. When an infant suffers extreme neurological damage, and is consequently not capable of experiencing either suffering or joy a decision may be made to withhold or withdraw life-sustaining treatment. When life-sustaining treatment is withheld or withdrawn, comfort care must not be discontinued.

When an infant's prognosis is largely uncertain, as is often the case with extremely premature newborns, all life-sustaining and life-enhancing treatment should be initiated. Decisions about life-sustaining treatment should be made once the prognosis becomes more certain. It is not necessary to attain absolute or near absolute prognostic certainty before life-sustaining treatment is withdrawn, since this goal is often unattainable and risks unnecessarily prolonging the infant's suffering.

Physicians must provide full information to parents of seriously ill newborns regarding the nature of treatments, therapeutic options and expected prognosis with and without therapy, so that parents can make informed decisions for their children about life-sustaining treatment. Counseling services and an opportunity to talk with persons who have had to make similar decisions should be available to parents. Ethics committees or infant review committees should also be utilized to facilitate parental decisionmaking. These committees should help mediate resolutions of conflicts that may arise among parents, physicians and others involved in the care of the infant. These committees should also be responsible for referring cases to the appropriate public agencies when it is concluded that the parents' decision is not a decision that could reasonably be judged to be in the best interests of the infant. (I, III, IV, V)

Issued June 1994 based on the report "Treatment Decisions for Seriously Ill Newborns," issued June 1992.

2.22    **Do-Not-Resuscitate Orders.** Efforts should be made to resuscitate patients who suffer cardiac or respiratory arrest except when circumstances indicate that cardiopulmonary resuscitation (CPR) would be inappropriate or not in accord with the desires or best interests of the patient.

Patients at risk of cardiac or respiratory failure should be encouraged to express in advance their preferences regarding the use of CPR and this should be documented in the patient's medical record. These discussions should include a description of the procedures encompassed by CPR and, when possible, should occur in an outpatient setting when general treatment preferences are discussed, or as early as possible during hospitalization. The physician has an ethical obligation to honor the resuscitation preferences expressed by the patient. Physicians should not permit their personal value judgments about qualify of life to obstruct the implementation of a patient's preferences regarding the use of CPR.

If a patient is incapable of rendering a decision regarding the use of CPR, a decision may be made by a surrogate decisionmaker, based upon the previously expressed preferences of the patient or, if such preferences are unknown, in accordance with the patient's best interests.

If, in the judgment of the attending physician, it would be inappropriate to pursue CPR, the attending physician may enter a do-not-resuscitate order into the patient's record. Resuscitative efforts should be considered inappropriate by the attending physician only if they cannot be expected either to restore cardiac or respiratory function to the patient or to meet established ethical criteria, as defined in the Principles of Medical Ethics and Opinions 2.03 and 2.095. When there is adequate time to do so, the physician must first inform the patient, or the incompetent patient's surrogate, of the content of the DNR order, as well as the basis for its implementation. The physician also should be prepared to discuss appropriate alternatives, such as obtaining a second opinion (e.g., consulting a bioethics committee) or arranging for transfer of care to another physician.

Do-Not-Resuscitate orders, as well as the basis for their implementation, should be entered by the attending physician in the patient's medical record.

DNR orders only preclude resuscitative efforts in the event of cardiopulmonary arrest and should not influence other therapeutic interventions that may be appropriate for the patient. (I, IV)

Issued March 1992 based on the report "Guidelines for the Appropriate Use of Do-Not-Resuscitate Orders," issued December 1990. (JAMA. 1991; 265: 1868–1871)

Updated June 1994.

2.23    **HIV Testing.** HIV testing is appropriate and should be encouraged for diagnosis and treatment of HIV infection or of medical conditions that may be affected by HIV. Treatment may prolong the lives of those with AIDS and prolong the symptom-free period in those with an asymptomatic HIV infection. Wider testing is imperative to ensure that individuals in need of treatment are identified and treated.

Physicians should ensure that HIV testing is conducted in a way that respects patient autonomy and assures patient confidentiality as much as possible.

The physician should secure the patient's informed consent specific for HIV testing before testing is performed. Because of the need for pretest counseling and the potential consequences of an HIV test on an individual's job, housing, insurability, and social relationships, the consent should be specific for HIV testing. Consent for HIV testing cannot be inferred from a general consent to treatment.

When a health care provider is at risk for HIV infection because of the occurrence of puncture injury or mucosal contact with potentially infected bodily fluids, it is acceptable to test the patient for HIV infection even if the patient refuses consent. When testing without consent is performed in accordance with the law, the patient should be given the customary pretest counseling.

The confidentiality of the results of HIV testing must be maintained as much as possible and the limits of a patient's confidentiality should be known to the patient before consent is given.

Exceptions to confidentiality are appropriate when necessary to protect the public health or when necessary to protect individuals, including health care workers, who are endangered by persons infected with HIV. If a physician knows that a seropositive individual is endangering a third party, the physician should, within the constraints of the law, (1) attempt to persuade the infected patient to cease endangering the third party; (2) if persuasion fails, notify authorities; and (3) if the authorities take no action, notify the endangered third party.

In order to limit the public spread of HIV infection, physicians should encourage voluntary testing of patients at risk for infection.

It is unethical to deny treatment to HIV-infected individuals because they are HIV seropositive or because they are unwilling to undergo HIV testing, except in the instance where knowledge of the patient's HIV status is vital to the appropriate treatment of the patient. When a patient refuses to be tested after being informed of the physician's medical opinion, the physician may transfer the patient to a second physician who is willing to manage the patient's care in accordance with the patient's preferences about testing. (I, IV)

Issued March 1992 based on the report "Ethical Issues Involved in the Growing AIDS Crisis," issued December 1987. (JAMA. 1988; 259: 1360–1361)
Updated June 1994.

## 3.00   Opinions on Interprofessional Relations

• • •

3.02   **Nurses.** The primary bond between the practices of medicine and nursing is mutual ethical concern for patients. One of the duties in providing reasonable care is fulfilled by a nurse who carries out the orders of the attending physician. Where orders appear to the nurse to be in error or contrary to customary medical and nursing practice, the physician has an ethical obligation to hear the nurse's concern and explain those orders to the nurse involved. The ethical physician should neither expect nor insist that nurses follow orders contrary to standards of good medical and nursing practice. In emergencies, when prompt action is necessary and the physician is not immediately available, a nurse may be justified in acting contrary to the physician's standing orders for the safety of the patient. Such occurrences should not be considered to be a breakdown in professional relations. (IV, V)

Issued June 1983.
Updated June 1994.

• • •

3.08   **Sexual Harassment and Exploitation Between Medical Supervisors and Trainees.** Sexual harassment may be defined as sexual advances, requests for sexual favors, and other verbal or physical conduct of a sexual nature when (1) such conduct interferes with an individual's work or academic performance or creates an intimidating, hostile, or offensive work or academic environment or (2) accepting or rejecting such conduct affects or may be perceived to affect employment decisions or academic evaluations concerning the individual. Sexual harassment is unethical.

Sexual relationships between medical supervisors and their medical trainees raise concerns because of inherent inequalities in the status and power that medical supervisors wield in relation to medical trainees and may adversely affect patient care. Sexual relationships between a medical trainee and a supervisor even when consensual are not acceptable regardless of the degree of supervision in any given situation. The supervisory role should be eliminated if the parties involved wish to pursue their relationship. (II, IV, VII)

Issued March 1992 based on the report "Sexual Harassment and Exploitation Between Medical Supervisors and Trainees," issued June 1989.
Updated June 1994

• • •

### 5.00    Opinions on Confidentiality, Advertising, and Communications Media Relations

• • •

5.05    **Confidentiality.** The information disclosed to a physician during the course of the relationship between physician and patient is confidential to the greatest possible degree. The patient should feel free to make a full disclosure of information to the physician in order that the physician may most effectively provide needed services. The patient should be able to make this disclosure with the knowledge that the patient will respect the confidential nature of the communication. The physician should not reveal confidential communications or information without the express consent of the patient, unless required to do so by law.

The obligation to safeguard patient confidences is subject to certain exceptions which are ethically and legally justified because of overriding social considerations. Where a patient threatens to inflict serious bodily harm to another person or to him or herself and there is a reasonable probability that the patient may carry out the threat, the physician should take reasonable precautions for the protection of the intended victim, including notification of law enforcement authorities. Also, communicable diseases, gun shot and knife wounds should be reported as required by applicable statutes or ordinances. (IV)

Issued December 1983.
Updated June 1994.

5.055    **Confidential Care for Minors.** Physicians who treat minors have an ethical duty to promote the autonomy of minor patients by involving them in the medical decisionmaking process to a degree commensurate with their abilities.

When minors request confidential services, physicians should encourage them to involve their parents. This includes making efforts to obtain the minor's reasons for not involving their parents and correcting misconceptions that may be motivating their objections.

Where the law does not require otherwise, physicians should permit a competent minor to consent to medical care and should not notify parents without the patient's consent. Depending on the seriousness of the decision, competence may be evaluated by physicians for most minors. When necessary, experts in adolescent medicine or child psychological development should be consulted. Use of the courts for competence determinations should be made only as a last resort.

When an immature minor requests contraceptive services, pregnancy-related care (including pregnancy testing, prenatal and postnatal care, and delivery services), or treatment for sexually transmitted disease, drug and alcohol abuse, or mental illness, physicians must recognize that requiring parental involvement may be counterproductive to the health of the patient. Physicians should encourage parental involvement in these situations. However, if the minor continues to object, his or her wishes ordinarily should be respected. If the physician is uncomfortable with providing services without parental involvement, and alternative confidential services are available, the minor may be referred to those services. In cases when the physician believes that without parental involvement and guidance, the minor will face a serious health threat, and there is reason to believe that the parents will be helpful and understanding, disclosing the problem to the parents is ethically justified. When the physician does breach confidentiality to the parents, he or she must discuss the reasons for the breach with the minor prior to the disclosure.

For minors who are mature enough to be unaccompanied by their parents for their examination, confidentiality of information disclosed during an exam, interview, or in counseling should be maintained. Such information may be disclosed to parents when the patient consents to disclosure. Confidentiality may be justifiably breached in situations for which confidentiality for adults may be breached. In addition, confidentiality for immature minors may be ethically breached when necessary to enable the parent to make an informed decision about treatment for the minor or when such a breach is necessary to avert serious harm to the minor. (IV)

Issued June 1994 based on the report "Confidential Care for Minors," issued June 1992.

• • •

5.07    **Confidentiality: Computers.** The utmost effort and care must be taken to protect the confidentiality of all medical records, including computerized medical records.

The guidelines below are offered to assist physicians and computer service organizations in maintaining the confidentiality of information in medical records when that information is stored in computerized data bases:

(1) Confidential medical information should be entered into the computer-based patient record only by authorized personnel. Additions to the record should be time and date stamped, and the person making the additions should be identified in the record.

(2) The patient and physician should be advised about the existence of computerized data bases in which medical information concerning the patient is stored. Such information should be communicated to the physician and patient prior to the physician's release of the medical information to the entity or entities maintaining the computer data bases. All individuals and organizations with some form of access to the computerized data bases, and the level of access permitted, should be specifically identified in advance. Full disclosure of this information to the patient is necessary in obtaining informed consent to treatment. Patient data should be assigned a security level appropriate for the data's degree of sensitivity, which should be used to control who has access to the information.

(3) The physician and patient should be notified of the distribution of all reports reflecting identifiable patient data prior to distribution of the reports by the computer facility. There should be approval by the patient and notification of the physician prior to the release of patient-identifiable clinical and administrative data to individuals or organizations external to the medical care environment. Such information should not be released without the express permission of the patient.

(4) The dissemination of confidential medical data should be limited to only those individuals or agencies with a bona fide use for the data. Only the data necessary for the bona fide use should be released. Patient identifiers should be omitted when appropriate. Release of confidential medical information from the data base should be confined to the specific purpose for which the information is requested and limited to the specific time frame requested. All such organizations or individuals should be advised that authorized release of data to them does not authorize their further release of the data to additional individuals or organizations, or subsequent use of the data for other purposes.

(5) Procedures for adding to or changing data on the computerized data base should indicate individuals authorized to make changes, time periods in which changes take place, and those individuals who will be informed about changes in the data from the medical records.

(6) Procedures for purging the computerized data base of archaic or inaccurate data should be established and the patient and physician should be notified before and after the data has been purged. There should be no commingling of a physician's computerized patient records with those of other computer service bureau clients. In addition, procedures should be developed to protect against inadvertent mixing of individual reports or segments thereof.

(7) The computerized medical data base should be on-line to the computer terminal only when authorized computer programs requiring the medical data are being used. Individuals and organizations external to the clinical facility should not be provided on-line access to a computerized data base containing identifiable data from medical records concerning patients. Access to the computerized data base should be controlled through security measures such as passwords, encryption (encoding) of information, and scannable badges or other user identification.

(8) Back-up systems and other mechanisms should be in place to prevent data loss and downtime as a result of hardware or software failure.

(9) Security:
   A. Stringent security procedures should be in place to prevent unauthorized access to computer-based patient records. Personnel audit procedures

should be developed to establish a record in the event of unauthorized disclosure of medical data. Terminated or former employees in the data processing environment should have no access to data from the medical records concerning patients.

B. Upon termination of computer services for a physician, those computer files maintained for the physician should be physically turned over to the physician. They may be destroyed (erased) only if it is established that the physician has another copy (in some form). In the event of file erasure, the computer service bureau should verify in writing to the physician that the erasure has taken place. (IV)

Issued prior to April 1977.
Updated June 1994.

• • •

6.00    **Opinions on Fees and Charges**

• • •

6.11    **Competition.** Competition between and among physicians and other health care practitioners on the basis of competitive factors such as quality of services, skill, experience, miscellaneous conveniences offered to patients, credit terms, fees charged, etc., is not only ethical but is encouraged. Ethical medical practice thrives best under free market conditions when prospective patients have adequate information and opportunity to choose freely between and among competing physicians and alternate systems of medical care. (VII)

Issued July 1983.

• • •

8.00    **Opinions on Practice Matters**

• • •

8.08    **Informed Consent.** The patient's right of self-decision can be effectively exercised only if the patient possesses enough information to enable an intelligent choice. The patient should make his or her own determination on treatment. The physician's obligation is to present the medical facts accurately to the patient or to the individual responsible for the patient's care and to make recommendations for management in accordance with good medical practice. The physician has an ethical obligation to help the patient make choices from among the therapeutic alternatives consistent with good medical practice. Informed consent is a basic social policy for which exceptions are permitted: (1) where the patient is unconscious or otherwise incapable of consenting and harm from failure to treat is imminent; or (2) when risk-disclosure poses such a serious psychological threat of detriment to the patient as to be medically contraindicated. Social policy does not accept the paternalistic view that the physician may remain silent because divulgence might prompt the patient to forego needed therapy. Rational, informed patients should not be expected to act uniformly, even under similar circumstances, in agreeing to or refusing treatment. (I, II, III, IV, V)

Issued March 1981.

• • •

8.11    **Neglect of Patient.** Physicians are free to choose whom they will serve. The physician should, however, respond to the best of his or her ability in cases of emergency where first aid treatment is essential. Once having undertaken a case, the physician should not neglect the patient, nor withdraw from the case without giving notice to the patient, the relatives, or responsible friends sufficiently long in advance of withdrawal to permit another medical attendant to be secured. (I, VI)

Issued prior to April 1977.

8.12    **Patient Information.** It is a fundamental ethical requirement that a physician should at all times deal honestly and openly with patients. Patients have a right to know their past and present medical status and to be free of any mistaken beliefs concerning their conditions. Situations occasionally occur in which a patient suffers significant medical complications that may have resulted from the physician's mistake or judgment. In these situations, the physician is ethically required to inform the patient of all the facts necessary to ensure understanding of what has occurred. Only through full disclosure is a patient able to make informed decisions regarding future medical care.

Ethical responsibility includes informing patients of changes in their diagnoses resulting from retrospective review of test results or any other information. This obligation holds even though the patient's medical treatment or therapeutic options may not be altered by the new information.

Concern regarding legal liability which might result following truthful disclosure should not affect the physician's honesty with a patient. (I, II, III, IV)

Issued March 1981.
Updated June 1994.

• • •

8.14    **Sexual Misconduct in the Practice of Medicine.** Sexual contact that occurs concurrent with the physician-patient relationship constitutes sexual misconduct. Sexual or romantic interactions between physicians and patients detract from the goals of the physician-patient relationship, may exploit the vulnerability of the patient, may obscure the physician's objective judgment concerning the patient's health care, and ultimately may be detrimental to the patient's well-being.

If a physician has reason to believe that non-sexual contact with a patient may be perceived as or may lead to sexual conduct, then he or she should avoid the non-sexual contact. At a minimum, a physician's ethical duties include terminating the physician-patient relationship before initiating a dating, romantic, or sexual relationship with a patient.

Sexual or romantic relationships between a physician and a former patient may be unduly influenced by the previous physician-patient relationship. Sexual or romantic relationships with former patients are unethical if the physician uses or exploits trust, knowledge, emotions, or influence derived from the previous professional relationship. (I, II, IV)

Issued December 1986.
Updated March 1992 based on the report "Sexual Misconduct in the Practice of Medicine," issued December 1990. (JAMA. 1991; 266: 2741–2745)

8.15    **Substance Abuse.** It is unethical for a physician to practice medicine while under the influence of a controlled substance, alcohol, or other chemical agents which impair the ability to practice medicine. (I)

Issued December 1986.

• • •

9.00    **Opinions on Professional Rights and Responsibilities**

• • •

9.031    **Reporting Impaired, Incompetent, or Unethical Colleagues.** Physicians have an ethical obligation to report impaired, incompetent, and unethical colleagues in accordance with the legal requirements in each state and assisted by the following guidelines:

*Impairment.* Impairment should be reported to the hospital's in-house impairment program, if available. Otherwise, either the chief of an appropriate clinical service or the chief of the hospital staff should be alerted. Reports may also be made directly to an external impaired physician program. Practicing physicians who do not have hospital privileges should be reported directly to an impaired physician program. If none of these steps would facilitate the entrance of the impaired physician into an impairment program, then the impaired physician should be reported directly to the state licensing board.

*Incompetence.* Initial reports of incompetence should be made to the appropriate clinical authority who would be empowered to assess the potential impact on patient welfare and to facilitate remedial action. The hospital peer review body should be notified where appropriate. Incompetence which poses an immediate threat to the health of patients should be reported directly to the state licensing board. Incompetence by physicians without a hospital affiliation should be reported to the local or state medical society and/or the state licensing or disciplinary board.

*Unethical conduct.* With the exception of incompetence or impairment, unethical behavior should be reported in accordance with the following guidelines:

Unethical conduct that threatens patient care or welfare should be reported to the appropriate authority for a particular clinical service. Unethical behavior which violates state licensing provisions should be reported to the state licensing board. Unethical conduct which violates criminal statutes must be reported to the appropriate law enforcement authorities. All other unethical conduct should be reported to the local or state medical society.

Where the inappropriate behavior of a physician continues despite the initial report(s), the reporting physician should report to a higher or additional authority. The person or body receiving the initial report should notify the reporting physician when appropriate action has been taken. Physicians who receive reports of inappropriate behavior have an ethical duty to critically and objectively evaluate the reported information and to assure that identified deficiencies are either remedied or further reported to a higher or additional authority. Anonymous reports should receive appropriate review and confidential investigation. Physicians who are under scrutiny or charge should be protected by the rules of confidentiality until such charges are proven or until the physician is exonerated. (II)

Issued March 1992 based on the report "Reporting Impaired, Incompetent, or Unethical Colleagues," issued January 1992.
Updated June 1994.

• • •

9.035    **Gender Discrimination in the Medical Profession.** Physician leaders in medical schools and other medical institutions should take immediate steps to increase the number of women in leadership positions as such positions become open. There is already a large enough pool of female physicians to provide strong candidates for such positions. Also, adjustments should be made to ensure that all physicians are equitably compensated for their work. Women and men in the same specialty with the same experience and doing the same work should be paid the same compensation.

Physicians in the workplace should actively develop the following: (1) Retraining or other programs which facilitate the reentry of physicians who take time away from their careers to have a family; (2) On-site child care services for dependent children; (3) Policies providing job security for physicians who are temporarily not in practice due to pregnancy or family obligations.

Physicians in the academic medical setting should strive to promote the following: (1) Extension of tenure decisions through "stop the clock" programs, relaxation of the seven year rule, or part-time appointments that would give faculty members longer to achieve standards for promotion and tenure; (2) More reasonable guidelines regarding the appropriate quantity and timing of published material needed for promotion or tenure that would emphasize quality over quantity and that would encourage the pursuit of careers based on individual talent rather than tenure standards that undervalue teaching ability and overvalue research; (3) Fair distribution of teaching, clinical, research, administrative responsibilities, and access to tenure tracks between men and women. Also, physicians in academic institutions should consider formally structuring the mentoring process, possibly matching students or faculty with advisors through a fair and visible system.

Where such policies do not exist or have not been followed, all medical workplaces and institutions should create strict policies to deal with sexual harassment. Grievance committees should have broad representation of both sexes and other groups. Such committees should have the power to enforce harassment policies and be accessible to those persons they are meant to serve.

Grantors of research funds and editors of scientific or medical journals should consider blind peer review of grant proposals and articles for publication to help prevent bias. However, grantors and editors will be able to consider the author's identity and give it appropriate weight. (II, VII)

Issued June 1994 based on the report "Gender Discrimination in the Medical Profession," issued June 1993. (*Women's Health Issues.* 1994; 4:1–11)

• • •

9.065    **Caring for the Poor.** Each physician has an obligation to share in providing care to the indigent. The measure of what constitutes an appropriate contribution may vary with circumstances such as community characteristics, geographic location, the nature of the physician's practice and specialty, and other conditions. All physicians should work to ensure that the needs of the poor in their communities are met. Caring for the poor should be a regular part of the physician's practice schedule.

In the poorest communities, it may not be possible to meet the needs of the indigent for physicians' services by relying solely on local physicians. The local physicians should be able to turn for assistance to their colleagues in prosperous communities, particularly those in close proximity.

Physicians are meeting their obligation, and are encouraged to continue to do so, in a number of ways such as seeing indigent patients in their offices at no cost or at reduced cost, serving at freestanding or hospital clinics that treat the poor, and participating in government programs that provide health care to the poor. Physicians can also volunteer their services at weekend clinics for the poor and at shelters for battered women or the homeless.

In addition to meeting their obligations to care for the indigent, physicians can devote their energy, knowledge, and prestige to designing and lobbying at all levels for better programs to provide care for the poor. (I, VII)

Issued June 1994 based on the report "Caring for the Poor," issued December 1992. (JAMA. 1993; 269: 2533–2537)

• • •

9.121    **Racial Disparities in Health Care.** Disparities in medical care based on immutable characteristics such as race must be avoided. Whether such disparities in health care are caused by treatment decisions, differences in income and education, sociocultural factors, or failures by the medical profession, they are unjustifiable and must be eliminated. Physicians should examine their own practices to ensure that racial prejudice does not affect clinical judgment in medical care. (I, IV)

Issued March 1992 based on the report "Black-White Disparities in Health Care," issued December 1989. (JAMA. 1990; 263: 2344–2346)
Updated June 1994.

9.122    **Gender Disparities in Health Care.** A patient's gender plays an appropriate role in medical decisionmaking when biological differences between the sexes are considered. However, some data suggest that gender bias may be playing a role in medical decisionmaking. Social attitudes, including stereotypes, prejudices and other evaluations based on gender role expectations may play themselves out in a variety of subtle ways. Physicians must ensure that gender is not used inappropriately as a consideration in clinical decisionmaking. Physicians should examine their practices and attitudes for influence of social or cultural biases which could be inadvertently affecting the delivery of medical care.

Research on health problems that affect both genders should include male and female subjects, and results of medical research done solely on males should not be generalized to females without evidence that results apply to both sexes. Medicine and society in general should ensure that resources for medical research should be distributed in a manner which promotes the health of both sexes to the greatest extent possible. (I, IV)

Issued March 1992 based on the report "Gender Disparities in Clinical Decisionmaking," issued December 1990. (JAMA. 1991; 266: 559–562)
Updated June 1994.

9.13    **Physicians and Infectious Diseases.** A physician who knows that he or she has an infectious disease, which if contracted by the patient would pose a significant risk to the patient, should not engage in any activity that creates a risk of transmission of that disease to the patient. The precautions taken to prevent the transmission of a contagious disease to a patient should be appropriate to the seriousness of the disease and must be particularly stringent in the case of a disease that is potentially fatal. (I, IV)

Issued August 1989.

9.131  **HIV-Infected Patients and Physicians.** A physician may not ethically refuse to treat a patient whose condition is within the physician's current realm of competence solely because the patient is seropositive for HIV. Persons who are seropositive should not be subjected to discrimination based on fear or prejudice.

When physicians are unable to provide the services required by an HIV-infected patient, they should make appropriate referrals to those physicians or facilities equipped to provide such services.

A physician who knows that he or she is seropositive should not engage in any activity that creates a risk of transmission of the disease to others. A physician who has HIV disease or who is seropositive should consult colleagues as to which activities the physician can pursue without creating a risk to patients. (I, II, IV)

Issued March 1992 based on the report "Ethical Issues in the Growing AIDS Crisis," issued December 1987. (*JAMA.* 1988; 259: 1360–1361)

# THE MORAL AND TECHNICAL COMPETENCE OF THE OPHTHALMOLOGIST
## American Academy of Ophthalmology
### 1991

*Although no other ethical directives from medical specialty organizations, including the American Academy of Ophthalmology's Code of Ethics, are printed in this Appendix, this document on the Moral and Technical Competence of the Ophthalmologist is included because of its unique focus on the notion of "moral competence" and the practice of "moral discernment." It was approved in 1991 by the Ethics Committee and the Board of Directors of the Academy.*

## Policy

The overall purpose of developing ophthalmologic competency is to improve the physician-patient relationship and the medical care that accompanies that relationship. Competent ophthalmologic practice requires both moral and technical capacities. Moral capacities are reflected in the practice of moral discernment, moral agency, and caring in relationships. Technical capacities are comprised of the knowledge and skills required to practice medicine, and especially ophthalmology, according to current standards of care.

## Background

• • •

Competence for medical (ophthalmologic) practice does not occur in the abstract. Physician competence exists for the purpose of advancing the best interests of the patient as a person—with sensitivity, and with respect for and understanding of their sovereignty, needs and wants.

Bioethicists generally agree that "moral" and "ethical" values are equivalent; these words are used synonymously here. Moral (and ethical) capacities are those which preserve, protect and advance the best interests of the patient through the practice (a process) of applying knowledge, skills and attitudes which resolve the human conflicts and dilemmas of clinical and scientific endeavor on principled bases.

## Ophthalmologic Competence

Ophthalmologic competence is comprised of both moral and technical capacities; both are necessary to establish ophthalmologic competence. Ophthalmologic competence is thus a continuing process of self-development; of acquiring and refining the knowledge, skills, values, and expectations to provide quality patient care.

This acquisition process, of necessity, must proceed along two paths:
1) an outer-directed process of study and instruction into the vocabulary, concepts, case studies, negotiation strategies, and so on, that concern moral and technical capacities, and
2) an inner-directed process of personal experience and insight that integrates personal and professional development and moral and technical capacities.

## Moral Competence

Moral competence follows from understanding the purpose of medical care and calls upon the physician to practice moral discernment, moral agency, and caring in relationships.

Moral discernment is the ability to confront, discuss, and resolve the ethical considerations in a clinical encounter. In particular, it is the ability to:
— use the vocabulary and concepts of ethical and moral reasoning to place a moral dilemma in perspective;
— respect the cultural, social, personal beliefs, expectations, and values that the patient brings to the therapeutic setting;
— respect the patient's chosen lifestyle and acknowledge the conditions and events that have helped to shape that lifestyle;
— confront one's own beliefs, expectations, and values when faced with different perspectives; and
— reflect on the causes and consequences of one's ethical decisions.

Moral Agency is the ability to act on behalf of the patient; to act with respect for social, religious, and cultural differences which may exist between physician and patient. It is the ability to:
— consider the possible consequences of one's actions and to act to affect consequences that are in accord with one's values and those of the patient;
— resolve differences on the basis of principle, rather than power;
— provide medical care that is both professionally appropriate and socially responsible;
— genuinely engage the patient as a fellow human being; and
— keep the confidences of the patient.

A caring and healing relationship between physician and patient is the foundation of medical care. Such a relationship is characterized by an ability to:
— acknowledge the patient's right to self-determination in the process of participating in his or her own care;
— avoid conflicts of interests in one's own personal, professional, and financial relationships with patients, colleagues, and other members of the health care community;
— provide the patient complete, accurate, and timely information about treatment options in the best spirit of informed consent;
— share one's weaknesses and limits as well as one's strengths and virtues; and
— strive for the experience of compassion through progressively deeper understandings of others' behavior.

## Technical Competence

Technical competence consists of the knowledge and skills necessary to diagnose and treat disease and disability according to the precepts of medical science and especially of ophthalmology, and to assist in the maintenance of health.

• • •

We acknowledge the importance of these moral commitments and technical capacities to the education, practice and credentialing of ophthalmologists. Further, the curriculum of ophthalmology should specifically address each of these two competencies and the two paths to developing them and should be defined further for purposes of assessment and accountability.

# CODE OF ETHICS
## American Osteopathic Association
revised 1985

*The 1965 revision of the American Osteopathic Association's (AOA) Code of Ethics appeared in the Appendix to the first edition of this encyclopedia. The 1985 revision of the AOA code, which is printed here, contains standards that address the osteopathic physician's responsibilities to other health-care providers, to patients, and to society. The code serves as a guide to all AOA members; wording that denotes masculine or feminine gender includes the other gender as well and imports no gender discrimination.*

*The more significant changes between the 1965 and 1985 revisions include: (1) addition of the nondiscrimination clause in Section 3; (2) elimination of the earlier ban on advertising, as required by law; (3) elimination of the previous requirement that degrees be acquired only from institutions sanctioned by the AOA; and (4) elimination of the prohibition on publicly commenting on the professional services of other physicians.*

**Section 1.** The physician shall keep in confidence whatever he may learn about a patient in the discharge of professional duties. Information shall be divulged by the physician when required by law or when authorized by the patient.

**Section 2.** The physician shall give a candid account of the patient's condition to the patient or to those responsible for the patient's care.

**Section 3.** A physician-patient relationship must be founded on mutual trust, cooperation, and respect. The patient, therefore, must have complete freedom to choose his physician. The physician must have complete freedom to choose patients whom he will serve. However, the physician should not refuse to accept patients because of the patient's race, creed, color, sex, national origin or handicap. In emergencies, a physician should make his services available.

**Section 4.** A physician is never justified in abandoning a patient. The physician shall give due notice to a patient or to those responsible for the patient's care when he withdraws from the case so that another physician may be engaged.

**Section 5.** A physician shall practice in accordance with the body of systematized and scientific knowledge related to the healing arts. A physician shall maintain competence in such systemized and scientific knowledge through study and clinical applications.

**Section 6.** The osteopathic profession has an obligation to society to maintain its high standards and, therefore, to continuously regulate itself. A substantial part of such regulation is due to the efforts and influence of the recognized local, state and national associations representing the osteopathic profession. A physician should maintain membership in and actively support such associations and abide by their rules and regulations.

**Section 7.** Under the law a physician may advertise, but no physician shall advertise or solicit patients directly or indirectly through the use of matters or activities which are false or misleading.

**Section 8.** A physician shall not hold forth or indicate possession of any degree recognized as the basis for licensure to practice the healing arts unless he is actually licensed on the basis of that degree in the state in which he practices. A physician shall designate his osteopathic school of practice in all professional uses of his name. Indications of specialty practice, membership in professional societies, and related matters shall be governed by rules promulgated by the American Osteopathic Association.

**Section 9.** A physician shall obtain consultation whenever requested to do so by the patient. A physician should not hesitate to seek consultation whenever he himself believes it advisable.

**Section 10.** In any dispute between or among physicians involving ethical or organizational matters, the matter in controversy should first be referred to the appropriate arbitrating bodies of the profession.

**Section 11.** In any dispute between or among physicians regarding the diagnosis and treatment of a patient, the attending physician has the responsibility for final decisions, consistent with any applicable osteopathic hospital rules or regulations.

**Section 12.** Any fee charged by a physician shall compensate the physician for services actually rendered. There shall be no division of professional fees for referrals of patients.

**Section 13.** A physician shall respect the law. When necessary a physician shall attempt to help to formulate the law by all proper means in order to improve patient care and public health.

**Section 14.** In addition to adhering to the foregoing ethical standards, a physician should whenever possible participate in community activities and services.

## CODE OF ETHICS AND GUIDE TO THE ETHICAL BEHAVIOUR OF PHYSICIANS
### Canadian Medical Association
revised 1990

*Revised by the Canadian Medical Association (CMA) in April 1990, the CMA Code of Ethics and Guide to the Ethical Behaviour of Physicians delineate standards of ethical behavior for Canadian physicians. The code offers seven principles of ethical conduct; the guide interprets the principles for use by individual physicians and provincial authorities.*

## Code of Ethics

Principles of Ethical Behaviour for all physicians, including those who may not be engaged directly in clinical practice.

### I
Consider first the well-being of the patient.

### II
Honour your profession and its traditions.

### III
Recognize your limitations and the special skills of others in the prevention and treatment of disease.

### IV
Protect the patient's secrets.

### V
Teach and be taught.

### VI
Remember that integrity and professional ability should be your best advertisement.

### VII
Be responsible in setting a value on your services.

## Guide to the Ethical Behaviour of Physicians

• • •

### Responsibilities to the Patient

*An Ethical Physician*

Standard of care

1. will practise the art and science of medicine to the best of his/her ability;
2. will continue self education to improve his/her standards of medical care;

Respect for patient

3. will practise in a fashion that is above reproach and will take neither physical, emotional nor financial advantage of the patient;

Patient's rights

4. will recognize his/her professional limitations and, when indicated, recommend to the patient that additional opinions and services be obtained;
5. will recognize that a patient has the right to accept or reject any physician and any medical care recommended. The patient having chosen a physician has the right to request of that physician opinions from other physicians of the patient's choice;
6. will keep in confidence information derived from a patient or from a colleague regarding a patient, and divulge it only with the permission of the patient except when otherwise required by law;
7. when acting on behalf of a third party will ensure that the patient understands the physician's legal responsibility to the third party before proceeding with the examination;
8. will recommend only diagnostic procedures that are believed necessary to assist in the care of the patient, and therapy that is believed necessary for the well-being of the patient. The physician will recognize a responsibility in advising the patient of the findings and recommendations and will exchange such information with the patient as is necessary for the patient to reach a decision;
9. will, upon a patient's request, supply the information that is required to enable the patient to receive any benefits to which the patient may be entitled;

10. will be considerate of the anxiety of the patient's next-of-kin and cooperate with them in the patient's interest;

### Choice of patient

11. will recognize the responsibility of a physician to render medical service to any person regardless of colour, religion or political belief;
12. shall, except in an emergency, have the right to refuse to accept a patient;
13. will render all possible assistance to any patient, where an urgent need for medical care exists;
14. will, when the patient is unable to give consent and an agent of the patient is unavailable to give consent, render such therapy as the physician believes to be in the patient's interest;

### Continuity of care

15. will, if absent, ensure the availability of medical care to his/her patients if possible; will, once having accepted professional responsibility for an acutely ill patient, continue to provide services until they are no longer required, or until arrangements have been made for the services of another suitable physician; may, in any other situation, withdraw from the responsibility for the care of any patient provided that the patient is given adequate notice of that intention;

### Personal morality

16. will inform the patient when personal morality or religious conscience prevent the recommendation of some form of therapy;

### Clinical research

17. will ensure that, before initiating clinical research involving humans, such research is appraised scientifically and ethically and approved by a responsible committee and is sufficiently planned and supervised that the individuals are unlikely to suffer any harm. The physician will ascertain that previous research and the purpose of the experiment justify this additional method of investigation. Before proceeding, the physician will obtain the consent of all involved persons or their agents, and will proceed only after explaining the purpose of the clinical investigation and any possible health hazard that can be reasonably foreseen;

### The dying patient

18. will allow death to occur with dignity and comfort when death of the body appears to be inevitable;
19. may support the body when clinical death of the brain has occurred, but need not prolong life by unusual or heroic means;

### Transplantation

20. may, when death of the brain has occurred, support cellular life in the body when some parts of the body might be used to prolong the life or improve the health of others;
21. will recognize a responsibility to a donor of organs to be transplanted and will give to the donor or the donor's relatives full disclosure of the intent and purpose of the procedure; in the case of a living donor, the physician will also explain the risks of the procedure;
22. will refrain from determining the time of death of the donor patient if there is a possibility of being involved as a participant in the transplant procedure, or when his/her association with the proposed recipient might improperly influence professional judgement;
23. may treat the transplant recipient subsequent to the transplant procedure in spite of having determined the time of death of the donor;

### Fees to patients

24. will consider, in determining professional fees, both the nature of the service provided and the ability of the patient to pay, and will be prepared to discuss the fee with the patient.

## Responsibilities to the Profession

*An Ethical Physician:*

### Personal conduct

25. will recognize that the profession demands integrity from each physician and dedication to its search for truth and to its service to mankind;
26. will recognize that self discipline of the profession is a privilege and that each physician has a continuing responsibility to merit the retention of this privilege;
27. will behave in a way beyond reproach and will report to the appropriate professional body any conduct by a colleague which might be generally considered as being unbecoming to the profession;

28. will behave in such a manner as to merit the respect of the public for members of the medical profession;

29. will avoid impugning the reputation of any colleague;

### Contracts

30. will, when aligned in practice with other physicians, insist that the standards enunciated in this Code of Ethics and the Guide to the Ethical Behaviour of Physicians be maintained;

31. will only enter into a contract regarding professional services which allows fees derived from physicians' services to be controlled by the physician rendering the services;

32. will enter a contract with an organization only if it will allow maintenance of professional integrity;

33. will only offer to a colleague a contract which has terms and conditions equitable to both parties;

### Reporting medical research

34. will first communicate to colleagues, through recognized scientific channels, the results of any medical research, in order that those colleagues may establish an opinion of its merits before they are presented to the public;

### Addressing the public

35. will recognize a responsibility to give the generally held opinions of the profession when interpreting scientific knowledge to the public; when presenting an opinion which is contrary to the generally held opinion of the profession, the physician will so indicate and will avoid any attempt to enhance his/her own personal professional reputation;

### Advertising

36. will build a professional reputation based on ability and integrity, and will only advertise professional services or make professional announcements as regulated by legislation or as permitted by the provincial medical licensing authority;

37. will avoid advocacy of any product when identified as a member of the medical profession;

38. will avoid the use of secret remedies;

### Consultation

39. will request the opinion of an appropriate colleague acceptable to the patient when diagnosis or treatment is difficult or obscure, or when the patient requests it. Having requested the opinion of a colleague, the physician will make available all relevant information and indicate clearly whether the consultant is to assume the continuing care of the patient during this illness;

40. will, when consulted by a colleague, report in detail all pertinent findings and recommendations to the attending physician and may outline an opinion to the patient. The consultant will continue with the care of the patient only at the specific request of the attending physician and with the consent of the patient;

### Patient care

41. will cooperate with those individuals who, in the opinion of the physician, may assist in the care of the patient;

42. will make available to another physician, upon the request of the patient, a report of pertinent findings and treatment of the patient;

43. will provide medical services to a colleague and dependent family without fee, unless specifically requested to render an account;

44. will limit self-treatment or treatment of family members to minor or emergency services only; such treatments should be without fee;

### Financial arrangements

45. will avoid any personal profit motive in ordering drugs, appliances or diagnostic procedures from any facility in which the physician has a financial interest;

46. will refuse to accept any commission or payment, direct or indirect, for any service rendered to a patient by other persons excepting direct employees and professional colleagues with whom there is a formal partnership or similar agreement.

### Responsibilities to Society

Physicians who act under the principles of this Guide to the Ethical Behaviour of Physicians will find that they have fulfilled many of their responsibilities to society.

*An Ethical Physician*

47. will strive to improve the standards of medical services in the community; will accept a share of the profession's responsibility to society in matters relating to the health

and safety of the public, health education, and legislation affecting the health or well-being of the community;

48. will recognize the responsibility as a witness to assist the court in arriving at a just decision;

49. will, in the interest of providing good and adequate medical care, support the opportunity of other physicians to obtain hospital privileges according to individual personal and professional qualifications.

*"The complete physician is not a man apart and cannot content himself with the practice of medicine alone, but should make his contribution, as does any other good citizen, towards the well-being and betterment of the community in which he lives."*

# CODE OF ETHICS AND GUIDE TO THE ETHICAL BEHAVIOUR OF PHYSICIANS
## New Zealand Medical Association
### 1989, last amended 1992

*The current New Zealand Medical Association (NZMA) Code of Ethics, which includes a Guide to the Ethical Behaviour of Physicians, was adopted in 1989 and last amended in December 1992 when paragraphs 47–49 were added, largely as a result of health reforms in New Zealand. There is great similarity, both in structure and content, between the NZMA code and the preceding code and guide of the Canadian Medical Association. The section of the NZMA entitled "Responsibilities to the Profession" and portions of the section entitled "Responsibilities to Society," not printed here, repeat some of the prescriptions of the Canadian code.*

## Code of Ethics

Principles of Ethical Behaviour applicable to all physicians including those who may not be engaged directly in clinical practice.

1. Consider the health and well-being of your patient to be your first priority.
2. Strive to improve your knowledge and skill so that the best possible advice and treatment can be afforded to your patient.
3. Honour your profession and its traditions.
4. Recognise both your own limitations and the special skills of others in the prevention and treatment of disease.
5. Protect the patient's secrets even after his or her death.
6. Let integrity and professional ability be your chief advertisement.

## Guide to the Ethical Behaviour of Physicians

• • •

### Responsibilities to the Patient

Standard of Care

1. Practise the science and art of medicine to the best of one's ability in full technical and moral independence and with compassion and respect for human dignity.
2. Continue self education to improve one's personal standards of medical care.
3. Ensure that every patient receives a complete and thorough examination into their complaint or condition.
4. Ensure that accurate records of fact are kept.

Respect for Patient

5. Ensure that all conduct in the practise of the profession is above reproach, and that neither physical, emotional nor financial advantage is taken of any patient.

Patient's Right

6. Recognize a responsibility to render medical service to any person regardless of colour, religion, political belief, and regardless of the nature of the illness so long as it lies within the limits of expertise as a practitioner.
7. Accepts the right of all patients to know the nature of any illness from which they are known to suffer, its probable cause, and the available treatments together with their likely benefits and risks.
8. Allow all patients the right to choose their doctors freely.
9. Recognize one's professional limitations and, when indicated, recommend to the patient that additional opinions and services be obtained.

10. Keep in confidence information derived from a patient, or from a colleague regarding a patient, and divulge it only with the permission of the patient except when the law requires otherwise.

11. Recommend only those diagnostic procedures which seem necessary to assist in the care of the patient and only that therapy which seems necessary for the well-being of the patient. Exchange such information with patients as is necessary for them to make informed choices where alternatives exist.

12. When requested, assist any patient by supplying the information required to enable the patient to receive any benefits to which he or she may be entitled.

13. Render all assistance possible to any patient where an urgent need for medical care exists.

Continuity of Care

14. Ensure that medical care is available to one's patients when one is personally absent, when professional responsibility for an acutely ill patient has been accepted, continue to provide services until they are no longer required, or until the services of another suitable physician have been obtained.

Personal Morality

15. When a personal moral judgement or religious conscience alone prevents the recommendation of some form of therapy, the patient must be so acquainted and an opportunity afforded the patient to seek alternative care.

Clinical Research    (This section summarises the principles outlined in the Declaration of Helsinki.)

• • •

Clinical Teaching

21. Recognize that clinical teaching is the basis on which sound clinical practice in the future is based. Before embarking on any clinical teaching involving patients ensure that they fully understand what is involved and have freely consented to what is proposed. Do not allow a refusal to participate in a study or in teaching to interfere with the doctor-patient relationship. In any teaching exercise ensure that every patient is assured of the best proven diagnostic and therapeutic methods.

The Dying Patient

22. Always bear in mind the obligation of preserving life, but allow death to occur with dignity and comfort when the death of the body appears to be inevitable.

Transplantation

23. Accept that when death of the brain has occurred cellular life in the body may be supported if some parts of the body might be used to prolong or improve the health of others.

24. Recognize full responsibility to the donor of organs that are to be transplanted to give to the donor or his or her relatives full disclosure of such an intent and the purpose of the procedure; in the case of a living donor also explain the risks of the procedure.

25. Ensure that the determination of the time of death of any donor patient is made by doctors who are in no way concerned with the transplant procedure or associated with any proposed recipient in a way that might exert any influence upon any decision made.

Fees to Patients

26. Be responsible in setting a value on your services and consider the personal service rendered when determining any fee. Be prepared to discuss any fee with the patient.

• • •

**Responsibilities to Society**

• • •

45. Accept that it is not an individual doctor's role to determine society's attitudes in matters such as abortion or invitro fertilization but attempt always both to protect any patient and safeguard the rights of the doctor within society.

46. Regardless of society's attitude, no doctor shall countenance, condone or participate in the practice of torture or other forms of cruel, inhuman, or degrading procedure whatever the offence of which the victim of such procedures is suspected, accused, or guilty.

Provision of Service in a Competitive Environment

47. Doctors must at all times regard their duty to a patient, or to patients collectively, as overriding any loyalty to an employer or other health provider entity. In partic-

ular, doctors must not allow the commercial interests of an employer or health provider to interfere with;

    a. the free exercise of clinical judgement in determining the best ways of meeting the needs of individual patients or the community, or

    b. cooperation with such other health providers as may be in the patient's interest, or

    c. the completion of any treatment or package of care, or

    d. the publication of regular and honest reports of their service provision, aims and achievements.

48. Doctors must not compete with each other, or allow the units that employ them to compete with each other, against the public interest.

49. Standards of care should not be compromised in order to meet financial or commercial targets whether these are set by a doctor personally or by an organisation.

# CODE OF ETHICS OF THE CHILEAN MEDICAL ASSOCIATION
### Chilean Medical Association
### 1983

*Approved by the Honorable General Council in November 1983, the Code of Ethics of the Chilean Medical Association sets moral standards for the conduct of members of the association and "should only be used by and for physicians." Articles of particular note include: (1) article 25, which proscribes physician participation in torture; (2) article 26, which permits abortion only for therapeutic reasons and, along with articles 27–28, reflects the prevalence of Catholicism in Chile; (3) articles 27 and 28, which pertain to euthanasia and death with dignity; and (4) article 44, which provides for a patient or the patient's family to request a review board to investigate the clinical findings and recommendations of the attending physician.*

## Declaration of Principles

• • •

A respect for life and the human person is the basic foundation for the professional practice of medicine.

The ethical principles that govern the conduct of physicians oblige them to protect the human being from pain, suffering, and death without any discrimination.

Decorum, dignity, honesty, and moral integrity, as imperative norms in the life of a doctor, are attributes the medical community deems fundamental in its professional practice.

• • •

## Title I
## General Resolutions

• • •

ARTICLE 10.—Doctor–patient confidentiality is both a right and an obligation of the profession. With respect to any patient this is imperative, even when the patient is no longer under a particular physician's care.

• • •

If a patient communicates to a physician the intent to commit a crime, such communication is not protected by the right and duty of doctor–patient confidentiality, and the physician must reveal any information necessary for the prevention of a crime or to protect any person(s) in danger.

• • •

## Title II
## On the Duties of the Doctor Toward Patients

ARTICLE 13.—The physician must attend to the needs of any person requiring his or her services and, in the absence of another colleague able to care for the patient, may not deny such attention.

ARTICLE 14.—Physicians may not, under any circumstances, directly or indirectly reveal facts, data, or information that they have learned or that have been revealed to them in the course of their professional work, except by judicial order, or by freely expressed authorization by a patient who is of legal age and of sound mind.

Doctor–patient confidentiality is an objective right of the patient that the physician must absolutely respect as a natural right, based neither on promise nor on pact. Doctor–patient confidentiality includes the patient's name.

ARTICLE 15.—In cases where it may be therapeutically necessary to have recourse to treatments involving known risk or serious disfiguring of the patient, the physician may not act without the express and informed consent of the patient or responsible family members when the patient is a minor or otherwise unable to make such decisions.

In emergency situations or in the absence of responsible family members and without the possibility of communication with them, or in the event that there be no next of kin, the physician may proceed without the above-mentioned authorization and without prejudice, after attempting to obtain the concurring opinion of another colleague in the treatment.

ARTICLE 16.—No physician may participate or advise in any transaction involving the transplantation of organs if said transaction involves monetary gain.

• • •

ARTICLE 22.—Scientific biomedical research on human beings is necessary; however, it is acceptable only when it does not involve serious health risks. It should always be carried out under direct medical supervision.

Its design and development should follow a strict protocol and be subject to scientific and ethical review. The patient or subject of the research must be informed of both potential risks and benefits, must give consent, and must reserve the right to abstain from any part of or withdraw from the study at any time.

• • •

ARTICLE 25.—A physician shall not support or participate in the practice of torture or the infliction of any other cruel, inhumane, or degrading procedures, regardless of the offense(s) of which the victim of such procedures is accused or guilty, and regardless of the beliefs or motivation of the accused or guilty victim of such procedures, including armed conflict or civil war.

A physician must not provide any rationale, instrument, substance, or knowledge/expertise that would facilitate the practice of torture or other forms of cruel, inhumane, or degrading treatment, or for the purpose of diminishing the victim's capacity to resist such treatment.

A physician must not be present before, during, or after any procedure in which torture or other forms of cruel, inhumane, or degrading treatment are used as a threat.

ARTICLE 26.—A physician must respect human life from the moment of conception. Abortion may be performed only under the following circumstances:

    a) it is performed for therapeutic reasons;
    b) the decision is approved in writing by two physicians chosen for their competence;
    c) the procedure is carried out by a specialist in the field.

If a physician considers that it is against his or her convictions to perform an abortion, he or she must withdraw, permitting the patient to continue medical care with another qualified physician.

ARTICLE 27.—A physician must not under any circumstances deliberately end the life of a patient. No authority may order or permit a physician to do so. Furthermore, no patient or person responsible for making decisions for the patient may request this of a physician.

ARTICLE 28.—Every person has the right to die with dignity. Thus, diagnostic and therapeutic procedures must be proportionate to the results that can be hoped for from such procedures.

A physician must relieve a patient's pain and suffering even though this may involve the risk of shortening the patient's life.

In the event of an imminent and inevitable death, were routine life support interrupted, a physician may in good faith make the decision to withhold any treatment that would prolong a precarious and painful condition. In a case where the patient is proven to be brain dead, the physician is authorized to withhold any and all types of treatment.

• • •

## Title III
## On Physicians' Relationship with Colleagues

• • •

ARTICLE 44.—Any and all physicians must consult with one or more colleagues whenever the making of a diagnosis, the type of illness, or treatment requires such collaboration.

A patient or patient's family, with the knowledge of the attending physician, may ask that a Review Board be arranged if they deem it necessary.

It is a moral duty of the attending physician to accept the collaboration of colleagues convened on the Review Board, who shall examine the patient in the presence of the attending physician and one after the other, except in special cases. The findings of the Board shall be discussed among the attending and collaborating physicians before the Chief Physician makes them known to the patient or to the patient's family.

· · ·

# CODE OF MEDICAL ETHICS, BRAZIL
**Federal Council of Medicine**
1988

*Brazil's Federal Council of Medicine approved the current Code of Medical Ethics in January 1988, rescinding the 1965 Code of Medical Ethics and the 1984 Brazilian Code of Medical Deontology. The preamble states that the code "contains the ethical standards governing physicians"; that "organizations delivering medical services are subject to the standards in this code"; and, interestingly, that "those who violate this code are subject to disciplinary action as stated by law." Other interesting features of the code include: (1) statements regarding occupational health and the natural environment (articles 12, 13); (2) the right of physicians to strike (article 24); and (3) the requirement that protocols for medical research be submitted to an independent committee for approval and monitoring (article 127).*

## Chapter I
## Basic Principles

· · ·

**Art. 6** - The physician shall have utmost respect for human life, always acting in the interest of the patient. He/she will never use his/her knowledge to inflict physical or moral suffering, to end the life of an individual, or to allow cover-ups against his dignity and integrity.

**Art. 7** - The physician shall practice his/her profession with ample autonomy and is not forced to provide professional services to an individual against his/her will, except in the absence of another physician, in emergency cases, or when his refusal could cause irreversible damage to the patient.

**Art. 8** - The physician may not, under any circumstance or pretext, renounce his professional freedom and shall disallow any restriction or imposition that could harm the efficacy and appropriateness of his/her work.

· · ·

**Art. 11** - The physician shall keep information, obtained during the practice of his profession, confidential. The same applies to his/her work with businesses, except in cases when such information damages or poses a risk to the health of an employee, or the community.

**Art. 12** - The physician shall promote an appropriate working environment for the individual, and the elimination, or control, of risks inherent in his/her work.

**Art. 13** - The physician shall inform competent authorities of any forms of pollution and deterioration of the environment, that pose a risk to health and life.

**Art. 14** - The physician shall promote the improvement of health conditions and medical service standards, and take part in responsibilities in relation to public health, health education, and health legislation.

· · ·

## Chapter II
## Rights of the Physician

The physician has the right to:

**Art. 20** - Practice Medicine without being discriminated against in terms of religion, race, sex, nationality, color, sexual choice, social status, political opinion, or for any other reason.

**Art. 21** - Recommend adequate procedures to the patient, observing regularly accepted practice and respecting legal standards in force in the country.

• • •

**Art. 24** - Suspend his/her activities, individually or collectively, when the public or private institution for which he/she works, does not offer minimal conditions for the practice of his/her profession, or does not pay accordingly, except in conditions of urgency and emergency. This decision shall be communicated immediately to the Regional Council of Medicine.

• • •

**Art. 27** - When employed, dedicate the time and professional experience recommended for the performance of his/her duties, to the patient, avoiding excessive workloads or consultations that could harm the patient.

**Art. 28** - Refuse to perform medical practices, although allowed by law, that are contrary to his/her conscience.

## Chapter III
## Professional Responsibility

The physician is forbidden:

• • •

**Art. 40** - Not to inform the individual about working conditions that could pose a risk to his/her health. These facts must be communicated to those in charge, the authorities, and the Regional Council of Medicine.

**Art. 41** - Not to inform the patient about social, environmental, or professional implications of his/her illness.

**Art. 42** - To practice or recommend medical procedures, not necessary or forbidden by local law.

**Art. 43** - Not to abide by specific legislation on organ or tissue transplants, sterilization, artificial insemination, and abortion.

• • •

## Chapter IV
## Human Rights

The physician is forbidden:

**Art. 46** - To perform any medical procedure without previous explanation and consent of the patient or his/her legal representative, except in cases of imminent threat to life.

**Art. 47** - To discriminate against a human being in any way or under any pretext.

**Art. 48** - To exercise his/her authority in such a way that it limits the right of the patient to decide freely for him/herself or on his/her well-being.

**Art. 49** - To participate in the practice of torture, or any other degrading procedures, that are inhuman or cruel; to be an accomplice in these kinds of practices, and not to denounce them when they come to his/her knowledge.

**Art. 50** - To provide means, instruments, substances, or knowledge that facilitate the practice of torture or other kinds of degrading, inhuman, and cruel procedures, in relation to the individual.

**Art. 51** - To force-feed any person on a hunger strike, who is considered capable, physically and mentally, of making perfect judgement of possible complications from this attitude. In these cases, the physician shall inform the individual of possible complications from prolonged lack of nutrition and treat him/her if there is imminent danger to life.

**Art. 52** - To use any process that might change the personality or conscience of an individual, to decrease his/her physical or mental resistance during a police investigation or of any other kind.

**Art. 53** - Not to respect the interest and integrity of an individual, by treating him/her in any institution where the person is being kept against his/her will.

**Single paragraph:** Any procedures damaging the personality or physical or mental health of an individual, while under the care of a physician, shall compel the physician in charge to denounce this fact to the competent authorities and to the Regional Council of Medicine.

**Art. 54** - To provide means, instruments, substances, knowledge, or to participate in any way, in the execution of a death penalty.

**Art. 55** - To use the profession to corrupt customs or to commit or favor crime.

## Chapter V
## Relation with Patients and Family Members

The physician is forbidden:

**Art. 56** - To disregard the right of the patient to decide freely about the performance of diagnostic or therapeutic practices, except in cases of imminent loss of life.

**Art. 57** - Not to use all available diagnostic and treatment means within his/her reach in favor of the patient.

**Art. 58** - Not to treat a patient, looking for his/her professional care, in an emergency, when there are no other physicians or medical services available.

**Art. 59** - Not to inform the patient of the diagnosis, prognosis, risks and objectives of treatment, except when direct communication may be harmful to the patient. In this case, communication shall take place with the legal representative of the patient.

**Art. 60** - To exaggerate the seriousness of a diagnosis or prognosis, to complicate treatment, or to exceed the number of visits, consultations, or any other medical procedures.

**Art. 61** - To abandon a patient under his/her care.

§1 - Under circumstances, that in his/her view are harmful to the doctor-patient relationship or that interfere with full professional performance, a physician has the right to renounce treatment, as long as this fact is previously communicated to the patient or his/her legal representative, with the assurance of continuity of care and supplying all necessary information to the substituting physician.

§2 - Except in cases of just cause, communicated to the patient or his/her family members, the physician may not abandon the patient for having a chronic or incurable disease. The physician shall continue to treat him/her, even if only to alleviate physical or psychological suffering.

**Art. 62** - To prescribe treatment or other procedures without examining the patient directly, except in emergency cases or the impossibility of performing such an examination. In this case, the examination shall be performed as soon as possible.

**Art. 63** - Not to respect the modesty of any individual in his/her professional care.

**Art. 64** - To oppose the realization of a medical inquiry requested by the patient or his legal representative.

**Art. 65** - To take advantage of the doctor–patient relationship to obtain physical, emotional, financial, or political advantages.

**Art. 66** - To use, in any case, means to shorten the life of a patient, even if requested to do so, by the patient or his legal representative.

**Art. 67** - Not to respect the right of the patient to decide freely on a contraceptive or conceptive method. The physician shall always explain indication, reliability, and reversibility, as well as the risk of each method.

**Art. 68** - To practice artificial insemination, without total consent by the participants, with the procedure duly explained.

**Art. 69** - Not to maintain medical records for each patient.

**Art. 70** - To deny the patient access to his/her medical records, clinical or similar records, as well as not to provide explanations necessary for their understanding, except when this incurs risks for the patient or third parties.

**Art. 71** - Not to provide a medical opinion to the patient, upon referral or transfer for the continuity of care, or upon release, if requested to do so.

• • •

## Chapter IX
## Medical Confidentiality

The physician is forbidden:

**Art. 102** - To reveal the fact that he is aware of information received during the practice of his/her profession, except for just cause, legal duty, or express authorization by the patient.

**Single paragraph:** this is maintained:

a) Even if the fact is public knowledge or if the patient is deceased.

b) When testifying. In this instance, the physician shall present him/herself and declare his/her constraint.

**Art. 103** - To reveal a professional secret relating to a minor, including to his/her parents or legal representatives, as long as the minor is capable of resolving his/her problem by his/her own means, except when the lack of revelation could imply damage to the patient.

**Art. 104** - To make reference to identifiable clinical cases, exhibit patients or their photographs in professional announcements or during medical programs on radio, television or movies, as well as in articles, interviews or newspaper reports, magazines or other publications not specific to Medicine.

**Art. 105** - To reveal confidential information obtained during the medical exam of workers, including upon demand by directors of businesses or institutions, except if silence poses a risk to the health of workers or the community.

**Art. 106** - To provide insurance companies with any information about the circumstances of the death of his/her patient, beyond that contained in the death certificate, except by express authorization of the legal representative or heir.

**Art. 107** - Not to inform his/her assistants and not to promote the respect of professional secrecy, as required by law.

**Art. 108** - To facilitate the handling and knowledge of medical records, forms, and other kinds of medical observations, subject to professional secrecy, by persons not obligated by this commitment.

**Art. 109** - Not to maintain professional secrecy when recovering professional fees by judicial or extra-judicial means.

• • •

## Chapter XII
## Medical Research

The physician is forbidden:

**Art. 122** - To participate in any type of experiment with human beings with warlike, political, racial, or eugenic reasons.

**Art. 123** - To perform research on an individual, without his/her express consent in writing, after having had the nature and consequence of research duly explained.
**Single paragraph:** If the patient is not in condition to give his/her consent, research shall only be performed, in his/her own benefit, after express authorization by his/her legal representative.

**Art. 124** - To use any type of experimental treatment, not approved for use in the country, without due authorization by competent authorities and without the consent of the patient or his legal representative, duly informed of the situation and possible consequences.

**Art. 125** - To promote medical research in the community without knowledge by the community and with a purpose not directed at public health, in consideration of local characteristics.

**Art. 126** - To obtain personal advantages or have any commercial interest or to renounce his/her professional independence in relation to medical research financing entities in which he/she participates.

**Art. 127** - To perform medical research on individuals without having submitted the protocol for approval and monitoring of a commission not subject to any entity related to the researcher.

**Art. 128** - To perform medical research on volunteers, healthy or not, who have a direct or indirect relation of dependency or subordination with the researcher.

**Art. 129** - To perform or participate in medical research in which there is a need to suspend or to stop using recognized treatment, thereby harming the patient.

**Art. 130** - To perform experiments with new clinical or surgical treatment on incurable or terminal patients, without reasonable hope for positive effects, imposing additional suffering.

• • •

## EUROPEAN CODE OF MEDICAL ETHICS
### Conférence Internationale des Ordres et des Organismes d'Attributions Similaires
### 1987

*Drafted in January 1987 by the Conférence Internationale des Ordres et des Organismes d'Attributions Similaires, this European Code of Medical Ethics represents one effort to articulate medical ethics guidelines for the European Community. The code represents a guide for the countries involved, each of which must decide whether further action at a national level is warranted. The twelve participating countries and their representative bodies include: Belgium, Conseil National de l'Ordre des Médecins Belges; Denmark, Danish Medical Association and*

*National Board of Health; Spain, Consejo General de Colegios Oficiales de Medicos; France, Conseil National de l'Ordre des Médecins Français; Luxembourg, Collège Médical; Ireland, Medical Council; Italy, Federazione Nazionale degli Ordini dei Medici; The Netherlands, Koninklijke Nederlandsche Maatschappij tot Bevordering der Geneeskunst; Portugal, Ordem dos Medicos; Germany, Bundesärztekammer; United Kingdom, General Medical Council; and observer for Sweden, Association Médicale Suédoise.*

This guide is intended to influence the professional conduct of doctors, in whatever branch of practice, in their contacts with patients, with society and between themselves. The guide also refers to the privileged position of doctors, upon which good medical practice depends. The Conference has recommended to its constituent regulatory bodies in each member state of the European Communities that they take such measures as may be necessary to ensure that their national requirements relating to the duties and privileges of doctors vis-à-vis their patients and society and in their professional relationships conform with the principles set out in this guide, and that there is provision within their legal systems for the effective enforcement of these principles.

Article 1

The doctor's vocation is to safeguard man's physical and mental health and relieve his suffering, while respecting human life and dignity with no discrimination on the grounds of age, race, religion, nationality, social status, political opinions or any other, whether in peace time or in war time.

## Undertakings by the Doctor

Article 2

A doctor engaging in medical practice undertakes to give priority to the medical interests of the patient. The doctor may use his professional knowledge only to improve or maintain the health of those who place their trust in him; in no circumstances may he act to their detriment.

Article 3

A doctor engaging in medical practice must refrain from imposing on a patient his personal philosophical, moral or political opinions.

## Enlightened Consent

Article 4

Except in an emergency, a doctor will explain to the patient the effects and the expected consequences of treatment. He will obtain the patient's consent, particularly when his proposed medical interventions present a serious risk.

The doctor may not substitute his own definition of the quality of life for that of his patient.

## Moral and Technical Independence

Article 5

Both when given advice and when giving treatment, a doctor must make best use of his complete professional freedom and the technical and moral circumstances which permit him to act in complete independence.

The patient should be informed if these conditions are not met.

Article 6

When a doctor is working for a private or public authority or when he is acting on behalf of a third party, be it an individual or institution, he must also inform the patient of this.

## Professional Confidentiality

Article 7

The doctor is necessarily the patient's confidant. He must guarantee to him complete confidentiality of all the information which he may have acquired and of the investigations which he may have undertaken in the course of his contacts with him.

The death of a patient does not absolve a doctor from the rule of professional secrecy.

Article 8

A doctor must respect the privacy of his patients and take all necessary steps to prevent the disclosure of anything which he may have learned in the course of his professional practice.

Where national law provides for exceptions to the principles of confidentiality, the doctor should be able to consult the Medical Council or equivalent professional authority.

Article 9

Doctors may not collaborate in the establishment of electronic medical data banks which could imperil or diminish the right of the patient to the safely protected confidentiality of his privacy. A nominated doctor should be responsible for ethical supervision and control of each computerised medical data bank.

Medical data banks must have no links with other data banks.

## Standards of Medical Care

Article 10

The doctor must have access to all the resources of medical knowledge in order to utilise them as necessary for the benefit of his patient.

Article 11

He should not lay claim to a competence which he does not possess.

Article 12

He must call upon a more experienced colleague in any case which requires an examination or method of treatment beyond his own competence.

## Care of the Terminally Ill

Article 13

While the practice of medicine must in all circumstances constantly respect the life, the moral autonomy and the free choice of the patient, the doctor may, in the case of an incurable and terminal illness, alleviate the physical and mental suffering of the patient by restricting his intervention to such treatment as is appropriate to preserve, so far as possible, the quality of a life which is drawing to its close.

It is essential to assist the dying patient right to the end and to take such action as will permit the patient to retain his dignity.

## Removal of Organs

Article 14

In a case where it is impossible to reverse the terminal processes leading to the cessation of a patient's vital functions, doctors will establish that death has occurred, taking account of the most recent scientific data.

At least two doctors, acting individually, should take meticulous steps to verify that this situation has occurred, and record their findings in writing.

They should be independent of the team which is to carry out the transplantation and must, in all respects, give priority to the care of the dying patient.

Article 15

Doctors removing an organ for transplantation may give particular treatment designed to maintain the condition of that organ.

Article 16

Doctors removing organs for transplantation and those carrying out transplantations should take all practicable steps to ensure that the donor had not expressed opposition or left instructions to this effect either in writing or with his family.

## Reproduction

Article 17

The doctor will furnish the patient, on request, with all relevant information on the subjects of reproduction and contraception.

Article 18

It is ethical for a doctor, by reason of his own beliefs, to refuse to intervene in the processes of reproduction or termination of pregnancy, and to suggest to the patients concerned that they consult other doctors.

## Experimentation on Humans

Article 19

Progress in the field of medicine is based on research which must finally lead to experiments which have a direct bearing on humans.

Article 20

Details of all proposed experimentation involving patients must first be submitted to an ethical committee which is independent of the research team for opinions and advice.

Article 21

The free and informed consent of any person who is to be involved in a research project must be obtained after he has first been sufficiently informed of the aims, methods and expected benefits as well as the risks and potential problems, and of his right not to take part in experiments (or other research) and to withdraw from participation at any time.

## Torture and Inhuman Treatment

Article 22

A doctor must never attend, take part in or carry out acts of torture or other kinds of cruel, inhuman or degrading treatment whatever the crime, accusation against, beliefs or motives of the victim or of those who commit these deeds, whatever the situation, including cases of civil or armed conflict.

Article 23

A doctor must never use his knowledge, his competence or his skills for the purpose of facilitating the use of torture or any other cruel, inhuman or degrading procedure for the purpose of weakening the resistance of a victim of these methods.

## The Doctor and Society

Article 24

In order to accomplish his humanitarian duties, every doctor has the right to legal protection of his professional independence and his standing in society, in times of peace as in times of war.

Article 25

It is the duty of a doctor, whether acting alone or in conjunction with other doctors, to draw the attention of society to any deficiencies in the quality of health care or in the professional independence of doctors.

Article 26

Doctors must be involved in the development and the implementation of all collective measures designed to improve the prevention, diagnosis and treatment of disease. In particular, they must provide a medical contribution to the organisation of rescue services, particularly in the event of public disaster.

Article 27

They must participate, so far as their competence and available facilities permit, in constant improvement of the quality of care through research and continual refinement of methods of treatment, in accordance with advances in medical knowledge.

## Relationships with Professional Colleagues

Article 28

The rules of professional etiquette were introduced in the interest of patients. They were designed to prevent patients becoming the victims of dishonest manoeuvres between doctors. The latter may, on the other hand, legitimately rely on their colleagues to adhere to the standards of conduct to which the profession as a whole subscribes.

Article 29

A doctor has a duty to inform the competent professional regulatory authorities of any lapses of which he may be aware on the part of his colleagues from the rules of medical ethics and good professional practice.

## Publication of Findings

Article 30

It is the duty of a doctor to publish, initially in professional journals, any discoveries that he may have made or conclusions that he may have drawn from his scientific studies relevant to diagnosis or treatment. He must submit his findings in the appropriate form for review by his colleagues before releasing them to the lay public.

Article 31

Any exploitation or advertisement of a medical success to the profit of an individual or of a group or of an institution is contrary to medical ethics.

## Continuity of Care

Article 32

A doctor, whatever his specialty, is obliged by his humanitarian duty to give emergency treatment to any patient in immediate danger, unless he is satisfied that other doctors will provide this care and are capable of doing so.

Article 33

The doctor who agrees to give care to a patient undertakes to ensure continuity of care when necessary with the help of assistants, locums or colleagues.

## Freedom of Choice

Article 34

Freedom of choice constitutes a fundamental principle of the patient:doctor relationship. The doctor must respect, and make sure that others respect, the patient's freedom of choice of doctors.

The doctor, for his part, may refuse to treat a particular patient, unless the patient is in immediate danger.

## Withdrawal of Services

Article 35

When a doctor decides to participate in an organised, collective withdrawal of services, he is not absolved of his ethical responsibilities vis-à-vis his patients to whom he must guarantee emergency services and such care as is required by those currently being treated.

## Fees

Article 36

In fixing his fees, the doctor will take account, in the absence of any contract or of individual or collective agreement, of the importance of the service which has been given, any special circumstances in a particular case, his own competence and the financial situation of the patient.

# CODE OF ETHICS FOR DOCTORS
**Norwegian Medical Association**
amended 1992

*Adopted in 1961 and most recently amended in 1992, the Norwegian Medical Association's Code of Ethics for Doctors is interesting in its freedom from the governmental intrusions that characterize U.S. codes, for example, the Norwegian code condemns advertising (I, §9). Other provisions of interest include the right to withhold information from patients (I, §13) and the admonition that physicians should take care of their own health (II, §3). Excerpts from the Norwegian code follow.*

## I. General Provisions

### §1.

A doctor's duty is to protect human health. He shall be careful and conscientious in the exercise of his profession, and help the ill to regain their health and the healthy to preserve theirs.

• • •

### §4.

Except in such cases as are mentioned above, a doctor is entitled to refuse to treat a patient provided the patient has reasonable access to treatment by another doctor.

### §5.

In examinations and treatment a doctor shall employ the means and methods indicated by sound medical practice. If an examination or treatment calls for methods for which the doctor lacks the appropriate knowledge or skill, he shall if at all possible ensure that the patient receives expert treatment.

### §6.

A doctor must not use methods which expose the patient to unnecessary risk. When new methods are being tried out, the welfare of the patient shall constantly be borne in mind.

### §7.

A doctor must not use or recommend methods which lack medical foundations in scientific research or sufficiently documented experience.

### §8.

A doctor must not conceal methods from other doctors or employ methods which are not available to any doctor.

### §9.

A doctor must not advertise medicaments, consumer goods, or methods. References in professional medical contexts in articles, lectures and the like, and involving no pecuniary gain, are not regarded as advertisements.

### §10.

A doctor shall take the greatest precautions when prescribing drugs on which the patient is or may become dependent.

### §11.

A doctor shall behave considerately and tactfully towards patients and their relatives. He must not involve himself in personal matters, family relations or the like unless the treatment of the patient justifies such involvement. Nor must he seek to exercise influence on patients or their relatives beyond that called for out of regard for the treatment.

### §12.

A doctor shall exercise discretion in respect of information he obtains in his professional capacity, even when it is not covered by statutory professional confidence.

### §13.

A doctor should generally inform a patient of his condition, but must have the right [based] on a conscientious assessment to withhold information which in his opinion may be harmful to the patient.

### §14.

Subject to the restrictions which follow from professional confidence, a doctor should give relatives the information concerning a patient's illness which the doctor finds necessary and helpful.

### §15.

A doctor shall in his practice have due regard for his patient's financial circumstances. Unnecessary or superfluous costly examinations or treatment must not take place.

### §16.

In relation to health insurance and other bodies which meet health expenses, a doctor shall be as economical as is compatible with sound medical practice.

• • •

### §19.

To whatever extent is reasonable in view of his age, specialisation and the like, a doctor should take part in collegiate arrangements aimed at providing the population with medical assistance or considered necessary to the maintenance of conditions favourable to public health.

## II. Rules Governing the Relations of Doctors with their Colleagues and Collaborators

### §1.

A doctor must show respect for colleagues and collaborators, and assist, advise and guide them.

### §2.

A doctor who sees signs of professional or ethical failings in a colleague or collaborator should first take the matter up directly with the person concerned. The approach should be tactful, especially towards students or doctors in training.

If this does not have the desired effect, the doctor should take the matter up with the person's administrative superior, bodies of the Norwegian Medical Association, or the competent health authority.

A doctor who sees signs of illness or abuse of intoxicants in a colleague or collaborator should offer his/her assistance.

### §3.

A doctor should take care of his own health and seek help if it fails.

### §4.

A doctor should take care not to criticise colleagues and collaborators in the presence of patients and their relatives, but must always keep the patient's interests in view.

• • •

# FINAL REPORT CONCERNING BRAIN DEATH AND ORGAN TRANSPLANTATION
## Japan Medical Association
### 1988

*Traditional religious and cultural values surrounding death and dying inform the Japanese public's reluctance to accept brain-based criteria for determining death and the subsequent harvesting of organs for transplantation. Generally, the medical profession has been more amenable to the use of brain criteria for determining death. In 1988, the Bioethics Council of the Japan Medical Association issued its Final Report Concerning Brain Death and Organ Transplantation. The report recognizes the legitimacy of brain criteria for determining death, in addition to the traditional cardiac criteria. However, it also includes a clause that emphasizes the need to consider the wishes of the patient and/or the patient's family and to obtain their consent when using brain criteria to determine death. This compromise position permits the introduction of brain criteria for death while not offending those individuals who oppose it.*

1. Definition of Death
   In addition to cardiac death heretofore, death of the brain (irreversible loss of brain function) can be considered as the state of death of the individual human being.
2. Brain Death Determination Criteria
   With the criteria of the Research Group of the Ministry of Health (Kazuo Takeuchi, Group Leader) as minimum required criteria, fundamental particulars should be determined by the ethics committees of university hospitals, etc., and determination should be carried out with certainty and circumspection according to these criteria in such a manner that no doubt remains.
3. Respecting the Wishes of the Patient Himself and His Family
   It is considered appropriate under present circumstances to carry out the determination of death resulting from brain death upon giving serious consideration to the wishes of the patient himself and his family and obtaining their consent.
4. Justifiability of the Determination of Death Resulting from Brain Death
   Together with being generally recognized by the Japan Medical Association and others, it is considered that the determination of death as a result of brain death is socially and legally justifiable when the consent on the part of the patient has been obtained and determination has been carried out by physicians in a reliable manner according to appropriate methods.
5. Time of Death as a Result of the Determination of Brain Death
   In regard to the time of a death as a result of a determination of brain death, it can be considered to be (1) the time when determination of brain death was first made

or (2) the time of confirmation of brain death six or more hours subsequent to that. The time of death indicated on the death certificate can be either (1) or (2) above; however, as a precaution in case of disputes over inheritance after death, the other of the two should be recorded in the records of the patient's treatment.

6. Organ Transplantation

The transplantation of organs is to be carried out in accordance with the guidelines established by the Japan Transplantation Association once the organ donor, organ recipient and the families involved have received thorough explanations and their consent given through their own free will has been obtained.

# SUMMARY OF THE REPORT ON INFORMATION FROM DOCTORS AND CONSENT OF PATIENTS
## Japan Medical Association
### 1991

*In 1951, the Japan Medical Association (JMA) issued a Physician's Code of Ethics, which is of historic interest for its emphasis on the Confucian concept of* jin, *"loving kindness," in the practice of medicine. Medicine is considered a* jin-jyutsu, *"humanitarian art." Traditionally, in Japanese medical practice, the combination of jin with the concept of* shinrai-kankei, *"fiduciary relationship," which is a positive value between people, correlated with a tendency for patients to trust and adhere to professional advice without question and a predilection toward medical paternalism. Since the 1960s, a gradual trend has emerged in Japan toward reassessing the nature of the patient–physician relationship. Exposure to contemporary Western bioethics and greater recognition of patients' rights is reflected in a movement among Japanese medical professionals to redefine the formerly paternalistic fiduciary relationship in light of a new emphasis on shared information and decision making with their patients. Although the JMA has never technically rescinded its 1951 code, the code has been superseded in practice by more recent documents from the JMA Bioethics Council that reflect the trend away from medical paternalism. One such document is the 1991 Summary of the Report on Information from Doctors and Consent of Patients, which follows.*

1. The Definition of Informed Consent

In strict terms, informed consent refers to the system of determining of the selection of medical procedures, which is carried out once the physician, as obliged, provides the patient with thorough explanations regarding feasible procedures within the course of medical treatment activities.

Informed consent is a concept which originated in U.S.A. as the principal statement of the rights of a patient and came to incorporate a specific content as a result of court-room judicial precedents and so forth in connection with mishaps during medical treatment.

It would seem necessary in the case of Japan, however, to examine its content independently and thereupon, with the opportunity offered by the informed consent, proceed with the structuring of a new relationship between physician and patient in the context of medical treatment.

2. The Relationship between the Physician's Explanation and Patient's Consent

As a general rule, the patient's consent is obtained on the occasion of direct or indirect invasions of the patient's body; carrying out such invasions without consent could, legally speaking, entail the possible occurrence of problems of the criminal infliction of bodily harm or those of civil justice involving injury compensation.

Thus, the consent of the patient is premised on explanations by the physician; the physician must provide thorough explanations to the patient necessary to allow the patient to make judgments or selections.

3. The Current Meaning of Informed Consent

In Japan up to the present, there has been a tendency on the part of the patient to leave everything up to the physician. However, more and more we are seeing an increase in the comprehension of patients relating to medical treatments, changes in the structure of present-day illnesses, together with subdivision and specialization taking place in treatment methods, resulting in an increased emphasis on the frank and open interaction between physician and patient. There has also been a deeper concern for the problem of informed consent.

At this point, instead of simply adopting the American style of informed consent intact, it is more reasonable that we should embrace one which is relevant to our own society, one which sufficiently takes into account the sentiments of the people, the history of medical treatment, cultural background, the character of the nation and so forth.

4. Specific Content of Informed Consent and Its Configuration

*The Physician's Explanation and the Patient's Consent*

The physician's explanations to the patient must be expressed in words which are easily understood, allowing effortless comprehension by the patient, with the minimum use of specialized terminology.

The patient's consent indicates that the patient has comprehended, is satisfied with and consents to the procedures which the physician proposes to take.

5. The Physician's Obligation to Explain and Its Limits

Explanations within the limits indicated below can be considered necessary under normal circumstances:

    1. The disease name and its present condition

    2. Proposed treatment methods for the disease

    3. The degree of risk involved in such treatment methods (the presence and extent of risk)

    4. Other possible choices of treatment methods and their relative advantages and disadvantages.

    5. Prognosis, that is, future assumptions relating to the patient's illness

Emergencies or cases in which the patient does not have the capacity to make judgments him or herself regarding consent after having been given explanations can be cited as exceptions to the general rule.

Cases in which the patient does not have the capacity to make judgments regarding consent after having been given explanations require that explanations be provided to the most appropriate next of kin and the patient's consent received by proxy. However, since the procedures in question are directed specifically to the patient, the inclinations of the patient should be taken into consideration when it is recognized that the patient does have judgmental capacity, though it may be impaired.

6. Informed Consent in Routine Diagnoses and Treatment

(1) Notification of Cancer

The following should be given thorough consideration as prior conditions upon the notification of cancer:

    1. The purpose of notification must be explicit.

    2. The family of the patient must be receptive.

    3. Physician or others in the practice of medicine must have a satisfactory relationship with the family of the patient.

    4. Mental care and support of the patient must be possible subsequent to notification.

(2) Living Wills

When a patient in terminal treatment has prepared a living will in advance and there is no hope of recovery, it is considered reasonable to respect the wishes of the patient not to engage in life-prolonging procedures, when such have been clearly stated.

(3) Others

If there is a necessity for blood transfusions in a patient who refuses such for religious reasons, the patient should be persuaded and then consent for transfusions obtained. However, if the patient persistently refuses, the will of the patient should be respected even though the outcome of not doing so would be disadvantageous to the patient. In such cases, it is considered that the physician does not assume any legal liability.

When the patient is a child, transfusions given contrary to the will of the parent can be considered permissible, even though the parent, as a follower of a religion, has refused such, since the child and the child's parents are fundamentally separate beings.

7. Informed Consent in Medical and Treatment Education

It cannot be denied that concern regarding informed consent among young physicians is lacking. It is of extreme importance that instruction regarding informed consent be promoted in the future both prior to graduation and thereafter through continuing education.

# OATH OF SOVIET PHYSICIANS
## 1971

*On 26 March 1971, the Presidium of the Supreme Soviet approved the text of the oath and ordered that all physicians and graduating medical students take the oath, sign a copy of it, and abide by it. The ruling went into effect on June 1, 1971. Distinctive features of this oath are: (1) dedication to preventive medicine; (2) commitment to the principles of communist morality; and (3) responsibility to the people and the Soviet government. The Soviet oath should be com-*

*pared to the 1988 Regulations on Criteria for Medical Ethics and Their Implementation, issued by the Ministry of Health, People's Republic of China, and included in this section.*

Having received the high title of physician and beginning a career in the healing arts, I solemnly swear:

to dedicate all my knowledge and all my strength to the care and improvement of human health, to treatment and prevention of disease, and to work conscientiously wherever the interests of the society will require it;

to be always ready to administer medical aid, to treat the patient with care and interest, and to keep professional secrets;

to constantly improve my medical knowledge and diagnostic and therapeutic skill, and to further medical science and the practice of medicine by my own work;

to turn, if the interests of my patients will require it, to my professional colleagues for advice and consultation, and to never refuse myself to give advice or help;

to keep and to develop the beneficial traditions of medicine in my country, to conduct all my actions according to the principles of the Communistic morale, to always keep in mind the high calling of the Soviet physician, and the high responsibility I have to my people and to the Soviet government.

I swear to be faithful to this Oath all my life long.

# SOLEMN OATH OF A PHYSICIAN OF RUSSIA
## 1992

*Approved by the Minister of Health and the Minister of Higher Education of the Russian Federation, this oath, which replaces the preceding Oath of Soviet Physicians, was first published in 1992. It is interesting to note the similarities between the new Russian oath and the Hippocratic Oath, indicating a conscious return to the Hippocratic tradition. While the Soviet oath bound physicians to the principles of communist morality and explicitly recognized their duty to the people and the Soviet state, the new oath focuses on the well-being of the individual patient.*

In the presence of my Teachers and colleagues in the great science of doctoring, accepting with deep gratitude the rights of a physician granted to me

### I SOLEMNLY PROMISE:

- to regard him who has taught me the art of doctoring as equal to my parents and to help him in his affairs and if he is in need;
- to impart any precepts, oral instruction, and all other learning to my pupils who are bound by the obligation of medical law but to no one else;
- I will conduct my life and my art purely and chastely, being charitable and not causing people harm;
- I will never deny medical assistance to anyone and will render it with equal diligence and patience to a patient of any means, nationality, religion, and conviction;
- no matter what house I may enter, I will go there for the benefit of the patient, remaining free of all intentional injustice and mischief, especially sexual relations;
- to prescribe dietetic measures and medical treatment for the patient's benefit according to my abilities and judgment, refraining from causing them any harm or injustice;
- I will never use my knowledge and skill to the detriment of anyone's health, even my enemy's;
- I will never give anyone a fatal drug if asked nor show ways to carry out such intentions;
- whatever I may see and hear during treatment or outside of treatment concerning a person's life, which should not be divulged, I will keep to myself, regarding such matters as secret;
- I promise to continue my study of the art of doctoring and do everything in my power to promote its advancement, reporting all my discoveries to the scientific world;
- I promise not to engage in the manufacture or sale of secret remedies;
- I promise to be just to my fellow doctors and not to insult their persons; however, if it is required for the benefit of a patient, I will speak the truth openly and impartially;
- in important cases I promise to seek the advice of doctors who are more versed and experienced than I; when I myself am summoned for consultation, I will acknowledge their merit and efforts according to my conscience.

If I fulfill this Oath without violating it, let me be given happiness in my life and art. If I transgress it and give a false Oath, let the opposite be my lot.

# REGULATIONS ON CRITERIA FOR MEDICAL ETHICS AND THEIR IMPLEMENTATION
### Ministry of Health, People's Republic of China
### 1988

*The following regulations on medical ethics for health-care providers were issued in December 1988 by the Ministry of Health of the People's Republic of China. The mention of socialist values in Article 1 may be compared to the statement regarding principles of communist morality found in the 1971 Soviet oath, which appears earlier in this section. It is notable, however, that these regulations do not mention responsibility to the State as did the Soviet oath. Also of note are the strong emphasis on education in medical ethics and the explicit application of the criteria to all health-care workers.*

Article 1. The purpose of the criteria is to strengthen the development of a society based on socialist values, to improve the quality of professional ethics of health-care workers and to promote health services.

Article 2. Medical ethics, which is also called professional ethics of health-care workers, guides the value system the health-care workers should have, covering all aspects from doctor-patient relationships to doctor-doctor relationships. The criteria for medical ethics form the code of conduct for health-care workers in their medical practice.

Article 3. The criteria for medical ethics include the following:

1. Heal the wounded, rescue the dying, and practice socialist humanitarianism. Keep the interests of the patient in your mind and try every means possible to relieve patient suffering.

2. Show respect to the patient's dignity and rights and treat all patients alike, whatever their nationality, race, sex, occupation, social position and economic status is.

3. Services should be provided in a civil, dignified, amiable, sympathetic, kind-hearted and courteous way.

4. Be honest in performing medical practice and conscious in observing medical discipline and law. Do not seek personal benefits through medical practice.

5. Keep the secrets related to the patient's illness and practice protective health-care service. In no case is one allowed to reveal the patient's health secret or compromise privacy.

6. Learn from other doctors and work together in cooperation. Handle professional relations between colleagues correctly.

7. Be rigorous in learning and practicing medicine and work hard to improve knowledge, ability, skills and service.

Article 4. Education in medical ethics is mandated for the implementation of these regulations and for supporting medical-ethical attitudes. Therefore, good control and assessment of medical ethics has to be introduced.

Article 5. Education on medical ethics and the promotion of medical ethics must be a part of managing and evaluating hospitals. Good and poor performance of working groups have to be judged and assessed according to these standards.

Article 6. Education in medical ethics should be conducted positively and unremittingly through linking theories with practice aiming to achieve actual and concrete results. It should be the rule to educate new health-care workers in medical ethics before they start their service; in no case are they allowed to practice before they get such an education.

Article 7. Every hospital should work out rules and regulations for the evaluation of medical ethics and should have a particular department to carry out the evaluation, regularly and irregularly. The results of the evaluation should be kept in record files.

Article 8. The evaluation of medical ethics should include self-evaluation, social evaluation, department evaluation and higher-level evaluation. Social evaluation is of particular importance and the opinions of the patients and public should be considered and health service should be offered under the surveillance of the masses.

Article 9. The result of the evaluation should be considered as an important standard in employment, promotion, payment and the hiring of health-care workers.

Article 10. Practice the rewarding of the best and the punishment of the worst. Those who observe medical ethics criteria should be rewarded and those who fail to observe criteria of medical ethics should be criticized and punished accordingly.

Article 11. These criteria are suitable for all health-care workers, including doctors, nurses, technicians and health-care administrators at all levels in all hospitals and clinics.

Article 12. Provincial health-care offices may work out detailed rules for the implementation of these criteria.

Article 13. These criteria become valid on the date they are issued.

# ETHICAL AND RELIGIOUS DIRECTIVES FOR CATHOLIC HEALTH FACILITIES
## United States Catholic Conference
### 1971, revised 1975

*The Catholic Church has published directives on medical ethics in several parts of the world, principally, though not exclusively, for use in its hospitals. These directives are considered binding not only on institutions but also on individuals: The medical staff, patients, and employees, regardless of their religion, are frequently expected to abide by such a code.*

*In the United States, a set of Ethical and Religious Directives for Catholic Hospitals was published in 1949 and revised in 1954. The directives printed here were originally approved as the national code by the National Conference of Catholic Bishops and the United States Catholic Conference in 1971 and were revised in 1975. Most distinctive are the directives on abortion, hysterectomy, sterilization, and artificial insemination. The preamble and a concluding section on the Religious Care of Patients have been omitted.*

*The directives were to be revised in 1994.*

## Section I
## Ethical and Religious Directives

### 1. General

*Directive*

1. The procedures listed in these *Directives* as permissible require the consent, at least implied or reasonably presumed, of the patient or his guardians. This condition is to be understood in all cases.
2. No person may be obliged to take part in a medical or surgical procedure which he judges in conscience to be immoral; nor may a health facility or any of its staff be obliged to provide a medical or surgical procedure which violates their conscience or these *Directives*.
3. Every patient, regardless of the extent of his physical or psychic disability, has a right to be treated with a respect consonant with his dignity as a person.
4. Man has the right and the duty to protect the integrity of his body together with all of its bodily functions.
5. Any procedure potentially harmful to the patient is morally justified only insofar as it is designed to produce a proportionate good.
6. Ordinarily the proportionate good that justifies a medical or surgical procedure should be the total good of the patient himself.
7. Adequate consultation is recommended, not only when there is doubt concerning the morality of some procedure, but also with regard to all procedures involving serious consequences, even though such procedures are listed here as permissible. The health facility has the right to insist on such consultations.
8. Everyone has the right and the duty to prepare for the solemn moment of death. Unless it is clear, therefore, that a dying patient is already well-prepared for death as regards both spiritual and temporal affairs, it is the physician's duty to inform him of his critical condition or to have some other responsible person impart this information.
9. The obligation of professional secrecy must be carefully fulfilled not only as regards the information on the patients' charts and records but also as regards confidential matters learned in the exercise of professional duties. Moreover, the charts and records must be duly safeguarded against inspection by those who have no right to see them.
10. The directly intended termination of any patient's life, even at his own request, is always morally wrong.
11. From the moment of conception, life must be guarded with the greatest care. Any deliberate medical procedure, the *purpose* of which is to deprive a fetus or an embryo of its life, is immoral.
12. Abortion, that is, the directly intended termination of pregnancy before viability, is never permitted nor is the directly intended destruction of a viable fetus. Every procedure whose sole immediate effect is the termination of pregnancy before viability is an abortion, which, in its moral context, includes the interval between conception and implantation of the embryo. Catholic hospitals are not to provide abortion services based upon the principle of material cooperation.
13. Operations, treatments, and medications, which do not directly intend termination of pregnancy but which have as their purpose the cure of a proportionately serious

pathological condition of the mother, are permitted when they cannot be safely postponed until the fetus is viable, even though they may or will result in the death of the fetus. If the fetus is not certainly dead, it should be baptized.

14. Regarding the treatment of hemorrhage during pregnancy and before the fetus is viable: Procedures that are designed to empty the uterus of a living fetus still effectively attached to the mother are not permitted; procedures designed to stop hemorrhage (as distinguished from those designed precisely to expel the living and attached fetus) are permitted insofar as necessary, even if fetal death is inevitably a side effect.

15. Cesarean section for the removal of a viable fetus is permitted, even with risk to the life of the mother, when necessary for successful delivery. It is likewise permitted, even with risk for the child, when necessary for the safety of the mother.

16. In extrauterine pregnancy the dangerously affected part of the mother (e.g., cervix, ovary, or fallopian tube) may be removed, even though fetal death is foreseen, provided that: (a) the affected part is presumed already to be so damaged and dangerously affected as to warrant its removal, and that (b) the operation is not just a separation of the embryo or fetus from its site within the part (which would be a direct abortion from a uterine appendage); and that (c) the operation cannot be postponed without notably increasing the danger to the mother.

17. Hysterectomy, in the presence of pregnancy and even before viability, is permitted when directed to the removal of a dangerous pathological condition of the uterus of such serious nature that the operation cannot be safely postponed until the fetus is viable.

### 2. Procedures Involving Reproductive Organs and Functions

*Directive*

18. Sterilization, whether permanent or temporary, for men or for women, may not be used as a means of contraception.

19. Similarly excluded is every action which, either in anticipation of the conjugal act, or in its accomplishment, or in the development of its natural consequences, proposes, whether as an end or as a means, to render procreation impossible.

20. Procedures that induce sterility, whether permanent or temporary, are permitted when: (a) They are immediately directed to the cure, diminution, or prevention of a serious pathological condition and are not directly contraceptive (that is, contraception is not the purpose); and (b) a simpler treatment is not reasonably available. Hence, for example, oophorectomy or irradiation of the ovaries may be allowed in treating carcinoma of the breast and metastasis therefrom; and orchidectomy is permitted in the treatment of carcinoma of the prostate.

21. Because the ultimate personal expression of conjugal love in the marital act is viewed as the only fitting context for the human sharing of the divine act of creation, donor insemination and insemination that is totally artificial are morally objectionable. However, help may be given to a normally performed conjugal act to attain its purpose. The use of the sex faculty outside the legitimate use by married partners is never permitted even for medical or other laudable purpose, e.g., masturbation as a means of obtaining seminal specimens.

22. Hysterectomy is permitted when it is sincerely judged to be a necessary means of removing some serious uterine pathological condition. In these cases, the pathological condition of each patient must be considered individually and care must be taken that a hysterectomy is not performed merely as a contraceptive measure, or as a routine procedure after any definite number of Cesarean sections.

23. For a proportionate reason, labor may be induced after the fetus is viable.

24. In all cases in which the presence of pregnancy would render some procedure illicit (e.g., curettage), the physician must make use of such pregnancy tests and consultation as may be needed in order to be reasonably certain that the patient is not pregnant. It is to be noted that curettage of the endometrium after rape to prevent implantation of a possible embryo is morally equivalent to abortion.

25. Radiation therapy of the mother's reproductive organs is permitted during pregnancy only when necessary to suppress a dangerous pathological condition.

### 3. Other Procedures

*Directive*

26. Therapeutic procedures which are likely to be dangerous are morally justifiable for proportionate reasons.

27. Experimentation on patients without due consent is morally objectionable, and even the moral right of the patient to consent is limited by his duties of stewardship.

28. Euthanasia ("mercy killing") in all its forms is forbidden. The failure to supply the ordinary means of preserving life is equivalent to euthanasia. However, neither the physician nor the patient is obliged to use extraordinary means.

29. It is not euthanasia to give a dying person sedatives and analgesics for the alleviation of pain, when such a measure is judged necessary, even though they may deprive the patient of the use of reason, or shorten his life.

30. The transplantation of organs from living donors is morally permissible when the anticipated benefit to the recipient is proportionate to the harm done to the donor, provided that the loss of such organ(s) does not deprive the donor of life itself nor of the functional integrity of his body.

31. Post-mortem examinations must not be begun until death is morally certain. Vital organs, that is, organs necessary to sustain life, may not be removed until death has taken place. The determination of the time of death must be made in accordance with responsible and commonly accepted scientific criteria. In accordance with current medical practice, to prevent any conflict of interest, the dying patient's doctor or doctors should ordinarily be distinct from the transplant team.

32. Ghost surgery, which implies the calculated deception of the patient as to the identity of the operating surgeon, is morally objectionable.

33. Unnecessary procedures, whether diagnostic or therapeutic, are morally objectionable. A procedure is unnecessary when no proportionate reason justifies it. *A fortiori*, any procedure that is contra-indicated by sound medical standards is unnecessary.

# HEALTH CARE ETHICS GUIDE
## Catholic Health Association of Canada
### 1991

*The Health Care Ethics Guide of the Catholic Health Association of Canada is designed for use by "all health care institutions and individuals who share an orientation toward morality based on human reason, enlivened by Christian faith and taught by the Roman Catholic Church." It replaces the Medico-Moral Guide used by the Catholic Health Association of Canada since 1971.*

*The full introduction to the guide includes a summary of the basic principles that shape Catholic medical ethics. Those principles, which can be found in textbooks, are: (1) the dignity of the person; (2) the social nature of the person; (3) the right to life; (4) a well-informed conscience; (5) the principle of double effect; (6) the principle of legitimate cooperation; (7) the principle of totality and integrity of the human person; (8) the principle of the common good, subsidiarity, and functionalism; (9) the principle of growth through suffering; and (10) the principle of stewardship and creativity.*

• • •

## Catholic Health Care Facilities

• • •

Catholic health care institutions are both communities of service and communities of work. Their raison d'être and the basic orientation of all their personnel are respect for the dignity of every person and concern for the total well-being of their patients/residents. They affirm the centrality of the resident/patient and recognize the importance of family, friends and the wider community in the health care endeavour. Underlying the care given is a comprehensive understanding of health that includes attention to the need for a balance of the biological, psychological, social and spiritual forces that interact within the person, the society and the ecosystem. Catholic health care institutions strive to provide for their personnel a milieu that is conducive to personal fulfillment.

The healing ministry of the Catholic health care facility is an expression of the ministry of Christ and of the church. Since we are creatures of body and spirit, we need visible, tangible, human institutions to assist us to work as a believing community bearing witness to the Good News. Physical, emotional, social and spiritual healing is to be a clear sign of the presence and compassion of Christ the Healer.

In order for this to happen, the total atmosphere of our institutions needs to be permeated with the love of Christ and with the visible signs of faith that characterize the authentic Catholic tradition. Some tangible signs of Catholic identity include availability of the sacraments and the prominence of various Christian symbols; a priority given to pastoral care and mission education; Catholic ownership and/or management and recognition by the bishop of the diocese of the institution as an integral part of the apostolate. It is hoped that the use of these ethical guidelines will become another tangible expression of the faith that permeates every aspect of our lives and of our health care institutions.

## Moral Reflection and Decision-Making

• • •

As Christians, we make our decisions as to what we ought to be and how we ought to act as believers in Jesus Christ. This means that our moral decisions should be based on an understanding of human life perceived by human reason and in conformity with the best medical information available, enlightened by what is revealed in the life, death and resurrection of Jesus Christ. The quality of our ethical decisions depends not merely on abstract reasoning, but on the lived faith, prudence and virtue of the decision maker.

The Catholic moral tradition is the fruit of an on-going dialogue between our understanding of human nature and our experience of God as revealed in Jesus Christ. It develops through study, reflection and a recognition of the working of the Spirit through various sources, such as, the experience of the health care and Christian communities, moral theologians, ethicists, the local bishop, church teachings and Sacred Scripture. No source of moral knowledge should be neglected in the making of moral decisions. This accumulated wisdom provides us with a firm foundation and direction for moral decision-making.

The local bishop has the responsibility to provide leadership and to collaborate with the mission of Catholic health care institutions. In fulfilling his role as the primary teacher and pastor of his community, with the assistance of specialists in different health care disciplines, he has the task to ensure that the constant teaching of the church is reflected faithfully in the context of rapidly developing medical advances and of the increasing complexity of the human sciences.

Since the Catholic moral tradition is a living tradition, our formulations of it are necessarily the product of a grasp of reality that is constantly being refined, of historically conditioned attitudes, and of limited philosophical concepts and language. At any given time in history, a particular formulation is only more or less adequate. Continued faithfulness to this living tradition presupposes growth in understanding of moral principles and their implications.

The tradition is not always clear or unanimous concerning all moral issues. In such cases, it is the teaching of the Catholic Church that obligations are not to be imposed unless they are certain. Thus, in moral questions debated by moral theologians in the church, Catholic tradition upholds a person's liberty to follow those opinions that seem to be consistent with the wishes of patients/residents and with the best standards of good health care.

• • •

## I. The Communal Nature of Health Care

• • •

### Fundamental Guideline

Catholic health care institutions are communities of service, united through collaborative activities and inspired by Roman Catholic moral principles, for the purpose of promoting a healthy society. The members of these professional and occupational communities seek fulfillment through the accomplishment of their particular responsibilities for this common end and receive just compensation for their services.

### Mission of the Catholic Health Care Institution

1. Every Catholic health care institution, in its mission statement, proclaims its religious identity that reflects a vision of life and of the world that is reasonable and in accordance with the Roman Catholic tradition. It commits itself to provide health care that is holistic and non-discriminatory. This mission will be kept in mind constantly if it is articulated clearly and reviewed regularly, with an opportunity provided for input from all members of the institution.

### Primary Purpose

2. Whatever its particular objectives, every Catholic health care institution aims primarily at the relief of suffering and the promotion of health. This leads to policies and programs that emphasize the care of people with acute or chronic illnesses, the prevention of disease and the promotion of health. Such a perspective on health care, that includes promoting a healthy social and physical environment, demands

collaboration among health care institutions and interactions between the health care system and other systems in society: education, housing, employment, religious bodies, professional organizations, and unions.

### An Atmosphere That Promotes Healing

3. The Catholic health care institution should be characterized by an atmosphere that promotes healing and by a spirit of compassion that is rooted in human solidarity and in fidelity to the healing mission of Christ. All persons within the institution are called to create an environment that is marked by mutual respect and sensitivity to the varied needs and concerns of others.

### Administrative Function

4. The administration coordinates the multiple functions in the health care institution in a way that encourages personnel and patients/residents to form a truly human community. At the heart of this community is a sense of unity of purpose expressed in collaboration involving patients/residents, families and health care givers.

• • •

### Allocation of Resources

6. Resource allocation is a primary responsibility of the health care facility in its roles as:
   • an agency commissioned to administer public funds in the health care system;
   • a human community of service expressing its solidarity with sick and infirm persons through specialized health care services directed to their needs;
   • a Christian community acting as a careful steward of God's gifts;
   • a church community following a preferential option for those who are poor.
7. Catholic health care institutions fulfill this responsibility of resource allocation in the following ways:
   • active participation in the formulation of policy for the equitable distribution of health care funds in society as a whole;
   • cooperation with other health care institutions to make limited resources available to more people;
   • planning for and appropriate distribution of funds among programs and services within the institution;
   • concern for the special needs of the most disadvantaged patients/residents.

### Evaluation of Developing Technologies

8. Critical analysis and evaluation of technology is a responsibility of each health care institution. This responsibility flows from four concerns:
   • the technologically possible is not necessarily the morally permissible;
   • the high financial cost of medical technology that benefits relatively few people limits resources for diagnosis, treatment, health promotion and disease prevention that benefit many people;
   • there are personal risks for the patients/residents involved;
   • the threat of depersonalized care can increase as technology becomes more sophisticated.

### Clinical Decision-Making

9. The patient/resident is the primary decision-maker with respect to decisions regarding treatment and care. Such decisions may, with the patient's/resident's consent, be collaborative in nature involving not only the patient/resident, but also care givers, and family or significant others where appropriate.

### Commitment to Education and Research

10. The health care institution recognizes the importance of education in its mandate, especially in the following areas: care and responsibility for one's own health; staff development; the education of students in the health care field and the education of the public in health promotion and disease prevention. This education is marked by ongoing reflection on the Christian meaning of suffering, illness, health, morality, life and death.
11. The health care institution, in keeping with its mission and purpose, recognizes the importance of research for advancing the science of health care and for improving the quality of care to its patients/residents. Research activities are guided by approved ethical standards.

### Respect for Different Cultures and Traditions

12. The health care facility recognizes the different cultures and religious traditions that are present in the institution. It respects and values these differences and strives to learn from the richness of such diversity.

### Employer/Employee Relationships

13. A special dimension of the health care community is the employer/employee relationship. This relationship calls for fairness and mutual accountability. There is a recognition of the rights and needs of the employer (represented by the board) and of the personnel.

14. Those who give direct care and those whose work enables care givers to function effectively are valued equally in the mission and operation of the institution. All persons are to be treated with respect and equal consideration in employment practices.

• • •

17. Women and men are to have equal opportunity for employment and career development and are entitled to fair compensation for their work.

• • •

### Conscientious Objection

20. No one may be required to participate in a health care procedure that in conscience the person considers to be immoral. The institution is to provide for and to facilitate the exercise of "conscientious objection" in order to protect individual freedom while at the same time continuing to fulfill its mission.

## II. Dignity of the Human Person

• • •

### Fundamental Guideline

The spiritual uniqueness and inherent dignity of each person are to be cherished by treating all persons with equal respect.

### Respect for Every Person

21. All persons, including those who are weak or sick, have value and dignity and are to be treated with respect at all times. All persons, therefore, are to be provided with the health care they need to the extent that the mission and resources of the institution allow.

### Emotional and Family Bonds

22. Each person's emotional and family ties are to be respected and fostered. These bonds create rights and duties for patients/residents as well as for their families and friends. Health care teams are to take these emotional and family ties into account in the making of decisions.

### Spiritual Care

23. The health care facility provides spiritual care for patients/residents, families and personnel, including spiritual support and an opportunity to participate in the full life of the faith community. All who work in the facility have a role to play in spiritual care, a care that is characterized by respect for the varying spiritual and religious needs of the recipients.

### Pastoral Care

24. The health care facility provides spiritual and religious care through the pastoral care department or service. Pastoral care could provide pastoral visiting, counselling, inservice education, spiritual direction, group prayer and opportunities for celebrating the sacraments.

### Knowledge of Health Status

25. The patients/residents have a right to know the state of their own health. This communication is to be given in an atmosphere of honesty and concern.

### Conscience

26. The patient's/resident's conscience is to be respected. The health care facility has the responsibility to provide the patients/residents with the information, counselling and spiritual support necessary to assist them to make decisions according to a well-formed conscience.

### Informed Consent

27. The informed consent of the patient/resident is necessary for any health care procedure. Informed consent requires that the patient/resident be given all information that would be useful to a reasonable person in the same circumstance, including the benefits, risks and harm of the proposed treatment, of its alternatives and of no treatment at all. Patients/residents must show that they understand what has been communicated to them. For the patient/resident who does not have decision-making capacity, consent is to be obtained from the guardian or others who are legally permitted to give such consent.

### Privacy

28. Every person has the right to privacy. This includes privacy of personal information, confidentiality and freedom in one's immediate situation from the unwanted intrusions of other people. Exceptions to the right of privacy must be clearly justified by those claiming them.

### Confidentiality of Information

29. Every person has the right to confidentiality of all information. In particular, special precautions are to be taken to protect the confidentiality of records, files and other information that could pose a serious threat of discrimination or other adverse social consequences. This right is limited when such confidentiality seriously endangers the health and well-being of others or when the law requires disclosure.

### Bodily Integrity

30. Surgical operations and medical interventions are justified only if the good it is hoped will be derived by the patient outweighs the foreseeable harm and risks of harm.

### Care of Those Violated or Abused

31. Health care personnel are to be trained to recognize the symptoms of violence and abuse. Institutions are to establish suitable protocols to deal with all forms of abuse, physical as well as psychological, with special attention to children, elderly persons, women and spouses.
32. The provision of special protocols in health care institutions to assist those who have been subjected to rape is highly recommended. Such protocols, however, may not approve the use of abortifacients. Institutions are also encouraged to cooperate in bringing the perpetrators of sexual assault to justice.
33. Health care facilities are to establish protocols to deal with sexual harassment within the institution. It is recommended that these protocols encompass situations among staff members and between staff members and patients/residents.

### Conflict Resolution

34. Each health care facility is to set up a mediating structure and process to deal with situations that involve conflicts between individuals or between individuals and the institution with respect to ethical issues. The intention is to initiate a dialogue that seeks to meet the needs of both the individual and the Catholic health care facility as fully as possible.

### Ethics Consultation Service

35. An ethics consultation service is to be established for every health care institution. This service can take many forms such as an ethics committee or an ethics consultant. This service exists to assist personnel, patients/residents and families with the discernment of ethical issues including those that pertain to patient/resident care.
36. This service may advise on particular ethical situations, review and recommend policies and promote education on ethical issues in the facility.

• • •

## III.  Human Reproduction

. . .

### Fundamental Guideline

The human actions directed to the transmission of human life possess a special significance and sacredness given to them by the Creator. Human life is to be respected and protected from conception to death.

### Responsible Parenthood Is to Be Fostered

39. Health care facilities are encouraged to foster responsible parenthood and to promote the various methods of the regulation of conception that respect a woman's natural fertility cycles.
40. Health professionals in relevant programs are to be well-informed on natural family planning methods. They are to provide instruction honestly and objectively about these and other methods so that couples can make free and informed decisions for responsible parenthood.
41. Any means that deliberately and intentionally frustrates the procreative aspect in sexual intercourse is morally unacceptable.

. . .

### Sterilization

42. Direct sterilization, whether it is permanent or temporary, for a man or a woman, may not be used for the regulation of conception.

. . .

### Conditions for Participation in Genetic Screening Programs

44  Individuals may participate voluntarily in a genetic screening program for research, education or genetic counselling, as long as their informed consent is obtained and there are no disproportionate risks involved.

### Conditions for Acceptability of Artificial Insemination

45. Artificial insemination (AIH) may be used appropriately within marriage as long as its use is to facilitate the natural act of marital intercourse in order to maintain the unitive and procreative meanings of marriage.

### Acceptable *In Vivo* Fertilizations

46. Certain *in vivo* fertilization procedures that respect the personal dimension of the marital act and protect every embryo, i.e. gamete intrafallopian transfer (GIFT), tubal ovum transfer (TOT), may be used to assist a married couple to achieve pregnancy.

### Unacceptable Forms of Artificial Insemination and Fertilization

47. Artificial insemination (AID) of a married woman with the sperm of a donor who is not her husband and fertilization with the husband's sperm of an ovum not from his wife are contrary to the covenant and unity of marriage.
48. *In vitro* fertilization is not permitted because it radically removes procreation from the personal, sexual act of love of the couple and because it can lead to the deliberate destruction of embryos.
49. Fertilization using the sperm and/or ovum from a deceased spouse(s) violates the natural aspect of the conjugal act as well as the dignity of the child by deliberately separating the child from the bonding and nurturing normally coming from the biological parent(s).

### Surrogate Mothers

50. Embryo or male gamete transfers to "surrogate mothers" are not permitted because such procedures violate the unity and dignity of marriage and the natural bonding involved in pregnancy.

### Disease Treatment of Pregnant Mothers

51. Medical means required to prevent or cure a grave illness in a pregnant woman that cannot be deferred until the newborn child is viable are permitted even though the pregnancy may be endangered.

### Abortions

52. Direct abortion, i.e. any deliberate action with the primary purpose of depriving an embryo or a fetus of its life, is immoral. All aborted embryos and fetuses are to be treated with the same respect owed to any other deceased human being.

53. Catholic health care institutions are to provide compassionate physical, psychological, emotional and spiritual care for those women and men who are distressed due to their involvement in abortions.

### Prenatal Diagnosis and Treatment

54. Prenatal diagnostic procedures with the informed and free consent of the parents are permitted as long as they respect the life and integrity of the embryo or fetus and are directed toward its protection or healing as an individual. The anticipated benefits for both the parents and the unborn must outweigh the risks involved in the diagnostic procedures.

55. The presentation of any diagnostic information is to be complete and objective. It is to be communicated in a supportive manner with no deliberate attempt to link prenatal diagnosis to direct abortion. Counselling and pastoral support are to be made available for the parents.

## IV. Organ Donation and Transplantation

• • •

### Fundamental Guideline

In the donation and transplantation of human organs the functional integrity of both donor and recipient is to be respected.

### Respect for Donor, Recipient and Common Good

56. In the donation and transplantation of human organs, respect is to be given to the rights of the donor, the recipient and the common good of society. In transplantation (autografts, allografts, and heterografts) the functional integrity of the individuals concerned is always to be respected. In addition, the transplanted organ is to fulfill the same essential function as it fulfilled in the donor's body. Organ or tissue donation by minors may be permitted in certain rare situations.

### Donors: Justification

57. The transplantation of an organ from one person to another is justified only if the good to be derived by the recipient is in proportion to the foreseeable damage to the donor. This requires that donors not be deprived of life or of the essential integrity of their bodily functions, that the transplanted organ be donated without coercion, and that the donor's consent or that of the parent or guardian, be free and informed.

### Recipients: Transplantation as Last Resort

58. The decision to transplant body organs is to be undertaken only after careful evaluation by health professionals of the availability and effectiveness of other possible therapies.

### Eligibility for Being a Recipient

59. The choice of transplant recipients is not to be based on criteria of personal or social worth. The recipients of organs are to be chosen according to principles of distributive justice. (Refer to article 21)

### Allocation of Resources: Social Justice

60. Basic health care needs are to be considered in the allocation of resources for transplantations, especially when it is a question of novel procedures involving scarce organs and expensive, limited medical facilities. (Refer to articles 5–8)

### Brain Cell Transplantations

61. Transplantations to the brain in order to restore functions lost through disease are permitted as long as the unique personal identity and abilities of the recipient are not compromised in any way.

### From Aborted Fetuses

62. Transplantations using organs and tissues from deliberately aborted fetuses are ethically objectionable. No fetus is ever to be conceived simply as a means to obtain tissue/organs for transplant purposes.

### From Dead Anencephalic Infants

63. The use of organs or tissue from an anencephalic infant after complete brain death has occurred may be justified. Pressure is not to be exerted on the parents for such a procedure.

### From Human Cadavers

64. Organ transplants from human cadavers based on the person's premortem-manifested wish, or in the absence of directions, such a wish expressed by the next of kin, are permissible for all organs. The previously expressed objections of the deceased are to be respected. No organs may be removed until the donor's death has been authenticated by a competent authority other than the recipient's physician or the transplant team. Particular attention should be taken to provide for the dying donor the usual care available to any dying person.

### No Monetary Remuneration

65. Monetary remuneration for tissues or organ donations contradicts the principle of charity which is part of the necessary justification for such transplantations. Organs, tissues and blood, therefore, should not be bought or sold.

### From Living Animals

66. Transplantations or implantations from living animals to humans and artificial substitutes for tissues or organs are permissible as long as these can fulfill an essentially beneficial human function in the recipient. The human dignity of the recipient is not to be compromised in any way and due respect is to be paid to the non-human donor in the whole transplant procedure.

### Distinct Teams for Health Care and Transplantation

• • •

### Evaluation and Communication of Medical Progress

• • •

## V.  Care of the Dying Person

• • •

### Fundamental Guideline

The dignity of the human person calls for respect through every stage of life. During the dying process and at the moment of death the patients/residents are to be surrounded by all appropriate healing and pastoral care resources.

### Care of the Dying Person

70. The Catholic health care facility is to provide dying persons with care, compassion and comfort. This ought to include the following: full information about their condition; the opportunity for discussion with health care personnel; full disclosure to the family of the patient's/resident's condition with the latter's consent, unless this is not possible because the patient/resident is non-competent; the provision of whatever social, emotional and spiritual support is needed and a degree of privacy that ensures death with dignity and peace.

### Palliative Care

71. Special care is to be extended to persons who are terminally ill and who are dying. For Christians and many others death can be the supreme moment of their final earthly encounter with God.
72. Catholic heath care facilities are encouraged to provide palliative care in specialized units and also by extension of this approach to the whole institution.

### Decision-Making and the Dying Person

73. In making the complex ethical decisions often required in the treatment of the dying person, the patient/resident is to be the primary decision-maker. Assistance

in decision-making is to be provided, as appropriate, by care givers, family, and other members of the dying person's personal community.

### The Competent Dying Person

74. The informed and voluntary decisions of competent persons, in consultation with their care givers and family, should determine whether life-sustaining treatment is to be undertaken or continued. Health care givers are to promote understanding of available treatment options and to facilitate the dying persons' making decisions on their own behalf.

### The Non-Competent Dying Person

75. When individuals are non-competent, that is, lack adequate decision-making capacity with respect to treatment, every effort is to be made to ensure that the choice of health care treatment is consistent with their known views. Care givers are to take into account the wishes that the patients/residents stated before they became incapacitated, giving due regard to those wishes expressed in writing. When their wishes are not known, family members or substitute decision-makers will act to promote the dying person's best interests.

### Proportionate Means of Treatment

76. Competent patients/residents are required to seek those measures for preserving life that offer a reasonable hope of benefit and that can be obtained and used without excessive pain, expense, or other serious inconvenience.

77. In deciding for non-competent persons whose wishes may not be known, those measures for preserving life that offer a reasonable hope of benefit and that can be obtained and used without excessive pain, expense, or other serious inconvenience, must be provided.

### Disproportionate Means of Treatment

78. Patients/residents are not obliged to seek treatment when it is of no benefit or when the burdens resulting from treatment are disproportionate to the benefits hoped for or obtained.

79. There is no obligation to provide treatment to patients/residents when it is of no benefit or when the burdens resulting from treatment are disproportionate to the benefits hoped for or obtained. Such a decision should include consultation with the patient/resident and/or family members or substitute decision-makers.

### Forgoing Life-Sustaining Treatment

80. Decisions to forgo providing life-sustaining measures are to be guided by a consideration of the benefits and burdens to the dying persons, taking into account their past and present expressed wishes, medical condition, age, personal values, religious convictions, psychological and economic resources and family support.

81. It is permitted, usually with the patient's/resident's consent, to forgo cardiopulmonary resuscitation, dialysis, or other medical procedure when it is judged that application of the procedure would impose on the person strain or suffering out of proportion with the benefits to be gained from the procedure.

82. Even when life-sustaining treatment has been undertaken, this treatment may be interrupted when the burdens outweigh the benefits. The competent patient/resident makes this decision. For such a decision to be made for non-competent patients/residents, account is to be taken of their prior wishes and the opinions of family or substitute decision-makers, physicians and other health care professionals who have special competence in the matter.

83. For persons in the final phase of a terminal illness it is morally permissible to forgo treatment, including artificially supplied nutrition and hydration, that secures only a precarious and burdensome prolongation of life.

84. A decision to forgo useless or burdensome treatment does not mean abandonment of the patients/residents. In all cases, their dignity and comfort as well as social, emotional and spiritual support must be maintained.

### Limits to Treatment

85. Treatment decisions for the patient/resident are never to include actions that intentionally cause death.

### Pain Relief

86. Patients/residents in the final phase of terminal illness may request and be given whatever analgesics are required to lessen their pain and suffering, even if such analgesics, though not intentionally, could shorten life.

### Suicide

87. Intentionally causing one's own death, or directly assisting in such action (suicide, or assisting suicide), is morally wrong.
88. Refusal to begin or to continue to use a medical procedure where the burdens, harm and risks of harm are out of proportion to any anticipated benefit is not the equivalent of suicide. It may be considered an acceptance of the human condition, a wish to avoid the application of a medical procedure that is disproportionate to the beneficial results that can be expected or it may reflect an acceptable desire not to impose excessive burden on the family or community.

### Infectious Diseases

89. Infectious diseases, especially ones with fatal outcomes or that are stigmatized such as AIDS, place special demands on care givers and require concerted efforts in education and prevention. Individuals with such infectious diseases deserve the same standards of care as other patients/residents: they are to be treated with compassion, respect and dignity.

• • •

## VI. Research on Human Subjects

• • •

### Fundamental Guideline

Research on human subjects should always ensure the highest respect for the human dignity of those participating in this research.

• • •

### Research on Competent Human Subjects

95. In all research involving competent individuals, subjects are to provide free and informed consent for their involvement. Volunteer patients who decline participation in experiments must be assured that their health care needs will not be compromised because of their refusal.

### Research on Vulnerable Groups

96. Research with children and with other subjects who lack competence to consent to participation involves special requirements:
    • For research that is of potentially direct benefit to the subject, consent is to be obtained from the appropriate guardian, and where possible, assent must be given by the subject.
    • For research that does not offer a potentially direct benefit to the subject the following conditions are to be met: there is no valid alternative to the specific population involved; the research involves no risk, or at the most, minimal risk; appropriate substitute consent is obtained and, to the extent possible, the subject assents.
    • In all situations, a subject's refusal to participate should be respected.

### Research on Embryos and Fetuses

97. Medical researchers must refrain from interventions on live embryos and fetuses, unless there is a moral certainty of not causing harm to the life or integrity of the unborn child and the mother, and on condition that the parents have given their free and informed consent to the procedure.
98. Experimentation on embryos and fetuses, whether viable or not, must respect them as human beings. Experimentation on them that is not therapeutic is not permitted.

### Cloning of Human Persons

99. Attempts to reproduce human life through cloning are contrary to human dignity.

### Preservation of Human Embryos

100. The practice of producing or keeping alive human embryos for commercial purposes or simply to be exploited as "biological material" is immoral because it is opposed to human dignity.

### Cryopreservation

101. The freezing of embryos, even when carried out to preserve the life of an embryo (cryopreservation) constitutes an offense against the respect due to human beings.

### Genetic Selection

102. Attempts to influence chromosomatic or genetic inheritance that are not therapeutic but aimed at selection of human beings according to predetermined categories, such as gender, are manipulations contrary to the personal dignity, integrity and identity of the human being. Such attempts are immoral and cannot be justified on the grounds of possible beneficial consequences for future humanity.

### Experimentation with Gametes

103. Any embryo research with the gametes of deceased spouses is not allowed.
104. Attempts to fertilize a human gamete with that of an animal are immoral because they are contrary to human dignity.

### Research on Non-Human Subjects

• • •

### Participation of Health Care Workers

• • •

### Access to and Use of Information

• • •

# THE OATH OF A MUSLIM PHYSICIAN
### Islamic Medical Association of North America
### 1977

*Adopted in 1977 by the Islamic Medical Association of North America, the Oath of a Muslim Physician is a composite drawn from the historical and contemporary writings of Muslim physicians.*

Praise be to Allah (God), the Teacher, the Unique, Majesty of the heavens, the Exalted, the Glorious, Glory be to Him, the Eternal Being Who created the Universe and all the creatures within, and the only Being Who containeth the infinity and the eternity. We serve no other god besides Thee and regard idolatry as an abominable injustice.

Give us the strength to be truthful, honest, modest, merciful and objective.

Give us the fortitude to admit our mistakes, to amend our ways and to forgive the wrongs of others.

Give us the wisdom to comfort and counsel all towards peace and harmony.

Give us the understanding that ours is a profession sacred that deals with your most precious gifts of life and intellect.

Therefore, make us worthy of this favoured station with honor, dignity and piety so that we may devote our lives in serving mankind, poor or rich, literate or illiterate, Muslim or non-Muslim, black or white with patience and tolerance with virtue and reverance, with knowledge and vigilance, with Thy love in our hearts and compassion for Thy servants, Thy most precious creation.

Hereby we take this oath in Thy name, the Creator of all the Heavens and the earth and follow Thy counsel as Thou hast revealed to Prophet Mohammad (pbuh).

"Whoever killeth a human being, not in lieu of another human being nor because of mischief on earth, it is as if he hath killed all mankind. And if he saveth a human life, he hath saved the life of all mankind." (Qur'an v/35)

# ISLAMIC CODE OF MEDICAL ETHICS
## KUWAIT DOCUMENT
### Islamic Organization of Medical Sciences
1981

*The First International Conference on Islamic Medicine, held in Kuwait in January 1981, endorsed this Islamic Code of Medical Ethics with the hope that every Muslim doctor would "find in it the guiding light to maintain his professional behaviour within the boundaries of Islamic teachings." As do other Muslim medical ethics texts, the code draws on passages from the Qur'an and demonstrates an explicitly religious tone, more so even than most contemporary Judaeo-Christian medical ethics directives. The code includes an oath for physicians.*

## The Oath of the Doctor

I swear by God . . . The Great

To regard God in carrying out my profession

To protect human life in all stages and under all circumstances, doing my utmost to rescue it from death, malady, pain and anxiety . . .

To keep people's dignity, cover their privacies and lock up their secrets . . .

To be, all the way, an instrument of God's mercy, extending my medical care to near and far, virtuous and sinner and friend and enemy . . .

To strive in the pursuit of knowledge and harnessing it for the benefit but not the harm of Mankind . . .

To revere my teacher, teach my junior, and be brother to members of the Medical Profession joined in piety and charity . . .

To live my Faith in private and in public, avoiding whatever blemishes me in the eyes of God, His apostle and my fellow Faithful.

And may God be witness to this Oath.

• • •

## Definition of Medical Profession

• "THERAPEUSIS" is a noble Profession. God honoured it by making it the miracle of Jesus son of Mary. Abraham enumerating his Lord's gifts upon him included "and if I fall ill He cures me."

• Like all aspects of knowledge, medical knowledge is part of the knowledge of God "who taught man what man never knew." The study of Medicine entails the revealing of God's signs in His creation. 'And in yourselves . . . do you not see?' The practice of Medicine brings God's mercy unto His subjects. Medical practice is therefore an act of worship and charity on top of being a career to make a living.

• But God's mercy is as accessible to all people including good and evil, virtuous and vicious and friend and foe—as are the rays of His sun, the comfort of His breeze, the coolness of His water and the bounty of His provision. And upon this basis must the medical profession operate, along the single track of God's mercy, never adversive and never punitive, never taking justice as its goal but mercy, under whatever situations and circumstances.

• In this respect the medical profession is unique. It shall never yield to social pressures motivated by enmity or feud be it personal, political or military. Enlightened statesmanship will do good by preserving the integrity of the medical profession and protecting its position beyond enmity or hostility.

• The provision of medical practice is a religious dictate upon the community, 'Fardh Kifaya,' that can be satisfied on behalf of the community by some citizens taking up medicine. It is the duty of the state to ensure the needs of the nation to doctors in the various needed specialities. In Islam, this is a duty that the ruler owes the nation.

• Need may arise to import from afar such medical expertise that is not locally available. It is the duty of the State to satisfy this need.

• It also behoves the State to recruit suitable candidates from the nation's youth to be trained as doctors. An ensuing duty therefore is to establish relevant schools, faculties, clinics, hospitals and institutions that are adequately equipped and manned to fulfill that purpose.

• "Medicine" is a religious necessity for society. In religious terms, whatever is necessary to satisfy that "necessity" automatically acquires the status of a "necessity." Exceptions shall therefore be made from certain general rules of jurisprudence for the sake of making medical education possible. One such example is the intimate inspection of the human body whether alive or dead, without in any way compromising the respect befitting the human body in life and death, and always in a climate of piety and awareness of the presence of God.

• The preservation of man's life should embrace also the utmost regard to his dignity, feelings, tenderness and the privacy of his sentiments and body parts. A patient is entitled to full attention, care and feeling of security while with his doctor. The doctor's privilege of being exempted from some general rules is only coupled with more responsibility and duty that he should carry out in conscientiousness and excellence in observing God, "excellence that entails that you worship God as if you see Him. For even though you don't see Him, He sees you."

• • •

## Characters of the Physician

• The physician should be amongst those who believe in God, fulfill His rights, are aware of His greatness, obedient to His orders, refraining from His prohibitions, and observing Him in secret and in public.

• The physician should be endowed with wisdom and graceful admonition. He should be cheering not dispiriting, smiling and not frowning, loving and not hateful, tolerant and not edgy. He should never succumb to a grudge or fall short of clemency. He should be an instrument of God's justice, forgiveness and not punishment, coverage and not exposure.

• He should be so tranquil as never to be rash even when he is right . . . chaste of words even when joking . . . tame of voice and not noisy or loud, neat and trim and not shabby or unkempt . . . conducive of trust and inspiring of respect . . . well mannered in his dealings with the poor or rich, modest or great . . . in perfect control of his composure . . . and never compromising his dignity, however modest and forebearing.

• The physician should firmly know that "life" is God's . . . awarded only by Him . . . and that "Death" is the conclusion of one life and the beginning of another. Death is a solid truth . . . and it is the end of all but God. In his profession the Physician is a soldier for "Life" only . . . defending and preserving it as best as it can be, to the best of his ability.

• The Physician should offer the good example by caring for his own health. It is not befitting for him that his "do's" and "don'ts" are not observed primarily by himself. He should not turn his back on the lessons of medical progress, because he will never convince his patients unless they see the evidence of his own conviction . . . God addresses us in the Qoran by saying "and make not your own hands throw you into destruction." The Prophet says "your body has a right on you" . . . and the known dictum is "no harm or harming in Islam."

• • •

• The role of Physician is that of a catalyst through whom God, the Creator, works to preserve life and health. He is merely an instrument of God in alleviating people's illness. For being so designated the Physician should be grateful and forever seeking God's help. He should be modest, free from arrogance and pride and never fall into boasting or hint at self glorification through speech, writing or direct or subtle advertisement.

• The Physician should strive to keep abreast of scientific progress and innovation. His zeal or complacency and knowledge or ignorance, directly bear on the health and well-being of his patients. Responsibility for others should limit his freedom to expend his time. As the poor and needy have a recognized right in the money of the capable, so the patients own a share of the Doctor's time spent in study and in following the progress of medicine.

• The Physician should also know that the pursuit of knowledge has a double indication in Islam. Apart from the applied therapeutic aspect, pursuit of knowledge is in itself worship, according to the Qoranic guidance: "And say . . . My Lord . . . advance me in knowledge." and: "Among His worshippers . . . the learned fear Him most" . . . and: "God will raise up the ranks of those of you who believed and those who have been given knowledge."

## Doctor–Doctor Relationship

• • •

• Physicians are jointly responsible for the health care of the Nation . . . and complement one another through the variety of their medical specialization be they preventive or therapeutic, in the private sector or in State employment . . . all abiding by the ethics and rules of their profession.

• • •

## Doctor–Patient Relationship

• For the sake of the patient the Doctor was . . . and not the other way round. Health is the goal and medical care is the means . . . the "patient" is master and the "Doctor" is at his service. As the Prophet says "The strongest should follow the pace of the weakest . . . for he is the one to be considered in deciding the pace of travel." Rules, schedules, time-tables and services should be so manipulated as to revolve around the patient and comply with his welfare and comfort as the top and overriding priority . . . other considerations coming next.

• • •

• The sphere of a Doctor's charity, nicety, tolerance and patience should be large enough to encompass the patient's relatives, friends and those who care for or worry about him . . . but without of course compromising the dictates of "Professional Secrecy".

• Health is a basic human necessity and is not a matter of luxury. It follows that the Medical Profession is unique in that the client is not denied the service even if he cannot afford the fee. Medical legislature should ensure medical help to all needy of it, by issuing and executing the necessary laws and regulations.

• • •

## Professional Secrecy

Keeping other persons' secrets is decreed on all the Faithful . . . the more so if these were Doctors, for people willfully disclose their secrets and feelings to their doctors, confident of the time old heritage of Professional Secrecy, that the medical profession embraced since the dawn of history. The Prophet (peace be upon Him) described the three signs of the hypocrite as: "He lies when he speaks, he breaks his promise and he betrays when confided in." The Doctor shall put the seal of confidentiality on all information acquired by him through sight, hearing or deduction. Islamic spirit also requires that the items of the Law should stress the right of the patient to protect his secrets that he confides to his Doctor. A breach thereof would be detrimental to the practice of medicine, beside precluding several categories of patients from seeking medical help.

## Doctor's Role During War

• Since the earliest battles of Islam it was decreed that the wounded is protected by his wound and the captive by his captivity. The faithful are praised in the Qoran as: "they offer food—dear as it is—to the needy, orphan or captive, (saying) we feed you for the sake of God without seeking any reward or gratitude from you." The Prophet (peace be upon Him) said to his companions: "I entrust the captives to your charity" . . . and they did . . . even giving them priority over themselves in the best of the food they shared. It is of interest to note that this was thirteen centuries prior to the Geneva Convention and the Red Cross.

• • •

• The Medical Profession shall not permit its technical, scientific or other resources to be utilized in any sort of harm or destruction or infliction upon man of physical, psychological, moral or other damage . . . regardless of all political or military considerations.

• • •

## The Sanctity of Human Life

• "On that account we decreed for the Children of Israel that whoever kills a human soul for other than manslaughter or corruption in the land, it shall be as if he killed all mankind, and who-so-ever saves the life of one, it shall be as if he saved the life of all mankind." 5-32

• Human Life is sacred . . . and should not be willfully taken except upon the indications specified in Islamic Jurisprudence, all of which are outside the domain of the Medical Profession.

• A Doctor shall not take away life even when motivated by mercy. This is prohibited because this is not one of the legitimate indications for killing. Direct guidance in this respect is given by the Prophet's tradition: "In old times there was a man with an ailment that taxed his endurance. He cut his wrist with a knife and bled to death. God was displeased and said 'My subject hastened his end . . . I deny him paradise.'"

• • •

• The sanctity of human Life covers all its stages including intrauterine life of the embryo and fetus. This shall not be compromised by the Doctor save for the absolute medical necessity recognised by Islamic Jurisprudence.

• • •

• In his defence of Life, however, the Doctor is well advised to realize his limit and not transgress it. If it is scientifically certain that life cannot be restored, then it is futile to diligently keep on the vegetative state of the patient by heroic means of animation or preserve him by deep-freezing or other artificial methods. It is the process of life that the Doctor aims to maintain and not the process of dying. In any case, the Doctor shall not take a positive measure to terminate the patient's life.

• To declare a person dead is a grave responsibility that ultimately rests with the Doctor. He shall appreciate the seriousness of his verdict and pass it in all honesty and only when sure of it. He may dispel any trace of doubt by seeking counsel and resorting to modern scientific gear.

• The Doctor shall do his best that what remains of the life of an incurable patient will be spent under good care, moral support and freedom from pain and misery.

• The Doctor shall comply with the patient's right to know his illness. The Doctor's particular way of answering should however be tailored to the particular patient in question. It is the Doctor's duty to thoroughly study the psychological acumen of his patient. He shall never fall short of suitable vocabulary if the situation warrants the deletion of frightening nomenclature or coinage of new names, expressions or descriptions.

• In all cases the Doctor should have the ability to bolster his patient's faith and endow him with tranquility and peace of mind.

## Doctor and Society

• • •

• The Medical Profession shall take it as duty to combat such health-destructive habits as smoking, uncleanliness, etc.

• • •

The combat and prevention of environmental pollution falls under this category.

• • •

# SECTION III

## Ethical Directives for Other Health-Care Professions

Code for Nurses, International Council of Nurses [1973, reaffirmed 1989]

Code for Nurses with Interpretive Statements, American Nurses' Association [1950, revised 1976, 1985]

Code of Ethics for Nursing, Canadian Nurses Association [1985, revised 1991]

Code of Ethics, American Chiropractic Association [1994–1995]

Principles of Ethics and Code of Professional Conduct with Advisory Opinions, American Dental Association [revised to May 1994]

Code of Ethics for the Profession of Dietetics, American Dietetic Association [1987]

Code of Ethics, American Association of Pastoral Counselors [last amended 1994]

Guidelines for the Chaplain's Role in Bioethics, College of Chaplains, American Protestant Health Association [1992]

Code of Ethics, American Pharmaceutical Association [1969, amended 1975, revised 1981]

Guidelines for Codes of Ethics for Pharmacists, Fédération Internationale Pharmaceutique [1988]

Code of Ethics and Guide for Professional Conduct, American Physical Therapy Association [1981, last amended 1991]

Occupational Therapy Code of Ethics, American Occupational Therapy Association [1988]

Code of Ethics of the Physician Assistant Profession, American Academy of Physician Assistants [1983, amended 1985, reaffirmed 1990]

Ethical Principles of Psychologists and Code of Conduct, American Psychological Association [1992]

Code of Ethics, National Association of Social Workers [1979, revised 1990]

Code of Ethics, American College of Healthcare Executives [amended 1990]

Ethical Conduct for Health Care Institutions, American Hospital Association [1992]

*This section demonstrates the great number and diversity of ethical directives for health-care professionals other than physicians. The section opens with several codes of ethics for nurses, followed by ethics directives for other professional groups from chiropractors and dentists to social workers and hospital administrators.*

*Most of the documents in this section represent professional organizations in the United States; the reader is referred to the bibliography to the Appendix for assistance in locating equivalent documents from other countries.*

# CODE FOR NURSES
### International Council of Nurses
### 1973, reaffirmed 1989

*The International Council of Nurses first adopted an international code of ethics for nurses in 1953 and revised it in 1965. In 1973, the council adopted a new code, which was reaffirmed in 1989.*

*The 1973 code includes several changes from the 1965 code. (1) The 1973 code makes explicit the nurse's responsibility and accountability for nursing care. It deletes the statement in the 1965 code, "The nurse is under an obligation to carry out the physician's orders intelligently and loyally," which tended to abrogate the nurse's judgment and personal responsibility. (2) The 1965 code stated that "the nurse believes in the . . . preservation of human life," adding: "The fundamental responsibility of the nurse is threefold: to conserve life, to alleviate suffering and to promote health." In its place, the 1973 code points to a fourfold responsibility: "to promote health, to prevent illness, to restore health and to alleviate suffering," adding that "respect for life, dignity and rights of man are inherent in nursing." (3) The traditional concept of the virtuous nurse was expressed in the 1965 code: "In personal conduct nurses should not knowingly disregard the accepted pattern of behavior of the community in which they live and work." In its place, the 1973 code incorporates a statement that places emphasis on the profession: "the nurse when acting in a professional capacity should at all times maintain the standards of personal conduct that would reflect credit upon the profession." The text of the International Code for Nurses follows.*

The fundamental responsibility of the nurse is fourfold: to promote health, to prevent illness, to restore health and to alleviate suffering.

The need for nursing is universal. Inherent in nursing is respect for life, dignity and rights of man. It is unrestricted by considerations of nationality, race, creed, colour, age, sex, politics or social status.

Nurses render health services to the individual, the family and the community and coordinate their services with those of related groups.

## Nurses and People

The nurse's primary responsibility is to those people who require nursing care.

The nurse, in providing care, promotes an environment in which the values, customs and spiritual beliefs of the individual are respected.

The nurse holds in confidence personal information and uses judgement in sharing this information.

## Nurses and Practice

The nurse carries personal responsibility for nursing practice and for maintaining competence by continual learning.

The nurse maintains the highest standards of nursing care possible within the reality of a specific situation.

The nurse uses judgement in relation to individual competence when accepting and delegating responsibilities.

The nurse when acting in a professional capacity should at all times maintain standards of personal conduct which reflect credit upon the profession.

## Nurses and Society

The nurse shares with other citizens the responsibility for initiating and supporting action to meet the health and social needs of the public.

## Nurses and Co-workers

The nurse sustains a cooperative relationship with co-workers in nursing and other fields.

The nurse takes appropriate action to safeguard the individual when his care is endangered by a co-worker or any other person.

## Nurses and the Profession

The nurse plays the major role in determining and implementing desirable standards of nursing practice and nursing education.

The nurse is active in developing a core of professional knowledge.

The nurse, acting through the professional organization, participates in establishing and maintaining equitable social and economic working conditions in nursing.

# CODE FOR NURSES WITH INTERPRETIVE STATEMENTS
### American Nurses' Association
### 1950, revised 1976, 1985

*The 1985 Code for Nurses is a revised version of the code adopted by the American Nurses' Association (ANA) in 1950. The eleven-point code and the accompanying interpretive statements provide a framework for ethical decision making that includes several noteworthy aspects: (1) It identifies the values and beliefs that undergird the ethical standards; (2) it encompasses a breadth of social and professional concerns; (3) it manifests an awareness of the ethical implications of shifting professional roles and of the complexity of modern health care; and (4) it goes beyond prescriptive statements regarding personal and professional conduct by advocating a sense of accountability to the client.*

*Although the text of the code remains essentially unchanged from the 1976 revision, both the organization and the text of the interpretive statements have been modified somewhat. Among the changes: (1) The discussion of human dignity following point 1 is expanded and includes specific statements that "the nurse does not act deliberately to terminate the life of any person," but that nurses may provide symptomatic intervention to dying clients "even when the interventions entail substantial risks of hastening death"; and (2) a statement under point 11 in the 1976 code, that "quality health care is mandated as a right to all citizens," has been deleted. The 1985 ANA Code for Nurses and the text of selected interpretive statements are printed here.*

1   **The nurse provides services with respect for human dignity and the uniqueness of the client, unrestricted by considerations of social or economic status, personal attributes, or the nature of health problems.**

## 1.1 Respect for Human Dignity

The fundamental principle of nursing practice is respect for the inherent dignity and worth of every client. Nurses are morally obligated to respect human existence and the individuality of all persons who are the recipients of nursing actions. Nurses therefore must take all reasonable means to protect and preserve human life when there is hope of recovery or reasonable hope of benefit from life-prolonging treatment.

Truth telling and the process of reaching informed choice underlie the exercise of self-determination, which is basic to respect for persons. Clients should be as fully involved as possible in the planning and implementation of their own health care. Clients have the moral right to determine what will be done with their own person; to be given accurate information, and all the information necessary for making informed judgments; to be assisted with weighing the benefits and burdens of options in their treatment; to accept, refuse, or terminate treatment without coercion; and to be given necessary emotional support. Each nurse has an obligation to be knowledgeable about the moral and legal rights of all clients and to protect and support those rights. In situations in which the client lacks the capacity to make a decision, a surrogate decision maker should be designated.

Individuals are interdependent members of the community. Taking into account both individual rights and the interdependence of persons in decision making, the nurse recognizes those situations in which individual rights to autonomy in health care may temporarily be overridden to preserve the life of the human community; for example, when a disaster demands triage or when an individual presents a direct danger to others. The many variables involved make it imperative that each case be considered with full awareness of the need to preserve the rights and responsibilities of clients and the demands of justice. The suspension of individual rights must always be considered a deviation to be tolerated as briefly as possible.

### 1.2  Status and Attributes of Clients

The need for health care is universal, transcending all national, ethnic, racial, religious, cultural, political, educational, economic, developmental, personality, role, and sexual differences. Nursing care is delivered without prejudicial behavior. Individual value systems and life-styles should be considered in the planning of health care with and for each client. Attributes of clients influence nursing practice to the extent that they represent factors the nurse must understand, consider, and respect in tailoring care to personal needs and in maintaining the individual's self-respect and dignity.

### 1.3  The Nature of Health Problems

The nurse's respect for the worth and dignity of the individual human being applies, irrespective of the nature of the health problem. It is reflected in care given the person who is disabled as well as one without disability, the person with long-term illness as well as one with acute illness, the recovering patient as well as one in the last phase of life. This respect extends to all who require the services of the nurse for the promotion of health, the prevention of illness, the restoration of health, the alleviation of suffering, and the provision of supportive care of the dying. The nurse does not act deliberately to terminate the life of any person.

The nurse's concern for human dignity and for the provision of high quality nursing care is not limited by personal attitudes or beliefs. If ethically opposed to interventions in a particular case because of the procedures to be used, the nurse is justified in refusing to participate. Such refusal should be made known in advance and in time for other appropriate arrangements to be made for the client's nursing care. If the nurse becomes involved in such a case and the client's life is in jeopardy, the nurse is obliged to provide for the client's safety, to avoid abandonment, and to withdraw only when assured that alternative sources of nursing care are available to the client.

The measures nurses take to care for the dying client and the client's family emphasize human contact. They enable the client to live with as much physical, emotional, and spiritual comfort as possible, and they maximize the values the client has treasured in life. Nursing care is directed toward the prevention and relief of the suffering commonly associated with the dying process. The nurse may provide interventions to relieve symptoms in the dying client even when the interventions entail substantial risks of hastening death.

### 1.4  The Setting for Health Care

The nurse adheres to the principle of nondiscriminatory, nonprejudicial care in every situation and endeavors to promote its acceptance by others. The setting shall not determine the nurse's readiness to respect clients and to render or obtain needed services.

### 2    The nurse safeguards the client's right to privacy by judiciously protecting information of a confidential nature.

### 2.1  The Client's Right to Privacy

The right to privacy is an inalienable human right. The client trusts the nurse to hold all information in confidence. This trust could be destroyed and the client's welfare jeopardized by injudicious disclosure of information provided in confidence. The duty of confidentiality, however, is not absolute when innocent parties are in direct jeopardy.

### 2.2  Protection of Information

The rights, well-being, and safety of the individual client should be the determining factors in arriving at any professional judgment concerning the disposition of confidential information received from the client relevant to his or her treatment. The standards of nursing practice and the nursing responsibility to provide high quality health services require that relevant data be shared with members of the health team. Only information pertinent to a client's treatment and welfare is disclosed, and it is disclosed only to those directly concerned with the client's care.

Information documenting the appropriateness, necessity, and quality of care required for the purposes of peer review, third-party payment, and other quality assurance mechanisms must be disclosed only under defined policies, mandates, or protocols. These written guidelines must assure that the rights, well-being, and safety of the client are maintained.

### 2.3 Access to Records

If in the course of providing care there is a need for the nurse to have access to the records of persons not under the nurse's care, the persons affected should be notified and, whenever possible, permission should be obtained first. Although records belong to the agency where the data are collected, the individual maintains the right of control over the information in the record. Similarly, professionals may exercise the right of control over information they have generated in the course of health care.

If the nurse wishes to use a client's treatment record for research or nonclinical purposes in which anonymity cannot be guaranteed, the client's consent must be obtained first. Ethically, this ensures the client's right to privacy; legally, it protects the client against unlawful invasion of privacy.

### 3   The nurse acts to safeguard the client and the public when health care and safety are affected by incompetent, unethical, or illegal practice by any person.

### 3.1 Safeguarding the Health and Safety of the Client

The nurse's primary commitment is to the health, welfare, and safety of the client. As an advocate for the client, the nurse must be alert to and take appropriate action regarding any instances of incompetent, unethical, or illegal practice by any member of the health care team or the health care system, or any action on the part of others that places the rights or best interests of the client in jeopardy. To function effectively in this role, nurses must be aware of the employing institution's policies and procedures, nursing standards of practice, the Code for Nurses, and laws governing nursing and health care practice with regard to incompetent, unethical, or illegal practice.

### 3.2 Acting on Questionable Practice

When the nurse is aware of inappropriate or questionable practice in the provision of health care, concern should be expressed to the person carrying out the questionable practice and attention called to the possible detrimental effect upon the client's welfare. When factors in the health care delivery system threaten the welfare of the client, similar action should be directed to the responsible administrative person. If indicated, the practice should then be reported to the appropriate authority within the institution, agency, or larger system.

There should be an established process for the reporting and handling of incompetent, unethical, or illegal practice within the employment setting so that such reporting can go through official channels without causing fear of reprisal. The nurse should be knowledgeable about the process and be prepared to use it if necessary. When questions are raised about the practices of individual practitioners or of health care systems, written documentation of the observed practices or behaviors must be available to the appropriate authorities. State nurses' associations should be prepared to provide assistance and support in the development and evaluation of such processes and in reporting procedures.

When incompetent, unethical, or illegal practice on the part of anyone concerned with the client's care is not corrected within the employment setting and continues to jeopardize the client's welfare and safety, the problem should be reported to other appropriate authorities such as practice committees of the pertinent professional organizations or the legally constituted bodies concerned with licensing of specific categories of health workers or professional practitioners. Some situations may warrant the concern and involvement of all such groups. Accurate reporting and documentation undergird all actions.

### 3.3 Review Mechanisms

The nurse should participate in the planning, establishment, implementation, and evaluation of review mechanisms that serve to safeguard clients, such as duly constituted peer review processes or committees and ethics committees. Such ongoing review mechanisms are based on established criteria, have stated purposes, include a process for making recommendations, and facilitate improved delivery of nursing and other health services to clients wherever nursing services are provided.

**4    The nurse assumes responsibilities and accountability for individual nursing judgments and actions.**

### 4.1 Acceptance of Responsibility and Accountability

The recipients of professional nursing services are entitled to high quality nursing care. Individual professional licensure is the protective mechanism legislated by the public to ensure the basic and minimum competencies of the professional nurse. Beyond that, society has accorded to the nursing profession the right to regulate its own practice. The regulation and control of nursing practice by nurses demand that individual practitioners of professional nursing must bear primary responsibility for the nursing care clients receive and must be individually accountable for their own practice.

### 4.2 Responsibility for Nursing Judgment and Action

Responsibility refers to the carrying out of duties associated with a particular role assumed by the nurse. Nursing obligations are reflected in the ANA publications *Nursing: A Social Policy Statement* and *Standards of Nursing Practice.* In recognizing the rights of clients, the standards describe a collaborative relationship between the nurse and the client through use of the nursing process. Nursing responsibilities include data collection and assessment of the health status of the client; formation of nursing diagnoses derived from client assessment; development of a nursing care plan that is directed toward designated goals, assists the client in maximizing his or her health capabilities, and provides for the client's participation in promoting, maintaining, and restoring his or her health; evaluation of the effectiveness of nursing care in achieving goals as determined by the client and the nurse; and subsequent reassessment and revision of the nursing care plan as warranted. In the process of assuming these responsibilities, the nurse is held accountable for them.

### 4.3 Accountability for Nursing Judgment and Action

Accountability refers to being answerable to someone for something one has done. It means providing an explanation or rationale to oneself, to clients, to peers, to the nursing profession, and to society. In order to be accountable, nurses act under a code of ethical conduct that is grounded in the moral principles of fidelity and respect for the dignity, worth, and self-determination of clients.

The nursing profession continues to develop ways to clarify nursing's accountability to society. The contract between the profession and society is made explicit through such mechanisms as (a) the Code for Nurses, (b) the standards of nursing practice, (c) the development of nursing theory derived from nursing research in order to guide nursing actions, (d) educational requirements for practice, (e) certification, and (f) mechanisms for evaluating the effectiveness of the nurse's performance of nursing responsibilities.

Nurses are accountable for judgments made and actions taken in the course of nursing practice. Neither physicians' orders nor the employing agency's policies relieve the nurse of accountability for actions taken and judgments made.

**5    The nurse maintains competence in nursing.**

### 5.1 Personal Responsibility for Competence

The profession of nursing is obligated to provide adequate and competent nursing care. Therefore it is the personal responsibility of each nurse to maintain competency in practice. For the client's optimum well-being and for the nurse's own professional development, the care of the client reflects and incorporates new techniques and knowledge in health care as these develop, especially as they relate to the nurse's particular field of practice. The nurse must be aware of the need for continued professional learning and must assume personal responsibility for currency of knowledge and skills.

• • •

**6     The nurse exercises informed judgment and uses individual competency and qualifications as criteria in seeking consultation, accepting responsibilities, and delegating nursing activities.**

## 6.1  Changing Functions

Nurses are faced with decisions in the context of the increased complexity of health care, changing patterns in the delivery of health services, and the development of evolving nursing practice in response to the health needs of clients. As the scope of nursing practice changes, the nurse must exercise judgment in accepting responsibilities, seeking consultation, and assigning responsibilities to others who carry out nursing care.

## 6.2  Accepting Responsibilities

The nurse must not engage in practices prohibited by law or delegate to others activities prohibited by practice acts of other health care personnel or by other laws. Nurses determine the scope of their practice in light of their education, knowledge, competency, and extent of experience. If the nurse concludes that he or she lacks competence or is inadequately prepared to carry out a specific function, the nurse has the responsibility to refuse that work and to seek alternative sources of care based on concern for the client's welfare. In that refusal, both the client and the nurse are protected. Inasmuch as the nurse is responsible for the continuous care of patients in health care settings, the nurse is frequently called upon to carry out components of care delegated by other health professionals as part of the client's treatment regimen. The nurse should not accept these interdependent functions if they are so extensive as to prevent the nurse from fulfilling the responsibility to provide appropriate nursing care to clients.

## 6.3  Consultation and Collaboration

The provision of health and illness care to clients is a complex process that requires a wide range of knowledge, skills, and collaborative efforts. Nurses must be aware of their own individual competencies. When the needs of the client are beyond the qualifications and competencies of the nurse, consultation and collaboration must be sought from qualified nurses, other health professionals, or other appropriate sources. Participation on intradisciplinary or interdisciplinary teams is often an effective approach to the provision of high quality total health services.

## 6.4  Delegation of Nursing Activities

Inasmuch as the nurse is accountable for the quality of nursing care rendered to clients, nurses are accountable for the delegation of nursing care activities to other health workers. Therefore, the nurse must assess individual competency in assigning selected components of nursing care to other nursing service personnel. The nurse should not delegate to any member of the nursing team a function for which that person is not prepared or qualified. Employer policies or directives do not relieve the nurse of accountability for making judgments about the delegation of nursing care activities.

**7     The nurse participates in activities that contribute to the ongoing development of the profession's body of knowledge.**

## 7.1  The Nurse and Development of Knowledge

Every profession must engage in scholarly inquiry to identify, verify, and continually enlarge the body of knowledge that forms the foundation for its practice. A unique body of verified knowledge provides both framework and direction for the profession in all of its activities and for the practitioner in the provision of nursing care. The accrual of scientific and humanistic knowledge promotes the advancement of practice and the well-being of the profession's clients. Ongoing scholarly activity such as research and the development of theory is indispensable to the full discharge of a profession's obligations to society. Each nurse has a role in this area of professional activity, whether as an investigator in furthering knowledge, as a participant in research, or as a user of theoretical and empirical knowledge.

## 7.2  Protection of Rights of Human Participants in Research

Individual rights valued by society and by the nursing profession that have particular application in research include the right of adequately informed consent, the right to freedom from risk of injury, and the right of privacy and preservation of dignity. Inherent in these rights is respect for each individual's rights to exercise self-determination, to choose to participate or not, to have full information, and to terminate participation in research without penalty.

It is the duty of the nurse functioning in any research role to maintain vigilance in protecting the life, health, and privacy of human subjects from both anticipated and unanticipated risks and in assuring informed consent. Subjects' integrity, privacy, and rights must be especially safeguarded if the subjects are unable to protect themselves because of incapacity or because they are in a dependent relationship to the investigator. The investigation should be discontinued if its continuance might be harmful to the subject.

## 7.3  General Guidelines for Participating in Research

Before participating in research conducted by others, the nurse has an obligation to (a) obtain information about the intent and the nature of the research and (b) ascertain that the study proposal is approved by the appropriate bodies, such as institutional review boards.

Research should be conducted and directed by qualified persons. The nurse who participates in research in any capacity should be fully informed about both the nurse's and the client's rights and obligations.

**8    The nurse participates in the profession's efforts to implement and improve standards of nursing.**

• • •

## 8.2  Responsibility to the Profession for Standards

Established standards reflect the practice of nursing grounded in ethical commitments and a body of knowledge. Professional standards or guidelines exist in nursing practice, nursing service, nursing education, and nursing research. The nurse has the responsibility to monitor these standards in daily practice and to participate actively in the profession's ongoing efforts to foster optimal standards of practice at the local, regional, state, and national levels of the health care system.

• • •

**9    The nurse participates in the profession's efforts to establish and maintain conditions of employment conducive to high quality nursing care.**

## 9.1  Responsibility for Conditions of Employment

The nurse must be concerned with conditions of employment that (a) enable the nurse to practice in accordance with the standards of nursing practice and (b) provide a care environment that meets the standards of nursing service. The provision of high quality nursing care is the responsibility of both the individual nurse and the nursing profession. Professional autonomy and self-regulation in the control of conditions of practice are necessary for implementing nursing standards.

## 9.2  Maintaining Conditions for High Quality Nursing Care

Articulation and control of nursing practice can be accomplished through individual agreement and collective action. A nurse may enter into an agreement with individuals or organizations to provide health care. Nurses may participate in collective action such as collective bargaining through their state nurses' association to determine the terms and conditions of employment conducive to high quality nursing care. Such agreements should be consistent with the profession's standards of practice, the state law regulating nursing practice, and the Code for Nurses.

**10** The nurse participates in the profession's efforts to protect the public from misinformation and misrepresentation and to maintain the integrity of nursing.

### 10.1 Protection from Misinformation and Misrepresentation

Nurses are responsible for advising clients against the use of products that endanger the clients' safety and welfare. The nurse shall not use any form of public or professional communication to make claims that are false, fraudulent, misleading, deceptive, or unfair.

The nurse does not give or imply endorsement to advertising, promotion, or sale of commercial products or services in a manner that may be interpreted as reflecting the opinion or judgment of the profession as a whole. The nurse may use knowledge of specific services or products in advising an individual client, since this may contribute to the client's health and well-being. In the course of providing information or education to clients or other practitioners about commercial products or services, however, a variety of similar products or services should be offered or described so the client or practitioner can make an informed choice.

### 10.2 Maintaining the Integrity of Nursing

• • •

Nurses should refrain from casting a vote in any deliberations involving health care services or facilities where the nurse has business or other interests that could be construed as a conflict of interest.

**11** The nurse collaborates with members of the health professions and other citizens in promoting community and national efforts to meet the health needs of the public.

### 11.1 Collaboration with Others to Meet Health Needs

The availability and accessibility of high quality health services to all people require collaborative planning at the local, state, national, and international levels that respects the interdependence of health professionals and clients in health care systems. Nursing care is an integral part of high quality health care, and nurses have an obligation to promote equitable access to nursing and health care for all people.

### 11.2 Responsibility to the Public

The nursing profession is committed to promoting the welfare and safety of all people. The goals and values of nursing are essential to effective delivery of health services. For the benefit of the individual client and the public at large, nursing's goals and commitments need adequate representation. Nurses should ensure this representation by active participation in decision making in institutional and political arenas to assure a just distribution of health care and nursing resources.

### 11.3 Relationships with Other Disciplines

The complexity of health care delivery systems requires a multidisciplinary approach to delivery of services that has the strong support and active participation of all the health professions. Nurses should actively promote the collaborative planning required to ensure the availability and accessibility of high quality health services to all persons whose health needs are unmet.

## CODE OF ETHICS FOR NURSING
**Canadian Nurses Association**
1985, revised 1991

*The introductory sections of the Canadian Nurses Association (CNA) code suggest a sophisticated view of the role of codes. For example, the code "provides clear direction for avoiding ethical violations," that is, "the neglect of moral obligation," but it cannot resolve "ethical dilem-*

*mas," in which there are "ethical reasons both for and against a particular course of action." The code also cannot relieve the "ethical distress" that occurs "when nurses experience the imposition of practices that provoke feelings of guilt, concern or distaste." The CNA code is unique in its explicit organization around values, which "express broad ideals of nursing"; obligations, which are "moral norms that have their basis in nursing values"; and limitations, which "describe exceptional circumstances in which a value or obligation cannot be applied."*

### Preamble

Nursing practice can be defined generally as a "dynamic, caring, helping relationship in which the nurse assists the client to achieve and maintain optimal health." Nurses in clinical practice, education, administration and research share the common goal of maintaining competent care and improving nursing practice. "Nurses direct their energies toward the promotion, maintenance and restoration of health, the prevention of illness, the alleviation of suffering and the ensuring of a peaceful death when life can no longer be sustained."

The nurse, by entering the profession, is committed to moral norms of conduct and assumes a professional commitment to health and the well-being of clients. As citizens, nurses continue to be bound by the moral and legal norms shared by all other participants in society. As individuals, nurses have a right to choose to live by their own values (their personal ethics) as long as those values do not compromise care of their clients.

• • •

### Ethical Problems

Situations often arise that present ethical problems for nurses in their practice. These situations tend to fall into three categories:

(a) **Ethical violations** involve the neglect of moral obligation; for example, a nurse who neglects to provide competent care to a client because of personal inconvenience has ethically failed the client.

(b) **Ethical dilemmas** arise where ethical reasons both for and against a particular course of action are present and one option must be selected. For example, a client who is likely to refuse some appropriate form of health care presents the nurse with an ethical dilemma. In this case, substantial moral reasons may be offered on behalf of several opposing options.

(c) **Ethical distress** occurs when nurses experience the imposition of practices that provoke feelings of guilt, concern or distaste. Such feelings may occur when nurses are ethically obliged to provide particular types of care despite their personal disagreement or discomfort with the course of treatment prescribed. For example, a nurse may think that continuing to tube feed an irreversibly unresponsive person is contrary to that client's well-being, but nonetheless is required to do so because that view is not shared by other caregivers.

This Code provides clear direction for avoiding ethical violations. When a course of action is mandated by the Code, and there exists no opposing ethical principle, ethical conduct requires that course of action.

This Code cannot serve the same function for all ethical dilemmas or for ethical distress. There is room within the profession of nursing for conscientious disagreement among nurses. The resolution of any dilemma often depends upon the specific circumstances of the case in question, and no particular resolution may be definitive of good nursing practice. Resolution may also depend upon the relative weight of the opposing principles, a matter about which reasonable people may disagree.

The Code cannot relieve ethical distress but it may serve as a guide for nurses to weigh and consider their responsibilities in the particular situation. Inevitably, nurses must reconcile their actions with their consciences in caring for clients.

The Code tries to provide guidance for those nurses who face ethical problems. Proper consideration of the Code should lead to better decision-making when ethical problems are encountered.

It should be noted that many problems or situations seen as ethical in nature are problems of miscommunication, failure of trust or management dilemmas in disguise. There is, therefore, a distinct need to clarify whether the problem is an ethical one or one of another sort.

### Elements of the Code

This Code contains different elements designed to help the nurse in its interpretation. The values and obligations are presented by topic and not in order of importance. There is intentional variation in the normative terminology used in the Code (the nurse **should** or **must**) to indicate differences in the moral force of the statements; the term **should** indicates a moral preference, while **must** indicates an obligation. A number of distinctions between ethics and morals may be found in the literature. Since no distinction has been uniformly adopted by writers on ethics, these terms are used interchangeably in this Code.

- **Values** express broad ideals of nursing. They establish correct directions for nursing. In the absence of a conflict of ethics, the fact that a particular action promotes a **value** of nursing may be decisive in some specific instances. Nursing behaviour can always be appraised in terms of values: How closely did the behaviour approach the value? How widely did it deviate from the value? The values expressed in this Code must be adhered to by all nurses in their practice. Because they are so broad, however, values may not give specific guidance in difficult instances.
- **Obligations** are moral norms that have their basis in nursing values. However, obligations provide more specific direction for conduct than do values; obligations spell out what a value requires under particular circumstances.
- **Limitations** describe exceptional circumstances in which a value or obligation cannot be applied. Limitations have been included separately to emphasize that, in the ordinary run of events, the values and obligations will be decisive.

It is also important to emphasize that even when a value or obligation must be limited, it nonetheless carries moral weight. For example, a nurse who is compelled to testify in a court of law on confidential matters is still subject to the values and obligations of confidentiality. While the requirement to testify is a justified limitation upon confidentiality, in other respects confidentiality must be observed. The nurse must only reveal that confidential information that is pertinent to the case at hand, and such revelation must take place within the appropriate context. The general obligation to preserve the client's confidences remains despite particular limiting circumstances.

## Rights and Responsibilities

Clients possess both legal and moral rights. These serve as one foundation for the responsibilities of nurses. However, for several reasons this Code emphasizes the obligations of nurses, rather than the rights of clients. Because the rights of clients do not depend upon professional acceptance of those rights, it would be presumptuous for a profession to claim to define the rights of clients. Emphasizing the rights of clients may also seem unduly legalistic and restrictive, ignoring the fact that sometimes ethics require nurses to go beyond the letter of the law. (For one example, see Value II, Obligation 3.) Finally, because it is sometimes beyond the power of a nurse to **secure** the rights of a client—an achievement that requires the cooperative and scrupulous efforts of all members of the health care team—it is better for a professional code of nursing to emphasize the responsibilities of nurses rather than to detail the entitlements of clients.

Nurses, too, possess legal and moral rights, as persons and as professionals. It is beyond the scope of this Code to address the personal rights of nurses. However, to the extent that conditions of employment have an impact on the establishment of ethical nursing, this Code must deal with that issue.

The satisfaction of some ethical responsibilities requires action taken by the nursing profession as a whole. The fourth section of the Code contains values and obligations concerned with those collective responsibilities of nursing; this section is particularly addressed to professional associations. Ethical reflection must be ongoing and its facilitation is a continuing responsibility of the Canadian Nurses Association.

• • •

## Clients

### Value I Respect for Needs and Values of Clients

*Value*

A nurse treats clients with respect for their individual needs and values.

*Obligations*

1. The client's perceived best interests must be a prime concern of the nurse.
2. Factors such as the client's race, religion or absence thereof, ethnic origin, social or marital status, sex or sexual orientation, age, or health status must not be permitted to compromise the nurse's commitment to that client's care.
3. The expectations and normal life patterns of clients are acknowledged. Individualized programs of nursing care are designed to accommodate the psychological, social, cultural and spiritual needs of clients, as well as their biological needs.
4. The nurse does more than respond to the requests of clients; the nurse accepts an

affirmative obligation within the context of health care to aid clients in their expression of needs and values, including their right to live at risk.

5. Recognizing the client's membership in a family and a community, the nurse, with the client's consent, should attempt to facilitate the participation of significant others in the care of the client.

### Value II   Respect for Client Choice

*Value*

Based upon respect for clients and regard for their right to control their own care, nursing care reflects respect for the right of choice held by clients.

*Obligations*

1. The competent client's consent is an essential precondition to the provision of health care. Nurses bear the primary responsibility to inform clients about the nursing care available to them.

2. Consent may be signified in many different ways. Verbal permission and knowledgeable cooperation are the usual forms by which clients consent to nursing care. In each case, however, a valid consent represents the free choice of the competent client to undergo that care.

3. Consent, properly understood, is the process by which a client becomes an active participant in care. All clients should be aided in becoming active participants in their care to the maximum extent that circumstances permit. Professional ethics may require of the nurse actions that exceed the legal requirements of consent. For example, although a child may be legally incompetent to consent, nurses should nevertheless attempt to inform and involve the child.

4. Force, coercion and manipulative tactics must not be employed in the obtaining of consent.

5. Illness or other factors may compromise the client's capacity for self-direction. Nurses have a continuing obligation to value autonomy in such clients; for example, by creatively providing clients with opportunities for choices within their capabilities, the nurse helps them to maintain or regain some degree of autonomy.

6. Whenever information is provided to a client, this must be done in a truthful, understandable and sensitive way. The nurse must proceed with an awareness of the individual client's needs, interests and values.

7. Nurses have a responsibility to assess the understanding of clients about their care and to provide information and explanation when in possession of the knowledge required to respond accurately. When the client's questions require information beyond that known to the nurse, the client must be informed of that fact and assisted to obtain the information from a health care practitioner who is in possession of the required facts.

### Value III   Confidentiality

*Value*

The nurse holds confidential all information about a client learned in the health care setting.

*Obligations*

1. The rights of persons to control the amount of personal information revealed applies with special force in the health care setting. It is, broadly speaking, up to clients to determine who shall be told of their condition, and in what detail.

2. In describing professional confidentiality to a client, its boundaries should be revealed:

   a) Competent care requires that other members of a team of health personnel have access to or be provided with the relevant details of a client's condition.

   b) In addition, discussions of the client's care may be required for the purpose of teaching or quality assurance. In this case, special care must be taken to protect the client's anonymity.

Whenever possible, the client should be informed of these necessities at the onset of care.

3. An affirmative duty exists to institute and maintain practices that protect client confidentiality—for example, by limiting access to records or by choosing the most secure method of communicating client information.

4. Nurses have a responsibility to intervene if other participants in the health care delivery system fail to respect the confidentiality of client information.

*Limitations*

The nurse is not morally obligated to maintain confidentiality when the failure to disclose information will place the client or third parties in danger. Generally, legal requirements or privileges to disclose are morally justified by these same criteria. In facing such a situation, the first concern of the nurse must be the safety of the client or the third party.

Even when the nurse is confronted with the necessity to disclose, confidentiality should be preserved to the maximum possible extent. Both the amount of information disclosed and the number of people to whom disclosure is made should be restricted to the minimum necessary to prevent the feared harm.

### Value IV    Dignity of Clients

*Value*

The nurse is guided by consideration for the dignity of clients.

*Obligations*

1. Nursing care must be done with consideration for the personal modesty of clients.
2. A nurse's conduct at all times should acknowledge the client as a person. For example, discussion of care in the presence of the client should actively involve or include that client.
3. Nurses have a responsibility to intervene when other participants in the health delivery system fail to respect any aspect of client dignity.
4. As ways of dealing with death and the dying process change, nursing is challenged to find new ways to preserve human values, autonomy and dignity. In assisting the dying client, measures must be taken to afford the client as much comfort, dignity and freedom from anxiety and pain as possible. Special consideration must be given to the need of the client's family or significant others to cope with their loss.

### Value V    Competent Nursing Care

*Value*

The nurse provides competent care to clients.

*Obligations*

1. Nurses should engage in continuing education and in the upgrading of knowledge and skills relevant to their area of practice, that is, clinical practice, education, research or administration.
2. In seeking or accepting employment, nurses must accurately state their area of competence as well as limitations.
3. Nurses assigned to work outside an area of present competence must seek to do what, under the circumstances, is in the best interests of their clients. The nurse manager on duty, or others, must be informed of the situation at the earliest possible moment so that protective measures can be instituted. As a temporary measure, the safety and welfare of clients may be better served by the best efforts of the nurse under the circumstances than by no nursing care at all. Nurse managers are obligated to support nurses who are placed in such difficult situations and to make every effort to remedy the problem.
4. When called upon outside an employment setting to provide emergency care, nurses fulfil their obligations by providing the best care that circumstances, experience and education permit.

*Limitations*

A nurse is not ethically obliged to provide requested care when compliance would involve a violation of her or his moral beliefs. When that request falls within recognized forms of health care, however, the client must be referred to a health care practitioner who is willing to provide the service. Nurses who have or are likely to encounter such situations are morally obligated to seek to arrange conditions of employment so that the care of clients will not be jeopardized.

## Nursing Roles and Relationships

### Value VI    Nursing Practice, Education, Research and Administration

*Value*

The nurse maintains trust in nurses and nursing.

*Obligations*

1. Nurses accepting professional employment must ascertain to the best of their ability that conditions will permit the provision of care consistent with the values and obligations of the Code. Prospective employers should be informed of the provisions of the Code so that realistic and ethical expectations may be established at the beginning of the nurse–employer relationship.

2. Nurse managers, educators and peers are morally obligated to provide timely and accurate feedback to nurses, nurse managers, students of nursing and nurse educators. Objective performance appraisal is essential to the growth of nurses and is required by a concern for present and future clients.

3. Nurse managers bear special ethical responsibilities that flow from a concern for present and future clients. The nurse manager must seek to ensure that the competencies of personnel are used efficiently. Working within available resources, the nurse manager must seek to ensure the welfare of clients. When competent care is threatened due to inadequate resources or for some other reason, the nurse manager must act to minimize the present danger and to prevent future harm.

4. Student–teacher and student–client encounters are essential elements of nursing education. These encounters must be conducted in accordance with ethical nursing practices. The nurse educator is obligated to treat students of nursing with respect and honesty and to provide fair guidance in developing nursing competence. The nurse educator should ensure that students of nursing are acquainted with and comply with the provisions of the Code. Student–client encounters must be conducted with client consent and require special attention to the dignity of the client.

5. Research is necessary to the development of the profession of nursing. Nurses should be acquainted with advances in research, so that established results may be incorporated into clinical practice, education and administration. The individual nurse's competencies may also be used to promote, to engage in or to assist health care research designed to enhance the health and welfare of clients.

The conduct of research must conform to ethical practice. The self-direction of clients takes on added importance in this context. Further direction is provided in the Canadian Nurses Association publication *Ethical Guidelines for Nursing Research Involving Human Subjects*.

### Value VII    Cooperation in Health Care

*Value*

The nurse recognizes the contribution and expertise of colleagues from nursing and other disciplines as essential to excellent health care.

*Obligations*

1. The nurse functions as a member of the health care team.
2. The nurse should participate in the assessment, planning, implementation and evaluation of comprehensive programs of care for individual clients and client groups. The scope of a nurse's responsibility should be based upon education and experience, as well as legal considerations of licensure or registration.
3. The nurse accepts responsibility to work with colleagues and other health care professionals, with nursing interest groups and through professional nurses' associations to secure excellent care for clients.

### Value VIII    Protecting Clients from Incompetence

*Value*

The nurse takes steps to ensure that the client receives competent and ethical care.

*Obligations*

1. The first consideration of the nurse who suspects incompetence or unethical conduct must be the welfare of present clients or potential harm to future clients. Subject to that principle, the following must be considered:
   a) The nurse is obliged to ascertain the facts of the situation before deciding upon the appropriate course of action.
   b) Relationships in the health care team should not be disrupted unnecessarily. If a situation can be resolved without peril to present or future clients by direct discussion with the colleague suspected of providing incompetent or unethical care, that discussion should be done.
   c) Institutional mechanisms for reporting incidents or risks of incompetent or unethical care must be followed.
   d) The nurse must report any reportable offence stipulated in provincial or territorial professional nursing legislation.
   e) It is unethical for a nurse to participate in efforts to deceive or mislead clients about the cause of alleged harm or injury resulting from unethical or incompetent conduct.

2. Guidance on activities that may be delegated by nurses to assistants and other health care workers is found in legislation and policy statements. When functions are delegated, the nurse should be satisfied about the competence of those who will be ful-

filling these functions. The nurse has a duty to provide continuing supervision in such a case.

3. The nurse who attempts to protect clients or colleagues threatened by incompetent or unethical conduct may be placed in a difficult position. Colleagues and professional associations are morally obliged to support nurses who fulfil their ethical obligations under the Code.

### Value IX   Conditions of Employment

*Value*

Conditions of employment should contribute in a positive way to client care and the professional satisfaction of nurses.

*Obligations*

1. Nurses accepting professional employment must ascertain, to the best of their ability, that employment conditions will permit provision of care consistent with the values and obligations of the Code.
2. Nurse managers must seek to ensure that the agencies where they are employed comply with all pertinent provincial or territorial legislation.
3. Nurse managers must seek to ensure the welfare of clients and nurses. When competent care is threatened due to inadequate resources or for some other reason, the nurse manager should act to minimize the present danger and to prevent future harm.
4. Nurse managers must seek to foster environments and conditions of employment that promote excellent care for clients and a good worklife for nurses.
5. Structures should exist in the work environment that provide nurses with means of recourse if conditions that promote a good worklife are absent.

### Value X   Job Action

*Value*

Job action by nurses is directed toward securing conditions of employment that enable safe and appropriate care for clients and contribute to the professional satisfaction of nurses.

*Obligations*

1. In the final analysis, the improvement of conditions of nursing employment is often to the advantage of clients. Over the short term, however, there is a danger that action directed toward this goal could work to the detriment of clients. In view of their ethical responsibility to current as well as future clients, nurses must respect the following principles:
   a) The safety of clients is the **first** concern in planning and implementing any job action.
   b) Individuals and groups of nurses participating in job actions share the ethical commitment to the safety of clients. However, their responsibilities may lead them to express this commitment in different but equally appropriate ways.
   c) Clients whose safety requires ongoing or emergency nursing care are entitled to have those needs satisfied throughout the duration of any job action. Individuals and groups of nurses participating in job actions have a duty through coordination and communication to take steps to ensure the safety of clients.
   d) Members of the public are entitled to know of the steps taken to ensure the safety of clients.

## Nursing Ethics and Society

### Value XI   Advocacy of the Interests of Clients, the Community and Society

*Value*

The nurse advocates the interests of clients.

*Obligations*

1. Advocating the interests of individual clients and groups of clients includes helping them to gain access to good health care. For example, by providing information to clients privately or publicly, the nurse enables them to satisfy their rights to health care.
2. When speaking in a public forum or in court, the nurse owes the public the same duties of accurate and relevant information as are owed to clients within the employment setting.

### Value XII    Representing Nursing Values and Ethics

*Value*

The nurse represents the values and ethics of nursing before colleagues and others.

*Obligations*

1. Nurses serving on committees concerned with health care or research should see their role as including the vigorous representation of nursing's professional ethics.
2. Many public issues include health as a major component. Involvement in public activities may give the nurse the opportunity to further the objectives of nursing as well as to fulfil the duties of a citizen.

## The Nursing Profession

### Value XIII    Responsibilities of Professional Nurses' Associations

*Value*

Professional nurses' organizations are responsible for clarifying, securing and sustaining ethical nursing conduct. The fulfilment of these tasks requires that professional nurses' organizations remain responsive to the rights, needs and legitimate interests of clients and nurses.

*Obligations*

1. Sustained communication and cooperation between the Canadian Nurses Association, provincial or territorial associations and other organizations of nurses are essential steps toward securing ethical nursing conduct.
2. Activities of professional nurses' associations must at all times reflect a prime concern for excellent client care.
3. Professional nurses's associations should represent nursing interests and perspectives before nonnursing bodies, including legislatures, employers, the professional organizations of other health disciplines and the public communication media.
4. Professional nurses' associations should provide and encourage organizational structures that facilitate ethical nursing conduct.
   a) Education in the ethical aspects of nursing should be available to nurses throughout their careers. Nurses' associations should actively support or develop structures to enhance sensitivity to, and application of, norms of ethical nursing conduct. Associations should also promote the development and dissemination of knowledge about ethical decision-making through nursing research.
   b) Changing circumstances call for ongoing review of this Code. Supplementation of the Code may be necessary to address special situations. Professional associations should consider the ethics of nursing on a regular and continuing basis and be prepared to provide assistance to those concerned with its implementation.

## CODE OF ETHICS
### American Chiropractic Association
### 1994–1995

*The current, 1994–1995 American Chiropractic Association (ACA) code differs significantly from an earlier, 1973 version. The current code rests on a single fundamental principle, "The greatest good for the patient," whereas the 1973 code also cited the Golden Rule—do unto others as you would have them do unto you—as a fundamental principle. In addition, the structure and language of the current code is much more modern than that of the 1973 code, which strongly resembled the American Medical Association Code of Medical Ethics of 1847 (see Section II) in the wording and ordering of its articles and subsections.*

*The 1994–1995 code is divided into four sections. Although the final section on "Administrative Procedures" is not printed below, it is noteworthy that two-thirds of the code is devoted to that section, which discusses the reporting and reviewing of alleged ethics violations.*

## Preamble

This Code of Ethics is based upon the fundamental principle that the ultimate end and object of the chiropractor's professional services and effort should be:

"The greatest good for the patient."

• • •

## A. Responsibility to the Patient

A(1)    Doctors of chiropractic should hold themselves ready at all times to respond to the call of those needing their professional services, although they are free to accept or reject a particular patient except in an emergency.

A(2)    Doctors of chiropractic should attend their patients as often as they consider necessary to ensure the well-being of their patients.

A(3)    Having once undertaken to serve a patient, doctors of chiropractic should not neglect the patient. Doctors of chiropractic should take reasonable steps to protect their patients prior to withdrawing their professional services; such steps shall include: due notice to them allowing a reasonable time for obtaining professional services of others and delivering to their patients all papers and documents in compliance with A(5) of this Code of Ethics.

A(4)    Doctors of chiropractic should be honest and endeavor to practice with the highest degree of professional competency and honesty in the proper care of their patients.

A(5)    Doctors of chiropractic should comply with a patient's authorization to provide records, or copies of such records, to those whom the patient designates as authorized to inspect or receive all or part of such records. A reasonable charge may be made for the cost of duplicating records.

A(6)    Subject to the foregoing Section A(5), doctors of chiropractic should preserve and protect the patient's confidences and records, except as the patient directs or consents or the law requires otherwise. They should not discuss a patient's history, symptoms, diagnosis, or treatment with any third party until they have received the written consent of the patient or the patient's personal representative. They should not exploit the trust and dependency of their patients.

A(7)    Doctors of chiropractic owe loyalty, compassion and respect to their patients. Their clinical judgment and practice should be objective and exercised solely for the patient's benefit.

A(8)    Doctors of chiropractic should recognize and respect the right of every person to free choice of chiropractors or other health care providers and to the right to change such choice at will.

A(9)    Doctors of chiropractic are entitled to receive proper and reasonable compensation for their professional services commensurate with the value of the services they have rendered taking into consideration their experience, time required, reputation and the nature of the condition involved. Doctors of chiropractic should terminate a professional relationship when it becomes reasonably clear that the patient is not benefiting from it. Doctors of chiropractic should support and participate in proper activities designed to enable access to necessary chiropractic care on the part of persons unable to pay such reasonable fees.

A(10)   Doctors of chiropractic should maintain the highest standards of professional and personal conduct, and should refrain from all illegal conduct.

A(11)   Doctors of chiropractic should be ready to consult and seek the talents of other health care professionals when such consultation would benefit their patients or when their patients express a desire for such consultation.

A(12)   Doctors of chiropractic should employ their best good faith efforts that the patient possesses enough information to enable an intelligent choice in regard to proposed chiropractic treatment. The patient should make his or her own determination on such treatment.

A(13)   Doctors of chiropractic should utilize only those laboratory and X-ray procedures, and such devices or nutritional products that are in the best interest of the patient and not in conflict with state statute or administrative rulings.

## B. Responsibility to the Public

B(1)    Doctors of chiropractic should act as members of a learned profession dedicated to the promotion of health, the prevention of illness and the alleviation of suffering.

B(2)    Doctors of chiropractic should observe and comply with all laws, decisions and regulations of state governmental agencies and cooperate with the pertinent activities and policies of associations legally authorized to regulate or assist in the regulation of the chiropractic profession.

B(3)    Doctors of chiropractic should comport themselves as responsible citizens in the public affairs of their local community, state and nation in order to improve law, administrative procedures and public policies that pertain to chiropractic and the system of health care delivery. Doctors of chiropractic should stand ready to take the initiative in the proposal and development of measures to benefit the general public health and well-being, and should cooperate in the administration and enforcement of such measures and programs to the extent consistent with law.

B(4)    Doctors of chiropractic may advertise but should exercise utmost care that such advertising is relevant to health awareness, is accurate, truthful, not misleading or false or deceptive, and scrupulously accurate in representing the chiropractor's professional status and area of special competence. Communications to the public should not appeal primarily to an individual's anxiety or create unjustified expectations of results. Doctors of chiropractic should conform to all applicable state laws, regulations and judicial decisions in connection with professional advertising.

B(5)    Doctors of chiropractic should continually strive to improve their skill and competency by keeping abreast of current developments contained in the health and scientific literature, and by participating in continuing chiropractic educational programs and utilizing other appropriate means.

B(6)    Doctors of chiropractic may testify either as experts or when their patients are involved in court cases, workers' compensation proceedings or in other similar administrative proceedings in personal injury or related cases.

B(7)    The chiropractic profession should address itself to improvements in licensing procedures consistent with the development of the profession and of relevant advances in science.

B(8)    Doctors of chiropractic who are public officers should not engage in activities which are, or may be reasonably perceived to be in conflict with their official duties.

B(9)    Doctors of chiropractic should protect the public and reputation of the chiropractic profession by bringing to the attention of the appropriate public or private organization the actions of chiropractors who engage in deception, fraud or dishonesty, or otherwise engage in conduct inconsistent with this Code of Ethics or relevant provisions of applicable law or regulations within their states.

## C. Responsibility to the Profession

C(1)    Doctors of chiropractic should assist in maintaining the integrity, competency and highest standards of the chiropractic profession.

C(2)    Doctors of chiropractic should by their behavior, avoid even the appearance of professional impropriety and should recognize that their public behavior may have an impact on the ability of the profession to serve the public. Doctors of chiropractic should promote public confidence in the chiropractic profession.

C(3)    As teachers, doctors of chiropractic should recognize their obligation to help others acquire knowledge and skill in the practice of the profession. They should maintain high standards of scholarship, education, training and objectivity in the accurate and full dissemination of information and ideas.

C(4)    Doctors of chiropractic should attempt to promote and maintain cordial relationships with other members of the chiropractic profession and other professions in an effort to promote information advantageous to the public's health and well-being.

• • •

# PRINCIPLES OF ETHICS AND CODE OF PROFESSIONAL CONDUCT WITH ADVISORY OPINIONS
### American Dental Association
revised to May 1994

*Although most of the topics addressed in the 1994 American Dental Association code are the same as those found twenty years ago in the 1974 version, the organization and details of the code have been modified. The twenty-two sections of the 1974 code have been reduced to five main principles, and many of the remaining original sections now appear as subsections, which constitute the "code of professional conduct." Some notable changes in content include the specification that dentists cannot ethically deny treatment to individuals who are HIV seropositive;*

*addition of the obligation to safeguard the confidentiality of patient records; and removal of the former prohibition on advertising.*

The ethical statements which have historically been subscribed to by the dental profession have had the benefit of the patient as their primary goal. Recognition of this goal, and of the education and training of a dentist, has resulted in society affording to the profession the privilege and obligation of self-government. The Association calls upon members of the profession to be caring and fair in their contact with patients. Although the structure of society may change, the overriding obligation of the dentist will always remain the duty to provide quality care in a competent and timely manner. All members must protect and preserve the high standards of oral health care provided to the public by the profession. They must strive to improve the care delivered—through education, training, research and, most of all, adherence to a stringent code of ethics, structured to meet the needs of the patient.

## Principle - Section 1

### Service to the Public and Quality of Care

The dentist's primary professional obligation shall be service to the public. The competent and timely delivery of quality care within the bounds of the clinical circumstances presented by the patient, with due consideration being given to the needs and desires of the patient, shall be the most important aspect of that obligation.

## Code of Professional Conduct

### 1-A. Patient Selection

While dentists, in serving the public, may exercise reasonable discretion in selecting patients for their practices, dentists shall not refuse to accept patients into their practice or deny dental service to patients because of the patient's race, creed, color, sex, or national origin.

*Advisory Opinion*

1. A dentist has the general obligation to provide care to those in need. A decision not to provide treatment to an individual because the individual has AIDS or is HIV seropositive, based solely on that fact, is unethical. Decisions with regard to the type of dental treatment provided or referrals made or suggested, in such instances, should be made on the same basis as they are made with other patients, that is, whether the individual dentist believes he or she has need of another's skills, knowledge, equipment or experience and whether the dentist believes, after consultation with the patient's physician if appropriate, the patient's health status would be significantly compromised by the provision of dental treatment.

### 1-B. Patient Records

Dentists are obliged to safeguard the confidentiality of patient records. Dentists shall maintain patient records in a manner consistent with the protection of the welfare of the patient. Upon request of a patient or another dental practitioner, dentists shall provide any information that will be beneficial for the future treatment of that patient. This obligation exists whether or not the patient's account is paid in full.

*Advisory Opinions*

1. A dentist has the ethical obligation on request of either the patient or the patient's new dentist to furnish, either gratuitously or for nominal cost, such dental records or copies or summaries of them, including dental X-rays or copies of them, as will be beneficial for the future treatment of that patient.

2. The dominant theme in Code Section 1-B is the protection of the confidentiality of a patient's records. The statement in this section that relevant information in the records shall be released to another dental practitioner assumes that the dentist requesting the information is the patient's present dentist. The former dentist should be free to provide the present dentist with relevant information from the patient's records. This may often be required for the protection of both the patient and the present dentist. There may be circumstances where the former dentist has an ethical obligation to inform the present dentist of certain facts. Dentists should be aware, however, that the laws of the various jurisdictions in the United States are not uniform, and some confidentiality laws appear to prohibit the transfer of pertinent information, such as HIV seropositivity. Absent certain knowledge that the laws of the dentist's jurisdiction permit the forwarding of this information, a dentist should obtain the patient's written permission before for-

warding health records which contain information of a sensitive nature, such as HIV seropositivity, chemical dependency or sexual preference. If it is necessary for a treating dentist to consult with another dentist or physician with respect to the patient, and the circumstances do not permit the patient to remain anonymous, the treating dentist should seek the permission of the patient prior to the release of data from the patient's records to the consulting practitioner. If the patient refuses, the treating dentist should then contemplate obtaining legal advice regarding the termination of the dentist/patient relationship.

### 1-C. Community Service

Since dentists have an obligation to use their skills, knowledge, and experience for the improvement of the dental health of the public and are encouraged to be leaders in their community, dentists in such service shall conduct themselves in such a manner as to maintain or elevate the esteem of the profession.

• • •

### 1-D. Emergency Service

Dentists shall be obliged to make reasonable arrangements for the emergency care of their patients of record.

Dentists shall be obliged when consulted in an emergency by patients not of record to make reasonable arrangements for emergency care. If treatment is provided, the dentist, upon completion of such treatment, is obliged to return the patient to his or her regular dentist unless the patient expressly reveals a different preference.

### 1-E. Consultation and Referral

Dentists shall be obliged to seek consultation, if possible, whenever the welfare of patients will be safeguarded or advanced by utilizing those who have special skills, knowledge, and experience. When patients visit or are referred to specialists or consulting dentists for consultation:

1. The specialists or consulting dentists upon completion of their care shall return the patient, unless the patient expressly reveals a different preference, to the referring dentist, or if none, to the dentist of record for future care.

2. The specialists shall be obliged when there is no referring dentist and upon a completion of their treatment to inform patients when there is a need for further dental care.

• • •

### 1-F. Child Abuse

Dentists shall be obliged to become familiar with the perioral signs of child abuse and to report suspected cases to the proper authorities consistent with state laws.

• • •

### 1-H. Justifiable Criticism

Dentists shall be obliged to report to the appropriate reviewing agency as determined by the local component or constituent society instances of gross or continual faulty treatment by other dentists.

Patients should be informed of their present oral health status without disparaging comment about prior services.

Dentists issuing a public statement with respect to the profession shall have a reasonable basis to believe that the comments made are true.

• • •

### 1-I. Expert Testimony

Dentists may provide expert testimony when that testimony is essential to a just and fair disposition of a judicial or administrative action.

• • •

### 1-J. Rebate and Split Fees

Dentists shall not accept or tender "rebates" or "split fees."

### 1-K. Representation of Care

Dentists shall not represent the care being rendered to their patients in a false or misleading manner.

• • •

### 1-L. Representation of Fees

Dentists shall not represent the fees being charged for providing care in a false or misleading manner.

• • •

### 1-M. Patient Involvement

The dentist should inform the patient of the proposed treatment, and any reasonable alternatives, in a manner that allows the patient to become involved in treatment decisions.

### 1-N. Chemical Dependency

It is unethical for a dentist to practice while abusing controlled substances, alcohol or other chemical agents which impair the ability to practice. All dentists have an ethical obligation to urge impaired colleagues to seek treatment. Dentists with first-hand knowledge that a colleague is practicing dentistry when so impaired have an ethical responsibility to report such evidence to the professional assistance committee of a dental society.

## Principle - Section 2

### Education

The privilege of dentists to be accorded professional status rests primarily in the knowledge, skill, and experience with which they serve their patients and society. All dentists, therefore, have the obligation of keeping their knowledge and skill current.

## Code of Professional Conduct

### 2-A. Disclosure of Conflict of Interest

A dentist who presents educational or scientific information in an article, seminar or other program shall disclose to the readers or participants any monetary or other special interest the dentist may have with a company whose products are promoted or endorsed in the presentation. Disclosure shall be made in any promotional material and in the presentation itself.

## Principle - Section 3

### Government of a Profession

Every profession owes society the responsibility to regulate itself. Such regulation is achieved largely through the influence of the professional societies. All dentists, therefore, have the dual obligation of making themselves a part of a professional society and of observing its rules of ethics.

## Principle - Section 4

### Research and Development

Dentists have the obligation of making the results and benefits of their investigative efforts available to all when they are useful in safeguarding or promoting the health of the public.

## Code of Professional Conduct

### 4-A. Devices and Therapeutic Methods

Except for formal investigative studies, dentists shall be obliged to prescribe, dispense, or promote only those devices, drugs, and other agents whose complete formulae are available to the dental profession. Dentists shall have the further obligation of not holding out as exclusive any device, agent, method, or technique.

### 4-B. Patents and Copyrights

Patents and copyrights may be secured by dentists provided that such patents and copyrights shall not be used to restrict research or practice.

### Principle - Section 5

#### Professional Announcement

In order to properly serve the public, dentists should represent themselves in a manner that contributes to the esteem of the profession. Dentists should not misrepresent their training and competence in any way that would be false or misleading in any material respect.

## Code of Professional Conduct

#### 5-A. Advertising

Although any dentist may advertise, no dentist shall advertise or solicit patients in any form of communication in a manner that is false or misleading in any material respect.

• • •

# CODE OF ETHICS FOR THE PROFESSION OF DIETETICS
## American Dietetic Association
### 1987

*The current Code of Ethics for the Profession of Dietetics was adopted by the American Dietetic Association (ADA) in October 1987. Whereas most professional codes apply only to members of the authoring organization, the ADA code applies both to members of the ADA and to nonmembers who are credentialed as "registered dieticians" (RDs) or "dietetic technicians, registered" (DTRs) by the Commission on Dietetic Registration, the ADA's credentialing agency. Certain provisions, however, apply only to one group or the other. The code is supplemented by a detailed Review Process for Alleged Violations.*
*The nineteen principles of the code are printed here.*

• • •

## Principles

1. The dietetic practitioner provides professional services with objectivity and with respect for the unique needs and values of individuals.
2. The dietetic practitioner avoids discrimination against other individuals on the basis of race, creed, religion, sex, age, and national origin.
3. The dietetic practitioner fulfills professional commitments in good faith.
4. The dietetic practitioner conducts him/herself with honesty, integrity, and fairness.
5. The dietetic practitioner remains free of conflict of interest while fulfilling the objectives and maintaining the integrity of the dietetic profession.
6. The dietetic practitioner maintains confidentiality of information.
7. The dietetic practitioner practices dietetics based on scientific principles and current information.
8. The dietetic practitioner assumes responsibility and accountability for personal competence in practice.
9. The dietetic practitioner recognizes and exercises professional judgment within the limits of his/her qualifications and seeks counsel or makes referrals as appropriate.
10. The dietetic practitioner provides sufficient information to enable clients to make their own informed decisions.
11. The dietetic practitioner who wishes to inform the public and colleagues of his/her services does so by using factual information. The dietetic practitioner does not advertise in a false or misleading manner.
12. The dietetic practitioner promotes or endorses products in a manner that is neither false nor misleading.
13. The dietetic practitioner permits use of his/her name for the purpose of certifying that dietetic services have been rendered only if he/she has provided or supervised the provision of those services.
14. The dietetic practitioner accurately presents professional qualifications and credentials.

• • •

15. The dietetic practitioner presents substantiated information and interprets controversial information without personal bias, recognizing that legitimate differences of opinion exist.

16. The dietetic practitioner makes all reasonable effort to avoid bias in any kind of professional evaluation. The dietetic practitioner provides objective evaluation of candidates for professional association membership, awards, scholarships, or job advancements.

17. The dietetic practitioner voluntarily withdraws from professional practice under the following circumstances:

    A. The dietetic practitioner has engaged in any substance abuse that could affect his/her practice;

    B. The dietetic practitioner has been adjudged by a court to be mentally incompetent;

    C. The dietetic practitioner has an emotional or mental disability that affects his/her practice in a manner that could harm the client.

18. The dietetic practitioner complies with all applicable laws and regulations concerning the profession. The dietetic practitioner is subject to disciplinary action under the following circumstances:

    A. The dietetic practitioner has been convicted of a crime under the laws of the United States which is a felony or a misdemeanor, an essential element of which is dishonesty, and which is related to the practice of the profession.

    B. The dietetic practitioner has been disciplined by a state, and at least one of the grounds for the discipline is the same or substantially equivalent to these principles.

    C. The dietetic practitioner has committed an act of misfeasance or malfeasance which is directly related to the practice of the profession as determined by a court of competent jurisdiction, a licensing board, or an agency of a governmental body.

19. The dietetic practitioner accepts the obligation to protect society and the profession by upholding the Code of Ethics for the Profession of Dietetics and by reporting alleged violations of the Code through the defined review process of The American Dietetic Association and its credentialing agency, the Commission on Dietetic Registration.

# CODE OF ETHICS
## American Association of Pastoral Counselors
last amended 1994

*Amended in 1994, the current Code of Ethics of the American Association of Pastoral Counselors contains many of the same elements as other professional codes, for example, statements pertaining to confidentiality, professional qualifications, and the welfare of the individuals they serve. In addition, the code contains aspects unique to the profession, such as avoiding the imposition of one's personal theology on clients and maintaining a responsible association with one's faith group.*

### Principle I - Prologue

As members of the American Association of Pastoral Counselors, we are committed to the various theologies, traditions, and values of our faith communities and to the dignity and worth of each individual. We are dedicated to advancing the welfare of those who seek our assistance and to the maintenance of high standards of professional conduct and competence. We are accountable for our ministry whatever its setting. This accountability is expressed in relationships to clients, colleagues, students, our faith communities, and through the acceptance and practice of the principles and procedures of this Code of Ethics.

In order to uphold our standards, as members of AAPC we covenant to accept the following foundational premises:

A. To maintain responsible association with the faith group in which we have ecclesiastical standing.

B. To avoid discriminating against or refusing employment, educational opportunity or professional assistance to anyone on the basis of race, gender, sexual orientation, religion, or national origin.

C. To remain abreast of new developments in the field through both educational activities and clinical experience. We agree at all levels of membership to continue postgraduate education and professional growth including supervision, consultation, and active participation in the meetings and affairs of the Association.

D. To seek out and engage in collegial relationships, recognizing that isolation can lead to a loss of perspective and judgement.

E. To manage our personal lives in a healthful fashion and to seek appropriate assistance for our own personal problems or conflicts.

F. To diagnose or provide treatment only for those problems or issues that are within the reasonable boundaries of our competence.

G. To establish and maintain appropriate professional relationship boundaries.

## Principle II - Professional Practices

In all professional matters members of AAPC maintain practices that protect the public and advance the profession.

A. We use our knowledge and professional associations for the benefit of the people we serve and not to secure unfair personal advantage.

B. We clearly represent our level of membership and limit our practice to that level.

C. Fees and financial arrangements, as with all contractual matters, are always discussed without hesitation or equivocation at the onset and are established in a straightforward, professional manner.

D. We are prepared to render service to individuals and communities in crisis without regard to financial remuneration when necessary.

E. We neither receive nor pay a commission for referral of a client.

F. We conduct our practice, agency, regional and Association fiscal affairs with due regard to recognized business and accounting procedures.

G. Upon the transfer of a pastoral counseling practice or the sale of real, personal, tangible or intangible property or assets used in such practice, the privacy and well being of the client shall be of primary concern.
   1. Client names and records shall be excluded from the transfer or sale.
   2. Any fees paid shall be for services rendered, consultation, equipment, real estate, and the name and logo of the counseling agency.

H. We are careful to represent facts truthfully to clients, referral sources, and third party payors regarding credentials and services rendered. We shall correct any misrepresentation of our professional qualifications or affiliations.

I. We do not malign colleagues or other professionals.

## Principle III - Client Relationships

It is the responsibility of members of AAPC to maintain relationships with clients on a professional basis.

A. We do not abandon or neglect clients. If we are unable, or unwilling for appropriate reasons, to provide professional help or continue a professional relationship, every reasonable effort is made to arrange for continuation of treatment with another professional.

B. We make only realistic statements regarding the pastoral counseling process and its outcome.

C. We show sensitive regard for the moral, social, and religious standards of clients and communities. We avoid imposing our beliefs on others, although we may express them when appropriate in the pastoral counseling process.

D. Counseling relationships are continued only so long as it is reasonably clear that the clients are benefiting from the relationship.

E. We recognize the trust placed in and unique power of the therapeutic relationship. While acknowledging the complexity of some pastoral relationships, we avoid exploiting the trust and dependency of clients. We avoid those dual relationships with clients (e.g., business or close personal relationships) which could impair our professional judgement, compromise the integrity of the treatment, and/or use the relationship for our own gain.

F. We do not engage in harassment, abusive words or actions, or exploitative coercion of clients or former clients.

G. All forms of sexual behavior or harassment with clients are unethical, even when a client invites or consents to such behavior or involvement. Sexual behavior is defined as, but not limited to, all forms of overt and covert seductive speech, gestures, and behavior as well as physical contact of a sexual nature; harassment is defined as but not limited to, repeated comments, gestures or physical contacts of a sexual nature.

H.  We recognize that the therapist/client relationship involves a power imbalance, the residual effects of which are operative following the termination of the therapy relationship. Therefore, all sexual behavior or harassment as defined in Principle III, G with former clients is unethical.

## Principle IV - Confidentiality

As members of AAPC we respect the integrity and protect the welfare of all persons with whom we are working and have an obligation to safeguard information about them that has been obtained in the course of the counseling process.

A.  All records kept on a client are stored or disposed of in a manner that assures security and confidentiality.

B.  We treat all communications from clients with professional confidence.

C.  Except in those situations where the identity of the client is necessary to the understanding of the case, we use only the first names of our clients when engaged in supervision or consultation. It is our responsibility to convey the importance of confidentiality to the supervisor/consultant; this is particularly important when the supervision is shared by other professionals, as in a supervisory group.

D.  We do not disclose client confidences to anyone, except: as mandated by law; to prevent a clear and immediate danger to someone; in the course of a civil, criminal or disciplinary action arising from the counseling where the pastoral counselor is a defendant; for purposes of supervision or consultation; or by previously obtained written permission. In cases involving more than one person (as client) written permission must be obtained from all legally accountable persons who have been present during the counseling before any disclosure can be made.

E.  We obtain informed written consent of clients before audio and/or video tape recording or permitting third party observation of their sessions.

F.  We do not use these standards of confidentiality to avoid intervention when it is necessary, e.g., when there is evidence of abuse of minors, the elderly, the disabled, the physically or mentally incompetent.

G.  When current or former clients are referred to in a publication, while teaching or in a public presentation, their identity is thoroughly disguised.

H.  We as members of AAPC agree that as an express condition of our membership in the Association, Association ethics communications, files, investigative reports, and related records are strictly confidential and waive their right to use same in a court of law to advance any claim against another member. Any member seeking such records for such purpose shall be subject to disciplinary action for attempting to violate the confidentiality requirements of the organization. This policy is intended to promote pastoral and confessional communications without legal consequences and to protect potential privacy and confidentiality interests of third parties.

## Principle V - Supervisee, Student & Employee Relationships

As members of AAPC we have an ethical concern for the integrity and welfare of our supervisees, students and employees. These relationships are maintained on a professional and confidential basis. We recognize our influential position with regard to both current and former supervisees, students and employees, and avoid exploiting their trust and dependency. We make every effort to avoid dual relationships with such persons that could impair our judgement or increase the risk of personal and/or financial exploitation.

A.  We do not engage in ongoing counseling relationships with current supervisees, students and employees.

B.  We do not engage in sexual or other harassment of supervisees, students, employees, research subjects or colleagues.

C.  All forms of sexual behavior, as defined in Principle III.G, with our supervisees, students, research subjects and employees (except in employee situations involving domestic partners) are unethical.

D.  We advise our students, supervisees, and employees against offering or engaging in, or holding themselves out as competent to engage in, professional services beyond their training, level of experience and competence.

E.  We do not harass or dismiss an employee who has acted in a reasonable, responsible and ethical manner to protect, or intervene on behalf of, a client or other member of the public or another employee.

### Principle VI - Interprofessional Relationships

As members of AAPC we relate to and cooperate with other professional persons in our community and beyond. We are part of a network of health care professionals and are expected to develop and maintain interdisciplinary and interprofessional relationships.

A. We do not offer ongoing clinical services to persons currently receiving treatment from another professional without prior knowledge of and in consultation with the other professional, with the clients' informed consent. Soliciting such clients is unethical.

B. We exercise care and interprofessional courtesy when approached for services by persons who claim or appear to have inappropriately terminated treatment with another professional.

### Principle VII - Advertising

Any advertising by or for a member of AAPC, including announcements, public statements and promotional activities, is undertaken with the purpose of helping the public make informed judgements and choices.

• • •

## GUIDELINES FOR THE CHAPLAINS' ROLE IN BIOETHICS
### College of Chaplains, American Protestant Health Association
### 1992

*This document differs from codes of ethics in its focus on the role of chaplains in clinical settings, particularly within health-care institutions. Certified chaplains are recognized to be essential members of the health-care team; they help to identify and integrate the spiritual and moral perspectives of patients with those of other health-care disciplines to form a holistic approach to bioethics.*

### Introduction

While rapid advances in medical science and technology have produced many benefits, they have also created new dilemmas in ethical decision-making. The formulation and strengthening of a process for ethical reflection in the clinical context has become a vital issue for all health care providers. Patients, family members, and health care team professionals increasingly face perplexing problems related to such issues as treatment choices, informed consent, surrogate decision-making, withholding or withdrawing treatment, personal autonomy and the preservation of personal dignity.

Certified chaplains are essential members of the health care team, and are committed to providing care at the highest possible level of quality. Chaplains assist patients, families and staff in exploring the human and religious values that inform their decisions and choices in treatment. In playing this multifaceted role, however, chaplains are committed to the Code of Ethics of the College of Chaplains, which forbids proselytizing of persons under care in health care institutions.

We take it as a primary assumption that any health care institution that has an official bioethics committee should include a certified chaplain on that committee. Bioethics committees normally serve three functions: 1) education, 2) consultation, and 3) review and recommendation of institutional policies and procedures. As members of bioethics committees, chaplains play a crucial role in bioethical reflection. The questions of philosophy, theology, human values and morals that are often raised in bioethics committees can be fully addressed only within context of the culture, religious or faith traditions, and the personalities and personal backgrounds of the patients, families or other decision-makers.

While some chaplains may have an education in ethics, their role as chaplain differs from that of ethicist. The chaplain identifies and focusses the patient's spiritual and moral perspectives as essential ingredients in the process of bioethical reflection. It is the integration of these perspectives with those of other health care disciplines that makes a wholistic approach to bioethics possible.

These Guidelines provide the essential components for the effective inclusion of pastoral care perspectives in the bioethical reflection process. While each health care institution has its own unique context within which ethical reflection is done, these guidelines are general enough to apply to a variety of clinical settings. The primary emphasis of these guidelines is that pastoral care's unique perspective should be an integral part of any health care institution's bioethical reflection process.

## Principle I

**The health care institution will include a certified chaplain on its bioethics committee.**

*Interpretation - Of the many contributions that a certified chaplain can make to a bioethics committee, one of the most important is to act as a liaison between the committee and community clergy. Representatives of the community's religious groups, given their professional relationship of trust with patients, residents or families, often have significant contributions to make both to the quality of patient care and to the process of ethical decision-making.*

### Guideline 1

In order to be knowledgeable about the potential contributions of community clergy to ethical decision- and policy-making, chaplains facilitate the pastoral ministry of community clergy to members of their congregations who are patients or residents in health care facilities.

### Guideline 2

Chaplains serve as resource persons concerning the spiritual dimensions of illness and health, both to community clergy and to the bioethics committee—even when patients or their families have no apparent religious affiliation.

## Principle II

**Chaplains will develop a continuing education plan, both for themselves and their colleagues, in bioethical principles as they relate to the spiritual, religious, cultural and philosophic values represented in the persons served by their health care institutions, and will contribute to the institution's educational program.**

*Interpretation - Certified Chaplains have a theological education on at least the master's level that has included formal training in the areas of pastoral theology, and clinical pastoral education. This theological and clinical grounding can provide a necessary mooring within a contemporary setting where multi-disciplines reflect and discuss bioethical dilemmas from the perspective of their own professional discipline.*

### Guideline 1

Chaplains are expected to regularly study the bioethical literature, have basic training in bioethical principles, and seek ways to learn and gain experience in integrating bioethical reflection with the spiritual dimensions and values which chaplains are called upon to address.

### Guideline 2

Chaplains participate and serve as resource persons to the institution's bioethics education program to patients, staff, and community, providing a forum for a discussion of various spiritual and religious perspectives about the bioethical issues.

### Guideline 3

Chaplains are included in peer review as the multi-disciplinary team seeks to teach bioethical principles and options that apply in specific situations.

### Guideline 4

Chaplains contribute as resource persons and speakers in the institution's patient, professional and public education programs.

### Guideline 5

Chaplains bring the discipline of theology and the practice of pastoral care and counseling to the multi-disciplinary team in the clinical setting.

### Guideline 6

Chaplains bring the expertise in spiritual, theological, ethical and moral values to the multi-disciplinary reflection and discourse concerning ethical issues, dilemmas, case studies and retrospective reviews.

### Principle III

**Chaplains will participate in the bioethics consultation services of the facility.**

*Interpretation - An institutional bioethics committee can provide the service of consultation to physicians, nurses, administration, patients and family. Consultation does not take the place of or interfere with the patient-physician relationship. Rather, it can help clarify various ethical options through reflective discussion in the context of bioethical principles and good medical practice.*

#### Guideline 1

Certified chaplains have the experience and training that relates to effective group process, an essential ingredient for effective ethical decision-making. Within the health care arena, there is potential for interdisciplinary tension and competition. There needs to be an open process that facilitates communication.

#### Guideline 2

Chaplains can provide substantive input by helping the patient, family, and staff identify competing spiritual, moral, religious, cultural, and philosophical values. These values underlie principles that inform the patient's and physician's treatment options and decisions.

### Principle IV

**Chaplains will participate in assisting the institution in reviewing and recommending policies having bioethical implications in the services provided by the facility.**

*Interpretation - Institutional bioethics committees in the process of reflection are usually responsible for reviewing existing or proposed policies and procedures for the institution, medical staff, nursing staff, etc. As members of the bioethics committee, chaplains provide input appropriate to their own discipline of pastoral care.*

#### Guideline 1

Chaplains are utilized as resource persons for understanding and interpreting faith communities and belief systems as they might relate to or be affected by proposed policies and procedures.

#### Guideline 2

Chaplains address the spiritual and religious concerns of the staff who are charged with the responsibility of implementing policies and procedures having bioethical ramifications.

### Principle V

**Chaplains will provide pastoral care to those involved in the bioethical reflection process.**

*Interpretation - The ministry of chaplains includes a wide repertoire of services including "pastoral presence", "pastoral conversation", pastoral care and pastoral counseling. Through experiencing such services, patients, families and staff feel affirmed, understood, and supported in their particular predicament and in the right to have a particular perspective. Then those involved in the process can be enabled to explore the relationships of the physical issues of health and illness, the psychological dimensions of the situation, i.e., anxiety, fear, trust, etc., and the spiritual issues, i.e. meaning, hope, ultimate concerns, and God's presence. The issues will vary tremendously from person to person depending upon the situation and belief system of the individual. The pastoral care process itself becomes therapeutic for all involved within the context of bioethical decision-making.*

#### Guideline 1

Chaplains provide appropriate religious resources and support from the patient's and family's own faith system and community as appropriate.

#### Guideline 2

Chaplains facilitate the ministry of community clergy for the purpose of offering support and the opportunity to patients and families to explore the important issues, values and meaning inherent in each patient situation.

## Principle VI

**Chaplains will provide specific evaluation of the process of bioethical reflection from a "spiritual perspective" as well as from a clinical perspective.**

Interpretation - *Evaluation of the bioethical process in each case in which there was a consultation, policy review, or educational event, is important so that the quality of care can be improved. Each discipline has its own perspective and responsibility to contribute to the evaluation process.*

### Guideline 1

Chaplains have the responsibility to be advocates for the particular spiritual values of the patient, family and also staff. The role of the chaplain is to help ensure that the bioethical reflection process is as respectful, attentive, and inclusive of their values and wishes as possible.

### Guideline 2

Pastoral intervention in the bioethics process will be evaluated through peer review with input from a clinically trained and experienced ethicist regularly. Opportunities and encouragement for attendance and participation by chaplains in regional and/or national bioethics workshops and other educational events are to be provided by the health care institution.

## Principle VII

**Chaplains will provide for alternate coverage of the chaplain's role in the bioethical reflection process when it is appropriate for the chaplain usually designated to contribute to the process to exclude her/himself.**

Interpretation - *There are times when it is appropriate for the chaplain usually charged with the responsibility to serve on the bioethics committee or participate in the consultation service to withdraw from participation so that objectivity and professionalism may be maintained in the process.*

### Guideline 1

In situations where the chaplain does not have adequate knowledge about a particular issue, particularly a patient's or family's spiritual perspective, the chaplain is to seek consultation or make an appropriate referral.

### Guideline 2

In situations where the chaplain has a personal relationship with one or more of the significant parties involved in the case under review, objective and professional integrity is maintained by designating another certified chaplain to participate in the process.

### Guideline 3

Chaplains will be familiar with the bioethics process of consultation in their institutions. When particular patients with whom they have pastoral relationships are brought to the attention of the bioethics program for consultation or for education purposes, other pastoral care staff persons or community clergy can be involved when and to the degree appropriate. In this process, confidentiality will be maintained.

# CODE OF ETHICS
## American Pharmaceutical Association
### 1969, amended 1975, revised 1981

*The current code of the American Pharmaceutical Association (APhA) was approved in 1969, amended in 1975, and last revised in 1981. Since the 1969 code, the Association has introduced gender-neutral language and removed the prohibition on advertising. The APhA code is currently undergoing significant revision, but approval of the revision was not expected before the end of 1994.*

## Preamble

These principles of professional conduct are established to guide pharmacists in relationships with patients, fellow practitioners, other health professionals, and the public.

A **Pharmacist** should hold the health and safety of patients to be of first consideration and should render to each patient the full measure of professional ability as an essential health practitioner.

A **Pharmacist** should never knowingly condone the dispensing, promoting, or distributing of drugs or medical devices, or assist therein, that are not of good quality, that do not meet standards required by law, or that lack therapeutic value for the patient.

A **Pharmacist** should always strive to perfect and enlarge professional knowledge. A pharmacist should utilize and make available this knowledge as may be required in accordance with the best professional judgment.

A **Pharmacist** has the duty to observe the law, to uphold the dignity and honor of the profession, and to accept its ethical principles. A pharmacist should not engage in any activity that will bring discredit to the profession and should expose, without fear or favor, illegal or unethical conduct in the profession.

A **Pharmacist** should seek at all times only fair and reasonable remuneration for professional services. A pharmacist should never agree to, or participate in, transactions with practitioners of other health professions or any other person under which fees are divided or that may cause financial or other exploitation in connection with the rendering of professional services.

A **Pharmacist** should respect the confidential and personal nature of professional records; except where the best interest of the patient requires or the law demands, a pharmacist should not disclose such information to anyone without proper patient authorization.

A **Pharmacist** should not agree to practice under terms or conditions that interfere with or impair the proper exercise of professional judgment and skill, that cause a deterioration of the quality of professional services, or that require consent to unethical conduct.

A **Pharmacist** should strive to provide information to patients regarding professional services truthfully, accurately, and fully and should avoid misleading patients regarding the nature, cost, or value of these professional services.

A **Pharmacist** should associate with organizations having for their objective the betterment of the profession of pharmacy and should contribute time and funds to carry on the work of these organizations.

## GUIDELINES FOR CODES OF ETHICS FOR PHARMACISTS
### Fédération Internationale Pharmaceutique
### 1988

*In 1988, the Fédération Internationale Pharmaceutique adopted sixteen guidelines for ethical behavior by pharmacists. The guidelines, which are deliberately broad so that nations may adapt them in creating their own ethics codes, mention several topics of particular note: (1) the independence of the profession, extending to the refusal to dispense medications, including prescriptions, if it serves the patient's health; (2) the role of pharmacists as health educators; and (3) respect for the freedom of choice of patients.*

1. Pharmacists who serve public health and individuals should carry out their professional role with respect for life and for the human being.
2. Pharmacists should show the same dedication to all their patients.
3. It is the duty of pharmacists to update their professional knowledge continually.
4. Pharmacists should respect professional confidentiality and should not divulge information except with the consent of the patient or on the rare occasion when it would be in the best interest of the patient.
5. Pharmacists should accomplish each pharmaceutical act with care and attention.
6. Pharmacists should not undermine, even partially, their professional independence in any way.
7. Pharmacists should abstain from any deed or any action which is liable to discredit the profession, even if it is unrelated to its practice. Under all circumstances they should see to it that the dignity and the independence of the profession are upheld and respected.
8. Pharmacists should respect the ethical standards of the profession and, if it exists, the national code of ethics.
9. Pharmacists should respect the freedom of choice of the patient, which is an inalienable right.
10. Pharmacists should, in all circumstances, ensure that charges for their services are both fair and reasonable. Any act which places the well-being of patients at risk,

and any sharing of remuneration for the services of a pharmacist, are considered to be contrary to ethical behavior and conventions.

11. Pharmacists should ensure that all publicity and information relating to their practice is accurate, truthful, and in conformity with professional ethics.
12. Pharmacists should maintain a relationship of trust with the administrative authorities.
13. Pharmacists should assist the appropriate authorities in their efforts to protect health. By way of advice to the authorities, the pharmacist should endeavor to promote measures designed to prevent ill health.
14. Pharmacists should act as health educators.
15. Pharmacists should participate in the activities of national and international professional organizations whose aim it is to improve the conditions of practice or the standards of the profession.
16. Pharmacists can, in the interest of the health of the patient, refuse to dispense, sell, or supply a medicament. If that medicament is ordered on prescription, the pharmacist should immediately advise the prescriber.

## CODE OF ETHICS AND GUIDE
## FOR PROFESSIONAL CONDUCT
### American Physical Therapy Association
1981, last amended 1991

*The American Physical Therapy Association Code of Ethics articulates eight ethical principles for the physical therapy profession, which are developed further in the Guide for Professional Conduct. The eight principles and selected interpretations from the guide are printed here.*

• • •

## Principle 1

*Physical therapists respect the rights and dignity of all individuals.*

### 1.1 Attitudes of Physical Therapists

A. Physical therapists shall recognize that each individual is different from all other individuals and shall respect and be responsive to those differences.

B. Physical therapists are to be guided at all times by concern for the physical, psychological, and socioeconomic welfare of those individuals entrusted to their care.

C. Physical therapists shall be responsive to and mutually supportive of colleagues and associates.

### 1.2 Confidential Information

A. Information relating to the physical therapist-patient relationship is confidential and may not be communicated to a third party not involved in that patient's care without the prior written consent of the patient, subject to applicable law.

B. Information derived from a component-sponsored peer review shall be held confidential by the reviewer unless written permission to release the information is obtained from the physical therapist who was reviewed.

C. Information derived from the working relationships of physical therapists shall be held confidential by all parties.

D. Information may be disclosed to appropriate authorities when it is necessary to protect the welfare of an individual or the community. Such disclosure shall be in accordance with applicable law.

## Principle 2

*Physical therapists comply with the laws and regulations governing the practice of physical therapy.*

• • •

## Principle 3

*Physical therapists accept responsibility for the exercise of sound judgement.*

### 3.1 Acceptance of Responsibility

A. Upon accepting an individual for provision of physical therapy services, physical therapists shall assume the responsibility for evaluating that individual; planning, implementing, and supervising the therapeutic program; reevaluating and changing that program; and maintaining adequate records of the case, including progress reports.

B.   When the individual's needs are beyond the scope of the physical therapist's expertise, the individual shall be so informed and assisted in identifying a qualified person to provide the necessary services.

C.   When physical therapists judge that benefit can no longer be obtained from their services, they shall so inform the individual receiving the services. It is unethical to initiate or continue services that, in the therapist's judgment, either cannot result in beneficial outcome or are contraindicated.

D.  Physical therapists shall maintain the ability to make independent judgments, which must not be limited or compromised by professional affiliations, including employment relationships.

• • •

## Principle 4

*Physical therapists maintain and promote high standards for physical therapy practice, education, and research.*

• • •

## Principle 5

*Physical therapists seek remuneration for their services that is deserved and reasonable.*

• • •

## Principle 6

*Physical therapists provide accurate information to the consumer about the profession and about those services they provide.*

• • •

## Principle 7

*Physical therapists accept the responsibility to protect the public and the profession from unethical, incompetent, or illegal acts.*

• • •

## Principle 8

*Physical therapists participate in efforts to address the health needs of the public.*

# OCCUPATIONAL THERAPY CODE OF ETHICS
## American Occupational Therapy Association
### 1988

*The Occupational Therapy Code of Ethics, approved in 1988, replaces the 1977/1979 Principles of Occupational Therapy Ethics. Although the code is enforceable only with respect to members of the association, it is interesting because it expressly applies to all "occupational therapy personnel," including therapists, assistants, and students.*

The American Occupational Therapy Association and its component members are committed to furthering people's ability to function fully within their total environment. To this end the occupational therapist renders service to clients in all stages of health and illness, to institutions, to other professionals and colleagues, to students, and to the general public.

• • •

## Principle 1 (Beneficence/Autonomy)

Occupational therapy personnel shall demonstrate a concern for the welfare and dignity of the recipient of their services.

A.  The individual is responsible for providing services without regard to race, creed, national origin, sex, age, handicap, disease entity, social status, financial status, or religious affiliation.

B.  The individual shall inform those people served of the nature and potential outcomes of treatment and shall respect the right of potential recipients of service to refuse treatment.

C. The individual shall inform subjects involved in education or research activities of the potential outcome of those activities.

D. The individual shall include those people served in the treatment planning process.

E. The individual shall maintain goal-directed and objective relationships with all people served.

F. The individual shall protect the confidential nature of information gained from educational, practice, and investigational activities unless sharing such information could be deemed necessary to protect the well-being of a third party.

G. The individual shall take all reasonable precautions to avoid harm to the recipient of services or detriment to the recipient's property.

H. The individual shall establish fees, based on cost analysis, that are commensurate with services rendered.

## Principle 2 (Competence)

Occupational therapy personnel shall actively maintain high standards of professional competence.

A. The individual shall hold the appropriate credential for providing service.

B. The individual shall recognize the need for competence and shall participate in continuing professional development.

C. The individual shall function within the parameters of his or her competence and the standards of the profession.

D. The individual shall refer clients to other service providers or consult with other service providers when additional knowledge and expertise is required.

## Principle 3 (Compliance With Laws and Regulations)

Occupational therapy personnel shall comply with laws and Association policies guiding the profession of occupational therapy.

A. The individual shall be acquainted with applicable local, state, federal, and institutional rules and Association policies and shall function accordingly.

B. The individual shall inform employers, employees, and colleagues about those laws and policies that apply to the profession of occupational therapy.

C. The individual shall require those whom they supervise to adhere to the Code of Ethics.

D. The individual shall accurately record and report information.

## Principle 4 (Public Information)

Occupational therapy personnel shall provide accurate information concerning occupational therapy services.

A. The individual shall accurately represent his or her competence and training.

B. The individual shall not use or participate in the use of any form of communication that contains a false, fraudulent, deceptive, or unfair statement or claim.

## Principle 5 (Professional Relationships)

Occupational therapy personnel shall function with discretion and integrity in relations with colleagues and other professionals, and shall be concerned with the quality of their services.

A. The individual shall report illegal, incompetent, and/or unethical practice to the appropriate authority.

B. The individual shall not disclose privileged information when participating in reviews of peers, programs, or systems.

C. The individual who employs or supervises colleagues shall provide appropriate supervision, as defined in AOTA guidelines or state laws, regulations, and institutional policies.

D. The individual shall recognize the contributions of colleagues when disseminating professional information.

## Principle 6 (Professional Conduct)

Occupational therapy personnel shall not engage in any form of conduct that constitutes a conflict of interest or that adversely reflects on the profession.

# CODE OF ETHICS OF THE PHYSICIAN ASSISTANT PROFESSION
## American Academy of Physician Assistants
### 1983, amended 1985, reaffirmed 1990

*The American Academy of Physician Assistants' (AAPA) current Code of Ethics was adopted in 1983, amended in 1985, and reaffirmed in 1990. In addition to standard features, the code explicitly recognizes that: (1) It is necessarily limited and does not preclude additional, equally imperative, obligations; (2) physician assistants should use their skills "to contribute to an improved community"; and (3) physician assistants "shall place service before material gain." The AAPA also has issued Guidelines for Professional Conduct, which interpret and elaborate upon the principles found in the code of ethics.*

The American Academy of Physician Assistants recognizes its responsibility to aid the profession in maintaining high standards in the provision of quality and accessible health care services. The following principles delineate the standards governing the conduct of physician assistants in their professional interactions with patients, colleagues, other health professionals and the general public. Realizing that no code can encompass all ethical responsibilities of the physician assistant, this enumeration of obligations in the Code of Ethics is not comprehensive and does not constitute a denial of the existence of other obligations, equally imperative, though not specifically mentioned.

**Physician assistants** shall be committed to providing competent medical care, assuming as their primary responsibility the health, safety, welfare and dignity of all humans.

**Physician assistants** shall extend to each patient the full measure of their ability as dedicated, empathetic health care providers and shall assume responsibility for the skillful and proficient transactions of their professional duties.

**Physician assistants** shall deliver needed health care services to health consumers without regard to sex, age, race, creed, socioeconomic and political status.

**Physician assistants** shall adhere to all state and federal laws governing informed consent concerning the patient's health care.

**Physician assistants** shall seek consultation with their supervising physician, other health providers, or qualified professionals having special skills, knowledge or experience whenever the welfare of the patient will be safeguarded or advanced by such consultation. Supervision should include ongoing communication between the physician and the physician assistant regarding the care of all patients.

**Physician assistants** shall take personal responsibility for being familiar with and adhering to all federal/state laws applicable to the practice of their profession.

**Physician assistants** shall provide only those services for which they are qualified via education and/or experience and by pertinent legal regulatory process.

**Physician assistants** shall not misrepresent in any manner, either directly or indirectly, their skills, training, professional credentials, identity, or services.

**Physician assistants** shall uphold the doctrine of confidentiality regarding privileged patient information, unless required to release such information by law or such information becomes necessary to protect the welfare of the patient or the community.

**Physician assistants** shall strive to maintain and increase the quality of individual health care service through individual study and continuing eduction.

**Physician assistants** shall have the duty to respect the law, to uphold the dignity of the physician assistant profession and to accept its ethical principles. The physician assistant shall not participate in or conceal any activity that will bring discredit or dishonor to the physician assistant profession and shall expose, without fear or favor, any illegal or unethical conduct in the medical profession.

**Physician assistants,** ever cognizant of the needs of the community, shall use the knowledge and experience acquired as professionals to contribute to an improved community.

**Physician assistants** shall place service before material gain and must carefully guard against conflicts of professional interest.

**Physician assistants** shall strive to maintain a spirit of cooperation with their professional organizations and the general public.

# ETHICAL PRINCIPLES OF PSYCHOLOGISTS AND CODE OF CONDUCT
### American Psychological Association
### 1992

*A substantially revised version of the Ethical Principles of Psychologists and Code of Conduct was adopted by the American Psychological Association (APA) in 1992. The 1992 revision, which is still current, consists of an introduction, a preamble, six general principles, and specific ethical standards. The preamble and general principles represent "aspirational goals to guide psychologists toward the highest ideals of psychology," whereas the ethical standards establish "enforceable rules for conduct." The standards are noteworthy for the scope of the topics addressed, including sexual harassment, misuse of influence, and informed consent, that pertain to therapeutic and research relationships, as well as those that pertain to the care and use of animals in research.*

*The preamble, general principles, and excerpts from the ethical standards follow.*

• • •

## Preamble

Psychologists work to develop a valid and reliable body of scientific knowledge based on research. They may apply that knowledge to human behavior in a variety of contexts. In doing so, they perform many roles, such as researcher, educator, diagnostician, therapist, supervisor, consultant, administrator, social interventionist, and expert witness. Their goal is to broaden knowledge of behavior and, where appropriate, to apply it pragmatically to improve the condition of both the individual and society. Psychologists respect the central importance of freedom of inquiry and expression in research, teaching, and publication. They also strive to help the public in developing informed judgments and choices concerning human behavior. This Ethics Code provides a common set of values upon which psychologists build their professional and scientific work.

This Code is intended to provide both the general principles and the decision rules to cover most situations encountered by psychologists. It has as its primary goal the welfare and protection of the individuals and groups with whom psychologists work. It is the individual responsibility of each psychologist to aspire to the highest possible standards of conduct. Psychologists respect and protect human and civil rights, and do not knowingly participate in or condone unfair discriminatory practices.

The development of a dynamic set of ethical standards for a psychologist's work-related conduct requires a personal commitment to a lifelong effort to act ethically; to encourage ethical behavior by students, supervisees, employees, and colleagues, as appropriate; and to consult with others, as needed, concerning ethical problems. Each psychologist supplements, but does not violate, the Ethics Code's values and rules on the basis of guidance drawn from personal values, culture, and experience.

## General Principles

### Principle A: Competence

Psychologists strive to maintain high standards of competence in their work. They recognize the boundaries of their particular competencies and the limitations of their expertise. They provide only those services and use only those techniques for which they are qualified by education, training, or experience. Psychologists are cognizant of the fact that the competencies required in serving, teaching, and/or studying groups of people vary with the distinctive characteristics of those groups. In those areas in which recognized professional standards do not yet exist, psychologists exercise careful judgment and take appropriate precautions to protect the welfare of those with whom they work. They maintain knowledge of relevant scientific and professional information related to the services they render, and they recognize the need for ongoing education. Psychologists make appropriate use of scientific, professional, technical, and administrative resources.

### Principle B: Integrity

Psychologists seek to promote integrity in the science, teaching, and practice of psychology. In these activities psychologists are honest, fair, and respectful of others. In describing or reporting their qualifications, services, products, fees, research, or teaching, they do not make statements that are false, misleading, or deceptive. Psychologists strive to be aware of their own belief systems, values, needs, and limitations and the effect of these on their work. To the extent feasible, they attempt to clarify for relevant parties the roles they are performing and to function appropriately in accordance with those roles. Psychologists avoid improper and potentially harmful dual relationships.

### Principle C: Professional and Scientific Responsibility

Psychologists uphold professional standards of conduct, clarify their professional roles and obligations, accept appropriate responsibility for their behavior, and adapt their methods to the needs of different populations. Psychologists consult with, refer to, or cooperate with other professionals and institutions to the extent needed to serve the best interests of their patients, clients, or other recipients of their services. Psychologists' moral standards and conduct are personal matters to the same degree as is true for any other person, except as psychologists' conduct may compromise their professional responsibilities or reduce the public's trust in psychology and psychologists. Psychologists are concerned about the ethical compliance of their colleagues' scientific and professional conduct. When appropriate, they consult with colleagues in order to prevent or avoid unethical conduct.

### Principle D: Respect for People's Rights and Dignity

Psychologists accord appropriate respect to the fundamental rights, dignity, and worth of all people. They respect the rights of individuals to privacy, confidentiality, self-determination, and autonomy, mindful that legal and other obligations may lead to inconsistency and conflict with the exercise of these rights. Psychologists are aware of cultural, individual, and role differences, including those due to age, gender, race, ethnicity, national origin, religion, sexual orientation, disability, language, and socioeconomic status. Psychologists try to eliminate the effect on their work of biases based on those factors, and they do not knowingly participate in or condone unfair discriminatory practices.

### Principle E: Concern for Others' Welfare

Psychologists seek to contribute to the welfare of those with whom they interact professionally. In their professional actions, psychologists weigh the welfare and rights of their patients or clients, students, supervisees, human research participants, and other affected persons, and the welfare of animal subjects of research. When conflicts occur among psychologists' obligations or concerns, they attempt to resolve these conflicts and to perform their roles in a responsible fashion that avoids or minimizes harm. Psychologists are sensitive to real and ascribed differences in power between themselves and others, and they do not exploit or mislead other people during or after professional relationships.

### Principle F: Social Responsibility

Psychologists are aware of their professional and scientific responsibilities to the community and the society in which they work and live. They apply and make public their knowledge of psychology in order to contribute to human welfare. Psychologists are concerned about and work to mitigate the causes of human suffering. When undertaking research, they strive to advance human welfare and the science of psychology. Psychologists try to avoid misuse of their work. Psychologists comply with the law and encourage the development of law and social policy that serve the interests of their patients and clients and the public. They are encouraged to contribute a portion of their professional time for little or no personal advantage.

## ETHICAL STANDARDS

### 1. General Standards

These General Standards are potentially applicable to the professional and scientific activities of all psychologists.

• • •

### 1.02 Relationship of Ethics and Law

If psychologists' ethical responsibilities conflict with law, psychologists make known their commitment to the Ethics Code and take steps to resolve the conflict in a responsible manner.

• • •

### 1.09 Respecting Others

In their work-related activities, psychologists respect the rights of others to hold values, attitudes, and opinions that differ from their own.

### 1.10 Nondiscrimination

In their work-related activities, psychologists do not engage in unfair discrimination based on age, gender, race, ethnicity, national origin, religion, sexual orientation, disability, socioeconomic status, or any basis proscribed by law.

### 1.11 Sexual Harassment

(a) Psychologists do not engage in sexual harassment. Sexual harassment is sexual solicitation, physical advances, or verbal or nonverbal conduct that is sexual in nature, that occurs in connection with the psychologist's activities or roles as a psychologist, and that either: (1) is unwelcome, is offensive, or creates a hostile workplace environment, and the psychologist knows or is told this; or (2) is sufficiently severe or intense to be abusive to a reasonable person in the context. Sexual harassment can consist of a single intense or severe act or of multiple persistent or pervasive acts.

(b) Psychologists accord sexual-harassment complainants and respondents dignity and respect. Psychologists do not participate in denying a person academic admittance or advancement, employment, tenure, or promotion, based solely upon their having made, or their being the subject of, sexual-harassment charges. This does not preclude taking action based upon the outcome of such proceedings or consideration of other appropriate information.

### 1.12 Other Harassment

Psychologists do not knowingly engage in behavior that is harassing or demeaning to persons with whom they interact in their work based on factors such as those persons' age, gender, race, ethnicity, national origin, religion, sexual orientation, disability, language, or socioeconomic status.

### 1.13 Personal Problems and Conflicts

(a) Psychologists recognize that their personal problems and conflicts may interfere with their effectiveness. Accordingly, they refrain from undertaking an activity when they know or should know that their personal problems are likely to lead to harm to a patient, client, colleague, student, research participant, or other person to whom they may owe a professional or scientific obligation.

(b) In addition, psychologists have an obligation to be alert to signs of, and to obtain assistance for, their personal problems at an early stage, in order to prevent significantly impaired performance.

(c) When psychologists become aware of personal problems that may interfere with their performing work-related duties adequately, they take appropriate measures, such as obtaining professional consultation or assistance, and determine whether they should limit, suspend, or terminate their work-related duties.

### 1.14 Avoiding Harm

Psychologists take reasonable steps to avoid harming their patients or clients, research participants, students, and others with whom they work, and to minimize harm where it is foreseeable and unavoidable.

### 1.15 Misuse of Psychologists' Influence

Because psychologists' scientific and professional judgments and actions may affect the lives of others, they are alert to and guard against personal, financial, social, organizational, or political factors that might lead to misuse of their influence.

### 1.16 Misuse of Psychologists' Work

(a) Psychologists do not participate in activities in which it appears likely that their skills or data will be misused by others, unless corrective mechanisms are available.

(b) If psychologists learn of misuse or misrepresentation of their work, they take reasonable steps to correct or minimize the misuse or misrepresentation.

### 1.17 Multiple Relationships

(a) In many communities and situations, it may not be feasible or reasonable for psychologists to avoid social or other nonprofessional contacts with persons such as patients, clients, students, supervisees, or research participants. Psychologists must always be sensitive to the potential harmful effects of other contacts on their work and on those persons with whom they deal. A psychologist refrains from entering into or promising another personal, scientific, professional, financial, or other relationship with such persons if it appears likely that such a relationship reasonably might impair the psychologist's objectivity or otherwise interfere with the psychologist's effectively performing his or her functions as a psychologist, or might harm or exploit the other party.

(b) Likewise, whenever feasible, a psychologist refrains from taking on professional or scientific obligations when preexisting relationships would create a risk of such harm.

(c) If a psychologist finds that, due to unforeseen factors, a potentially harmful multiple relationship has arisen, the psychologist attempts to resolve it with due regard for the best interests of the affected person and maximal compliance with the Ethics Code.

• • •

### 1.19 Exploitative Relationships

(a) Psychologists do not exploit persons over whom they have supervisory, evaluative, or other authority such as students, supervisees, employees, research participants, and clients or patients.

(b) Psychologists do not engage in sexual relationships with students or supervisees in training over whom the psychologist has evaluative or direct authority, because such relationships are so likely to impair judgment or be exploitative.

### 1.20 Consultations and Referrals

(a) Psychologist arrange for appropriate consultations and referrals based principally on the best interests of their patients or clients, with appropriate consent, and subject to other relevant considerations, including applicable law and contractual obligations.

• • •

### 1.21 Third-Party Requests for Services

(a) When a psychologist agrees to provide services to a person or entity at the request of a third party, the psychologist clarifies to the extent feasible, at the outset of the service, the nature of the relationship with each party. This clarification includes the role of the psychologist (such as therapist, organizational consultant, diagnostician, or expert witness), the probable uses of the services provided or the information obtained, and the fact that there may be limits to confidentiality.

(b) If there is a foreseeable risk of the psychologist's being called upon to perform conflicting roles because of the involvement of a third party, the psychologist clarifies the nature and direction of his or her responsibilities, keeps all parties appropriately informed as matters develop, and resolves the situation in accordance with this Ethics Code.

• • •

### 3. Advertising and Other Public Statements

• • •

### 3.03 Avoidance of False or Deceptive Statements

(a) Psychologists do not make public statements that are false, deceptive, misleading, or fraudulent, either because of what they state, convey, or suggest or because of what they omit, concerning their research, practice, or other work activities or those of persons or organizations with which they are affiliated.

• • •

### 4. Therapy

### 4.01 Structuring the Relationship

(a) Psychologists discuss with clients or patients as early as is feasible in the therapeutic relationship appropriate issues, such as the nature and anticipated course of therapy, fees, and confidentiality.

(b) When the psychologist's work with clients or patients will be supervised, the above discussion includes that fact, and the name of the supervisor, when the supervisor has legal responsibility for the case.

(c) When the therapist is a student intern, the client or patient is informed of that fact.

(d) Psychologists make reasonable efforts to answer patients' questions and to avoid apparent misunderstandings about therapy. Whenever possible, psychologists provide oral and/or written information, using language that is reasonably understandable to the patient or client.

### 4.02  Informed Consent to Therapy

(a) Psychologists obtain appropriate informed consent to therapy or related procedures, using language that is reasonably understandable to participants. The content of informed consent will vary depending on many circumstances; however, informed consent generally implies that the person (1) has the capacity to consent, (2) has been informed of significant information concerning the procedure, (3) has freely and without undue influence expressed consent, and (4) consent has been appropriately documented.

(b) When persons are legally incapable of giving informed consent, psychologists obtain informed permission from a legally authorized person, if such substitute consent is permitted by law.

(c) In addition, psychologists (1) inform those persons who are legally incapable of giving informed consent about the proposed interventions in a manner commensurate with the persons' psychological capacities, (2) seek their assent to those interventions, and (3) consider such persons' preferences and best interests.

### 4.03  Couple and Family Relationships

(a) When a psychologist agrees to provide services to several persons who have a relationship (such as husband and wife or parents and children), the psychologist attempts to clarify at the outset (1) which of the individuals are patients or clients and (2) the relationship the psychologist will have with each person. This clarification includes the role of the psychologist and the probable uses of the services provided or the information obtained.

(b) As soon as it becomes apparent that the psychologist may be called on to perform potentially conflicting roles (such as marital counselor to husband and wife, and then witness for one party in a divorce proceeding), the psychologist attempts to clarify and adjust, or withdraw from, roles appropriately.

### 4.04  Providing Mental Health Services to Those Served by Others

In deciding whether to offer or provide services to those already receiving mental health services elsewhere, psychologists carefully consider the treatment issues and the potential patient's or client's welfare. The psychologist discusses these issues with the patient or client, or another legally authorized person on behalf of the client, in order to minimize the risk of confusion and conflict, consults with the other service providers when appropriate, and proceeds with caution and sensitivity to the therapeutic issues.

### 4.05  Sexual Intimacies With Current Patients or Clients

Psychologists do not engage in sexual intimacies with current patients or clients.

### 4.06  Therapy With Former Sexual Partners

Psychologists do not accept as therapy patients or clients persons with whom they have engaged in sexual intimacies.

### 4.07  Sexual Intimacies With Former Therapy Patients

(a) Psychologists do not engage in sexual intimacies with a former therapy patient or client for at least two years after cessation or termination of professional services.

(b) Because sexual intimacies with a former therapy patient or client are so frequently harmful to the patient or client, and because such intimacies undermine public confidence in the psychology profession and thereby deter the public's use of needed services, psychologists do not engage in sexual intimacies with former therapy patients and clients even after a two-year interval except in the most unusual circumstances. The psychologist who engages in such activity after the two years following cessation or termination of treatment bears the burden of demonstrating that there has been no exploitation, in light of all relevant factors, including (1) the amount of time that has passed since therapy terminated, (2) the nature and duration of the therapy, (3) the circumstances of termination, (4) the patient's or client's personal history, (5) the patient's or client's current mental status, (6) the likelihood of adverse impact on the patient or client and others, and (7) any statements or actions made by the therapist during the course of therapy suggesting or inviting the possibility of a posttermination sexual or romantic relationship with the patient or client.

### 4.08  Interruption of Services

(a) Psychologists make reasonable efforts to plan for facilitating care in the event that psychological services are interrupted by factors such as the psychologist's illness, death, unavailability, or relocation or by the client's relocation or financial limitations.

(b) When entering into employment or contractual relationships, psychologists provide for orderly and appropriate resolution of responsibility for patient or client care in the event that the employment or contractual relationship ends, with paramount consideration given to the welfare of the patient or client.

### 4.09  Terminating the Professional Relationship

(a) Psychologists do not abandon patients or clients.

(b) Psychologists terminate a professional relationship when it becomes reasonably clear that the patient or client no longer needs the service, is not benefiting, or is being harmed by continued service.

(c) Prior to termination for whatever reason, except where precluded by the patient's or client's conduct, the psychologist discusses the patient's or client's views and needs, provides appropriate pretermination counseling, suggests alternative service providers as appropriate, and takes other reasonable steps to facilitate transfer of responsibility to another provider if the patient or client needs one immediately.

### 5. Privacy and Confidentiality

These Standards are potentially applicable to the professional and scientific activities of all psychologists.

### 5.01  Discussing the Limits of Confidentiality

(a) Psychologists discuss with persons and organizations with whom they establish a scientific or professional relationship (including, to the extent feasible, minors and their legal representatives) (1) the relevant limitations on confidentiality, including limitations where applicable in group, marital, and family therapy or in organizational consulting, and (2) the foreseeable uses of the information generated throughout their services.

(b) Unless it is not feasible or is contraindicated, the discussion of confidentiality occurs at the outset of the relationship and thereafter as new circumstances may warrant.

(c) Permission for electronic recording of interviews is secured from clients and patients.

### 5.02  Maintaining Confidentiality

Psychologists have a primary obligation and take reasonable precautions to respect the confidentiality rights of those with whom they work or consult, recognizing that confidentiality may be established by law, institutional rules, or professional or scientific relationships.

### 5.03  Minimizing Intrusions on Privacy

(a) In order to minimize intrusions on privacy, psychologists include in written and oral reports, consultations, and the like, only information germane to the purpose for which the communication is made.

(b) Psychologists discuss confidential information obtained in clinical or consulting relationships, or evaluative data concerning patients, individual or organizational clients, students, research participants, supervisees, and employees, only for appropriate scientific or professional purposes and only with persons clearly concerned with such matters.

### 5.04  Maintenance of Records

Psychologists maintain appropriate confidentiality in creating, storing, accessing, transferring, and disposing of records under their control, whether these are written, automated, or in any other medium. Psychologists maintain and dispose of records in accordance with law and in a manner that permits compliance with the requirements of this Ethics Code.

### 5.05  Disclosures

(a) Psychologists disclose confidential information without the consent of the individual only as mandated by law, or where permitted by law for a valid purpose, such as (1) to provide needed professional services to the patient or the individual or organizational client, (2) to obtain appropriate professional consultations, (3) to protect the patient or client or others from harm, or (4) to obtain payment for services, in which instance disclosure is limited to the minimum that is necessary to achieve the purpose.

(b) Psychologists also may disclose confidential information with the appropriate consent of the patient or the individual or organizational client (or of another legally authorized person on behalf of the patient or client), unless prohibited by law.

### 5.06  Consultations

When consulting with colleagues, (1) psychologists do not share confidential information that reasonably could lead to the identification of a patient, client, research participant, or other person or organization with whom they have a confidential relationship unless they have obtained the prior consent of the person or organization or the disclosure cannot be avoided, and (2) they share information only to the extent necessary to achieve the purposes of the consultation. (See also Standard 5.02, Maintaining Confidentiality.)

### 5.07  Confidential Information in Databases

(a) If confidential information concerning recipients of psychological services is to be entered into databases or systems of records available to persons whose access has not been consented to by the recipient, then psychologists use coding or other techniques to avoid the inclusion of personal identifiers.

(b) If a research protocol approved by an institutional review board or similar body requires the inclusion of personal identifiers, such identifiers are deleted before the information is made accessible to persons other than those of whom the subject was advised.

(c) If such deletion is not feasible, then before psychologists transfer such data to others or review such data collected by others, they take reasonable steps to determine that appropriate consent of personally identifiable individuals has been obtained.

### 5.08  Use of Confidential Information for Didactic or Other Purposes

(a) Psychologists do not disclose in their writings, lectures, or other public media, confidential, personally identifiable information concerning their patients, individual or organizational clients, students, research participants, or other recipients of their services that they obtained during the course of their work, unless the person or organization has consented in writing or unless there is other ethical or legal authorization for doing so.

(b) Ordinarily, in such scientific and professional presentations, psychologists disguise confidential information concerning such persons or organizations so that they are not individually identifiable to others and so that discussions do not cause harm to subjects who might identify themselves.

### 5.09  Preserving Records and Data

A psychologist makes plans in advance so that confidentiality of records and data is protected in the event of the psychologist's death, incapacity, or withdrawal from the position or practice.

### 5.10  Ownership of Records and Data

Recognizing that ownership of records and data is governed by legal principles, psychologists take reasonable and lawful steps so that records and data remain available to the extent needed to serve the best interests of patients, individual or organizational clients, research participants, or appropriate others.

### 5.11  Withholding Records for Nonpayment

Psychologists may not withhold records under their control that are requested and imminently needed for a patient's or client's treatment solely because payment has not been received, except as otherwise provided by law.

### 6. Teaching, Training Supervision, Research, and Publishing

• • •

### 6.06  Planning Research

(a) Psychologists design, conduct, and report research in accordance with recognized standards of scientific competence and ethical research.

(b) Psychologists plan their research so as to minimize the possibility that results will be misleading.

(c) In planning research, psychologists consider its ethical acceptability under the Ethics Code. If an ethical issue is unclear, psychologists seek to resolve the issue through consultation with institutional review boards, animal care and use committees, peer consultations, or other proper mechanisms.

(d) Psychologists take reasonable steps to implement appropriate protections for the rights and welfare of human participants, other persons affected by the research, and the welfare of animal subjects.

### 6.07 Responsibility

(a) Psychologists conduct research competently and with due concern for the dignity and welfare of the participants.

(b) Psychologists are responsible for the ethical conduct of research conducted by them or by others under their supervision or control.

(c) Researchers and assistants are permitted to perform only those tasks for which they are appropriately trained and prepared.

(d) As part of the process of development and implementation of research projects, psychologists consult those with expertise concerning any special population under investigation or most likely to be affected.

### 6.08 Compliance With Law and Standards

Psychologists plan and conduct research in a manner consistent with federal and state law and regulations, as well as professional standards governing the conduct of research, and particularly those standards governing research with human participants and animal subjects.

### 6.09 Institutional Approval

Psychologists obtain from host institutions or organizations appropriate approval prior to conducting research, and they provide accurate information about their research proposals. They conduct the research in accordance with the approved research protocol.

### 6.10 Research Responsibilities

Prior to conducting research (except research involving only anonymous surveys, naturalistic observations, or similar research), psychologists enter into an agreement with participants that clarifies the nature of the research and the responsibilities of each party.

### 6.11 Informed Consent to Research

(a) Psychologists use language that is reasonably understandable to research participants in obtaining their appropriate informed consent (except as provided in Standard 6.12, Dispensing With Informed Consent). Such informed consent is appropriately documented.

(b) Using language that is reasonably understandable to participants, psychologists inform participants of the nature of the research; they inform participants that they are free to participate or to decline to participate or to withdraw from the research; they explain the foreseeable consequences of declining or withdrawing; they inform participants of significant factors that may be expected to influence their willingness to participate (such as risks, discomfort, adverse effects, or limitations on confidentiality, except as provided in Standard 6.15, Deception in Research); and they explain other aspects about which the prospective participants inquire.

(c) When psychologists conduct research with individuals such as students or subordinates, psychologists take special care to protect the prospective participants from adverse consequences of declining or withdrawing from participation.

(d) When research participation is a course requirement or opportunity for extra credit, the prospective participant is given the choice of equitable alternative activities.

(e) For persons who are legally incapable of giving informed consent, psychologists nevertheless (1) provide an appropriate explanation, (2) obtain the participant's assent, and (3) obtain appropriate permission from a legally authorized person, if such substitute consent is permitted by law.

### 6.12 Dispensing With Informed Consent

Before determining that planned research (such as research involving only anonymous questionnaires, naturalistic observations, or certain kinds of archival research) does not require the informed consent of research participants, psychologists consider applicable regulations and institutional review board requirements, and they consult with colleagues as appropriate.

### 6.13 Informed Consent in Research Filming or Recording

Psychologists obtain informed consent from research participants prior to filming or recording them in any form, unless the research involves simply naturalistic observations in public places and it is not anticipated that the recording will be used in a manner that could cause personal identification or harm.

### 6.14 Offering Inducements for Research Participants

(a) In offering professional services as an inducement to obtain research participants, psychologists make clear the nature of the services, as well as the risks, obligations, and limitations.

(b) Psychologists do not offer excessive or inappropriate financial or other inducements to obtain research participants, particularly when it might tend to coerce participation.

### 6.15 Deception in Research

(a) Psychologists do not conduct a study involving deception unless they have determined that the use of deceptive techniques is justified by the study's prospective scientific, educational, or applied value and that equally effective alternative procedures that do not use deception are not feasible.

(b) Psychologists never deceive research participants about significant aspects that would affect their willingness to participate, such as physical risks, discomfort, or unpleasant emotional experiences.

(c) Any other deception that is an integral feature of the design and conduct of an experiment must be explained to participants as early as is feasible, preferably at the conclusion of their participation, but no later than at the conclusion of the research. (See also Standard 6.18, Providing Participants With Information About the Study.)

### 6.16 Sharing and Utilizing Data

Psychologists inform research participants of their anticipated sharing or further use of personally identifiable research data and of the possibility of unanticipated future uses.

### 6.17 Minimizing Invasiveness

In conducting research, psychologists interfere with the participants or milieu from which data are collected only in a manner that is warranted by an appropriate research design and that is consistent with psychologists' roles as scientific investigators.

### 6.18 Providing Participants With Information About the Study

(a) Psychologists provide a prompt opportunity for participants to obtain appropriate information about the nature, results, and conclusions of the research, and psychologists attempt to correct any misconceptions that participants may have.

(b) If scientific or humane values justify delaying or withholding this information, psychologists take reasonable measures to reduce the risk of harm.

### 6.19 Honoring Commitments

Psychologists take reasonable measures to honor all commitments they have made to research participants.

### 6.20 Care and Use of Animals in Research

(a) Psychologists who conduct research involving animals treat them humanely.

(b) Psychologists acquire, care for, use, and dispose of animals in compliance with current federal, state, and local laws and regulations, and with professional standards.

(c) Psychologists trained in research methods and experienced in the care of laboratory animals supervise all procedures involving animals and are responsible for ensuring appropriate consideration of their comfort, health, and humane treatment.

(d) Psychologists ensure that all individuals using animals under their supervision have received instruction in research methods and in the care, maintenance, and handling of the species being used, to the extent appropriate to their role.

(e) Responsibilities and activities of individuals assisting in a research project are consistent with their respective competencies.

(f) Psychologists make reasonable efforts to minimize the discomfort, infection, illness, and pain of animal subjects.

(g) A procedure subjecting animals to pain, stress, or privation is used only when an alternative procedure is unavailable and the goal is justified by its prospective scientific, educational, or applied value.

(h) Surgical procedures are performed under appropriate anesthesia; techniques to avoid infection and minimize pain are followed during and after surgery.

(i) When it is appropriate that the animal's life be terminated, it is done rapidly, with an effort to minimize pain, and in accordance with accepted procedures.

### 6.21 Reporting of Results

(a) Psychologists do not fabricate data or falsify results in their publications.

(b) If psychologists discover significant errors in their published data, they take reasonable steps to correct such errors in a correction, retraction, erratum, or other appropriate publication means.

### 6.22 Plagiarism

Psychologists do not present substantial portions or elements of another's work or data as their own, even if the other work or data source is cited occasionally.

### 6.23 Publication Credit

(a) Psychologists take responsibility and credit, including authorship credit, only for work they have actually performed or to which they have contributed.

(b) Principal authorship and other publication credits accurately reflect the relative scientific or professional contributions of the individuals involved, regardless of their relative status. Mere possession of an institutional position, such as Department Chair, does not justify authorship credit. Minor contributions to the research or to the writing for publications are appropriately acknowledged, such as in footnotes or in an introductory statement.

• • •

### 6.24 Duplicate Publication of Data

Psychologists do not publish, as original data, data that have been previously published. This does not preclude republishing data when they are accompanied by proper acknowledgment.

### 6.25 Sharing Data

After research results are published, psychologists do not withhold the data on which their conclusions are based from other competent professionals who seek to verify the substantive claims through reanalysis and who intend to use such data only for that purpose, provided that the confidentiality of the participants can be protected and unless legal rights concerning proprietary data preclude their release.

### 6.26 Professional Reviewers

Psychologists who review material submitted for publication, grant, or other research proposal review respect the confidentiality of and the proprietary rights in such information of those who submitted it.

• • •

### 8. Resolving Ethical Issues

### 8.01 Familiarity With Ethics Code

Psychologists have an obligation to be familiar with this Ethics Code, other applicable ethics codes, and their application to psychologists' work. Lack of awareness or misunderstanding of an ethical standard is not itself a defense to a charge of unethical conduct.

### 8.02 Confronting Ethical Issues

When a psychologist is uncertain whether a particular situation or course of action would violate this Ethics Code, the psychologist ordinarily consults with other psychologists knowledgeable about ethical issues, with state or national psychology ethics committees, or with other appropriate authorities in order to choose a proper response.

### 8.03 Conflicts Between Ethics and Organizational Demands

If the demands of an organization with which psychologists are affiliated conflict with this Ethics Code, psychologists clarify the nature of the conflict, make known their commitment to the Ethics Code, and to the extent feasible, seek to resolve the conflict in a way that permits the fullest adherence to the Ethics Code.

### 8.04 Informal Resolution of Ethical Violations

When psychologists believe that there may have been an ethical violation by another psychologist, they attempt to resolve the issue by bringing it to the attention of that individual if an informal resolution appears appropriate and the intervention does not violate any confidentiality rights that may be involved.

#### 8.05  Reporting Ethical Violations

If an apparent ethical violation is not appropriate for informal resolution under Standard 8.04 or is not resolved properly in that fashion, psychologists take further action appropriate to the situation, unless such action conflicts with confidentiality rights in ways that cannot be resolved. Such action might include referral to state or national committees on professional ethics or to state licensing boards.

• • •

# CODE OF ETHICS
### National Association of Social Workers
1979, revised 1990

*The current Code of Ethics of the National Association of Social Workers (NASW) was adopted by the NASW Delegate Assembly in 1979 and revised in 1990. The preamble states that the code "is based on the fundamental values of the social work profession that include the worth, dignity, and uniqueness of all persons as well as their rights and opportunities." The code "does not represent a set of rules that will prescribe all the behaviors of social workers. . . [r]ather, it offers general principles to guide conduct, and the judicious appraisal of conduct, in situations that have ethical implications."*

*Elements of particular interest for their uniqueness include directives for the social worker relative to discriminatory or other practices of employing organizations, and directives toward improving social conditions and promoting justice in society.*

## I.  The Social Worker's Conduct and Comportment as a Social Worker

**A.** Propriety—The Social worker should maintain high standards of personal conduct in the capacity or identity as social worker.
  1. The private conduct of the social worker is a personal matter to the same degree as is any other person's, except when such conduct compromises the fulfillment of professional responsibilities.
  2. The social worker should not participate in, condone, or be associated with dishonesty, fraud, deceit, or misrepresentation.
  3. The social worker should distinguish clearly between statements and actions made as a private individual and as a representative of the social work profession or an organization or group.
**B.** Competence and Professional Development—The social worker should strive to become and remain proficient in professional practice and the performance of professional functions.
  1. The social worker should accept responsibility or employment only on the basis of existing competence or the intention to acquire the necessary competence.
  2. The social worker should not misrepresent professional qualifications, education, experience, or affiliations.
**C.** Service—The social worker should regard as primary the service obligation of the social work profession.
  1. The social worker should retain ultimate responsibility for the quality and extent of the service that individual assumes, assigns, or performs.
  2. The social worker should act to prevent practices that are inhumane or discriminatory against any person or group of persons.
**D.** Integrity—The social worker should act in accordance with the highest standards of professional integrity and impartiality.
  1. The social worker should be alert to and resist the influences and pressures that interfere with the exercise of professional discretion and impartial judgement required for the performance of professional functions.
  2. The social worker should not exploit professional relationships for personal gain.
**E.** Scholarship and Research—The social worker engaged in study and research should be guided by the conventions of scholarly inquiry.
  1. The social worker engaged in research should consider carefully its possible consequences for human beings.
  2. The social worker engaged in research should ascertain that the consent of participants in the research is voluntary and informed, without any implied deprivation or penalty for refusal to participate, and with due regard for participants' privacy and dignity.

3. The social worker engaged in research should protect participants from unwarranted physical or mental discomfort, distress, harm, danger, or deprivation.
4. The social worker who engages in the evaluation of services or cases should discuss them only for the professional purposes and only with persons directly and professionally concerned with them.
5. Information obtained about participants in research should be treated as confidential.
6. The social worker should take credit only for work actually done in connection with scholarly and research endeavors and credit contributions made by others.

## II. The Social Worker's Ethical Responsibility to Clients

F. Primacy of Clients' Interests—The social worker's primary responsibility is to clients.
   1. The social worker should serve clients with devotion, loyalty, determination, and the maximum application of professional skill and competence.
   2. The social worker should not exploit relationships with clients for personal advantage.
   3. The social worker should not practice, condone, facilitate or collaborate with any form of discrimination on the basis of race, color, sex, sexual orientation, age, religion, national origin, marital status, political belief, mental or physical handicap, or any other preference or personal characteristic, condition or status.
   4. The social worker should avoid relationships or commitments that conflict with the interests of clients.
   5. The social worker should under no circumstances engage in sexual activities with clients.
   6. The social worker should provide clients with accurate and complete information regarding the extent and nature of the services available to them.
   7. The social worker should apprise clients of their risks, rights, opportunities, and obligations associated with social service to them.
   8. The social worker should seek advice and counsel of colleagues and supervisors whenever such consultation is in the best interest of clients.
   9. The social worker should terminate service to clients, and professional relationships with them, when such service and relationships are no longer required or no longer serve the clients' needs or interests.
   10. The social worker should withdraw services precipitously only under unusual circumstances, giving careful consideration to all factors in the situation and taking care to minimize possible adverse effects.
   11. The social worker who anticipates the termination or interruption of service to clients should notify clients promptly and seek the transfer, referral, or continuation of service in relation to the clients' needs and preferences.
G. Rights and Prerogatives of Clients—The social worker should make every effort to foster maximum self-determination on the part of clients.
   1. When the social worker must act on behalf of a client who has been adjudged legally incompetent, the social worker should safeguard the interests and rights of that client.
   2. When another individual has been legally authorized to act in behalf of a client, the social worker should deal with that person always with the client's best interest in mind.
   3. The social worker should not engage in any action that violates or diminishes the civil or legal rights of clients.
H. Confidentiality and Privacy—The social worker should respect the privacy of clients and hold in confidence all information obtained in the course of professional service.
   1. The social worker should share with others confidences revealed by clients, without their consent, only for compelling professional reasons.
   2. The social worker should inform clients fully about the limits of confidentiality in a given situation, the purposes for which information is obtained, and how it may be used.
   3. The social worker should afford clients reasonable access to any official social work records concerning them.
   4. When providing clients with access to records, the social worker should take due care to protect the confidences of others contained in those records.
   5. The social worker should obtain informed consent of clients before taping, recording, or permitting third party observation of their activities.
I. Fees—When setting fees, the social worker should ensure that they are fair, reasonable, considerate, and commensurate with the service performed and with due regard for the clients' ability to pay.
   1. The social worker should not accept anything of value for making a referral.

### III. The Social Worker's Ethical Responsibility to Colleagues

**J.** Respect, Fairness, and Courtesy—The social worker should treat colleagues with respect, courtesy, fairness, and good faith.

1. The social worker should cooperate with colleagues to promote professional interests and concerns.
2. The social worker should respect confidences shared by colleagues in the course of their professional relationships and transactions.
3. The social worker should create and maintain conditions of practice that facilitate ethical and competent professional performance by colleagues.
4. The social worker should treat with respect, and represent accurately and fairly, the qualifications, views, and findings of colleagues and use appropriate channels to express judgements on these matters.
5. The social worker who replaces or is replaced by a colleague in professional practice should act with consideration for the interest, character, and reputation of that colleague.
6. The social worker should not exploit a dispute between a colleague and employers to obtain a position or otherwise advance the social worker's interest.
7. The social worker should seek arbitration or mediation when conflicts with colleagues require resolution for compelling professional reasons.
8. The social worker should extend to colleagues of other professions the same respect and cooperation that is extended to social work colleagues.
9. The social worker who serves as an employer, supervisor, or mentor to colleagues should make orderly and explicit arrangements regarding the conditions of their continuing professional relationship.
10. The social worker who has the responsibility for employing and evaluating the performance of other staff members, should fulfill such responsibility in a fair, considerate, and equitable manner, on the basis of clearly enunciated criteria.
11. The social worker who has the responsibility for evaluating the performance of employees, supervisees, or students should share evaluations with them.

**K.** Dealing with Colleagues' Clients—The social worker has the responsibility to relate to the clients of colleagues with full professional consideration.

1. The social worker should not assume professional responsibility for the clients of another agency or a colleague without appropriate communication with that agency or colleague.
2. The social worker who serves the clients of colleagues, during a temporary absence or emergency, should serve those clients with the same consideration as that afforded any client.

### IV. The Social Worker's Ethical Responsibility to Employers and Employing Organizations

**L.** Commitments to Employing Organization—The social worker should adhere to commitments made to the employing organization.

1. The social worker should work to improve the employing agency's policies and procedures, and the efficiency and effectiveness of its services.
2. The social worker should not accept employment or arrange student field placements in an organization which is currently under public sanction by NASW for violating personnel standards, or imposing limitations on or penalties for professional actions on behalf of clients.
3. The social worker should act to prevent and eliminate discrimination in the employing organization's work assignments and in its employment policies and practices.
4. The social worker should use with scrupulous regard, and only for the purpose for which they are intended, the resources of the employing organization.

### V. The Social Worker's Ethical Responsibility to the Social Work Profession

**M.** Maintaining the Integrity of the Profession—The social worker should uphold and advance the values, ethics, knowledge, and mission of the profession.

1. The social worker should protect and enhance the dignity and integrity of the profession and should be responsible and vigorous in discussion and criticism of the profession.
2. The social worker should take action through appropriate channels against unethical conduct by any other member of the profession.
3. The social worker should act to prevent the unauthorized and unqualified practice of social work.
4. The social worker should make no misrepresentation in advertising as to qualifications, competence, service, or results to be achieved.

N. Community Service—The social worker should assist the profession in making social services available to the general public.
1. The social worker should contribute time and professional expertise to activities that promote respect for the utility, the integrity, and the competence of the social work profession.
2. The social worker should support the formulation, development, enactment and implementation of social policies of concern to the profession.
O. Development of Knowledge—The social worker should take responsibility for identifying, developing, and fully utilizing knowledge for professional practice.
1. The social worker should base practice upon recognized knowledge relevant to social work.
2. The social worker should critically examine, and keep current with emerging knowledge relevant to social work.
3. The social worker should contribute to the knowledge base of social work and share research knowledge and practice wisdom with colleagues.

## VI. The Social Worker's Ethical Responsibility to Society

P. Promoting the General Welfare—The social worker should promote the general welfare of society.
1. The social worker should act to prevent and eliminate discrimination against any person or group on the basis of race, color, sex, sexual orientation, age, religion, national origin, marital status, political belief, mental or physical handicap, or any other preference or personal characteristic, condition, or status.
2. The social worker should act to ensure that all persons have access to the resources, services, and opportunities which they require.
3. The social worker should act to expand choice and opportunity for all persons, with special regard for disadvantaged or oppressed groups and persons.
4. The social worker should promote conditions that encourage respect for the diversity of cultures which constitute American society.
5. The social worker should provide appropriate professional services in public emergencies.
6. The social worker should advocate changes in policy and legislation to improve social conditions and to promote social justice.
7. The social worker should encourage informed participation by the public in shaping social policies and institutions.

# CODE OF ETHICS
## American College of Healthcare Executives
amended 1990

*The American College of Healthcare Executives' Code of Ethics sets standards for the ethical behavior of health-care executives both in their professional relationships and in their personal behavior, particularly when it relates to their professional role and identity. Of particular note are statements about assuring "all people . . . reasonable access to healthcare services" and establishing "a resource allocation process that considers ethical ramifications," as well as a section addressing conflicts of interest.*

• • •

## Preamble

• • •

The fundamental objectives of the healthcare management profession are to enhance overall quality of life, dignity and well-being of every individual needing healthcare services; and to create a more equitable, accessible, effective and efficient healthcare system.

Healthcare executives have an obligation to act in ways that will merit the trust, confidence and respect of healthcare professionals and the general public. To do so, healthcare executives must lead lives that embody an exemplary system of values and ethics.

In fulfilling their commitments and obligations to patients, clients or others they serve, healthcare executives function as moral agents. Since every management decision affects the health and well-being of both individuals and communities, healthcare executives must evaluate the possible outcomes of their decisions and accept full responsibility for the consequences. In organizations that deliver healthcare services, they must safeguard and foster the rights, interests and prerogatives of patients, clients or others served. The role of moral agent requires that healthcare executives speak out and take actions necessary to promote such rights, interests and prerogatives if they are threatened.

## I. The Healthcare Executive's Responsibilities to the Profession of Healthcare Management

The healthcare executive shall:

A. Uphold the values, ethics and mission of the healthcare management profession;
B. Conduct all personal and professional activities with honesty, integrity, respect, fairness and good faith in a manner that will reflect well upon the profession;
C. Comply with all laws in the jurisdictions in which the healthcare executive is located, or conducts professional or personal activities;
D. Maintain competence and proficiency in healthcare management by implementing a personal program of assessment and continuing professional education;
E. Avoid the exploitation of professional relationships for personal gain;
F. Use this code to further the interests of the profession and not for selfish reasons;
G. Respect professional confidences;
H. Enhance the dignity and image of the healthcare management profession through positive public information programs;
I. Refrain from participating in any endorsement or publicity that demeans the credibility and dignity of the healthcare management profession; and
J. Refrain from using the College's credential or affiliation with the College to promote or endorse external commercial products or services.

## II. The Healthcare Executive's Obligations to the Organization and to Patients, Clients or Others Served

### A. Commitments to the Organization

The healthcare executive shall:

1. Provide healthcare services consistent with available resources and assure the existence of a resource allocation process that considers ethical ramifications;
2. Conduct both competitive and cooperative activities in ways that improve community healthcare services;
3. Lead the organization in the use and improvement of standards of management and sound business practices;
4. Respect the customs and practices of patients, clients or others served, consistent with the organization's philosophy; and
5. Be truthful in all forms of professional and organizational communication and avoid information that is false, misleading, and deceptive or information that would create unreasonable expectations.

### B. Commitments to Patients, Clients or Others Served

The healthcare executive shall:

1. Assure the existence of a process to evaluate the quality of care or service rendered;
2. Avoid exploitation of relationships for personal advantage;
3. Avoid practicing or facilitating discrimination and institute safeguards to prevent discriminatory organizational practices;
4. Assure the existence of a process that will advise patients, clients or others served of the rights, opportunities, responsibilities and risks regarding available healthcare services;
5. Provide a process which assures the autonomy and self-determination of patients, clients or others served; and
6. Assure the existence of procedures that will safeguard the confidentiality and privacy of patients, clients and others served.

### C. Conflicts of Interest

A conflict of interest may be only a matter of degree, but exists when the healthcare executive:

• Is in a position to benefit directly or indirectly by using authority or inside information, or allows a friend, relative or associate to benefit from such authority or information.
• Uses authority or information to make a decision to intentionally affect the organization in an adverse manner.

The healthcare executive shall:

1. Conduct all personal and professional relationships in such a way that all those affected are assured that management decisions are made in the best interests of the organization and the individuals served by it;
2. Disclose to the appropriate authority any direct or indirect financial or personal interests that might pose potential conflicts of interest;
3. Accept no gifts or benefits offered with the expectation of influencing a management decision; and
4. Inform the appropriate authority and other involved parties of potential conflicts of interest related to appointments or elections to boards or committees inside or outside the healthcare executive's organization.

### III. The Healthcare Executive's Responsibilities to Community and Society

The healthcare executive shall:
A. Work to identify and meet the healthcare needs of the community;
B. Work to assure that all people have reasonable access to healthcare services;
C. Participate in public dialogue on healthcare policy issues and advocate solutions that will improve health status and promote quality healthcare;
D. Consider the short-term and long-term impact of management decisions on both the community and on society; and
E. Provide prospective consumers with adequate and accurate information, enabling them to make enlightened judgments and decisions regarding services.

### IV. The Healthcare Executive's Duty to Report Violations of the Code

An affiliate of the College who has reasonable grounds to believe that another affiliate has violated this Code has a duty to communicate such facts to the Committee on Ethics.

# ETHICAL CONDUCT FOR HEALTH CARE INSTITUTIONS
### American Hospital Association
### 1992

*In 1973, the American Hospital Association (AHA) developed its Guidelines on Ethical Conduct and Relationships for Health Care Institutions, the precursor to the present document, as a complement to the preceding code of ethics for health-care executives. This AHA code of ethics for health-care institutions, which addresses the major areas affecting their ethical conduct, is different because it is written for institutions, that is, their "mission, programs, and services," rather than for people.*

*Points of interest include (1) responsibility for "fair and effective use" of available resources and helping to resolve the problem of providing care to medically indigent individuals; (2) respect for the spiritual needs and cultural beliefs of patients and families; (3) accommodation, to the extent possible, of "the desire of employees and medical staff to embody religious and/or moral values in their professional activities"; and (4) sensitivity to "institutional decisions that employees might interpret as compromising their ability to provide high-quality health care."*

## Introduction

Health care institutions, by virtue of their roles as health care providers, employers, and community health resources, have special responsibilities for ethical conduct and ethical practices that go beyond meeting minimum legal and regulatory standards. Their broad range of patient care, education, public health, social service, and business functions is essential to the health and well being of their communities. These roles and functions demand that health care organizations conduct themselves in an ethical manner that emphasizes a basic community service orientation and justifies the public trust. The health care institution's mission and values should be embodied in all its programs, services, and activities.

Because health care organizations must frequently seek a balance among the interests and values of individuals, the institution, and society, they often face ethical dilemmas in meeting the needs of their patients and their communities. This advisory is intended to assist members of the American Hospital Association to better identify and understand the ethical aspects and implications of institutional policies and practices. It is offered with the understanding that each institution's leadership in making policy and decisions must take into account the needs and values of the institution, its physicians, other caregivers, and employees and those of individual patients, their families, and the community as a whole.

$\bullet$ $\bullet$ $\bullet$

## Community Role

- Health care institutions should be concerned with the overall health status of their communities while continuing to provide direct patient services. They should take a leadership role in enhancing public health and continuity of care in the community by communicating and working with other health care and social agencies to improve the availability and provision of health promotion, education, and patient care services.
- Health care institutions are responsible for fair and effective use of available health care delivery resources to promote access to comprehensive and affordable health care services of high quality. This responsibility extends beyond the resources of the given institution to include efforts to coordinate with other health care organizations and professionals and to share in community solutions for providing care for the medically indigent and others in need of specific health services.
- All health care institutions are responsible for meeting community service obligations which may include special initiatives for care for the poor and uninsured, provision of needed medical or social services, education, and various programs designed to meet the specific needs of their communities.
- Health care institutions, being dependent upon community confidence and support, are accountable to the public, and therefore their communications and disclosure of information and data related to the institution should be clear, accurate, and sufficiently complete to assure that it is not misleading. Such disclosure should be aimed primarily at better public understanding of health issues, the services available to prevent and treat illness, and patient rights and responsibilities relating to health care decisions.
- Advertising may be used to advance the health care organization's goals and objectives and should, in all cases, support the mission of the health care organization. Advertising may be used to educate the public, to report to the community, to increase awareness of available services, to increase support for the organization, and to recruit employees. Health care advertising should be truthful, fair, accurate, complete, and sensitive to the health care needs of the public. False or misleading statements, or statements that might lead the uninformed to draw false conclusions about the health care facility, its competitors, or other health care providers are unacceptable and unethical.
- As health care institutions operate in an increasingly challenging environment, they should consider the overall welfare of their communities and their own missions in determining their activities, service mixes, and business. Health care organizations should be particularly sensitive to potential conflicts of interests involving individuals or groups associated with the medical staff, governing board, or executive management. Examples of such conflicts include ownership or other financial interests in competing provider organizations or groups contracting with the health care institution.

## Patient Care

- Health care institutions are responsible for providing each patient with care that is both appropriate and necessary for the patient's condition. Development and maintenance of organized programs for utilization review and quality improvement and of procedures to verify the credentials of physicians and other health professionals are basic to this obligation.
- Health care institutions in conjunction with attending physicians are responsible for assuring reasonable continuity of care and for informing patients of patient care alternatives when acute care is no longer needed.
- Health care institutions should ensure that the health care professionals and organizations with which they are formally or informally affiliated have appropriate credentials and/or accreditation and participate in organized programs to assess and assure continuous improvement in quality of care.
- Health care institutions should have policies and practices that assure that patient transfers are medically appropriate and legally permissible. Health care institutions should inform patients of the need for and alternatives to such transfers.
- Health care institutions should have policies and practices that support informed consent for diagnostic and therapeutic procedures and use of advance directives. Policies and practices must respect and promote the patient's responsibility for decision making.

- Health care institutions are responsible for assuring confidentiality of patient-specific information. They are responsible for providing safeguards to prevent unauthorized release of information and establishing procedures for authorizing release of data.
- Health care institutions should assure that the psychological, social, spiritual, and physical needs and cultural beliefs and practices of patients and families are respected and should promote employee and medical staff sensitivity to the full range of such needs and practices. The religious and social beliefs and customs of patients should be accommodated whenever possible.
- Health care institutions should have specific mechanisms or procedures to resolve conflicting values and ethical dilemmas as well as complaints and disputes among patients/their families, medical staff, employees, the institution, and the community.

## Organizational Conduct

- The policies and practices of health care institutions should respect and support the professional ethical codes and responsibilities of their employees and medical staff members and be sensitive to institutional decisions that employees might interpret as compromising their ability to provide high-quality health care.
- Health care institutions should provide for fair and equitably-administered employee compensation, benefits, and other policies and practices.
- To the extent possible and consistent with the ethical commitments of the institution, health care institutions should accommodate the desires of employees and medical staff to embody religious and/or moral values in their professional activities.
- Health care institutions should have written policies on conflict of interest that apply to officers, governing board members, and medical staff, as well as others who may make or influence decisions for or on behalf of the institution, including contract employees. Particular attention should be given to potential conflicts related to referral sources, vendors, competing health care services, and investments. These policies should recognize that individuals in decision-making or administrative positions often have duality of interests that may not always present conflicts. But they should provide mechanisms for identifying and addressing dualities when they do exist.
- Health care institutions should communicate their mission, values, and priorities to their employees and volunteers, whose patient care and service activities are the most visible embodiment of the institution's ethical commitments and values.

• • •

# SECTION IV
## Ethical Directives for Human Research

German Guidelines on Human Experimentation [1931]

Nuremberg Code [1947]

Principles for Those in Research and Experimentation, World Medical
Association [1954]

Article Seven, International Covenant on Civil and Political Rights, General
Assembly of the United Nations [1958]

Declaration of Helsinki, World Medical Association [1964, revised 1975,
1983, 1989]

The Belmont Report: Ethical Principles and Guidelines for the Protection of
Human Subjects of Research, National Commission for the Protection of
Human Subjects of Biomedical and Behavioral Research [1979]

DHHS Regulations for the Protection of Human Subjects (45 CFR 46) [June
18, 1991]

Summary Report of the International Summit Conference on Bioethics [1987]

Recommendation No. R (90) 3 of the Committee of Ministers to Member
States Concerning Medical Research on Human Beings, Council of
Europe [1990]

International Ethical Guidelines for Biomedical Research Involving Human
Subjects, Council for International Organizations of Medical Sciences
(CIOMS) in collaboration with the World Health Organization [1993]

*Directives pertaining to the ethics of research on human subjects generally fall into two categories: (1) national or international policies and/or laws and (2) policies of professional groups, e.g., medicine, nursing, epidemiology, and psychology. In addition, directives may pertain either to research in general or to specific types of research. For example, the U.S. Food and Drug Administration (FDA), the Recombinant DNA Advisory Committee of the National Institutes of Health, and the Medical Research Council of Canada all have guidelines governing gene therapy, investigational drugs, or reproductive technologies; and the Ethics Committee of the American Fertility Society has issued a comprehensive document, "Ethical Considerations of the New Reproductive Technologies."*

*Due to space limitations, research directives issued by professional associations and those pertaining to specific areas of research are not printed in this section; but a selection of such documents are listed in the bibliography to the Appendix. In addition, some of the professional codes included in other sections contain guidelines on research.*

*The documents in this section are organized chronologically except for the 1991 United States DHHS regulations, which follow The Belmont Report because of the two documents' interdependence.*

# GERMAN GUIDELINES ON HUMAN EXPERIMENTATION
## 1931

*The following guidelines for therapeutic and scientific research on human subjects, which are thought to be the first of their kind, were published originally as a Circular of the Reich Minister of the Interior dated February 28, 1931. The guidelines remained in force until 1945, but were not included in the Reich legislation validated at the end of World War II. It is interesting to note the disjunction between the guidelines and the practice of the Nazi researchers.*

1. In order that medical science may continue to advance, the initiation in appropriate cases of therapy involving new and as yet insufficiently tested means and procedures cannot be avoided. Similarly, scientific experimentation involving human subjects cannot be completely excluded as such, as this would hinder or even prevent progress in the diagnosis, treatment, and prevention of diseases.

The freedom to be granted to the physician accordingly shall be weighed against his special duty to remain aware at all times of his major responsibility for the life and health of any person on whom he undertakes innovative therapy or performs an experiment.

2. For the purposes of these Guidelines, "innovative therapy" means interventions and treatment methods that involve humans and serve a therapeutic purpose, in other words that are carried out in a particular, individual case in order to diagnose, treat, or prevent a disease or suffering or to eliminate a physical defect, although their effects and consequences cannot be sufficiently evaluated on the basis of existing experience.

3. For the purposes of these Guidelines, "scientific experimentation" means interventions and treatment methods that involve humans and are undertaken for research purposes without serving a therapeutic purpose in an individual case, and whose effects and consequences cannot be sufficiently evaluated on the basis of existing experience.

4. Any innovative therapy must be justified and performed in accordance with the principles of medical ethics and the rules of medical practice and theory.

In all cases, the question of whether any adverse effects which may occur are proportionate to the anticipated benefits shall be examined and assessed.

Innovative therapy may be carried out only it if has been tested in advance in animal trials (where these are possible).

5. Innovative therapy may be carried out only after the subject or his legal representative has unambiguously consented to the procedure in the light of relevant information provided in advance.

Where consent is refused, innovative therapy may be initiated only if it constitutes an urgent procedure to preserve life or prevent serious damage to health and prior consent could not be obtained under the circumstances.

6. The question of whether to use innovative therapy must be examined with particular care where the subject is a child or a person under 18 years of age.

7. Exploitation of social hardship in order to undertake innovative therapy is incompatible with the principles of medical ethics.

8. Extreme caution shall be exercised in connexion with innovative therapy involving live microorganisms, especially live pathogens. Such therapy shall be considered permissible only if the procedure can be assumed to be relatively safe and similar benefits are unlikely to be achieved under the circumstances by any other method.

9. In clinics, policlinics, hospitals, or other treatment and care establishments, innovative therapy may be carried out only by the physician in charge or by another physician acting in accordance with his express instructions and subject to his complete responsibility.

10. A report shall be made in respect of any innovative therapy, indicating the purpose of the procedure, the justification for it, and the manner in which it is carried out. In particular, the report shall include a statement that the subject or, where appropriate, his legal representative has been provided in advance with relevant information and has given his consent.

Where therapy has been carried out without consent, under the conditions referred to in the second paragraph of Section 5, the statement shall give full details of these conditions.

11. The results of any innovative therapy may be published only in a manner whereby the patient's dignity and the dictates of humanity are fully respected.

12. Sections 4–11 of these Guidelines shall be applicable, *mutatis mutandis*, to scientific experimentation (cf. Section 3).

The following additional requirements shall apply to such experimentation:

(*a*) experimentation shall be prohibited in all cases where consent has not been given;

(*b*) experimentation involving human subjects shall be avoided if it can be replaced by animal studies. Experimentation involving human subjects may be carried out only after all data that can be collected by means of those biological methods (laboratory testing and animal studies) that are available to medical science for purposes of clarification and confirmation of the validity of the experiment have been obtained. Under these circumstances, motiveless and unplanned experimentation involving human subjects shall obviously be prohibited;

(*c*) experimentation involving children or young persons under 18 years of age shall be prohibited if it in any way endangers the child or young person;

(*d*) experimentation involving dying subjects is incompatible with the principles of medical ethics and shall therefore be prohibited.

13. While physicians and, more particularly, those in charge of hospital establishments may thus be expected to be guided by a strong sense of responsibility towards their patients, they should at the same time not be denied the satisfying responsibility (verantwortungsfreudigkeit) of seeking new ways to protect or treat patients or alleviate or remedy their suffering where they are convinced, in the light of their medical experience, that known methods are likely to fail.

14. Academic training courses should take every suitable opportunity to stress the physician's special duties when carrying out a new form of therapy or a scientific experiment as well as when publishing his results.

# NUREMBERG CODE
## 1947

*The Nuremberg Military Tribunal's decision in the case of the* United States *v.* Karl Brandt *et al. includes what is now called the Nuremberg Code, a ten-point statement delimiting permissible medical experimentation on human subjects. According to this statement, human experimentation is justified only if its results benefit society and it is carried out in accord with basic principles that "satisfy moral, ethical, and legal concepts."*

1. The voluntary consent of the human subject is absolutely essential.

This means that the person involved should have legal capacity to give consent; should be so situated as to be able to exercise free power of choice, without the intervention of any element of force, fraud, deceit, duress, over-reaching, or other ulterior form of constraint or coercion; and should have sufficient knowledge and comprehension of the elements of the subject matter involved as to enable him to make an understanding and enlightened decision. This latter element requires that before the acceptance of an affirmative decision by the experimental subject there should be made known to him the nature, duration, and purpose of the experiment; the method and means by which it is to be conducted; all inconveniences and hazards reasonably to be expected; and the effects upon his health or person which may possibly come from his participation in the experiment.

The duty and responsibility for ascertaining the quality of the consent rests upon each individual who initiates, directs or engages in the experiment. It is a personal duty and responsibility which may not be delegated to another with impunity.

2. The experiment should be such as to yield fruitful results for the good of society, unprocurable by other methods or means of study, and not random and unnecessary in nature.

3. The experiment should be so designed and based on the results of animal experimentation and a knowledge of the natural history of the disease or other problem under study that the anticipated results will justify the performance of the experiment.

4. The experiment should be so conducted as to avoid all unnecessary physical and mental suffering and injury.

5. No experiment should be conducted where there is an *a priori* reason to believe that death or disabling injury will occur; except, perhaps, in those experiments where the experimental physicians also serve as subjects.

6. The degree of risk to be taken should never exceed that determined by the humanitarian importance of the problem to be solved by the experiment.

7. Proper preparations should be made and adequate facilities provided to protect the experimental subject against even remote possibilities of injury, disability, or death.

8. The experiment should be conducted only by scientifically qualified persons. The highest degree of skill and care should be required through all stages of the experiment of those who conduct or engage in the experiment.

9. During the course of the experiment the human subject should be at liberty to bring the experiment to an end if he has reached the physical or mental state where continuation of the experiment seems to him to be impossible.

10. During the course of the experiment the scientist in charge must be prepared to terminate the experiment at any stage, if he has probable cause to believe, in the exercise of the good faith, superior skill and careful judgment required of him that a continuation of the experiment is likely to result in injury, disability, or death to the experimental subject.

## PRINCIPLES FOR THOSE IN RESEARCH AND EXPERIMENTATION
### World Medical Association
### 1954

*Formulated by the Committee on Medical Ethics and adopted by the Eighth General Assembly of the World Medical Association (WMA), this document is the first set of guidelines governing research issued by the WMA and is the historical predecessor of the Declaration of Helsinki.*

1. Scientific and Moral Aspects of Experimentation
The word experimentation applies not only to experimentation itself but also to the experimenter. An individual cannot and should not attempt any kind of experimentation. Scientific qualities are indisputable and must always be respected. Likewise, there must be strict adherence to the general rules of respect of the individual.

2. Prudence and Discretion in the Publication of the First Results of Experimentation
This principle applies primarily to the medical press and we are proud to note that in the majority of cases this rule has been adhered to by the editors of our journals. Then there is the general press which does not in every instance have the same rules of prudence and discretion as the medical press. The World Medical Association draws attention to the detrimental effects of premature or unjustified statements. In the interest of the public, each national association should consider methods of avoiding this danger.

3. Experimentation on Healthy Subjects
Every step must be taken in order to make sure that those who submit themselves to experimentation be fully informed. The paramount factor in experimentation on human beings is the responsibility of the research worker and not the willingness of the person submitting to the experiment.

4. Experimentation on Sick Subjects
Here it may be that in the presence of individual and desperate cases one may attempt an operation or a treatment of a rather daring nature. Such exceptions will be rare and require the approval either of the person or his next of kin. In such a situation it is the doctor's conscience which will make the decision.

5. Necessity of Informing the Person Who Submits to Experimentation of the Nature of the Experimentation, the Reasons for the Experiment, and the Risks Involved
It should be required that each person who submits to experimentation be informed of the nature of, the reason for, and the risk of the proposed experiment. If the patient is irresponsible, consent should be obtained from the individual who is legally responsible for the individual. In both instances, consent should be obtained in writing.

# ARTICLE SEVEN, INTERNATIONAL COVENANT ON CIVIL AND POLITICAL RIGHTS
### General Assembly of the United Nations
### 1958

*Prepared by the Commission on Human Rights, the draft Covenant on Civil and Political Rights was first considered by the Third (Social, Humanitarian, and Cultural) Committee of the General Assembly of the United Nations in 1954. Article Seven of the draft covenant was adopted in 1958. Discussion of the article focused primarily on the second sentence. Some members argued that emphasis on one type of cruel and inhuman treatment weakened the article. However, it was generally agreed that that sentence was directed against criminal experimentation, such as that conducted by Nazi physician-researchers, and should be retained. The difficulty lay in prohibiting criminal experimentation without hindering legitimate research.*

*The committee entertained many amendments. Two notable discussions involved the "free consent" requirement and the phrase ". . . involving risk, where such is not required by his state of physical or mental health," which appeared at the end of the second sentence in the original draft. The committee ultimately retained the "free consent" requirement as an important criterion for determining when experimentation amounted to "cruel, inhuman, or degrading treatment." The committee also deleted the final phrase on the grounds that the term "experimentation" did not cover medical treatment that was required in the interest of an individual's health, and inclusion of the phrase would confuse the meaning of the provision by implying that scientific or medical practices directed toward an individual's welfare came within the scope of the article.*

*Article 7.*
No one shall be subjected to torture or to cruel, inhuman or degrading treatment or punishment. In particular, no one shall be subjected without his free consent to medical or scientific experimentation.

# DECLARATION OF HELSINKI
### World Medical Association
### 1964, revised 1975, 1983, 1989

*The Declaration of Helsinki, which offers recommendations for conducting experiments using human subjects, was adopted in 1962 and revised by the 18th World Medical Assembly at Helsinki, Finland, in 1964. Subsequent revisions were approved in Tokyo (1975), Venice (1983), and Hong Kong (1989). The 1989 version is reprinted below; the citations for earlier versions appear in the bibliography.*

*The only significant changes between the 1975 revision, which was the most extensive, and the 1989 version are the addition in 1983 of the requirement that, whenever possible, the consent of a minor child "must be obtained in addition to the consent of the minor's legal guardian" (I. 11) and the 1989 specification that the "specially appointed [independent] committee" (I. 2) be "independent of the investigator and the sponsor" and "in conformity with the laws and regulations of the country in which the research experiment is performed."*

## Introduction

It is the mission of the physician to safeguard the health of the people. His or her knowledge and conscience are dedicated to the fulfillment of this mission.

The Declaration of Geneva of the World Medical Association binds the physician with the words, "The health of my patient will be my first consideration," and the International Code of Medical Ethics declares that, "A physician shall act only in the patient's interest when providing medical care which might have the effect of weakening the physical and mental condition of the patient."

The purpose of biomedical research involving human subjects must be to improve diagnostic, therapeutic and prophylactic procedures and the understanding of the aetiology and pathogenesis of disease.

In current medical practice most diagnostic, therapeutic or prophylactic procedures involve hazards. This applies especially to biomedical research.

Medical progress is based on research which ultimately must rest in part on experimentation involving human subjects.

In the field of biomedical research a fundamental distinction must be recognized between medical research in which the aim is essentially diagnostic or therapeutic for a patient, and medical research, the essential object of which is purely scientific and without implying direct diagnostic or therapeutic value to the person subjected to the research.

Special caution must be exercised in the conduct of research which may affect the environment, and the welfare of animals used for research must be respected.

Because it is essential that the results of laboratory experiments be applied to human beings to further scientific knowledge and to help suffering humanity, the World Medical Association has prepared the following recommendations as a guide to every physician in biomedical research involving human subjects. They should be kept under review in the future. It must be stressed that the standards as drafted are only a guide to physicians all over the world. Physicians are not relieved from criminal, civil and ethical responsibilities under the laws of their own countries.

## I. Basic Principles

1. Biomedical research involving human subjects must conform to generally accepted scientific principles and should be based on adequately performed laboratory and animal experimentation and a thorough knowledge of the scientific literature.

2. The design and performance of each experimental procedure involving human subjects should be clearly formulated in an experimental protocol which should be transmitted for consideration, comment and guidance to a specially appointed committee independent of the investigator and the sponsor, provided that this independent committee is in conformity with the laws and regulations of the country in which the research experiment is performed.

3. Biomedical research involving human subjects should be conducted only by scientifically qualified persons and under the supervision of a clinically competent medical person. The responsibility for the human subject must always rest with a medically qualified person and never rest on the subject of the research, even though the subject has given his or her consent.

4. Biomedical research involving human subjects cannot legitimately be carried out unless the importance of the objective is in proportion to the inherent risk to the subject.

5. Every biomedical research project involving human subjects should be preceded by careful assessment of predictable risks in comparison with foreseeable benefits to the subject or to others. Concern for the interests of the subject must always prevail over the interests of science and society.

6. The right of the research subject to safeguard his or her integrity must always be respected. Every precaution should be taken to respect the privacy of the subject and to minimize the impact of the study on the subject's physical and mental integrity and on the personality of the subject.

7. Physicians should abstain from engaging in research projects involving human subjects unless they are satisfied that the hazards involved are believed to be predictable. Physicians should cease any investigation if the hazards are found to outweigh the potential benefits.

8. In publication of the results of his or her research, the physician is obliged to preserve the accuracy of the results. Reports of experimentation not in accordance with the principles laid down in this Declaration should not be accepted for publication.

9. In any research on human beings, each potential subject must be adequately informed of the aims, methods, anticipated benefits and potential hazards of the study and the discomfort it may entail. He or she should be informed that he or she is at liberty to abstain from participation in the study and that he or she is free to withdraw his or her consent to participation at any time. The physician should then obtain the subject's freely-given informed consent, preferably in writing.

10. When obtaining informed consent for the research project the physician should be particularly cautious if the subject is in a dependent relationship to him or her or may consent under duress. In that case the informed consent should be obtained by a physician who is not engaged in the investigation and who is completely independent of this official relationship.

11. In case of legal incompetence, informed consent should be obtained from the legal guardian in accordance with national legislation. Where physical or mental incapacity makes it impossible to obtain informed consent, or when the subject is a minor, permission from the responsible relative replaces that of the subject in accordance with national legislation. Whenever the minor child is in fact able to

give a consent, the minor's consent must be obtained in addition to the consent of the minor's legal guardian.

12. The research protocol should always contain a statement of the ethical considerations involved and should indicate that the principles enunciated in the present Declaration are complied with.

## II. Medical Research Combined with Professional Care (Clinical research)

1. In the treatment of the sick person, the physician must be free to use a new diagnostic and therapeutic measure, if in his or her judgement it offers hope of saving life, reestablishing health or alleviating suffering.

2. The potential benefits, hazards and discomfort of a new method should be weighed against the advantages of the best current diagnostic and therapeutic methods.

3. In any medical study, every patient—including those of a control group, if any—should be assured of the best proven diagnostic and therapeutic method.

4. The refusal of the patient to participate in a study must never interfere with the physician-patient relationship.

5. If the physician considers it essential not to obtain informed consent, the specific reasons for this proposal should be stated in the experimental protocol for transmission to the independent committee (1, 2).

6. The physician can combine medical research with professional care, the objective being the acquisition of new medical knowledge, only to the extent that medical research is justified by its potential diagnostic or therapeutic value for the patient.

## III. Non-Therapeutic Biomedical Research Involving Human Subjects (Non-clinical biomedical research)

1. In the purely scientific application of medical research carried out on a human being, it is the duty of the physician to remain the protector of the life and health of that person on whom biomedical research is being carried out.

2. The subjects should be volunteers—either healthy persons or patients for whom the experimental design is not related to the patient's illness.

3. The investigator or the investigating team should discontinue the research if in his/her or their judgement it may, if continued, be harmful to the individual.

4. In research on man, the interest of science and society should never take precedence over considerations related to the well-being of the subject.

# THE BELMONT REPORT: ETHICAL PRINCIPLES AND GUIDELINES FOR THE PROTECTION OF HUMAN SUBJECTS OF RESEARCH
### National Commission for the Protection of Human Subjects of Biomedical and Behavioral Research
### 1979

*The National Commission for the Protection of Human Subjects of Biomedical and Behavioral Research was created when the National Research Act (P.L. 93-348) became law on July 12, 1974. One of its mandates was to identify the basic ethical principles that should underlie research involving human subjects and to develop guidelines to ensure that such research is conducted in accordance with those principles. Since the first set of federal guidelines for human experimentation applicable to all programs under the auspices of what was then the Department of Health, Education, and Welfare (DHEW) was enacted in 1971, the National Commission's task, in part, was to identify and articulate the theoretical principles upon which those already existing guidelines were based.*

*After nearly four years of deliberation, the commission published its findings as the Belmont Report, which is printed below. The current, 1991 revision of the 1971 federal guidelines for human experimentation are also included in this section of the Appendix. Federal regulations require that every U.S. research institution that receives federal funds for research involving human subjects adopt a statement of principles to govern the protection of human subjects of research, and virtually all such institutions have endorsed the Belmont principles. Many research institutions outside of the United States also endorse the Belmont principles; however, the majority of foreign institutions cite the Declaration of Helsinki as their core ethical standard.*

Scientific research has produced substantial social benefits. It has also posed some troubling ethical questions. Public attention was drawn to these questions by reported abuses of human subjects in biomedical experiments, especially during the Second World War. During the Nuremberg War Crime Trials, the Nuremberg code was drafted as a set of standards for judging physicians and scientists who had conducted biomedical experiments on concentration camp prisoners. This code became the prototype of many later codes intended to assure that research involving human subjects would be carried out in an ethical manner.

The codes consist of rules, some general, others specific, that guide the investigators or the reviewers of research in their work. Such rules often are inadequate to cover complex situations; at times they come into conflict, and they are frequently difficult to interpret or apply. Broader ethical principles will provide a basis on which specific rules may be formulated, criticized and interpreted.

Three principles, or general prescriptive judgments, that are relevant to research involving human subjects are identified in this statement. Other principles may also be relevant. These three are comprehensive, however, and are stated at a level of generalization that should assist scientists, subjects, reviewers and interested citizens to understand the ethical issues inherent in research involving human subjects. These principles cannot always be applied so as to resolve beyond dispute particular ethical problems. The objective is to provide an analytical framework that will guide the resolution of ethical problems arising from research involving human subjects.

This statement consists of a distinction between research and practice, a discussion of the three basic ethical principles, and remarks about the application of these principles.

## A. Boundaries Between Practice and Research

It is important to distinguish between biomedical and behavioral research, on the one hand, and the practice of accepted therapy on the other, in order to know what activities ought to undergo review for the protection of human subjects of research. The distinction between research and practice is blurred partly because both often occur together (as in research designed to evaluate a therapy) and partly because notable departures from standard practice are often called "experimental" when the terms "experimental" and "research" are not carefully defined.

For the most part, the term "practice" refers to interventions that are designed solely to enhance the well-being of an individual patient or client and that have a reasonable expectation of success. The purpose of medical or behavioral practice is to provide diagnosis, preventive treatment or therapy to particular individuals. By contrast, the term "research" designates an activity designed to test an hypothesis, permit conclusions to be drawn, and thereby to develop or contribute to generalizable knowledge (expressed, for example, in theories, principles, and statements of relationships). Research is usually described in a formal protocol that sets forth an objective and a set of procedures designed to reach that objective.

When a clinician departs in a significant way from standard or accepted practice, the innovation does not, in and of itself, constitute research. The fact that a procedure is "experimental," in the sense of new, untested or different, does not automatically place it in the category of research. Radically new procedures of this description should, however, be made the object of formal research at an early stage in order to determine whether they are safe and effective. Thus, it is the responsibility of medical practice committees, for example, to insist that a major innovation be incorporated into a formal research project.

Research and practice may be carried on together when research is designed to evaluate the safety and efficacy of a therapy. This need not cause any confusion regarding whether or not the activity requires review; the general rule is that if there is any element of research in an activity, that activity should undergo review for the protection of human subjects.

## B. Basic Ethical Principles

The expression "basic ethical principles" refers to those general judgments that serve as a basic justification for the many particular ethical prescriptions and evaluations of human actions. Three basic principles, among those generally accepted in our cultural tradition, are particularly relevant to the ethics of research involving human subjects: the principles of respect for persons, beneficence and justice.

1. *Respect for Persons.*—Respect for persons incorporates at least two ethical convictions: first, that individuals should be treated as autonomous agents, and second, that persons with diminished autonomy are entitled to protection. The principle of respect

for persons thus divides into two separate moral requirements: the requirement to acknowledge autonomy and the requirement to protect those with diminished autonomy.

An autonomous person is an individual capable of deliberation about personal goals and of acting under the direction of such deliberation. To respect autonomy is to give weight to autonomous persons' considered opinions and choices while refraining from obstructing their actions unless they are clearly detrimental to others. To show lack of respect for an autonomous agent is to repudiate that person's considered judgments, to deny an individual the freedom to act on those considered judgments, or to withhold information necessary to make a considered judgment, when there are no compelling reasons to do so.

However, not every human being is capable of self-determination. The capacity for self-determination matures during an individual's life, and some individuals lose this capacity wholly or in part because of illness, mental disability, or circumstances that severely restrict liberty. Respect for the immature and the incapacitated may require protecting them as they mature or while they are incapacitated.

Some persons are in need of extensive protection, even to the point of excluding them from activities which may harm them; other persons require little protection beyond making sure they undertake activities freely and with awareness of possible adverse consequences. The extent of protection afforded should depend upon the risk of harm and the likelihood of benefit. The judgment that any individual lacks autonomy should be periodically reevaluated and will vary in different situations.

In most cases of research involving human subjects, respect for persons demands that subjects enter into the research voluntarily and with adequate information. In some situations, however, application of the principle is not obvious. The involvement of prisoners as subjects of research provides an instructive example. On the one hand, it would seem that the principle of respect for persons requires that prisoners not be deprived of the opportunity to volunteer for research. On the other hand, under prison conditions they may be subtly coerced or unduly influenced to engage in research activities for which they would not otherwise volunteer. Respect for persons would then dictate that prisoners be protected. Whether to allow prisoners to "volunteer" or to "protect" them presents a dilemma. Respecting persons, in most hard cases, is often a matter of balancing competing claims urged by the principle of respect itself.

2. *Beneficence.*—Persons are treated in an ethical manner not only by respecting their decisions and protecting them from harm, but also by making efforts to secure their well-being. Such treatment falls under the principle of beneficence. The term "beneficence" is often understood to cover acts of kindness or charity that go beyond strict obligation. In this document, beneficence is understood in a stronger sense, as an obligation. Two general rules have been formulated as complementary expressions of beneficent actions in this sense: (1) do not harm and (2) maximize possible benefits and minimize possible harms.

The Hippocratic maxim "do no harm" has long been a fundamental principle of medical ethics. Claude Bernard extended it to the realm of research, saying that one should not injure one person regardless of the benefits that might come to others. However, even avoiding harm requires learning what is harmful; and, in the process of obtaining this information, persons may be exposed to risk of harm. Further, the Hippocratic Oath requires physicians to benefit their patients "according to their best judgment." Learning what will in fact benefit may require exposing persons to risk. The problem posed by these imperatives is to decide when it is justifiable to seek certain benefits despite the risks involved, and when the benefits should be foregone because of the risks.

The obligations of beneficence affect both individual investigators and society at large, because they extend both to particular research projects and to the entire enterprise of research. In the case of particular projects, investigators and members of their institutions are obliged to give forethought to the maximization of benefits and the reduction of risk that might occur from the research investigation. In the case of scientific research in general, members of the larger society are obliged to recognize the longer term benefits and risks that may result from the improvement of knowledge and from the development of novel medical, psychotherapeutic, and social procedures.

The principle of beneficence often occupies a well-defined justifying role in many areas of research involving human subjects. An example is found in research involving children. Effective ways of treating childhood diseases and fostering healthy development are benefits that serve to justify research involving children—even when individual research subjects are not direct beneficiaries. Research also makes it possible to avoid the harm that may result from the application of previously accepted routine practices that on closer investigation turn out to be dangerous. But the role of the principle of beneficence is not always so unambiguous. A difficult ethical problem remains, for example, about research that presents more than minimal risk without immediate prospect of direct benefit to the children involved. Some have argued that such research is inadmissible, while others have pointed out that this limit would rule out much research promising great benefit to children in the future. Here again, as with all hard cases, the different claims covered by the principle of beneficence may come into conflict and force difficult choices.

3. *Justice.*—Who ought to receive the benefits of research and bear its burdens? This is a question of justice, in the sense of "fairness in distribution" or "what is deserved." An injustice occurs when some benefit to which a person is entitled is denied without good reason or when some burden is imposed unduly. Another way of conceiving the principle of justice is that equals ought to be treated equally. However, this statement requires explication. Who is equal and who is unequal? What considerations justify departure from equal distribution? Almost all commentators allow that distinctions based on experience, age, deprivation, competence, merit and position do sometimes constitute criteria justifying differential treatment for certain purposes. It is necessary, then, to explain in what respects people should be treated equally. There are several widely accepted formulations of just ways to distribute burdens and benefits. Each formulation mentions some relevant property on the basis of which burdens and benefits should be distributed. These formulations are (1) to each person an equal share, (2) to each person according to individual need, (3) to each person according to individual effort, (4) to each person according to societal contribution, and (5) to each person according to merit.

Questions of justice have long been associated with social practices such as punishment, taxation and political representation. Until recently these questions have not generally been associated with scientific research. However, they are foreshadowed even in the earliest reflections on the ethics of research involving human subjects. For example, during the 19th and early 20th centuries the burdens of serving as research subjects fell largely upon poor ward patients, while the benefits of improved medical care flowed primarily to private patients. Subsequently, the exploitation of unwilling prisoners as research subjects in Nazi concentration camps was condemned as a particularly flagrant injustice. In this country, in the 1940's, the Tuskegee syphilis study used disadvantaged, rural black men to study the untreated course of a disease that is by no means confined to that population. These subjects were deprived of demonstrably effective treatment in order not to interrupt the project, long after such treatment became generally available.

Against this historical background, it can be seen how conceptions of justice are relevant to research involving human subjects. For example, the selection of research subjects needs to be scrutinized in order to determine whether some classes (e.g., welfare patients, particularly racial and ethnic minorities, or persons confined to institutions) are being systematically selected simply because of their easy availability, their compromised position, or their manipulability, rather than for reasons directly related to the problem being studied. Finally, whenever research supported by public funds leads to the development of therapeutic devices and procedures, justice demands both that these not provide advantages only to those who can afford them and that such research should not unduly involve persons from groups unlikely to be among the beneficiaries of subsequent applications of the research.

## C. Applications

Applications of the general principles to the conduct of research leads to consideration of the following requirements: informed consent, risk/benefit assessment, and the selection of subjects of research.

1. *Informed Consent.*—Respect for persons requires that subjects, to the degree that they are capable, be given the opportunity to choose what shall or shall not happen to them. This opportunity is provided when adequate standards for informed consent are satisfied.

While the importance of informed consent is unquestioned, controversy prevails over the nature and possibility of an informed consent. Nonetheless, there is widespread agreement that the consent process can be analyzed as containing three elements: information, comprehension and voluntariness.

*Information.* Most codes of research establish specific items for disclosure intended to assure that subjects are given sufficient information. These items generally include: the research procedure, their purposes, risks and anticipated benefits, alternative procedures (where therapy is involved), and a statement offering the subject the opportunity to ask questions and to withdraw at any time from the research. Additional items have been proposed, including how subjects are selected, the person responsible for the research, etc.

However, a simple listing of items does not answer the question of what the standard should be for judging how much and what sort of information should be provided. One standard frequently invoked in medical practice, namely the information commonly provided by practitioners in the field or in the locale, is inadequate since research takes place precisely when a common understanding does not exist. Another standard, currently popular in malpractice law, requires the practitioner to reveal the information that reasonable persons would wish to know in order to make a decision regarding their care. This, too, seems insufficient since the research subject, being in essence a volunteer, may wish to know considerably more about risks gratuitously undertaken than do patients who deliver themselves into the hand of a clinician for needed care. It may be that a standard of "the reasonable volunteer" should be proposed: the extent and nature of information should be such that persons, knowing that the procedure is neither necessary for their care nor perhaps fully understood, can decide whether they wish to participate in the furthering of knowledge. Even when some direct benefit to them is anticipated, the subjects should understand clearly the range of risk and the voluntary nature of participation.

A special problem of consent arises where informing subjects of some pertinent aspect of the research is likely to impair the validity of the research. In many cases, it is sufficient to indicate to subjects that they are being invited to participate in research of which some features will not be revealed until the research is concluded. In all cases of research involving incomplete disclosure, such research is justified only if it is clear that (1) incomplete disclosure is truly necessary to accomplish the goals of the research, (2) there are no undisclosed risks to subjects that are more than minimal, and (3) there is an adequate plan for debriefing subjects, when appropriate, and for dissemination of research results to them. Information about risks should never be withheld for the purpose of eliciting the cooperation of subjects, and truthful answers should always be given to direct questions about the research. Care should be taken to distinguish cases in which disclosure would destroy or invalidate the research from cases in which disclosure would simply inconvenience the investigator.

*Comprehension.* The manner and context in which information is conveyed is as important as the information itself. For example, presenting information in a disorganized and rapid fashion, allowing too little time for consideration or curtailing opportunities for questioning, all may adversely affect a subject's ability to make an informed choice.

Because the subject's ability to understand is a function of intelligence, rationality, maturity and language, it is necessary to adapt the presentation of the information to the subject's capacities. Investigators are responsible for ascertaining that the subject has comprehended the information. While there is always an obligation to ascertain that the information about risk to subjects is complete and adequately comprehended, when the risks are more serious, that obligation increases. On occasion, it may be suitable to give some oral or written tests of comprehension.

Special provision may need to be made when comprehension is severely limited—for example, by conditions of immaturity or mental disability. Each class of subjects that one might consider as incompetent (e.g., infants and young children, mentally disabled patients, the terminally ill and the comatose) should be considered on its own terms. Even for these persons, however, respect requires giving them the opportunity to choose to the extent they are able, whether or not to participate in research. The objections of these subjects to involvement should be honored, unless the research entails providing them a therapy unavailable elsewhere. Respect for persons also requires seeking the permission of other parties in order to protect the subjects from harm. Such persons are thus respected both by acknowledging their own wishes and by the use of third parties to protect them from harm.

The third parties chosen should be those who are most likely to understand the incompetent subject's situation and to act in that person's best interest. The person authorized to act on behalf of the subject should be given an opportunity to observe the research as it proceeds in order to be able to withdraw the subject from the research, if such action appears in the subject's best interest.

*Voluntariness.* An agreement to participate in research constitutes a valid consent only if voluntarily given. This element of informed consent requires conditions free of coercion and undue influence. Coercion occurs when an overt threat of harm is intentionally presented by one person to another in order to obtain compliance. Undue influence, by contrast, occurs through an offer of an excessive, unwarranted, inappropriate or improper reward or other overture in order to obtain compliance. Also, inducements that would ordinarily be acceptable may become undue influences if the subject is especially vulnerable.

Unjustifiable pressures usually occur when persons in positions of authority or commanding influence—especially where possible sanctions are involved—urge a course of action for a subject. A continuum of such influencing factors exists, however, and it is impossible to state precisely where justifiable persuasion ends and undue influence begins. But undue influence would include actions such as manipulating a person's choice through the controlling influence of a close relative and threatening to withdraw health services to which an individual would otherwise be entitled.

2. *Assessment of Risks and Benefits.*—The assessment of risks and benefits requires a careful arrayal of relevant data, including, in some cases, alternative ways of obtaining the benefits sought in the research. Thus, the assessment presents both an opportunity and a responsibility to gather systematic and comprehensive information about proposed research. For the investigator, it is a means to examine whether the proposed research is properly designed. For a review committee, it is a method for determining whether the risks that will be presented to subjects are justified. For prospective subjects, the assessment will assist the determination whether or not to participate.

*The Nature and Scope of Risks and Benefits.* The requirement that research be justified on the basis of a favorable risk/benefit assessment bears a close relation to the principle of beneficence, just as the moral requirement that informed consent be obtained is derived primarily from the principle of respect for persons. The term "risk" refers to a possibility that harm may occur. However, when expressions such as "small risk" or "high risk" are used, they usually refer (often ambiguously) both to the chance (probability) of experiencing a harm and the severity (magnitude) of the envisioned harm.

The term "benefit" is used in the research context to refer to something of positive value related to health or welfare. Unlike "risk," "benefit" is not a term that expresses probabilities. Risk is properly contrasted to probability of benefits, and benefits are properly contrasted with harms rather than risks of harm. Accordingly, so-called risk benefit assessments are concerned with the probabilities and magnitudes of possible harms and anticipated benefits. Many kinds of possible harms and benefits need to be taken into account. There are, for example, risks of psychological harm, physical harm, legal harm, social harm and economic harm and the corresponding benefits. While the most likely types of harms to research subjects are those of psychological or physical pain or injury, other possible kinds should not be overlooked.

Risks and benefits of research may affect the individual subjects, the families of the individual subjects, and society at large (or special groups of subjects in society). Previous codes and Federal regulations have required that risks to subjects be outweighed by the sum of both the anticipated benefit to the subject, if any, and the anticipated benefit to society in the form of knowledge to be gained from the research. In balancing these different elements, the risks and benefits affecting the immediate research subject will normally carry special weight. On the other hand, interests other than those of the subject may on some occasions be sufficient by themselves to justify the risks involved in the research, so long as the subjects' rights have been protected. Beneficence thus requires that we protect against risk of harm to subjects and also that we be concerned about the loss of the substantial benefits that might be gained from research.

*The Systematic Assessment of Risks and Benefits.* It is commonly said that benefits and risks must be "balanced" and shown to be "in a favorable ratio." The metaphorical character of these terms draws attention to the difficulty of making precise judgments. Only on rare occasions will quantitative techniques be available for the scrutiny of research protocols. However, the idea of systematic, nonarbitrary analysis of risks and benefits should be emulated insofar as possible. This ideal requires those making decisions about the justifiability of research to be thorough in the accumulation and assessment of information about all aspects of the research, and to consider alternatives systematically. This procedure renders the assessment of research more rigorous and precise, while making communication between review board members and investigators less subject to misinterpretation, misinformation and conflicting judgments. Thus, there should first be a determination of the validity of the presuppositions of the research; then the nature, probability and magnitude of risk should be distinguished with as much clarity as possible. The method of ascertaining risks should be explicit, especially where there is no alternative to the use of such vague categories as small or slight risk. It should also be determined whether an investigator's estimates of the probability of harm or benefits are reasonable, as judged by known facts or other available studies.

Finally, assessment of the justifiability of research should reflect at least the following considerations: (i) Brutal or inhumane treatment of human subjects is never morally justified. (ii) Risks should be reduced to those necessary to achieve the research objective. It should be determined whether it is in fact necessary to use human subjects at all. Risk can perhaps never be entirely eliminated, but it can often be reduced by careful attention to alternative procedures. (iii) When research involves significant risk of serious impairment, review committees should be extraordinarily insistent on the justification of the risk (looking usually to the likelihood of benefit to the subject—or, in some rare cases, to the manifest voluntariness of the participation). (iv) When vulnerable populations are involved in research, the appropriateness of involving them should itself be demonstrated. A number of variables go into such judgments, including the nature and degree of risk, the condition of the particular population involved, and the nature and level of the anticipated benefits. (v) Relevant risks and benefits must be thoroughly arrayed in documents and procedures used in the informed consent process.

3. *Selection of Subjects.*—Just as the principle of respect for persons finds expression in the requirements for consent, and the principle of beneficence in risk benefit assessment, the principle of justice gives rise to moral requirements that there be fair procedures and outcomes in the selection of research subjects.

Justice is relevant to the selection of subjects of research at two levels: the social and the individual. Individual justice in the selection of subjects would require that researchers exhibit fairness: thus, they should not offer potentially beneficial research only to some patients who are in their favor or select only "undesirable" persons for risky research. Social justice requires that distinction be drawn between classes of subjects that ought, and ought not, to participate in any particular kind of research, based on the ability of members of that class to bear burdens and on the appropriateness of placing further burdens on already burdened persons. Thus, it can be considered a matter of social justice that there is an order of preference in the selection of classes of subjects (e.g., adults before children) and that some classes of potential subjects (e.g., the institutionalized mentally infirm or prisoners) may be involved as research subjects, if at all, only on certain conditions.

Injustice may appear in the selection of subjects, even if individual subjects are selected fairly by investigators and treated fairly in the course of research. Thus injustice arises from social, racial, sexual and cultural biases institutionalized in society. Thus, even if individual researchers are treating their research subjects fairly, and even if IRBs are taking care to assure that subjects are selected fairly within a particular institution, unjust social patterns may nevertheless appear in the overall distribution of the burdens and benefits of research. Although individual institutions or investigators may not be able to resolve a problem that is pervasive in their social setting, they can consider distributive justice in selecting research subjects.

Some populations, especially institutionalized ones, are already burdened in many ways by their infirmities and environments. When research is proposed that involves risks and does not include a therapeutic component, other less burdened classes of persons should be called upon first to accept these risks of research, except where the research is directly related to the specific conditions of the class involved. Also, even though public funds for research may often flow in the same directions as public funds for health care, it seems unfair that populations dependent on public health care constitute a pool of preferred research subjects if more advantaged populations are likely to be the recipients of the benefits.

One special instance of injustice results from the involvement of vulnerable subjects. Certain groups, such as racial minorities, the economically disadvantaged, the very sick, and the institutionalized may continually be sought as research subjects, owing to their ready availability in settings where research is conducted. Given their dependent status and their frequently compromised capacity for free consent, they should be protected against the danger of being involved in research solely for administrative convenience, or because they are easy to manipulate as a result of their illness or socioeconomic condition.

# DHHS REGULATIONS FOR THE PROTECTION
## OF HUMAN SUBJECTS (45 CFR 46)
### June 18, 1991

*Between 1953 and 1971 various agencies within the U.S. Department of Health, Education, and Welfare (DHEW), now the Department of Health and Human Services (DHHS), issued their own guidelines on human experimentation. Finally, in 1971, the first set of federal guidelines for human experimentation applicable to all DHEW programs was established. Those guidelines were revised slightly and officially published (May 30, 1974) as part of the Code of Federal Regulations (Title 45, Subtitle A, Part 46).*

*In 1981, the regulations underwent a major revision in light of various reports by the National Commission for the Protection of Human Subjects of Biomedical and Behavioral Research, which also issued the Belmont Report (see preceding document). The regulations were expanded to include guidelines for research involving fetuses, pregnant women, and human in vitro fertilization (Subpart B); children (Subpart C); and prisoners (Subpart D).*

*In June 1991, a revised Federal Policy for the Protection of Human Subjects (Subpart A) was adopted as "the Common Rule" by fifteen federal departments and agencies and the Office of Science and Technology Policy. Subparts B, C, and D remain directly applicable only to DHHS-supported human subjects research. The 1991 regulations, which are printed here, took effect on August 19, 1991.*

### Subpart A—Federal Policy for the Protection of Human Subjects (Basic DHHS Policy for Protection of Human Research Subjects)

• • •

#### §46.101  To What Does This Policy Apply?

(a) Except as provided in paragraph (b) of this section, this policy applies to all re-search involving human subjects conducted, supported or otherwise subject to regulation by any Federal Department or Agency which takes appropriate administrative action to make the policy applicable to such research. This includes research conducted by Federal civilian employees or military personnel, except that each Department or Agency head may adopt such procedural modifications as may be appropriate from an administrative standpoint. It also includes research conducted, supported, or otherwise subject to reg-ulation by the Federal Government outside the United States.

(1) Research that is conducted or supported by a Federal Department or Agency, whether or not it is regulated as defined in §46.102(e) must comply with all sections of this policy.

(2) Research that is neither conducted nor supported by a Federal Department or Agency but is subject to regulation as defined in §46.102(e) must be reviewed and ap-proved, in compliance with §46.101, §46.102, and §46.107 through §46.117 of this policy, by an Institutional Review Board (IRB) that operates in accordance with the pertinent requirements of this policy.

(b) Unless otherwise required by Department or Agency heads, research activities in which the only involvement of human subjects will be in one or more of the following categories are exempt from this policy:

(1) Research conducted in established or commonly accepted educational settings, involving normal educational practices, such as (i) research on regular and special edu-cation instructional strategies, or (ii) research on the effectiveness of or the comparison among instructional techniques, curricula, or classroom management methods.

(2) Research involving the use of educational tests (cognitive, diagnostic, aptitude, achievement), survey procedures, interview procedures or observation of public behav-ior, unless:

(i) information obtained is recorded in such a manner that human subjects can be identified, directly or through identifiers linked to the subjects; and (ii) any disclosure of the human subjects' responses outside the research could reasonably place the subjects at risk of criminal or civil liability or be damaging to the subjects' financial standing, em-ployability, or reputation.

(3) Research involving the use of educational tests (cognitive, diagnostic, aptitude, achievement), survey procedures, interview procedures, or observation of public behav-ior that is not exempt under paragraph (b)(2) of this section, if:

(i) the human subjects are elected or appointed public officials or candidates for public office; or (ii) Federal statute(s) require(s) without exception that the confidentiality of the personally identifiable information will be maintained throughout the research and thereafter.

(4) Research involving the collection or study of existing data, documents, records, pathological specimens, or diagnostic specimens, if these sources are publicly available or if the information is recorded by the investigator in such a manner that subjects cannot be identified, directly or through identifiers linked to the subjects.

(5) Research and demonstration projects which are conducted by or subject to the approval of Department or Agency heads, and which are designed to study, evaluate, or otherwise examine:

(i) Public benefit or service programs; (ii) procedures for obtaining benefits or services under those programs; (iii) possible changes in or alternatives to those programs or pro-cedures; or (iv) possible changes in methods or levels of payment for benefits or services under those programs.

(6) Taste and food quality evaluation and consumer acceptance studies, (i) if whole-some foods without additives are consumed or (ii) if a food is consumed that contains a food ingredient at or below the level and for a use found to be safe, or agricultural chemical or environmental contaminant at or below the level found to be safe, by the

Food and Drug Administration or approved by the Environmental Protection Agency or the Food Safety and Inspection Service of the U.S. Department of Agriculture.

(c) Department or Agency heads retain final judgment as to whether a particular activity is covered by this policy.

(d) Department or Agency heads may require that specific research activities or classes of research activities conducted, supported, or otherwise subject to regulation by the Department or Agency but not otherwise covered by this policy, comply with some or all of the requirements of this policy.

(e) Compliance with this policy requires compliance with pertinent Federal laws or regulations which provide additional protection for human subjects.

(f) This policy does not affect any state or local laws or regulations which may otherwise be applicable and which provide additional protections for human subjects.

(g) This policy does not affect any foreign laws or regulations which may otherwise be applicable and which provide additional protections to human subjects of research.

(h) When research covered by this policy takes place in foreign countries, procedures normally followed in the foreign countries to protect human subjects may differ from those set forth in this policy. [An example is a foreign institution which complies with guidelines consistent with the World Medical Assembly Declaration (Declaration of Helsinki amended 1989) issued either by sovereign states or by an organization whose function for the protection of human research subjects is internationally recognized.] In these circumstances, if a Department or Agency head determines that the procedures prescribed by the institution afford protections that are at least equivalent to those provided in this policy, the Department or Agency head may approve the substitution of the foreign procedures in lieu of the procedural requirements provided in this policy. Except when otherwise required by statute, Executive Order, or the Department or Agency head, notices of these actions as they occur will be published in the **Federal Register** or will be otherwise published as provided in Department or Agency procedures.

(i) Unless otherwise required by law, Department or Agency heads may waive the applicability of some or all of the provisions of this policy to specific research activities or classes of research activities otherwise covered by this policy. Except when otherwise required by statute or Executive Order, the Department or Agency head shall forward advance notices of these actions to the Office for Protection from Research Risks, National Institutes of Health, Department of Health and Human Services (DHHS), and shall also publish them in the **Federal Register** or in such other manner as provided in Department or Agency procedures.

### §46.102 Definitions

(a) *Department or Agency head* means the head of any Federal Department or Agency and any other officer or employee of any Department or Agency to whom authority has been delegated.

(b) *Institution* means any public or private entity or Agency (including Federal, State, and other agencies).

(c) *Legally authorized representative* means an individual or judicial or other body authorized under applicable law to consent on behalf of a prospective subject to the subject's participation in the procedure(s) involved in the research.

(d) *Research* means a systematic investigation, including research development, testing and evaluation, designed to develop or contribute to generalizable knowledge. Activities which meet this definition constitute research for purposes of this policy, whether or not they are conducted or supported under a program which is considered research for other purposes. For example, some demonstration and service programs may include research activities.

(e) *Research subject to regulation,* and similar terms are intended to encompass those research activities for which a Federal Department or Agency has specific responsibility for regulating as a research activity, (for example, Investigational New Drug requirements administered by the Food and Drug Administration). It does not include research activities which are incidentally regulated by a Federal Department or Agency solely as part of the Department's or Agency's broader responsibility to regulate certain types of activities whether research or non-research in nature (for example, Wage and Hour requirements administered by the Department of Labor).

(f) *Human subject* means a living individual about whom an investigator (whether professional or student) conducting research obtains

(1) data through intervention or interaction with the individual, or

(2) identifiable private information. *Intervention* includes both physical procedures by which data are gathered (for example, venipuncture) and manipulations of the subject or the subject's environment that are performed for research purposes. Interaction in-

cludes communication or interpersonal contact between investigator and subject. *Private information* includes information about behavior that occurs in a context in which an individual can reasonably expect that no observation or recording is taking place, and information which has been provided for specific purposes by an individual and which the individual can reasonably expect will not be made public (for example, a medical record). Private information must be individually identifiable (i.e., the identity of the subject is or may readily be ascertained by the investigator or associated with the information) in order for obtaining the information to constitute research involving human subjects.

(g) *IRB* means an Institutional Review Board established in accord with and for the purposes expressed in this policy.

(h) *IRB approval* means the determination of the IRB that the research has been reviewed and may be conducted at an institution within the constraints set forth by the IRB and by other institutional and Federal requirements.

(i) *Minimal risk* means that the probability and magnitude of harm or discomfort anticipated in the research are not greater in and of themselves than those ordinarily encountered in daily life or during the performance of routine physical or psychological examinations or tests.

(j) *Certification* means the official notification by the institution to the supporting Department or Agency, in accordance with the requirements of this policy, that a research project or activity involving human subjects has been reviewed and approved by an IRB in accordance with an approved assurance.

### §46.103 Assuring Compliance With This Policy—Research Conducted or Supported By Any Federal Department or Agency

(a) Each institution engaged in research which is covered by this policy and which is conducted or supported by a Federal Department or Agency shall provide written assurance satisfactory to the Department or Agency head that it will comply with the requirements set forth in this policy. In lieu of requiring submission of an assurance, individual Department or Agency heads shall accept the existence of a current assurance, appropriate for the research in question, on file with the Office for Protection from Research Risks, National Institutes Health, DHHS, and approved for Federalwide use by that office. When the existence of an DHHS-approved assurance is accepted in lieu of requiring submission of an assurance, reports (except certification) required by this policy to be made to Department and Agency heads shall also be made to the Office for Protection from Research Risks, National Institutes of Health, DHHS.

(b) Department and agencies will conduct or support research covered by this policy only if the institution has an assurance approved as provided in this section, and only if the institution has certified to the Department or Agency head that the research has been reviewed and approved by an IRB provided for in the assurance, and will be subject to continuing review by the IRB. Assurances applicable to federally supported or conducted research shall at a minimum include:

(1) A statement of principles governing the institution in the discharge of its responsibilities for protecting the rights and welfare of human subjects of research conducted at or sponsored by the institution, regardless of whether the research is subject to Federal regulation. This may include an appropriate existing code, declaration, or statement of ethical principles, or a statement formulated by the institution itself. This requirement does not preempt provisions of this policy applicable to Department- or Agency-supported or regulated research and need not be applicable to any research exempted or waived under §46.101 (b) or (i).

(2) Designation of one or more IRBs established in accordance with the requirements of this policy, and for which provisions are made for meeting space and sufficient staff to support the IRB's review and recordkeeping duties.

(3) A list of IRB members identified by name; earned degrees; representative capacity; indications of experience such as board certifications, licenses, etc., sufficient to describe each member's chief anticipated contributions to IRB deliberations; and any employment or other relationship between each member and the institution; for example: full-time employee, part-time employee, member of governing panel or board, stockholder, paid or unpaid consultant. Changes in IRB membership shall be reported to the Department or Agency head, unless in accord with §46.103(a) of this policy, the existence of a DHHS-approved assurance is accepted. In this case, change in IRB membership shall be reported to the Office for Protection from Research Risks, National Institutes of Health, DHHS.

(4) Written procedures which the IRB will follow (i) for conducting its initial and continuing review of research and for reporting its findings and actions to the investigator

and the institution; (ii) for determining which projects require review more often than annually and which projects need verification from sources other than the investigators that no material changes have occurred since previous IRB review; and (iii) for ensuring prompt reporting to the IRB of proposed changes in a research activity, and for ensuring that such changes in approved research, during the period for which IRB approval has already been given, may not be initiated without IRB review and approval except when necessary to eliminate apparent immediate hazards to the subject.

(5) Written procedures for ensuring prompt reporting to the IRB, appropriate institutional officials, and the Department or Agency head of (i) any unanticipated problems involving risks to subjects or others or any serious or continuing noncompliance with this policy or the requirements or determinations of the IRB: and (ii) any suspension or termination of IRB approval.

(c) The assurance shall be executed by an individual authorized to act for the institution and to assume on behalf of the institution the obligations imposed by this policy and shall be filed in such form and manner as the Department or Agency head prescribes.

(d) The Department or Agency head will evaluate all assurances submitted in accordance with this policy through such officers and employees of the Department or Agency and such experts or consultants engaged for this purpose as the Department or Agency head determines to be appropriate. The Department or Agency head's evaluation will take into consideration the adequacy of the proposed IRB in light of the anticipated scope of the institution's research activities and the types of subject populations likely to be involved, the appropriateness of the proposed initial and continuing review procedures in light of the probable risks, and the size and complexity of the institution.

(e) On the basis of this evaluation, the Department or Agency head may approve or disapprove the assurance, or enter into negotiations to develop an approvable one. The Department or Agency head may limit the period during which any particular approved assurance or class of approved assurances shall remain effective or otherwise condition or restrict approval.

(f) Certification is required when the research is supported by a Federal Department or Agency and not otherwise exempted or waived under §46.101 (b) or (i). An institution with an approved assurance shall certify that each application or proposal for research covered by the assurance and by §46.103 of this policy has been reviewed and approved by the IRB. Such certification must be submitted with the application or proposal or by such later date as may be prescribed by the Department or Agency to which the application or proposal is submitted. Under no condition shall research covered by §46.103 of the policy be supported prior to receipt of the certification that the research has been reviewed and approved by the IRB. Institutions without an approved assurance covering the research shall certify within 30 days after receipt of a request for such a certification from the Department or Agency, that the application or proposal has been approved by the IRB. If the certification is not submitted within these time limits, the application or proposal may be returned to the institution.
(Approved by the Office of Management and Budget under Control Number 9999–0020.)

### §§46.104–46.106 [Reserved]

### §46.107 IRB Membership

(a) Each IRB shall have at least five members, with varying backgrounds to promote complete and adequate review of research activities commonly conducted by the institution. The IRB shall be sufficiently qualified through the experience and expertise of its members, and the diversity of the members, including consideration of race, gender, and cultural backgrounds and sensitivity to such issues as community attitudes, to promote respect for its advice and counsel in safeguarding the rights and welfare of human subjects. In addition to possessing the professional competence necessary to review specific research activities, the IRB shall be able to ascertain the acceptability of proposed research in terms of institutional commitments and regulations, applicable law, and standards of professional conduct and practice. The IRB shall therefore include persons knowledgeable in these areas. If an IRB regularly reviews research that involves a vulnerable category of subjects, such as children, prisoners, pregnant women, or handicapped or mentally disabled persons, consideration shall be given to the inclusion of one or more individuals who are knowledgeable about and experienced in working with these subjects.

(b) Every nondiscriminatory effort will be made to ensure that no IRB consists entirely of men or entirely of women, including the institution's consideration of qualified persons of both sexes, so long as no selection is made to the IRB on the basis of gender. No IRB may consist entirely of members of one profession.

(c) Each IRB shall include at least one member whose primary concerns are in scientific areas and at least one member whose primary concerns are in nonscientific areas.

(d) Each IRB shall include at least one member who is not otherwise affiliated with the institution and who is not part of the immediate family of a person who is affiliated with the institution.

(e) No IRB may have a member participate in the IRB's initial or continuing review of any project in which the member has a conflicting interest, except to provide information requested by the IRB.

(f) An IRB may, in its discretion, invite individuals with competence in special areas to assist in the review of issues which require expertise beyond or in addition to that available on the IRB. These individuals may not vote with the IRB.

### §46.108  IRB Functions and Operations

In order to fulfill the requirements of this policy each IRB shall:

(a) Follow written procedures in the same detail as described in §46.103(b)(4) and to the extent required by §46.103(b)(5).

(b) Except when an expedited review procedure is used (see §46.110), review proposed research at convened meetings at which a majority of the members of the IRB are present, including at least one member whose primary concerns are in nonscientific areas. In order for the research to be approved, it shall receive the approval of a majority of those members present at the meeting.

### §46.109  IRB Review of Research

(a) An IRB shall review and have authority to approve, require modifications in (to secure approval), or disapprove all research activities covered by this policy.

(b) An IRB shall require that information given to subjects as part of informed consent is in accordance with §46.116. The IRB may require that information, in addition to that specifically mentioned in §46.116, be given to the subjects when in the IRB's judgment the information would meaningfully add to the protection of the rights and welfare of subjects.

(c) An IRB shall require documentation of informed consent or may waive documentation in accordance with §46.117.

(d) An IRB shall notify investigators and the institution in writing of its decision to approve or disapprove the proposed research activity, or of modifications required to secure IRB approval of the research activity. If the IRB decides to disapprove a research activity, it shall include in its written notification a statement of the reasons for its decision and give the investigator an opportunity to respond in person or in writing.

(e) An IRB shall conduct continuing review of research covered by this policy at intervals appropriate to the degree of risk, but not less than once per year, and shall have authority to observe or have a third party observe the consent process and the research. (Approved by the Office of Management and Budget under Control Number 9999–0020.)

### §46.110  Expedited Review Procedures For Certain Kinds of Research Involving No More Than Minimal Risk, and For Minor Changes in Approved Research

(a) The Secretary, HHS, has established, and published as a Notice in the **Federal Register,** a list of categories of research that may be reviewed by the IRB through an expedited review procedure. The list will be amended, as appropriate, after consultation with other departments and agencies, through periodic republication by the Secretary, HHS, in the **Federal Register.** A copy of the list is available from the Office for Protection from Research Risks, National Institutes of Health, DHHS, Bethesda, Maryland 20892.

(b) An IRB may use the expedited review procedure to review either or both of the following:

(1) some or all of the research appearing on the list and found by the reviewer(s) to involve no more than minimal risk,

(2) minor changes in previously approved research during the period (of one year or less) for which approval is authorized.

Under an expedited review procedure, the review may be carried out by the IRB chairperson or by one or more experienced reviewers designated by the chairperson from among members of the IRB. In reviewing the research, the reviewers may exercise all of the authorities of the IRB except that the reviewers may not disapprove the research. A research activity may be disapproved only after review in accordance with the non-expedited procedure set forth in §46.108(b).

(c) Each IRB which uses an expedited review procedure shall adopt a method for keeping all members advised of research proposals which have been approved under the procedure.

(d) The Department or Agency head may restrict, suspend, terminate, or choose not to authorize an institution's or IRB's use of the expedited review procedure.

### §46.111 Criteria for IRB Approval of Research

(a) In order to approve research covered by this policy the IRB shall determine that all of the following requirements are satisfied:

(1) Risks to subjects are minimized: (i) by using procedures which are consistent with sound research design and which do not unnecessarily expose subjects to risk, and (ii) whenever appropriate, by using procedures already being performed on the subjects for diagnostic or treatment purposes.

(2) Risks to subjects are reasonable in relation to anticipated benefits, if any, to subjects, and the importance of the knowledge that may reasonably be expected to result. In evaluating risks and benefits, the IRB should consider only those risks and benefits that may result from the research (as distinguished from risks and benefits of therapies subjects would receive even if not participating in the research). The IRB should not consider possible long-range effects of applying knowledge gained in the research (for example, the possible effects of the research on public policy) as among those research risks that fall within the purview of its responsibility.

(3) Selection of subjects is equitable. In making this assessment the IRB should take into account the purposes of the research and the setting in which the research will be conducted and should be particularly cognizant of the special problems of research involving vulnerable populations, such as children, prisoners, pregnant women, mentally disabled persons, or economically or educationally disadvantaged persons.

(4) Informed consent will be sought from each prospective subject or the subject's legally authorized representative, in accordance with, and to the extent required by §46.116.

(5) Informed consent will be appropriately documented, in accordance with, and to the extent required by §46.117.

(6) When appropriate, the research plan makes adequate provision for monitoring the data collected to ensure the safety of subjects.

(7) When appropriate, there are adequate provisions to protect the privacy of subjects and to maintain the confidentiality of data.

(b) When some or all of the subjects are likely to be vulnerable to coercion or undue influence, such as children, prisoners, pregnant women, mentally disabled persons, or economically or educationally disadvantaged persons, additional safeguards have been included in the study to protect the rights and welfare of these subjects.

### §46.112 Review by Institution

Research covered by this policy that has been approved by an IRB may be subject to further appropriate review and approval or disapproval by officials of the institution. However, those officials may not approve the research if it has not been approved by an IRB.

### §46.113 Suspension or Termination of IRB Approval of Research

An IRB shall have authority to suspend or terminate approval of research that is not being conducted in accordance with the IRB's requirements or that has been associated with unexpected serious harm to subjects. Any suspension or termination of approval shall include a statement of the reasons for the IRB's action and shall be reported promptly to the investigator, appropriate institutional officials, and the Department or Agency head.
(Approved by the Office of Management and Budget under Control Number 9999–0020.)

### §46.114 Cooperative Research

Cooperative research projects are those projects covered by this policy which involve more than one institution. In the conduct of cooperative research projects, each institution is responsible for safeguarding the rights and welfare of human subjects and for complying with this policy. With the approval of the Department or Agency head, an institution participating in a cooperative project may enter into a joint review arrangement, rely upon the review of another qualified IRB, or make similar arrangements for avoiding duplication of effort.

### §46.115 IRB Records

(a) An institution, or when appropriate an IRB, shall prepare and maintain adequate documentation of IRB activities, including the following:

(1) Copies of all research proposals reviewed, scientific evaluations, if any, that accompany the proposals, approved sample consent documents, progress reports submitted by investigators, and reports of injuries to subjects.

(2) Minutes of IRB meetings which shall be in sufficient detail to show attendance at the meetings; actions taken by the IRB; the vote on these actions including the number of members voting for, against, and abstaining; the basis for requiring changes in or disapproving research; and a written summary of the discussion of controverted issues and their resolution.

(3) Records of continuing review activities.

(4) Copies of all correspondence between the IRB and the investigators.

(5) A list of IRB members in the same detail as described in §46.103(b)(3).

(6) Written procedures for the IRB in the same detail as described in §46.103(b)(4) and §46.103(b)(5).

(7) Statements of significant new findings provided to subjects, as required by §46.116(b)(5).

(b) The records required by this policy shall be retained for at least 3 years, and records relating to research which is conducted shall be retained for at least 3 years after completion of the research. All records shall be accessible for inspection and copying by authorized representatives of the Department or Agency at reasonable times and in a reasonable manner.

(Approved by the Office of Management and Budget under Control Number 9999–0020.)

### §46.116 General Requirements for Informed Consent

Except as provided elsewhere in this policy, no investigator may involve a human being as a subject in research covered by this policy unless the investigator has obtained the legally effective informed consent of the subject or the subject's legally authorized representative. An investigator shall seek such consent only under circumstances that provide the prospective subject or the representative sufficient opportunity to consider whether or not to participate and that minimize the possibility of coercion or undue influence. The information that is given to the subject or the representative shall be in language understandable to the subject or the representative. No informed consent, whether oral or written, may include any exculpatory language through which the subject or the representative is made to waive or appear to waive any of the subject's legal rights, or releases or appears to release the investigator, the sponsor, the institution or its agents from liability for negligence.

(a) Basic elements of informed consent. Except as provided in paragraph (c) or (d) of this section, in seeking informed consent the following information shall be provided to each subject:

(1) a statement that the study involves research, an explanation of the purposes of the research and the expected duration of the subject's participation, a description of the procedures to be followed, and identification of any procedures which are experimental;

(2) a description of any reasonably foreseeable risks or discomforts to the subject;

(3) a description of any benefits to the subject or to others which may reasonably be expected from the research;

(4) a disclosure of appropriate alternative procedures or courses of treatment, if any, that might be advantageous to the subject;

(5) a statement describing the extent, if any, to which confidentiality of records identifying the subject will be maintained;

(6) for research involving more than minimal risk, an explanation as to whether any compensation and an explanation as to whether any medical treatments are available if injury occurs and, if so, what they consist of, or where further information may be obtained;

(7) an explanation of whom to contact for answers to pertinent questions about the research and research subjects' rights, and whom to contact in the event of a research-related injury to the subject; and

(8) a statement that participation is voluntary, refusal to participate will involve no penalty or loss of benefits to which the subject is otherwise entitled, and the subject may discontinue participation at any time without penalty or loss of benefits to which the subject is otherwise entitled.

(b) additional elements of informed consent. When appropriate, one or more of the following elements of information shall also be provided to each subject:

(1) a statement that the particular treatment or procedure may involve risks to the subject (or to the embryo or fetus, if the subject is or may become pregnant) which are currently unforeseeable;

(2) anticipated circumstances under which the subject's participation may be terminated by the investigator without regard to the subject's consent;

(3) any additional costs to the subject that may result from participation in the research;

(4) the consequences of a subject's decision to withdraw from the research and procedures for orderly termination of participation by the research;

(5) a statement that significant new findings developed during the course of the research which may relate to the subject's willingness to continue participation will be provided to the subject; and

(6) the approximate number of subjects involved in the study.

(c) An IRB may approve a consent procedure which does not include, or which alters, some or all of the elements of informed consent set forth above, or waive the requirement to obtain informed consent provided the IRB finds and documents that:

(1) the research or demonstration project is to be conducted by or subject to the approval of state or local government officials and is designed to study, evaluate, or otherwise examine: (i) public benefit or service programs; (ii) procedures for obtaining benefits or services under those programs; (iii) possible changes in or alternatives to those programs or procedures; or (iv) possible changes in methods or levels of payment for benefits or services under those programs; and

(2) the research could not practically be carried out without the waiver or alteration.

(d) An IRB may approve a consent procedure which does not include, or which alters, some or all of the elements of informed consent set forth in this section, or waive the requirements to obtain informed consent provided the IRB finds and documents that:

(1) the research involves no more than minimal risk to the subjects;

(2) the waiver or alteration will not adversely affect the rights and welfare of the subjects;

(3) the research could not practically be carried out without the waiver or alteration; and

(4) whenever appropriate, the subjects will be provided with additional pertinent information after participation.

(e) The informed consent requirements in this policy are not intended to preempt any applicable Federal, State, or local laws which require additional information to be disclosed in order for informed consent to be legally effective.

(f) Nothing in this policy is intended to limit the authority of a physician to provide emergency medical care, to the extent the physician is permitted to do so under applicable Federal, State, or local law.

(Approved by the Office of Management and Budget under Control Number 9999–0020.)

### §46.117 Documentation of Informed Consent

(a) Except as provided in paragraph (c) of this section, informed consent shall be documented by the use of a written consent form approved by the IRB and signed by the subject or the subject's legally authorized representative. A copy shall be given to the person signing the form.

(b) Except as provided in paragraph (c) of this section, the consent form may be either of the following:

(1) A written consent document that embodies the elements of informed consent required by §46.116. This form may be read to the subject or the subject's legally authorized representative, but in any event, the investigator shall give either the subject or the representative adequate opportunity to read it before it is signed; or

(2) A short form written consent document stating that the elements of informed consent required by §46.116 have been presented orally to the subject or the subject's legally authorized representative. When this method is used, there shall be a witness to the oral presentation. Also, the IRB shall approve a written summary of what is to be said to the subject or the representative. Only the short form itself is to be signed by the subject or the representative. However, the witness shall sign both the short form and a copy of the summary, and the person actually obtaining consent shall sign a copy of the summary. A copy of the summary shall be given to the subject or the representative, in addition to a copy of the short form.

(c) An IRB may waive the requirement for the investigator to obtain a signed consent form for some or all subjects if it finds either:

(1) That the only record linking the subject and the research would be the consent document and the principal risk would be potential harm resulting from a breach of

confidentiality. Each subject will be asked whether the subject wants documentation linking the subject with the research, and the subject's wishes will govern; or

(2) That the research presents no more than minimal risk of harm to subjects and involves no procedures for which written consent is normally required outside of the research context.

In cases in which the documentation requirement is waived, the IRB may require the investigator to provide subjects with a written statement regarding the research. (Approved by the Office of Management and Budget under Control Number 9999–0020.)

### §46.118 Applications and Proposals Lacking Definite Plans for Involvement of Human Subjects

Certain types of applications for grants, cooperative agreements, or contracts are submitted to departments or agencies with the knowledge that subjects may be involved within the period of support, but definite plans would not normally be set forth in the application or proposal. These include activities such as institutional type grants when selection of specific projects is the institution's responsibility; research training grants in which the activities involving subjects remain to be selected; and projects in which human subjects' involvement will depend upon completion of instruments, prior animal studies, or purification of compounds. These applications need not be reviewed by an IRB before an award may be made. However, except for research exempted or waived under §46.101 (b) or (i), no human subjects may be involved in any project supported by these awards until the project has been reviewed and approved by the IRB, as provided in this policy, and certification submitted, by the institution, to the Department or Agency.

### §46.119 Research Undertaken Without the Intention of Involving Human Subjects

In the event research is undertaken without the intention of involving human subjects, but it is later proposed to involve human subjects in the research, the research shall first be reviewed and approved by an IRB, as provided in this policy, a certification submitted, by the institution, to the Department or Agency, and final approval given to the proposed change by the Department or Agency.

### §46.120 Evaluation and Disposition of Applications and Proposals for Research to be Conducted or Supported by a Federal Department or Agency

(a) The Department or Agency head will evaluate all applications and proposals involving human subjects submitted to the Department or Agency through such officers and employees of the Department or Agency and such experts and consultants as the Department or Agency head determines to be appropriate. This evaluation will take into consideration the risks to the subjects, the adequacy of protection against these risks, the potential benefits of the research to the subjects and others, and the importance of the knowledge gained or to be gained.

(b) On the basis of this evaluation, the Department or Agency head may approve or disapprove the application or proposal, or enter into negotiations to develop an approvable one.

### §46.121 [Reserved]

### §46.122 Use of Federal Funds

Federal funds administered by a Department or Agency may not be expended for research involving human subjects unless the requirements of this policy have been satisfied.

### §46.123 Early Termination of Research Support: Evaluation of Applications and Proposals

(a) The Department or Agency head may require that Department or Agency support for any project be terminated or suspended in the manner prescribed in applicable program requirements, when the Department or Agency head finds an institution has materially failed to comply with the terms of this policy.

(b) In making decisions about supporting or approving applications or proposals covered by this policy the Department or Agency head may take into account, in addition to all other eligibility requirements and program criteria, factors such as whether the applicant has been subject to a termination or suspension under paragraph (a) of this section and whether the applicant or the person or persons who would direct or has/have directed the scientific and technical aspects of an activity has/have, in the judgment of the Department or Agency head, materially failed to discharge responsibility for the protection of the rights and welfare of human subjects (whether or not the research was subject to Federal regulation).

### §46.124  Conditions

With respect to any research project or any class of research projects the Department or Agency head may impose additional conditions prior to or at the time of approval when in the judgment of the Department or Agency head additional conditions are necessary for the protection of human subjects.

## Subpart B—Additional DHHS Protections Pertaining to Research, Development, and Related Activities Involving Fetuses, Pregnant Women, and Human In Vitro Fertilization

• • •

### §46.201  Applicability

(a) The regulations in this subpart are applicable to all Department of Health and Human Services grants and contracts supporting research, development, and related activities involving: (1) the fetus, (2) pregnant women, and (3) human *in vitro* fertilization.

(b) Nothing in this subpart shall be construed as indicating that compliance with the procedures set forth herein will in any way render inapplicable pertinent State or local laws bearing upon activities covered by this subpart.

(c) The requirements of this subpart are in addition to those imposed under the other subparts of this part.

### §46.202  Purpose

It is the purpose of this subpart to provide additional safeguards in reviewing activities to which this subpart is applicable to assure that they conform to appropriate ethical standards and relate to important societal needs.

### §46.203  Definitions

As used in this subpart:

(a) "Secretary" means the Secretary of Health and Human Services and any other officer or employee of the Department of Health and Human Services (DHHS) to whom authority has been delegated.

(b) "Pregnancy" encompasses the period of time from confirmation of implantation (through any of the presumptive signs of pregnancy, such as missed menses, or by a medically acceptable pregnancy test), until expulsion or extraction of the fetus.

(c) "Fetus" means the product of conception from the time of implantation (as evidenced by any of the presumptive signs of pregnancy, such as missed menses, or a medically acceptable pregnancy test), until a determination is made, following expulsion or extraction of the fetus, that it is viable.

(d) "Viable" as it pertains to the fetus means being able, after either spontaneous or induced delivery, to survive (given the benefit of available medical therapy) to the point of independently maintaining heart beat and respiration. The Secretary may from time to time, taking into account medical advances, publish in the **Federal Register** guidelines to assist in determining whether a fetus is viable for purposes of this subpart. If a fetus is viable after delivery, it is a premature infant.

(e) "Nonviable fetus" means a fetus *ex utero* which, although living, is not viable.

(f) "Dead fetus" means a fetus *ex utero* which exhibits neither heartbeat, spontaneous respiratory activity, spontaneous movement of voluntary muscles, nor pulsation of the umbilical cord (if still attached).

(g) "In vitro fertilization" means any fertilization of human ova which occurs outside the body of a female, either through admixture of donor human sperm and ova or by any other means.

### §46.204  Ethical Advisory Boards

(a) One or more Ethical Advisory Boards shall be established by the Secretary. Members of these Board(s) shall be so selected that the Board(s) will be competent to deal with medical, legal, social, ethical, and related issues and may include, for example, research scientists, physicians, psychologists, sociologists, educators, lawyers, and ethicists, as well as representatives of the general public. No Board member may be a regular, full-time employee of the Department of Health and Human Services.

(b) At the request of the Secretary, the Ethical Advisory Board shall render advice consistent with the policies and requirements of this part as to ethical issues, involving activities covered by this subpart, raised by individual applications or proposals. In addition, upon request by the Secretary, the Board shall render advice as to classes of applications or proposals and general policies, guidelines, and procedures.

(c) A Board may establish, with the approval of the Secretary, classes of applications or proposals which: (1) must be submitted to the Board, or (2) need not be submitted to the Board. Where the Board so establishes a class of applications or proposals which must be submitted, no application or proposal within the class may be funded by the Department or any component thereof until the application or proposal has been reviewed by the Board and the Board has rendered advice as to its acceptability from an ethical standpoint.

(d) No application or proposal involving human *in vitro* fertilization may be funded by the Department or any component thereof until the application or proposal has been reviewed by the Ethical Advisory Board and the Board has rendered advice as to its acceptability from an ethical standpoint.

### §46.205 Additional Duties of the Institutional Review Boards in Connection with Activities Involving Fetuses, Pregnant Women, or Human In Vitro Fertilization

(a) In addition to the responsibilities prescribed for Institutional Review Boards under Subpart A of this part, the applicant's or offeror's Board shall, with respect to activities covered by this subpart, carry out the following additional duties:

(1) determine that all aspects of the activity meet the requirements of this subpart;

(2) determine that adequate consideration has been given to the manner in which potential subjects will be selected, and adequate provision has been made by the applicant or offeror for monitoring the actual informed consent process (e.g., through such mechanisms, when appropriate, as participation by the Institutional Review Board or subject advocates in: (i) overseeing the actual process by which individual consents required by this subpart are secured either by approving induction of each individual into the activity or verifying, perhaps through sampling, that approved procedures for induction of individuals into the activity are being followed, and (ii) monitoring the progress of the activity and intervening as necessary through such steps as visits to the activity site and continuing evaluation to determine if any unanticipated risks have arisen);

(3) carry out such other responsibilities as may be assigned by the Secretary.

(b) No award may be issued until the applicant or offeror has certified to the Secretary that the Institutional Review Board has made the determinations required under paragraph (a) of this section and the Secretary has approved these determinations, as provided in §46.120 of Subpart A of this part.

(c) Applicants or offerors seeking support for activities covered by this subpart must provide for the designation of an Institutional Review Board, subject to approval by the Secretary, where no such Board has been established under Subpart A of this part.

### §46.206 General Limitations

(a) No activity to which this subpart is applicable may be undertaken unless:

(1) appropriate studies on animals and nonpregnant individuals have been completed;

(2) except where the purpose of the activity is to meet the health needs of the mother or the particular fetus, the risk to the fetus is minimal and, in all cases, is the least possible risk for achieving the objectives of the activity;

(3) individuals engaged in the activity will have no part in: (i) any decisions as to the timing, method, and procedures used to terminate the pregnancy, and (ii) determining the viability of the fetus at the termination of the pregnancy; and

(4) no procedural changes which may cause greater than minimal risk to the fetus or the pregnant woman will be introduced into the procedure for terminating the pregnancy solely in the interest of the activity.

(b) No inducements, monetary or otherwise, may be offered to terminate pregnancy for purposes of the activity.

• • •

### §46.207 Activities Directed Toward Pregnant Women as Subjects

(a) No pregnant woman may be involved as a subject in an activity covered by this subpart unless: (1) the purpose of the activity is to meet the health needs of the mother and the fetus will be placed at risk only to the minimum extent necessary to meet such needs, or (2) the risk to the fetus is minimal.

(b) An activity permitted under paragraph (a) of this section may be conducted only if the mother and father are legally competent and have given their informed consent after having been fully informed regarding possible impact on the fetus, except that the father's informed consent need not be secured if: (1) the purpose of the activity is to meet the health needs of the mother; (2) his identity or whereabouts cannot reasonably be ascertained; (3) he is not reasonably available; or (4) the pregnancy resulted from rape.

### §46.208 Activities Directed Toward Fetuses *In Utero* as Subjects

(a) No fetus *in utero* may be involved as a subject in any activity covered by this subpart unless: (1) the purpose of the activity is to meet the health needs of the particular fetus and the fetus will be placed at risk only to the minimum extent necessary to meet such needs, or (2) the risk to the fetus imposed by the research is minimal and the purpose of the activity is the development of important biomedical knowledge which cannot be obtained by other means.

(b) An activity permitted under paragraph (a) of this section may be conducted only if the mother and father are legally competent and have given their informed consent, except that the father's consent need not be secured if: (1) his identity or whereabouts cannot reasonably be ascertained, (2) he is not reasonably available, or (3) the pregnancy resulted from rape.

### §46.209 Activities Directed Toward Fetuses *Ex Utero*, Including Nonviable Fetuses, as Subjects

(a) Until it has been ascertained whether or not a fetus *ex utero* is viable, a fetus *ex utero* may not be involved as a subject in an activity covered by this subpart unless:

(1) there will be no added risk to the fetus resulting from the activity, and the purpose of the activity is the development of important biomedical knowledge which cannot be obtained by other means, or

(2) the purpose of the activity is to enhance the possibility of survival of the particular fetus to the point of viability.

(b) No nonviable fetus may be involved as a subject in an activity covered by this subpart unless:

(1) vital functions of the fetus will not be artificially maintained,

(2) experimental activities which of themselves would terminate the heartbeat or respiration of the fetus will not be employed, and

(3) the purpose of the activity is the development of important biomedical knowledge which cannot be obtained by other means.

(c) In the event the fetus *ex utero* is found to be viable, it may be included as a subject in the activity only to the extent permitted by and in accordance with the requirements of other subparts of this part.

(d) An activity permitted under paragraph (a) or (b) of this section may be conducted only if the mother and father are legally competent and have given their informed consent, except that the father's informed consent need not be secured if: (1) his identity or whereabouts cannot reasonably be ascertained, (2) he is not reasonably available, or (3) the pregnancy resulted from rape.

### §46.210 Activities Involving the Dead Fetus, Fetal Material, or the Placenta

Activities involving the dead fetus, mascerated fetal material, or cells, tissue, or organs excised from a dead fetus shall be conducted only in accordance with any applicable State or local laws regarding such activities.

### §46.211 Modification or Waiver of Specific Requirements

Upon the request of an applicant or offeror (with the approval of its Institutional Review Board), the Secretary may modify or waive specific requirements of this subpart, with the approval of the Ethical Advisory Board after such opportunity for public comment as the Ethical Advisory Board considers appropriate in the particular instance. In making such decisions, the Secretary will consider whether the risks to the subject are so outweighed by the sum of the benefit to the subject and the importance of the knowledge to be gained as to warrant such modification or waiver and that such benefits cannot be gained except through a modification or waiver. Any such modifications or waivers will be published as notices in the **Federal Register.**

### Subpart C—Additional DHHS Protections Pertaining to Biomedical and Behavioral Research Involving Prisoners as Subjects

• • •

#### §46.301  Applicability

(a) The regulations in this subpart are applicable to all biomedical and behavioral research conducted or supported by the Department of Health and Human Services involving prisoners as subjects.

(b) Nothing in this subpart shall be construed as indicating that compliance with the procedures set forth herein will authorize research involving prisoners as subjects, to the extent such research is limited or barred by applicable State or local law.

(c) The requirements of this subpart are in addition to those imposed under the other subparts of this part.

#### §46.302  Purpose

Inasmuch as prisoners may be under constraints because of their incarceration which could affect their ability to make a truly voluntary and uncoerced decision whether or not to participate as subjects in research, it is the purpose of this subpart to provide additional safeguards for the protection of prisoners involved in activities to which this subpart is applicable.

#### §46.303  Definitions

As used in this subpart:

(a) "Secretary" means the Secretary of Health and Human Services and any other officer or employee of the Department of Health and Human Services to whom authority has been delegated.

(b) "DHHS" means the Department of Health and Human Services.

(c) "Prisoner" means any individual involuntarily confined or detained in a penal institution. The term is intended to encompass individuals sentenced to such an institution under a criminal or civil statute, individuals detained in other facilities by virtue of statutes or commitment procedures which provide alternatives to criminal prosecution or incarceration in a penal institution, and individuals detained pending arraignment, trial, or sentencing.

(d) "Minimal risk" is the probability and magnitude of physical or psychological harm that is normally encountered in the daily lives, or in the routine medical, dental, or psychological examination of healthy persons.

#### §46.304  Composition of Institutional Review Boards Where Prisoners are Involved

In addition to satisfying the requirements in §46.107 of this part, an Institutional Review Board, carrying out responsibilities under this part with respect to research covered by this subpart, shall also meet the following specific requirements:

(a) A majority of the Board (exclusive of prisoner members) shall have no association with the prison(s) involved, apart from their membership on the Board.

(b) At least one member of the Board shall be a prisoner, or a prisoner representative with appropriate background and experience to serve in that capacity, except that where a particular research project is reviewed by more than one Board only one Board need satisfy this requirement.

#### §46.305  Additional Duties of the Institutional Review Boards Where Prisoners are Involved

(a) In addition to all other responsibilities prescribed for Institutional Review Boards under this part, the Board shall review research covered by this subpart and approve such research only if it finds that:

(1) the research under review represents one of the categories of research permissible under §46.306(a)(2);

(2) any possible advantages accruing to the prisoner through his or her participation in the research, when compared to the general living conditions, medical care, quality of food, amenities and opportunity for earnings in the prison, are not of such a magnitude that his or her ability to weigh the risks of the research against the value of such advantages in the limited choice environment of the prison is impaired;

(3) the risks involved in the research are commensurate with risks that would be accepted by nonprisoner volunteers;

(4) procedures for the selection of subjects within the prison are fair to all prisoners and immune from arbitrary intervention by prison authorities or prisoners. Unless the

principal investigator provides to the Board justification in writing for following some other procedures, control subjects must be selected randomly from the group of available prisoners who meet the characteristics needed for that particular research project;

(5) the information is presented in language which is understandable to the subject population;

(6) adequate assurance exists that parole boards will not take into account a prisoner's participation in the research in making decisions regarding parole, and each prisoner is clearly informed in advance that participation in the research will have no effect on his or her parole; and

(7) where the Board finds there may be a need for follow-up examination or care of participants after the end of their participation, adequate provision has been made for such examination or care, taking into account the varying lengths of individual prisoners' sentences, and for informing participants of this fact.

(b) The Board shall carry out such other duties as may be assigned by the Secretary.

(c) The institution shall certify to the Secretary, in such form and manner as the Secretary may require, that the duties of the Board under this section have been fulfilled.

### §46.306  Permitted Research Involving Prisoners

(a) Biomedical or behavioral research conducted or supported by DHHS may involve prisoners as subjects only if:

(1) the institution responsible for the conduct of the research has certified to the Secretary that the Institutional Review Board has approved the research under §46.305 of this subpart; and

(2) in the judgment of the Secretary the proposed research involves solely the following:

(A) study of the possible causes, effects, and processes of incarceration, and of criminal behavior, provided that the study presents no more than minimal risk and no more than inconvenience to the subjects;

(B) study of prisons as institutional structures or of prisoners as incarcerated persons, provided that the study presents no more than minimal risk and no more than inconvenience to the subjects;

(C) research on conditions particularly affecting prisoners as a class (for example, vaccine trials and other research on hepatitis which is much more prevalent in prisons than elsewhere; and research on social and psychological problems such as alcoholism, drug addiction, and sexual assaults) provided that the study may proceed only after the Secretary has consulted with appropriate experts including experts in penology, medicine, and ethics, and published notice, in the **Federal Register,** of his intent to approve such research; or

(D) research on practices, both innovative and accepted, which have the intent and reasonable probability of improving the health or well-being of the subject. In cases in which those studies require the assignment of prisoners in a manner consistent with protocols approved by the IRB to control groups which may not benefit from the research, the study may proceed only after the Secretary has consulted with appropriate experts, including experts in penology, medicine, and ethics, and published notice, in the **Federal Register,** of the intent to approve such research.

(b) Except as provided in paragraph (a) of this section, biomedical or behavioral research conducted or supported by DHHS shall not involve prisoners as subjects.

## Subpart D—Additional DHHS Protections for Children Involved as Subjects in Research

• • •

### §46.401  To What Do These Regulations Apply?

(a) This subpart applies to all research involving children as subjects, conducted or supported by the Department of Health and Human Services.

(1) This includes research conducted by Department employees, except that each head of an Operating Division of the Department may adopt such nonsubstantive, procedural modifications as may be appropriate from an administrative standpoint.

(2) It also includes research conducted or supported by the Department of Health and Human Services outside the United States, but in appropriate circumstances, the Secretary may, under paragraph (e) of §46.101 of Subpart A, waive the applicability of some or all of the requirements of these regulations for research of this type.

(b) Exemptions at §46.101(b)(1) and (b)(3) through (b)(6) are applicable to this subpart. The exemption at §46.101(b)(2) regarding educational tests is also applicable to this subpart. However, the exemption at §46.101(b)(2) for research involving survey or interview procedures or observations of public behavior does not apply to research covered by this subpart, except for research involving observation of public behavior when the investigator(s) do not participate in the activities being observed.

(c) The exceptions, additions, and provisions for waiver as they appear in paragraphs (c) through (i) of §46.101 of Subpart A are applicable to this subpart.

### §46.402  Definitions

The definitions in §46.102 of Subpart A shall be applicable to this subpart as well. In addition, as used in this subpart:

(a) "Children" are persons who have not attained the legal age for consent to treatments or procedures involved in the research, under the applicable law of the jurisdiction in which the research will be conducted.

(b) "Assent" means a child's affirmative agreement to participate in research. Mere failure to object should not, absent affirmative agreement, be construed as assent.

(c) "Permission" means the agreement of parent(s) or guardian to the participation of their child or ward in research.

(d) "Parent" means a child's biological or adoptive parent.

(e) "Guardian" means an individual who is authorized under applicable State or local law to consent on behalf of a child to general medical care.

### §46.403  IRB Duties

In addition to other responsibilities assigned to IRBs under this part, each IRB shall review research covered by this subpart and approve only research which satisfies the conditions of all applicable sections of this subpart.

### §46.404  Research Not Involving Greater Than Minimal Risk

DHHS will conduct or fund research in which the IRB finds that no greater than minimal risk to children is presented, only if the IRB finds that adequate provisions are made for soliciting the assent of the children and the permission of their parents or guardians, as set forth in §46.408.

### §46.405  Research Involving Greater Than Minimal Risk But Presenting the Prospect of Direct Benefit to the Individual Subjects

DHHS will conduct or fund research in which the IRB finds that more than minimal risk to children is presented by an intervention or procedure that holds out the prospect of direct benefit for the individual subject, or by a monitoring procedure that is likely to contribute to the subject's well-being, only if the IRB finds that:

(a) the risk is justified by the anticipated benefit to the subjects;

(b) the relation of the anticipated benefit to risk is at least as favorable to the subjects as that presented by available alternative approaches; and

(c) adequate provisions are made for soliciting the assent of the children and permission of their parents or guardians, as set forth in §46.408.

### §46.406  Research Involving Greater Than Minimal Risk and No Prospect of Direct Benefit to Individual Subjects, But Likely to Yield Generalizable Knowledge About the Subject's Disorder or Condition

DHHS will conduct or fund research in which the IRB finds that more than minimal risk to children is presented by an intervention or procedure that does not hold out the prospect of direct benefit for the individual subject, or by a monitoring procedure which is not likely to contribute to the well-being of the subject, only if the IRB finds that:

(a) the risk represents a minor increase over minimal risk;

(b) the intervention or procedure presents experiences to subjects that are reasonably commensurate with those inherent in their actual or expected medical, dental, psychological, social, or educational situations;

(c) the intervention or procedure is likely to yield generalizable knowledge about the subjects' disorder or condition which is of vital importance for the understanding or amelioration of the subjects' disorder or condition; and

(d) adequate provisions are made for soliciting assent of the children and permission of their parents or guardians, as set forth in §46.408.

### §46.407  Research Not Otherwise Approvable Which Presents an Opportunity to Understand, Prevent, or Alleviate a Serious Problem Affecting the Health or Welfare of Children

DHHS will conduct or fund research that the IRB does not believe meets the requirements of §46.404, §46.405, or §46.406 only if:

(a) the IRB finds that the research presents a reasonable opportunity to further the understanding, prevention, or alleviation of a serious problem affecting the health or welfare of children; and

(b) the Secretary, after consultation with a panel of experts in pertinent disciplines (for example: science, medicine, education, ethics, law) and following opportunity for public review and comment, has determined either:

(1) that the research in fact satisfies the conditions of §46.404, §46.405, or §46.406, as applicable, or (2) the following:

(i) the research presents a reasonable opportunity to further the understanding, prevention, or alleviation of a serious problem affecting the health or welfare of children;

(ii) the research will be conducted in accordance with sound ethical principles;

(iii) adequate provisions are made for soliciting the assent of children and the permission of their parents or guardians, as set forth in §46.408.

### §46.408 Requirements for Permission by Parents or Guardians and for Assent by Children

(a) In addition to the determinations required under other applicable sections of this subpart, the IRB shall determine that adequate provisions are made for soliciting the assent of the children, when in the judgment of the IRB the children are capable of providing assent. In determining whether children are capable of assenting, the IRB shall take into account the ages, maturity, and psychological state of the children involved. This judgment may be made for all children to be involved in research under a particular protocol, or for each child, as the IRB deems appropriate. If the IRB determines that the capability of some or all of the children is so limited that they cannot reasonably be consulted or that the intervention or procedure involved in the research holds out a prospect of direct benefit that is important to the health or well-being of the children and is available only in the context of the research, the assent of the children is not a necessary condition for proceeding with the research. Even where the IRB determines that the subjects are capable of assenting, the IRB may still waive the assent requirement under circumstances in which consent may be waived in accord with §46.116 of Subpart A.

(b) In addition to the determinations required under other applicable sections of this subpart, the IRB shall determine, in accordance with and to the extent that consent is required by §46.116 of Subpart A, that adequate provisions are made for soliciting the permission of each child's parents or guardian. Where parental permission is to be obtained, the IRB may find that the permission of one parent is sufficient for research to be conducted under §46.404 or §46.405. Where research is covered by §46.406 and §46.407 and permission is to be obtained from parents, both parents must give their permission unless one parent is deceased, unknown, incompetent, or not reasonably available, or when only one parent has legal responsibility for the care and custody of the child.

(c) In addition to the provisions for waiver contained in §46.116 of Subpart A, if the IRB determines that a research protocol is designed for conditions or for a subject population for which parental or guardian permission is not a reasonable requirement to protect the subjects (for example, neglected or abused children), it may waive the consent requirements in Subpart A of this part and paragraph (b) of this section, provided an appropriate mechanism for protecting the children who will participate as subjects in the research is substituted, and provided further that the waiver is not inconsistent with Federal, State, or local law. The choice of an appropriate mechanism would depend upon the nature and purpose of the activities described in the protocol, the risk and anticipated benefit to the research subjects, and their age, maturity, status, and condition.

(d) Permission by parents or guardians shall be documented in accordance with and to the extent required by §46.117 of Subpart A.

(e) When the IRB determines that assent is required, it shall also determine whether and how assent must be documented.

### §46.409 Wards

(a) Children who are wards of the State or any other agency, institution, or entity can be included in research approved under §46.406 or §46.407 only if such research is:

(1) related to their status as wards; or

(2) conducted in schools, camps, hospitals, institutions, or similar settings in which the majority of children involved as subjects are not wards.

(b) If the research is approved under paragraph (a) of this section, the IRB shall require appointment of an advocate for each child who is a ward, in addition to any other individual acting on behalf of the child as guardian or in loco parentis. One individual may serve as advocate for more than one child. The advocate shall be an individual who has the background and experience to act in, and agrees to act in, the best interests of the child for the duration of the child's participation in the research and who is not associated in any way (except in the role as advocate or member of the IRB) with the research, the investigator(s), or the guardian organization.

• • •

# SUMMARY REPORT OF THE INTERNATIONAL SUMMIT CONFERENCE ON BIOETHICS TOWARDS AN INTERNATIONAL ETHIC FOR RESEARCH INVOLVING HUMAN SUBJECTS
1987

*Twenty-six delegates, nominated by the heads of state of the Economic Summit nations, by the European Economic Community, and by the World Health Organization, met at the fourth Bioethics Summit Conference in Ottawa, Canada, on April 5–10, 1987. The Summary Report addresses the major areas discussed at the conference and presents both the background and the major recommendations of the delegates for improving the protection of research subjects throughout the world. The recommendations are shown in boldface within the text.*

## 1. Introduction

Rapid progress in bioscience has created an urgent need for continuing development of national standards of ethics in research with human subjects. The growing interdependence of nations throughout the world has stimulated a need for internationally agreed upon standards and practices based on a careful continuing dialogue and reflection on values. The delegates at the fourth International Summit Conference on Bioethics worked towards these goals. They focused not only on the principles, but more specifically on the practice and procedures guaranteeing their implementation.

The fourth in a series of annual bioethics summit meetings initiated by Prime Minister Nakasone in 1984, this meeting reflected deeply on an area important to the entire practice of bioscience and medical research. It is hoped that the discussions and recommendations will benefit national practices, and contribute to improved international standards.

We, the delegates to this meeting, invite the Prime Minister of Canada, the Right Honourable Brian Mulroney, to present this report to the next Economic Summit Conference, to be held in Italy in June, 1987.

## 2. Underlying Principles and Practices: Development and Implementation of National Ethics Standards

The underlying principles for the ethics of research with human subjects are defined in national and international codes. These include respect for individuals, contribution to the well-being of peoples, and the equitable distribution of potential risks and benefits throughout society. Even though only very general international guidelines have been accepted, as yet, uniform practices are not widely accepted due to national and cultural differences.

Though need for societal review of research proposals is generally accepted, there are great differences in how countries and even institutions within some countries carry out this review. Only some of these variations can be ascribed to the cultural differences which are an essential background to societal standards.

As national standards are established, consideration must be given to evolving international guidelines for research involving human subjects. These will permit research jointly undertaken between nations and amongst groups of nations using common protocols, stimulate sharing of research results amongst nations and avoid unnecessary duplication and multiplication of research efforts.

The question of how common standards can best be developed and implemented considering the present diversity in practice and the complexity of the biomedical research enterprise occupied much of the discussion.

For that reason, the delegates recommend that, **in order to safeguard the rights and well-being of patients and research subjects, research ethics committees should be established in all countries. All research projects involving human subjects must be submitted for approval to a research ethics committee.**

It is further recommended that **these committees should be comprised of medical experts, and of experts outside the medical profession (e.g. theologians, moral philosophers, lawyers and lay members who represent the general public). Lawyers acting professionally for an institution, and others having a financial interest or potentially conflicting interest in the institution or the research in question should not serve on the ethics committee adjudicating that research. Furthermore, the committees should be of a size which is sufficient to allow for the inclusion of the three groups (medical experts, outside experts and lay members) and small enough to make efficient work possible.**

Delegates also considered the means of operation, freedoms and accountabilities of the research ethics committees. The decisions which they must take often reflect fine-tuning of competing values, and the scientific, technical or cultural environments within which they work may vary. Therefore, some differences of views between research ethics committees should be expected. Delegates were of the view that, while there may well be a need for nations to monitor the functioning of local research ethics committees, the highest standards can best be assured if they are given responsibility and authority for the review of research ethics in their institutions; as well, their effect will be enhanced if seen by researchers and society as working with the research process in a collegial sense rather than in an adversarial mode.

### 3. Sharing the Risks

Three groups in society can be identified as carrying risks and benefits. The researchers or clinicians who carry out the trials and other research carry the primary burdens of ethical responsibility for protection of the research subjects. In the context of drug testing, the risks and costs of developing a new drug or device remain with the manufacturer. Nevertheless, the human beings on whom the research is performed carry the most direct risks of research, but can gain the benefits of the higher standards. Society or mankind as a whole is the ultimate beneficiary from research towards improved health standards, and for that reason, the delegates recommend **that human research subjects be fully informed concerning the availability or the lack of availability of mechanisms of care and compensation to subjects who are injured as a result of their participation in research.** The delegates encourage member nations to establish and implement appropriate mechanisms for care and compensation in areas where they do not presently exist.

### 4. Public Participation

The delegates agreed that the imposition of societal standards on the sensitive areas raised by medical research demand the involvement of the general public. Public involvement is required not only in the development of consensus but also in consideration of individual research proposals to ensure full and open discussion which might otherwise be uncritical or too narrowly based. The multi-disciplinary character of research ethics committees provides for both public accountability and credibility.

### 5. Research with Those with Restricted Ability to Give Consent

The overriding purpose of ethics review is the protection of the research subjects. An essential component of this protection, enunciated in all international codes of ethics, is that each research subject must consent freely, and with full information, to participate in the research. However, those who are legally incompetent cannot, by definition, give their consent. Delegates focused their discussion of this issue on research with children, while recognizing that similar concerns arise with adults who are mentally handicapped and with other vulnerable populations.

All delegates accepted the need for therapeutic research with children. Such research would be of potentially direct benefit to the well-being of the individual subjects.

Non-therapeutic research with children poses special problems. While such research is necessary if treatment of childhood diseases is to advance, there was agreement that such research could only be considered under the following conditions: the specific project must be approved by a research ethics committee; all needed knowledge must have been obtained through research with adults or animals; there must be no valid alternative to the use of children in the research; a valid proxy consent (by family, guardians, ombudsman, those with power of attorney or others) must have been obtained for each research subject; and, to the extent possible, the child should have given assent. Thus, it was the view of most delegates that needed non-therapeutic research on children, if within the limitations just mentioned and if involving minimal or no risk to such children, should not be precluded.

## 6. Research with Embryos

The integrity and uniqueness of human life in its earliest embryonic stages of formation must be accorded great respect. Generally, current forms of control of research procedures and manipulation of human embryos are not legislative in nature. In fact, in the almost total absence of legislation, research on the embryo is presently, for the most part, governed by the self-regulatory efforts of scientific and professional bodies, the centres themselves, and the review by ethics committees, local and national. Voluntary licensing control exists, for example in England, but there was consensus on the need to regulate the current anarchic proliferation and operation of *in vitro* fertilization centres in some countries as an interim measure while acquiring the experience necessary for effective legislation. Thus the delegates recommended **the need to keep in balance the professional liberty for clinical treatment and for scientific inquiry in the interest of progress in medical knowledge and skill while upholding regard for the human interest in the embryo.** To this end, the delegates recommend **the supervision and control of centres offering** *in vitro* **fertilization, of related treatments for infertility and of those conducting embryo research. Procedure should be regulated according to appropriate guidelines administered by a competent authority.**

All delegates recognized the preciousness of the human embryo. Nevertheless, different positions were taken with respect to the possibility of permitting research on the human embryo.

Several questions were raised with respect to the applicability of legal concepts of "ownership" (more properly discussed in terms of legitimate interest in) and control of human embryos during storage or after the death of the donors. Questions were also raised concerning penal sanction as opposed to professional regulation.

Considering the experimental nature of *in vitro* fertilization, its low success rate and the unknown long term effect of these procedures, which though "therapeutic" in nature for the infertile have implications for the manipulation and control of human life, **any work with embryos even as a treatment for infertility should be regarded as developmental procedures that are experimental in nature and therefore should be closely monitored.**

## 7. Pilot Studies and the Introduction of Novel Therapies

Delegates debated the special problem of ethics review of pilot studies or preliminary studies of medical innovations. Such studies were viewed as a phase between the initial observations on one or a few patients and the start of a full fledged protocol-based program.

Delegates recognized that it is often not easy to be sure whether an intervention by a physician should be regarded as a treatment undertaken only in the patient's best interest, or whether it is guided also by an intent to gain scientific knowledge.

The decision on when a research intent is present in therapy is a determination to be made by the physician. It was the opinion of the delegates that, if the health professional has any doubt whether the intervention is in fact research, the issue would best be brought to the attention of the ethics committee.

In reviewing the novel therapy of research, delegates recommended that **they should be subject to the same ethical judgements that apply to all research protocols. Special consideration should be given to limiting the number of subjects entered into pilot studies and to monitoring closely and frequently.**

In ethics review of pilot studies as in that of other proposed research, the delegates agreed that provision should be made for a mechanism to re-examine a research project rejected by a research ethics committee if the investigator should request it. Such a mechanism should be of a sort which would not invite the overriding of local decisions by a higher or distant authority. It should maintain the collaborative nature of the relationship between the researcher and the ethics committee, rather than encourage an adversarial relationship. It was also agreed that there should be a greater exchange of information between research ethics committees.

## 8. Industrial Research

Industries are a major source of medical innovation. Also much of their research is mandated by national standards for licensing drugs or devices. This research involves both animals and human beings and is often carried out in a number of countries. For that reason, the interactions between industries, governments and sometimes universities are of great concern.

Differences in the way ethics standards are interpreted and implemented can have direct economic effects. Lack of consistency can adversely affect national and commercial interests as well as the safety of research subjects. Delegates recommended that, at the very least, **a nation should not allow or support, in other countries, research which does not conform to ethics review standards at least equivalent to those in force within the nation.** Nations and industries should develop international accords which strive for common attitudes and the exchangeability of standards and for mutual trust. Nations and industries should also identify emerging technologies to foster early discussion of the ethical concerns. Such interaction might help the equitable distribution of effort in research and development.

Delegates also discussed the ethical concerns raised by the growing pace of commercialization of biomedical products. The increasingly close links between university-based and industry-based research mean that academic physicians or institutions may have financial interests in the outcome of the research; any such potential conflicts of interest should be declared in the research ethics review process. Moreover, it was the opinion of some delegates that we should develop and implement values which integrate ethics and economic interests.

Delegates also discussed the effects of confidentiality, and of compensation of research subjects. The confidentiality of commercially sensitive material may not be consistent with the requirements for ethics review. In addition, payment can induce subjects, especially those of more limited means, to participate in research, and may lead to financial competition for research subjects. With respect to both industrial and other research, concern was expressed over whether patients will be compensated for adverse effects which may on rare occasions arise from research.

Much industrial research and other biomedical research depends on research with animals. Delegates recommended that **in all research we must continue to insist that animal research precede research on humans, while recognizing the obligation to reduce the number of animals required to a minimum wherever possible and to encourage alternative methods for assessing safety and efficacy.**

Much of the regulatory testing of new drugs still requires the use of animals. In this regard, delegates recommended that **governmental agencies continuously modernize their own regulatory requirements to ensure that they do not demand test results of safety and toxicology which are no longer relevant or which can be replaced by satisfactory alternatives requiring fewer animals.**

## 9. The Selection of Research Topics and Directed Research

Researchers consider many scientific, social and other factors when choosing research topics; choices are also made in the context of national policies and systems of support as well as national policies and practices in respect to ethics. In some instances, this results in an apparent imbalance between the research topics being chosen and major global needs for research in fields such as fertility regulation and tropical diseases.

International research programs can provide a successful mechanism to promote and carry out research in those areas which are neglected, sensitive and/or economically unattractive to national researchers. These programs can make extensive use of the international scientific community and can apply high standards of scientific and ethical review to carry out research in the areas of high global priority which are difficult to address on a national basis. Those nations with the means to support research have an obligation to devote some of those resources to the research needs of nations without such means.

The group recommended that **research should focus upon the development of knowledge in broad fields of science with the aim of achieving a fundamental understanding of biological processes, even those which might not appear to have direct application over the short or longer term.** It is seen as a scientific infrastructure of further advance. It was also recommended that **the results of research should be applied as rapidly and as effectively as possible.**

Large scale support for narrowly focussed research on specific diseases without the necessary foundation of scientific knowledge was seen as rarely, if ever, successful. Also the failure to implement the results of research for the benefit of mankind has, in itself, serious ethical implications.

## 10. Towards Improved Ethics Standards: Biomedical Research in an Interdependent World

The last decade has witnessed profound growth in improved communication and common endeavor among nations. As well, movement has begun towards international agreement on research with human subjects.

Delegates are certain that meaningful international agreement is not only possible but necessary, and urge the Heads of States to work toward ensuring that practice accords with principles in all aspects of research involving human subjects.

The delegates accept that society should make the human subject an active and educated participant in a process in which he or she contributes from a sense of basic human altruism and a desire to serve the common good, rather than as a "subject of research" as has sometimes been the case in the past.

The further refinement and expansion of national standards of research ethics with human subjects across political and cultural boundaries demand continuing investigation into the ethical problems of biomedical research. Furthermore while agreeing on the necessity for this ethical review process, the delegates recommended that **these committees themselves, their operations and their functions be studied.**

According to the delegates, research ethics should always be integrated into clinical decision making. The delegates recommended that **education in medical ethics for physicians, investigators and medical students be intensified and that the media and public be informed.**

Delegates also recommended that **special attention be given to the ethical issues involved in epidemiological studies which can be as intrusive of human dignity and privacy as medical intervention.** In particular, the regulation of confidentiality, which may both restrict the exchange and gathering of information and may at the same time fail adequately to protect the subject of such epidemiological studies, requires examination.

In regard to dissemination of principles, statements by way of declaration are laudable and necessary. However, if such statements are to have proper binding power, they must be known and an effort made to ensure compliance with them. To assist in this endeavor and in view of the importance of continuing dialogue, delegates recommended the **establishment of appropriate fora devoted to the issues arising in research with human subjects.**

## Conclusions

This conference affirmed the growing importance of international agreement and cooperation on both the elaboration of principle and on the implementation of ethics review processes in medical research involving human subjects. To this end, the establishment of multi-disciplinary research ethics review bodies for the examination of research protocols was considered essential, as was further study and communication among nations.

Implementation of effective ethics review processes demands the enhanced education in medical ethics both of those involved in research and of the greater public.

The development of national and international standards for research with human subjects and their implementation must continue to aim at the protection of more vulnerable subjects.

The promulgation of ethics standards for research across nations and cultures should focus on areas of concern, as well as on international needs that are not being met.

# RECOMMENDATION NO. R (90) 3
## OF THE COMMITTEE OF MINISTERS TO MEMBER STATES CONCERNING MEDICAL RESEARCH ON HUMAN BEINGS
### Council of Europe
#### 1990

*In their recommendation concerning medical research on human beings, adopted February 6, 1990, the Committee of Ministers of the Council of Europe recommended that the governments of member states adopt legislation or take any other measures to ensure the implementation of the principles articulated as well as ensuring that the provisions adopted be brought to the knowledge of all persons concerned. When the recommendation was adopted, the representative of the Federal Republic of Germany reserved the right of his government to comply with it or not. Although delegates from other countries were not so explicit, other European countries are entitled to the same reservation.*

The Committee of Ministers, under the terms of Article 15.*b* of the Statute of the Council of Europe,

• • •

Being aware of the fact that the advancement of medical science and practice is dependent on knowledge and discovery which necessitate, as a last resort, experimentation on human beings;

Being convinced that medical research should never be carried out contrary to human dignity;

Considering the paramount concern to be the protection of the person undergoing medical research;

Considering that particular protection should be given to certain groups of persons;

Considering that every person has a right to accept or to refuse to undergo medical research and that no one should be forced to undergo it;

Considering that medical research on human beings should take into account ethical principles, and should also be subject to legal provisions;

Realising that in member states existing legal provisions are either divergent or insufficient in this field;

Noting the wish and the need to harmonise legislation,

Recommends the governments of member states:

a. to adopt legislation in conformity with the principles appended to this recommendation, or to take any other measures in order to ensure their implementation;

b. to ensure that the provisions so adopted are brought to the knowledge of all persons concerned.

## Principles Concerning Medical Research on Human Beings

### Scope and Definition

For the purpose of application of these principles, medical research means any trial and experimentation carried out on human beings, the purpose of which or one of the purposes of which is to increase medical knowledge.

### Principle 1

Any medical research must be carried out within the framework of a scientific plan and in accordance with the following principles.

### Principle 2

1. In medical research the interests and well-being of the person undergoing medical research must always prevail over the interests of science and society.

2. The risks incurred by a person undergoing medical research must be kept to a minimum. The risks should not be disproportionate to the benefits to that person or the importance of the aims pursued by the research.

### Principle 3

1. No medical research may be carried out without the informed, free, express and specific consent of the person undergoing it. Such consent may be freely withdrawn at any phase of the research and the person undergoing the research should be informed, before being included in it, of his right to withdraw his consent.

2. The person who is to undergo medical research should be given information on the purpose of the research and the methodology of the experimentation. He should also be informed of the foreseeable risks and inconveniences to him of the proposed research. This information should be sufficiently clear and suitably adapted to enable consent to be given or refused in full knowledge of the relevant facts.

3. The provisions of this principle should apply also to a legal representative and to a legally incapacitated person having the capacity of understanding, in the situations described in Principles 4 and 5.

### Principle 4

A legally incapacitated person may only undergo medical research where authorized by Principle 5 and if his legal representative, or an authority or an individual authorised or designated under his national law, consents. If the legally incapacitated person is capable of understanding, his consent is also required and no research may be undertaken if he does not give his consent.

### Principle 5

1. A legally incapacitated person may not undergo medical research unless it is expected to produce a direct and significant benefit to his health.

2. However, by way of exception, national law may authorise research involving a legally incapacitated person which is not of direct benefit to his health when that person offers no objection, provided that the research is to the benefit of persons in the same category and that the same scientific results cannot be obtained by research on persons who do not belong to this category.

### Principle 6

Pregnant or nursing women may not undergo medical research where their health and/or that of the child would not benefit directly unless this research is aimed at benefiting other women and children who are in the same position and the same scientific results cannot be obtained by research on women who are not pregnant or nursing.

### Principle 7

Persons deprived of liberty may not undergo medical research unless it is expected to produce a direct and significant benefit to their health.

### Principle 8

In an emergency situation, notwithstanding Principle 3, where a patient is unable to give a prior consent, medical research can be carried out only when the following conditions are fulfilled:
—the research must have been planned to be carried out in the emergency in question;
—the systematic research plan must have been approved by an ethics committee;
—the research must be intended for the direct health benefit of the patient.

### Principle 9

Any information of a personal nature obtained during medical research should be treated as confidential.

### Principle 10

Medical research may not be carried out unless satisfactory evidence as to its safety for the person undergoing research is furnished.

### Principle 11

Medical research that is not in accordance with scientific criteria in its design and cannot answer the questions posed is unacceptable even if the way it is to be carried out poses no risk to the person undergoing research.

### Principle 12

1. Medical research must be carried out under the responsibility of a doctor or a person who exercises full clinical responsibility and who possesses appropriate knowledge and qualifications to meet any clinical contingency.
2. The responsible doctor or other person referred to in the preceding paragraph should enjoy full professional independence and should have the power to stop the research at any time.

### Principle 13

1. Potential subjects of medical research should not be offered any inducement which compromises free consent. Persons undergoing medical research should not gain any financial benefit. However, expenses and any financial loss may be refunded and in appropriate cases a modest allowance may be given for any inconvenience inherent in the medical research.
2. If the person undergoing research is legally incapacitated, his legal representatives should not receive any form of remuneration whatever, except for the refund of their expenses.

### Principle 14

1. Persons undergoing medical research and/or their dependents should be compensated for injury and loss caused by the medical research.
2. Where there is no existing system providing compensation for the persons concerned, states should ensure that sufficient guarantees for such compensation are provided.
3. Terms and conditions which exclude or limit, in advance, compensation to the victim should be considered to be null and void.

**Principle 15**

All proposed medical research plans should be the subject of an ethical examination by an independent and multidisciplinary committee.

**Principle 16**

Any medical research which is:
—unplanned, or
—contrary to any of the preceding principles, or
—in any other way contrary to ethics or law, or
—not in accordance with scientific methods in its design and cannot answer the questions posed should be prohibited or, if it has already begun, stopped or revised, even if it poses no risk to the person(s) undergoing the research.

# INTERNATIONAL ETHICAL GUIDELINES FOR BIOMEDICAL RESEARCH INVOLVING HUMAN SUBJECTS
### Council for International Organizations of Medical Sciences (CIOMS) in collaboration with the World Health Organization
### 1993

*These guidelines replace the Proposed International Guidelines for Biomedical Research Involving Human Subjects issued by CIOMS in 1982. Like the 1982 document, the current guidelines are intended to help inform national policies on the ethics of biomedical research, apply ethical standards at the local level, and define adequate mechanisms for the ethical review of human subjects research, particularly in developing countries. The steering committee that oversaw the revisions decided that emphasis should be placed on epidemiological studies, which ultimately resulted in the "International Guidelines for Ethical Review of Epidemiological Studies," issued by CIOMS in 1991. Preparation of the epidemiological guidelines greatly influenced the 1993 Guidelines for Biomedical Research Involving Human Subjects.*

*In addition to a statement of general ethical principles, a preamble, and fifteen guidelines with extensive interpretive commentary on each, the full text includes an introduction and brief account of earlier international declarations and guidelines. The statement of general ethical principles and the fifteen guidelines are excerpted below.*

• • •

## General Ethical Principles

All research involving human subjects should be conducted in accordance with three basic ethical principles, namely respect for persons, beneficence and justice. It is generally agreed that these principles, which in the abstract have equal moral force, guide the conscientious preparation of proposals for scientific studies. In varying circumstances they may be expressed differently and given different moral weight, and their application may lead to different decisions or courses of action. The present guidelines are directed at the application of these principles to research involving human subjects.

**Respect for persons** incorporates at least two fundamental ethical considerations, namely:
   a) respect for autonomy, which requires that those who are capable of deliberation about their personal choices should be treated with respect for their capacity for self-determination; and
   b) protection of persons with impaired or diminished autonomy, which requires that those who are dependent or vulnerable be afforded security against harm or abuse.

**Beneficence** refers to the ethical obligation to maximize benefits and to minimize harms and wrongs. This principle gives rise to norms requiring that the risks of research be reasonable in the light of the expected benefits, that the research design be sound, and that the investigators be competent both to conduct the research and to safeguard the welfare of the research subjects. Beneficence further proscribes the deliberate infliction of harm on persons; this aspect of beneficence is sometimes expressed as a separate principle, **nonmaleficence** (do no harm).

**Justice** refers to the ethical obligation to treat each person in accordance with what is morally right and proper, to give each person what is due to him or her. In the ethics of research involving human subjects the principle refers primarily to **distributive justice,** which requires the equitable distribution of both the burdens and the benefits of participation in research. Differences in distribution of burdens and benefits are justifiable only if they are based on morally relevant distinctions between persons; one such distinction is vulnerability. "Vulnerability" refers to a substantial incapacity to protect one's own interests owing to such impediments as lack of capability to give informed consent, lack of alternative means of obtaining medical care or other expensive necessities, or being a junior or subordinate member of a hierarchical group. Accordingly, special provisions must be made for the protection of the rights and welfare of vulnerable persons.

. . .

## The Guidelines

### Informed Consent of Subjects

*Guideline 1: Individual informed consent*
For all biomedical research involving human subjects, the investigator must obtain the informed consent of the prospective subject or, in the case of an individual who is not capable of giving informed consent, the proxy consent of a properly authorized representative.

. . .

*Guideline 2: Essential information for prospective research subjects*
Before requesting an individual's consent to participate in research, the investigator must provide the individual with the following information, in language that he or she is capable of understanding:
- —that each individual is invited to participate as a subject in research, and the aims and methods of the research;
- —the expected duration of the subject's participation;
- —the benefits that might reasonably be expected to result to the subject or to others as an outcome of the research;
- —any foreseeable risks or discomfort to the subject, associated with participation in the research;
- —any alternative procedures or courses of treatment that might be as advantageous to the subject as the procedure or treatment being tested;
- —the extent to which confidentiality of records in which the subject is identified will be maintained;
- —the extent of the investigator's responsibility, if any, to provide medical services to the subject;
- —that therapy will be provided free of charge for specified types of research-related injury;
- —whether the subject or the subject's family or dependents will be compensated for disability or death resulting from such injury; and
- —that the individual is free to refuse to participate and will be free to withdraw from the research at any time without penalty or loss of benefits to which he or she would otherwise be entitled.

. . .

*Guideline 3: Obligations of investigators regarding informed consent*
The investigator has a duty to:
- —communicate to the prospective subject all the information necessary for adequately informed consent;
- —give the prospective subject full opportunity and encouragement to ask questions;
- —exclude the possibility of unjustified deception, undue influence and intimidation;
- —seek consent only after the prospective subject has adequate knowledge of the relevant facts and of the consequences of participation, and has had sufficient opportunity to consider whether to participate;
- —as a general rule, obtain from each prospective subject a signed form as evidence of informed consent; and
- —renew the informed consent of each subject if there are material changes in the conditions or procedures of the research.

. . .

*Guideline 4: Inducement to participate*
Subjects may be paid for inconvenience and time spent, and should be reimbursed for expenses incurred, in connection with their participation in research; they may also receive free medical services. However, the payments should not be so large or the medical services so extensive as to induce prospective subjects to consent to participate in

the research against their better judgment ("undue inducement"). All payments, reimbursements and medical services to be provided to research subjects should be approved by an ethical review committee.

• • •

*Guideline 5: Research involving children*
Before undertaking research involving children, the investigator must ensure that:
—children will not be involved in research that might equally well be carried out with adults;
—the purpose of the research is to obtain knowledge relevant to the health needs of children;
—a parent or legal guardian of each child has given proxy consent;
—the consent of each child has been obtained to the extent of the child's capabilities;
—the child's refusal to participate in research must always be respected unless according to the research protocol the child would receive therapy for which there is no medically-acceptable alternative;
—the risk presented by interventions not intended to benefit the individual child-subject is low and commensurate with the importance of the knowledge to be gained; and
—interventions that are intended to provide therapeutic benefit are likely to be at least as advantageous to the individual child-subject as any available alternative.

• • •

*Guideline 6: Research involving persons with mental or behavioural disorders*
Before undertaking research involving individuals who by reason of mental or behavioural disorders are not capable of giving adequately informed consent, the investigator must ensure that:
—such persons will not be subjects of research that might equally well be carried out on persons in full possession of their mental faculties;
—the purpose of the research is to obtain knowledge relevant to the particular health needs of persons with mental or behavioural disorders;
—the consent of each subject has been obtained to the extent of that subject's capabilities, and a prospective subject's refusal to participate in non-clinical research is always respected;
—in the case of incompetent subjects, informed consent is obtained from the legal guardian or other duly authorized person;
—the degree of risk attached to interventions that are not intended to benefit the individual subject is low and commensurate with the importance of the knowledge to be gained; and
—interventions that are intended to provide therapeutic benefit are likely to be at least as advantageous to the individual subject as any alternative.

• • •

*Guideline 7: Research involving prisoners*
Prisoners with serious illness or at risk of serious illness should not arbitrarily be denied access to investigational drugs, vaccines or other agents that show promise of therapeutic or preventive benefit.

• • •

*Guideline 8: Research involving subjects in underdeveloped communities*
Before undertaking research involving subjects in underdeveloped communities, whether in developed or developing countries, the investigator must ensure that:
—persons in underdeveloped communities will not ordinarily be involved in research that could be carried out reasonably well in developed communities;
—the research is responsive to the health needs and the priorities of the community in which it is to be carried out;
—every effort will be made to secure the ethical imperative that the consent of individual subjects be informed; and
—the proposals for the research have been reviewed and approved by an ethical review committee that has among its members or consultants persons who are thoroughly familiar with the customs and traditions of the community.

• • •

*Guideline 9: Informed consent in epidemiological studies*
For several types of epidemiological research individual informed consent is either impracticable or inadvisable. In such cases the ethical review committee should determine

whether it is ethically acceptable to proceed without individual informed consent and whether the investigator's plans to protect the safety and respect the privacy of research subjects and to maintain the confidentiality of the data are adequate.

• • •

### Selection of Research Subjects

*Guideline 10: Equitable distribution of burdens and benefits*
Individuals or communities to be invited to be subjects of research should be selected in such a way that the burdens and benefits of the research will be equitably distributed. Special justification is required for inviting vulnerable individuals and, if they are selected, the means of protecting their rights and welfare must be particularly strictly applied.

• • •

*Guideline 11: Selection of pregnant or nursing (breastfeeding) women as research subjects*
Pregnant or nursing women should in no circumstances be the subjects of non-clinical research unless the research carries no more than minimal risk to the fetus or nursing infant and the object of the research is to obtain new knowledge about pregnancy or lactation. As a general rule, pregnant or nursing women should not be subjects of any clinical trials except such trials as are designed to protect or advance the health of pregnant or nursing women or fetuses or nursing infants, and for which women who are not pregnant or nursing would not be suitable subjects.

• • •

### Confidentiality of Data

*Guideline 12: Safeguarding confidentiality*
The investigator must establish secure safeguards of the confidentiality of research data. Subjects should be told of the limits to the investigators' ability to safeguard confidentiality and of the anticipated consequences of breaches of confidentiality.

• • •

### Compensation of Research Subjects for Accidental Injury

*Guideline 13: Right of subjects to compensation*
Research subjects who suffer physical injury as a result of their participation are entitled to such financial or other assistance as would compensate them equitably for any temporary or permanent impairment or disability. In the case of death, their dependents are entitled to material compensation. The right to compensation may not be waived.

• • •

### Review Procedures

*Guideline 14: Constitution and responsibilities of ethical review committees*
All proposals to conduct research involving human subjects must be submitted for review and approval to one or more independent ethical and scientific review committees. The investigator must obtain such approval of the proposal to conduct research before the research is begun.

• • •

### Externally Sponsored Research

*Guideline 15: Obligations of sponsoring and host countries*
Externally sponsored research entails two ethical obligations:
- An external sponsoring agency should submit the research protocol to ethical and scientific review according to the standards of the country of the sponsoring agency, and the ethical standards applied should be no less exacting than they would be in the case of research carried out in that country.
- After scientific and ethical approval in the country of the sponsoring agency, the appropriate authorities of the host country, including a national or local ethical review committee or its equivalent, should satisfy themselves that the proposed research meets their own ethical requirements.

• • •

# SECTION V

## Ethical Directives Pertaining to the Welfare and Use of Animals

### 1. Veterinary Medicine

Veterinarian's Oath, American Veterinary Medical Association (AVMA)
[1954, revised 1969]

Principles of Veterinary Medical Ethics, American Veterinary Medical Association (AVMA) [revised 1993]

### 2. Research Involving Animals

International Guiding Principles for Biomedical Research Involving Animals,
Council for International Organizations of Medical Sciences (CIOMS),
World Health Organization [1984]

Principles for the Utilization and Care of Vertebrate Animals Used in Testing,
Research, and Education, U.S. Interagency Research Animal Committee
[1985]

Ethics of Animal Investigation, Canadian Council on Animal Care [revised
1989]

Australian Code of Practice for the Care and Use of Animals for Scientific
Purposes, National Health and Medical Research Council, Commonwealth Scientific and Industrial Research Organization, and Australian
Agricultural Council [revised 1989]

World Medical Association Statement on Animal Use in Biomedical Research, World Medical Association [1989]

Guidelines for Ethical Conduct in the Care and Use of Animals, American
Psychological Association [1985, revised 1992]

Principles and Guidelines for the Use of Animals in Precollege Education, Institute of Laboratory Animal Resources, National Research Council
[1989]

*Concern for the humane treatment of animals was expressed in the nineteenth century in both the United Kingdom and the United States through societies organized for the prevention of cruelty to animals. The Cruelty to Animals Act, enacted by the British Parliament in 1876, was among the earliest and most comprehensive laws for the protection of animals. Antivivisection proposals were made to the New York State legislature in the nineteenth century, but it was not until 1966 that the United States government enacted the Animal Welfare Act (7 U.S.C. 2131 et seq.), which, with accompanying regulations administered by the U.S. Department of Agriculture (USDA), is the most comprehensive code for the promotion of animal welfare in the United States.*

## 1. Veterinary Medicine

*Documents focusing on the ethics of veterinary medicine are similar to those pertaining to human health care except that they are concerned both with the patient (animal) and the client (owner).*

# VETERINARIAN'S OATH
### American Veterinary Medical Association (AVMA)
1954, revised 1969

*Originally adopted by the AVMA House of Delegates in 1954, the Veterinarian's Oath was revised in 1969. Phrases regarding "the promotion of public health, and the advancement of medical knowledge" were added to the oath. Others were dropped, including a specific pledge to "temper pain with anesthesia where indicated" and one not to use professional knowledge "contrary to the laws of humanity." The 1969 version of the oath, printed below, is administered to the graduating classes at many veterinary colleges.*

Being admitted to the profession of veterinary medicine,

I solemnly swear to use my scientific knowledge and skills for the benefit of society through the protection of animal health, the relief of animal suffering, the conservation of livestock resources, the promotion of public health, and the advancement of medical knowledge.

I will practice my profession conscientiously, with dignity, and in keeping with the principles of veterinary medical ethics.

I accept as a lifelong obligation the continual improvement of my professional knowledge and competence.

# PRINCIPLES OF VETERINARY MEDICAL ETHICS
### American Veterinary Medical Association (AVMA)
revised 1993

*Whereas animal research guidelines focus on the treatment of animals being used primarily for human purposes, veterinary medicine is concerned with balancing the interests and welfare of the patient (animal) and those of the client (owner). As a professionally generated ethics document, the AVMA's Principles of Veterinary Medical Ethics in many ways parallels the structure, content, and function of professional documents in human health care. The following are excerpts from the principles.*

• • •

## Attitude and Intent

The *Principles of Veterinary Medical Ethics* are purposely constructed in a general and broad manner, but veterinarians who accept the Golden Rule as a guide for general conduct and make a reasonable effort to abide by the *Principles of Veterinary Medical Ethics* in professional life will have little difficulty with ethics.

The honor and dignity of our profession rest in our obedience to a just and reasonable code of ethics set forth as a guide to the members. The object of this code, however, is more far-reaching, for exemplary professional conduct not only upholds honor and dignity, but also enlarges our sphere of usefulness, exalts our social standards, and promotes the science we cultivate. Briefly stated, our code of ethics is the foundation of our individual and collective efforts. It is the solemn duty of all members of the Association to deport themselves in accordance with the spirit of this code.

These *Principles of Veterinary Medical Ethics* are intended as aspirational goals. This code is not intended to cover the entire field of veterinary medical ethics. Professional life is too complex to classify one's duties and obligations to clients, colleagues, and fellow citizens into a set of rules.

## General Concepts

The *Principles of Veterinary Medical Ethics* are intended to aid veterinarians individually and collectively in maintaining a high level of ethical conduct. They are standards by which an individual may determine the propriety of conduct in relationships with clients, colleagues, and the public. A high standard of professional behavior is expected of all members of the profession.

Veterinarians should be good citizens and participate in activities to advance community welfare. They should conduct themselves in a manner that will enhance the worthiness of their profession.

Professional associations of veterinarians should adopt the AVMA *Principles of Veterinary Medical Ethics* or a similar code, and each should establish an active committee on ethics.

State veterinary associations should include reports or discussions on professional ethics in the programs of their meetings.

Teaching of ethics and professional concepts should be intensified in the educational programs of the colleges of veterinary medicine.

The *Principles of Veterinary Medical Ethics* should be subjected to review with the object of clarification of any obscure parts and the amendment of any inadequate or inappropriate items. A determined effort should be made to encourage compliance with the *Principles* in their entirety.

## Guidelines for Professional Behavior

1. In their relations with others, veterinarians should speak and act on the basis of honesty and fairness.

2. Veterinarians should consider first the welfare of the patient for the purpose of relieving suffering and disability while causing a minimum of pain or fright. Benefit to the patient should transcend personal advantage or monetary gain in decisions concerning therapy.

3. Veterinarians should not employ professional knowledge and attainments nor render services under terms and conditions which tend to interfere with the free exercise of judgment and skill or tend to cause a deterioration of the quality of veterinary service.

4. Veterinarians should seek for themselves and their profession the respect of their colleagues, their clients, and the public through courteous verbal interchange, considerate treatment, professional appearances, professionally acceptable procedures, and the utilization of current professional and scientific knowledge. Veterinarians should be concerned with the affairs and welfare of their communities, including the public health.

5. Veterinarians should respect the rights of clients, colleagues, and other health professionals. No member shall belittle or injure the professional standing of another member of the profession or unnecessarily condemn the character of that person's professional acts in such a manner as to be false or misleading.

6. Veterinarians may choose whom they will serve. Once they have undertaken care of a patient they must not neglect the patient. In an emergency, however, they should render service to the best of their ability.

7. Veterinarians should strive continually to improve veterinary knowledge and skill, making available to their colleagues the benefit of their professional attainments, and seeking, through consultation, assistance of others when it appears that the quality of veterinary service may be enhanced thereby.

8. Advertising or solicitation of clients by veterinarians should adhere to the Advertising Regulations, and should in no case be false, misleading, or deceptive.

9. The veterinary profession should safeguard the public and itself against veterinarians deficient in moral character or professional competence. Veterinarians should observe all laws, uphold the honor and dignity of the profession, and accept its self-imposed discipline.

10. The responsibilities of the veterinary profession extend not only to the patient but also to society. The health of the community as well as the patient deserves the veterinarian's interest and participation in nonprofessional activities and organizations.

• • •

### Referrals, Consultations, and Relationships with Clients

Consultations and referrals should be offered or sought whenever it appears that the quality of veterinary service will be enhanced thereby.

Consultations should be conducted in a spirit of professional cooperation between the consultant and the attending veterinarian to assure the client's confidence in and respect for veterinary medicine.

When a fellow practitioner or a diagnostic laboratory, research, academic, or regulatory veterinarian is called into consultation by an attending veterinarian, findings and discussions with the client shall be handled in such a manner as to avoid criticism of the attending veterinarian by the consultant or the client, if that criticism is false or misleading.

When in the course of authorized official duty it is necessary for a veterinarian to render service in the field of another veterinarian, it will be considered unethical to offer free or compensated service or advice other than that which comes strictly within the scope of the official duty, unless the client and attending veterinarian agree.

Consultants must not revisit the patient or communicate in person with the client without the knowledge of the attending veterinarian.

Diagnostic laboratory, research, academic, or regulatory veterinarians in the role of consultants shall deport themselves in the same manner as fellow practitioners whether they are private, commercial, or public functionaries.

In dealing with referrals, veterinarians acting as consultants should not take charge of a case or problem without the consent of the client and notification of the referring veterinarian.

The first veterinarian to handle a case has an obligation to other veterinarians that the client may choose to consult about the same case. The first veterinarian should readily withdraw from the case, indicating the circumstances on the records, and should be willing to forward copies of the medical records to other veterinarians who request them.

A veterinarian may refuse to accept a client or a patient, but should not do so solely because the client has previously contacted another veterinarian.

If for any reason a client requests referral to another veterinarian or veterinary institution, the attending veterinarian should be willing to honor the request and facilitate the necessary arrangements.

The following suggestions are offered for consideration by veterinarians in dealing with clients with whom they are not acquainted or for whom they have not previously rendered service:

1) Conduct yourself in word and action as if the person had been referred to you by a colleague. Try to determine by careful questioning whether the client has consulted another veterinarian and if so, the veterinarian's name, diagnosis, and treatment. It may be advisable to contact the previous veterinarian to ascertain the original diagnosis and treatment before telling the client how you plan to handle the case.

2) Describe your diagnosis and intended treatment carefully so that the client will be generally satisfied with the professional contact.

3) Consider the advisability of notifying the previous veterinarian(s) of your diagnosis and therapy.

4) If your colleague's actions reflect professional incompetence or neglect or abuse of the patient, call it to your colleague's attention and, if appropriate, to the attention of officers or practice committees of the local or state veterinary associations or the proper regulatory agency. Remember that a client who is abruptly changing veterinarians is often under severe stress and is likely to overstate or mis-state the causes for differences with the other practitioner.

### Confidentiality

The ethical ideals of the veterinary profession imply that a doctor of veterinary medicine and the veterinarian's staff will protect the personal privacy of clients, unless the veterinarian is required, by law, to reveal the confidences or unless it becomes necessary in order to protect the health and welfare of the individual, the animals, and/or others whose health and welfare may be endangered.

### Emergency Service

Every practitioner has a moral and ethical responsibility to provide service when because of accidents or other emergencies involving animals it is necessary to save life or relieve suffering. Since veterinarians cannot always be available to provide this service, veterinarians should cooperate with colleagues to assure that emergency services are provided consistent with the needs of the locality.

## Frauds

Members of the Association shall avoid the impropriety of employing misrepresentations to attract public attention.

When employed by the buyer to examine an animal for purchase, it is unethical to accept a fee from the seller. The acceptance of such a fee is prima facie evidence of fraud. On the other hand, it is deemed unethical to criticize unfairly an animal about to be sold. The veterinarian's duty in this connection is to be a just and honest referee.

When veterinarians know that surgery has been requested with intent to deceive a third party, they will have engaged in an unethical practice if they perform or participate in the operation.

## Secret Remedies

It is unethical and unprofessional for veterinarians to promote, sell, prescribe, or use any product the ingredient formula of which has not been revealed to them.

## Genetic Defects

Performance of surgical procedures in all species for the purpose of concealing genetic defects in animals to be shown, raced, bred, or sold as breeding animals is unethical. However, should the health or welfare of the individual patient require correction of such genetic defects, it is recommended that the patient be rendered incapable of reproduction.

## Alliance with Unqualified Persons

No member shall willfully place professional knowledge, attainments, or services at the disposal of any lay body, organization, group, or individual by whatever name called, or however organized, for the purpose of encouraging unqualified groups and individuals to diagnose and prescribe for the ailments and diseases of animals.

• • •

## Therapy, Determination of

Determination of therapy must not be relegated to secondary consideration with remuneration of the veterinarian being the primary interest. The veterinarian's obligation to uphold the dignity and honor of the profession precludes entering into an arrangement whereby, through commission or rebates, judgment on choice of treatment would be influenced by considerations other than needs of the patient, welfare of the client, or safety to the public.

• • •

## Vaccination Clinics

Definition: The term vaccination clinics applies to either privately or publicly supported activities in which veterinarians are engaged in mass immunization of pet animals. Usually, animals are brought into points of assembly by their owners or caretakers in response to a notification that immunization services will be available. Characteristically, these clinics do not provide the opportunity for the participating veterinarians to (1) conduct a physical examination of the individual animals to be immunized, (2) obtain a history of past immunization or prior disease, or (3) advise individual owners on follow-up immunization and health care.

Scientific and Technical Considerations - Rabies vaccination for the purpose of protecting the public health may be achieved in a rabies vaccination clinic.

When the primary objective is to protect the animal patient's health, clinical examination of the patient including proper history taking, is an essential and necessary part of a professionally acceptable immunization procedure.

Such a clinical examination is expected to be provided without regard to where the vaccination procedure is performed.

• • •

### Drugs, Practitioner's Responsibility in the Choice of

Practitioners of veterinary medicine, in common with practitioners in other branches of medicine, are fully responsible for their actions with respect to a patient from the time they accept the case until it is released from their care. In the choice of drugs, biologics, or other treatments, they are expected to use their professional judgment in the interests of the patient, based upon their knowledge of the condition, the probable effects of the treatment, and the available scientific evidence which may affect these decisions. If the preponderance of professional judgement is, or seems to be, contrary to theirs, the burden upon the practitioners to sustain their judgment becomes heavier. Nevertheless, the judgment is theirs and theirs alone.

• • •

### Dispensing, Marketing, and Merchandising

Dispensing is the direct distribution of veterinary products to clients for their use on the supposition that the veterinarian has knowledge of the particular case or general conditions relating to the current health status of the animals involved and has established a veterinarian client patient relationship. A veterinarian client patient relationship is characterized by these attributes:

1) The veterinarian has assumed the responsibility for making medical judgments regarding the health of the animal(s) and the need for medical treatment, and the client (owner or other caretaker) has agreed to follow the instructions of the veterinarian; and when

2) There is sufficient knowledge of the animal(s) by the veterinarian to initiate at least a general or preliminary diagnosis of the medical condition of the animal(s). This means that the veterinarian has recently seen and is personally acquainted with the keeping and care of the animal(s) by virtue of an examination of the animal(s) and/or by medically appropriate and timely visits to the premises where the animal(s) are kept; and when

3) The practicing veterinarian is readily available for follow-up in case of adverse reactions or failure of the regimen of therapy.

In the veterinarian's office dispensing becomes the distributing of professional veterinary products by virtue of verbal information presented by the owner, as an adjunct to the knowledge gained previously by the practitioner. This is in contrast to a written prescription involving a pharmacist.

Marketing is interpreted to mean those efforts directed at stimulating and encouraging animal owners to make use of veterinary services and products for the purpose of improving animal health and welfare.

Merchandising is buying and selling of professional veterinary products without a veterinarian client patient relationship. Merchandising as defined here is unethical.

• • •

## 2. Research Involving Animals

*Guidelines and regulations addressing the ethical treatment of animals, especially their use in scientific research, include those developed by groups involved in animal use and those generated by nonresearch groups.*

# INTERNATIONAL GUIDING PRINCIPLES FOR BIOMEDICAL RESEARCH INVOLVING ANIMALS
### Council for International Organizations of Medical Sciences (CIOMS), World Health Organization
#### 1984

*The purpose of the guiding principles, approved in 1984, is to provide a conceptual and ethical framework for whatever regulations governing animal research a country chooses to adopt. The guiding principles reflect consultation with a large, representative sample of the international biomedical community as well as with representatives of animal welfare groups. They have gained general international acceptance and have served as a model for similar guidelines in specific countries, including the United States and Canada.*

### Basic Principles

I. The advancement of biological knowledge and the development of improved means for the protection of the health and wellbeing both of man and of animals require recourse to experimentation on intact live animals of a wide variety of species.

II. Methods such as mathematical models, computer simulation and *in vitro* biological systems should be used wherever appropriate.

III. Animal experiments should be undertaken only after due consideration of their relevance for human or animal health and the advancement of biological knowledge.

IV. The animals selected for an experiment should be of an appropriate species and quality, and the minimum number required, to obtain scientifically valid results.

V. Investigators and other personnel should never fail to treat animals as sentient, and should regard their proper care and use and the avoidance or minimization of discomfort, distress, or pain as ethical imperatives.

VI. Investigators should assume that procedures that would cause pain in human beings cause pain in other vertebrate species although more needs to be known about the perception of pain in animals.

VII. Procedures with animals that may cause more than momentary or minimal pain or distress should be performed with appropriate sedation, analgesia, or anaesthesia in accordance with accepted veterinary practice. Surgical or other painful procedures should not be performed on unanaesthetized animals paralysed by chemical agents.

VIII. Where waivers are required in relation to the provisions of article VII, the decisions should not rest solely with the investigators directly concerned but should be made, with due regard to the provisions of articles IV, V, and VI, by a suitably constituted review body. Such waivers should not be made solely for the purposes of teaching or demonstration.

IX. At the end of, or when appropriate during, an experiment, animals that would otherwise suffer severe or chronic pain, distress, discomfort, or disablement that cannot be relieved should be painlessly killed.

X. The best possible living conditions should be maintained for animals kept for biomedical purposes. Normally the care of animals should be under the supervision of veterinarians having experience in laboratory animal science. In any case, veterinary care should be available as required.

XI. It is the responsibility of the director of an institute or department using animals to ensure that investigators and personnel have appropriate qualifications or experience for conducting procedures on animals. Adequate opportunities shall be provided for in-service training, including the proper and humane concern for the animals under their care.

# PRINCIPLES FOR THE UTILIZATION AND CARE OF VERTEBRATE ANIMALS USED IN TESTING, RESEARCH, AND EDUCATION
### U.S. Interagency Research Animal Committee
#### 1985

*Developed in 1984 by the U.S. Interagency Research Animal Committee, which serves as a focal point for the discussion by federal agencies of issues involving the use of animals in research and testing, these principles are based on the CIOMS Guiding Principles. The U.S. principles are endorsed, implemented, and supplemented by the National Institutes of Health's Public Health Service Policy on Humane Care and Use of Laboratory Animals, which was revised in 1986, and the Guide for the Care and Use of Laboratory Animals, prepared by the Institute of Laboratory Animal Resources, National Academy of Sciences, in 1985. The Public Health Service (PHS) policy applies to all PHS researchers, grantees, and contractors who use warm-blooded vertebrates in research and testing. The policy requires compliance with the Animal Welfare Act (AWA) (7 U.S.C. 2131 et seq.) and the USDA regulations that implement it (9 CFR, Subchapter A—Animal Welfare).*

*The AWA was originally enacted in 1966 to impose civil and criminal penalties on persons who stole household pets and sold them to biomedical research facilities. It has been amended many times to provide additional protections for warm-blooded animals used in agriculture, the food and fiber industry, circuses, pet shops, and research. In 1985, the AWA was amended by*

*P.L. 99-198 to require, among other provisions, the establishment of Animal Care and Use Committees to oversee animal housing and care and to review proposed research. Both the USDA regulations implementing the act and the PHS policy reference the Guide for the Care and Use of Laboratory Animals as the standard according to which programs for the care and use of laboratory animals will be judged.*

*The AWA and its accompanying regulations and the correlative Public Health Service Act and its accompanying PHS policy together with the guide constitute the fundamental documents that govern the care and use of animals used for research, testing, and teaching in the United States. Additionally, the Food and Drug Administration's Good Laboratory Practices regulations include similar provisions for the care and use of animals in testing sites used by the industry.*

The development of knowledge necessary for the improvement of the health and well-being of humans as well as other animals requires *in vivo* experimentation with a wide variety of animal species. Whenever U.S. Government agencies develop requirements for testing, research, or training procedures involving the use of vertebrate animals, the following principles shall be considered; and whenever these agencies actually perform or sponsor such procedures, the responsible institutional official shall ensure that these principles are adhered to:

I.    The transportation, care, and use of animals should be in accordance with the Animal Welfare Act (7 U.S.C. 2131 et seq.) and other applicable Federal laws, guidelines and policies.

II.   Procedures involving animals should be designed and performed with due consideration of their relevance to human or animal health, the advancement of knowledge, or the good of society.

III.  The animals selected for a procedure should be of an appropriate species and quality and the minimum number required to obtain valid results. Methods such as mathematical models, computer simulation, and *in vitro* biological systems should be considered.

IV.   Proper use of animals, including the avoidance or minimization of discomfort, distress, and pain when consistent with sound scientific practices, is imperative. Unless the contrary is established, investigators should consider that procedures that cause pain or distress in human beings may cause pain or distress in other animals.

V.    Procedures with animals that may cause more than momentary or slight pain or distress should be performed with appropriate sedation, analgesia, or anesthesia. Surgical or other painful procedures should not be performed on unanesthetized animals paralyzed by chemical agents.

VI.   Animals that would otherwise suffer severe or chronic pain or distress that cannot be relieved should be painlessly killed at the end of the procedure or, if appropriate, during the procedure.

VII.  The living conditions of animals should be appropriate for their species and contribute to their health and comfort. Normally, the housing, feeding, and care of all animals used for biomedical purposes must be directed by a veterinarian or other scientist trained and experienced in the proper care, handling, and use of the species being maintained or studied. In any case, veterinary care shall be provided as indicated.

VIII. Investigators and other personnel shall be appropriately qualified and experienced for conducting procedures on living animals. Adequate arrangements shall be made for their in-service training, including the proper and humane care and use of laboratory animals.

IX.   Where exceptions are required in relation to the provision of these Principles, the decisions should not rest with the investigators directly concerned but should be made, with due regard to Principle II, by an appropriate review group such as an institutional animal research committee. Such exceptions should not be made solely for the purposes of teaching or demonstration.

## ETHICS OF ANIMAL INVESTIGATION
### Canadian Council on Animal Care
revised 1989

*More detailed than the CIOMS and U.S. government principles, the Canadian Council on Animal Care's Ethics of Animal Investigation includes nine principles designed to be used in association with the CCAC's Guide to the Care and Use of Experimental Animals, a highly respected, two-volume document that provides detailed requirements for the humane use of animals in research, teaching, and testing.*

The use of animals in research, teaching, and testing is acceptable only if it promises to contribute to understanding of fundamental biological principles, or to the development of knowledge that can reasonably be expected to benefit humans or animals.

Animals should be used only if the researcher's best efforts to find an alternative have failed. A continuing sharing of knowledge, review of the literature, and adherence to the Russell-Burch "3R" tenet of "Replacement, Reduction and Refinement" are also requisites. Those using animals should employ the most humane methods on the smallest number of appropriate animals required to obtain valid information.

The following principles incorporate suggestions from members of both the scientific and animal welfare communities, as well as the organizations represented on Council. They should be applied in conjunction with CCAC's "Guide to the Care and Use of Experimental Animals."

1. If animals must be used, they should be maintained in a manner that provides for their physical comfort and psychological well-being, according to CCAC's "Policy Statement on Social and Behavioural Requirements of Experimental Animals."

2. Animals must not be subjected to unnecessary pain or distress. The experimental design must offer them every practicable safeguard, whether in research, in teaching or in testing procedures; cost and convenience must not take precedence over the animal's physical and mental well-being.

3. Expert opinion must attest to the potential value of studies with animals. The following procedures, which are restricted, require independent, external evaluation to justify their use:

   i)  burns, freezing injuries, fractures, and other types of trauma investigation in anesthetized animals, concomitant to which must be acceptable veterinary practices for the relief of pain, including adequate analgesia during the recovery period;

   ii) staged encounters between predator and prey or between conspecifics where prolonged fighting and injury are probable.

4. If pain or distress are necessary concomitants to the study, these must be minimized both in intensity and duration. Investigators, animal care committees, grant review committees and referees must be especially cautious in evaluating the proposed use of the following procedures:

   a)  experiments involving withholding pre- and post-operative pain-relieving medication;

   b)  paralyzing and immobilizing experiments where there is no reduction in the sensation of pain;

   c)  electric shock as negative reinforcement;

   d)  extreme environmental conditions such as low or high temperatures, high humidity, modified atmospheres, etc., or sudden changes therein;

   e)  experiments studying stress and pain;

   f)  experiments requiring withholding of food and water for periods incompatible with the species specific psychological needs; such experiments should have no detrimental effect on the health of the animal;

   g)  injection of Freund's Complete Adjuvant (FCA). This must be carried out in accordance with "CCAC Guidelines on Immunization Procedures."

5. An animal observed to be experiencing severe, unrelievable pain or discomfort should immediately be humanely killed, using a method providing initial rapid unconsciousness.

6. While non-recovery procedures involving anesthetized animals, and studies involving no pain or distress are considered acceptable; the following experimental procedures inflict excessive pain and are thus unacceptable:

   a)  utilization of muscle relaxants or paralytics (curare and curare-like) alone, without anesthetics, during surgical procedures;

   b)  traumatizing procedures involving crushing, burning, striking or beating in unanesthetized animals.

7. Studies such as toxicological and biological testing, cancer research and infectious disease investigation may, in the past, have required continuation until the death of the animal. However, in the face of distinct signs that such processes are causing irreversible pain or distress, alternative endpoints should be sought to satisfy both the requirements of the study and the needs of the animal.

8. Physical restraint should only be used after alternative procedures have been fully considered and found inadequate. Animals so restrained must receive exceptional care

and attention, in compliance with species specific and general requirements as set forth in the "Guide."

9.  Painful experiments or multiple invasive procedures on an individual animal, conducted solely for the instruction of students in the classroom, or for the demonstration of established scientific knowledge, cannot be justified. Audiovisual or other alternative techniques should be employed to convey such information.

# AUSTRALIAN CODE OF PRACTICE FOR THE CARE AND USE OF ANIMALS FOR SCIENTIFIC PURPOSES
### National Health and Medical Research Council, Commonwealth Scientific and Industrial Research Organization, and Australian Agricultural Council
revised 1989

*The first Australian code was issued in 1969 and revised in 1979, 1982, 1985, and 1989. The current code encompasses all aspects of the care and use of animals for scientific purposes in medicine, biology, agriculture, veterinary and other animal sciences, industry, and teaching. Section 1 of the code, "General Principles for the Care and Use of Animals for Scientific Purposes," which is printed below, is similar to the CIOMS principles, but is unique in its inclusion of the principle that animals must not be taken from their natural habitats if others, bred in captivity, are available. In addition to general principles for the care and use of animals, the code specifies the responsibilities of researchers and institutions and the composition and function of Animal Experimentation Ethics Committees. It also provides guidelines for the acquisition and care of animals.*

For the guidance of Investigators, Institutions and Animal Experimentation Ethics Committees and all involved in the care and use of animals for scientific purposes.

1.1  Experiments on animals may be performed only when they are essential to obtain and establish significant information relevant to the understanding of humans or animals, to the maintenance and improvement of human or animal health and welfare, to the improvement of animal management or production, or to the achievement of educational objectives.

1.2  People who use animals for scientific purposes have an obligation to treat the animals with respect and to consider their welfare as an essential factor when planning and conducting experiments.

1.3  Investigators have direct and ultimate responsibility for all matters relating to the welfare of the animals they use in experiments.

1.4  Techniques which replace or complement animal experiments must be used wherever possible.

1.5  Experiments using animals may be performed only after a decision has been made that they are justified, weighing the scientific or educational value of the experiment against the potential effects on the welfare of the animals.

1.6  Animals chosen must be of an appropriate species with suitable biological characteristics, including behavioural characteristics, genetic constitution and nutritional, microbiological and general health status.

1.7  Animals must not be taken from their natural habitats if animals bred in captivity are available and suitable.

1.8  Experiments must be scientifically valid, and must use no more than the minimum number of animals needed.

1.9  Experiments must use the best available scientific techniques and must be carried out only by persons competent in the procedures they perform.

1.10  Experiments must not be repeated unnecessarily.

1.11  Experiments must be as brief as possible.

1.12  Experiments must be designed to avoid pain or distress to animals. If this is not possible, pain or distress must be minimised.

1.13  Pain and distress cannot be evaluated easily in animals and therefore investigators must assume that animals experience pain in a manner similar to humans. Decisions regarding the animals' welfare must be based on this assumption unless there is evidence to the contrary.

1.14  Experiments which may cause pain or distress of a kind and degree for which anaesthesia would normally be used in medical or veterinary practice must be carried out using anaesthesia appropriate to the species and the procedure. When it is not possible to use anaesthesia, such as in certain toxicological or animal production experiments or in animal models of disease, the end-point of the experiments must be as early as possible to avoid or minimise pain or distress to the animals.

1.15 Investigators must avoid using death as an experimental end-point whenever possible.

1.16 Analgesic and tranquilliser usage must be appropriate for the species and should at least parallel usage in medical or veterinary practice.

1.17 An animal which develops signs of pain or distress of a kind and degree not predicted in the proposal, must have the pain or distress alleviated promptly. If severe pain cannot be alleviated without delay, the animal must be killed humanely forthwith. Alleviation of such pain or distress must take precedence over finishing an experiment.

1.18 Neuromuscular blocking agents must not be used without appropriate general anaesthesia, except in animals where sensory awareness has been eliminated. If such agents are used, continuous or frequent intermittent monitoring of paralysed animals is essential to ensure that the depth of anaesthesia is adequate to prevent pain or distress.

1.19 Animals must be transported, housed, fed, watered, handled and used under conditions which are appropriate to the species and which ensure a high standard of care.

1.20 Institutions using animals for scientific purposes must establish Animal Experimentation Ethics Committees (AEECs) to ensure that all animal use conforms with the standards of this Code.

1.21 Investigators must submit written proposals for all animal experimentation to an AEEC which must take into account the expected value of the knowledge to be gained, the validity of the experiments, and all ethical and animal welfare aspects.

1.22 Experiments must not commence until written approval has been obtained from the AEEC.

1.23 The care and use of animals for all scientific purposes in Australia must be in accord with this Code of Practice, and with Commonwealth, State and Territory legislation.

# WORLD MEDICAL ASSOCIATION STATEMENT ON ANIMAL USE IN BIOMEDICAL RESEARCH
## World Medical Association
### 1989

*Adopted by the Forty-first World Medical Assembly in Hong Kong, September 1989, the World Medical Association Statement on Animal Use in Biomedical Research includes principles that affirm not only the need to respect the welfare of animals used for research but also the continued use of animals in biomedical research as essential, and it condemns the harassment of scientists by animal rights activitists.*

## Preamble

Biomedical research is essential to the health and well-being of every person in our society. Advances in biomedical research have dramatically improved the quality and prolonged the duration of life throughout the world. However, the ability of the scientific community to continue its efforts to improve personal and public health is being threatened by a movement to eliminate the use of animals in biomedical research. This movement is spearheaded by groups of radical animal rights activists whose views are far outside mainstream public attitudes and whose tactics range from sophisticated lobbying, fund raising, propaganda and misinformation campaigns to violent attacks on biomedical research facilities and individual scientists.

The magnitude of violent animal rights activities is staggering. In the United States alone, since 1980, animal rights groups have staged more than 29 raids on U.S. research facilities, stealing over 2,000 animals, causing more than 7 million dollars in physical damages and ruining years of scientific research in the process. Animal activist groups have engaged in similar activities in Great Britain, Western Europe, Canada and Australia. Various groups in these countries have claimed responsibility for the bombing of cars, institutions, stores, and the private homes of researchers.

Animal rights violence has had a chilling effect on the scientific community internationally. Scientists, research organizations, and universities have been intimidated into altering or even terminating important research efforts that depend on the use of animals.

Laboratories have been forced to divert thousands of research dollars for the purchase of sophisticated security equipment. Young people who might otherwise pursue a career in biomedical research are turning their sights to alternative professions.

Despite the efforts of many groups striving to protect biomedical research from animal activism, the response to the animal rights movement has been fragmented, under-funded, and primarily defensive. Many groups within the biomedical community are hesitant to take a public stand about animal activism because of fear of reprisal. As a result, the research establishment has been backed into a defensive posture. Its motiva-tions are questioned, and the need for using animals in research is repeatedly challenged.

While research involving animals is necessary to enhance the medical care of all per-sons, we recognized also that humane treatment of research animals must be ensured. Appropriate training for all research personnel should be prescribed and adequate vet-erinary care should be available. Experiments must comply with any rules or regulations promulgated to govern human handling, housing, care, treatment and transportation of animals.

International medical and scientific organizations must develop a stronger and more cohesive campaign to counter the growing threat to public health posed by animal activ-ists. Leadership and coordination must be provided.

The World Medical Association therefore affirms the following principles:

1. Animal use in biomedical research is essential for continued medical progress.
2. The WMA Declaration of Helsinki requires that biomedical research involving hu-man subjects should be based on animal experimentation, but also requires that the welfare of animals used for research be respected.
3. Humane treatment of animals used in biomedical research is essential.
4. All research facilities should be required to comply with all guiding principles for humane treatment of animals.
5. Medical Societies should resist any attempt to deny the appropriate use of animals in biomedical research because such denial would compromise patient care.
6. Although rights to free speech should not be compromised, the anarchistic element among animal right activists should be condemned.
7. The use of threats, intimidation, violence, and personal harassment of scientists and their families should be condemned internationally.
8. A maximum coordinated effort from international law enforcement agencies should be sought to protect researchers and research facilities from activities of a terrorist nature.

# GUIDELINES FOR ETHICAL CONDUCT IN THE CARE AND USE OF ANIMALS
## American Psychological Association
### 1985, revised 1992

*Some professional associations, such as the American Psychological Association (APA), have developed their own guidelines governing research with animals, which reinforce and/or supple-ment all pertinent laws and other regulations. The APA produced one of the earliest and most complete sets of association guidelines pertaining to research on animals. Like other professional groups, the APA requires that individuals publishing research in APA journals attest to the fact that animal research was conducted in accordance with its guidelines.*

## I. Justification of the Research

A. Research should be undertaken with a clear scientific purpose. There should be a reasonable expectation that the research will a) increase knowledge of the processes un-derlying the evolution, development, maintenance, alteration, control, or biological sig-nificance of behavior; b) increase understanding of the species under study; or c) provide results that benefit the health or welfare of humans or other animals.

B. The scientific purpose of the research should be of sufficient potential significance to justify the use of animals. Psychologists should act on the assumption that procedures that would produce pain in humans will also do so in other animals.

C. The species chosen for study should be best suited to answer the question(s) posed. The psychologist should always consider the possibility of using other species, nonanimal alternatives, or procedures that minimize the number of animals in research, and should be familiar with the appropriate literature.

D. Research on animals may not be conducted until the protocol has been reviewed by the institutional animal care and use committee (IACUC) to ensure that the procedures are appropriate and humane.

E. The psychologist should monitor the research and the animals' welfare throughout the course of an investigation to ensure continued justification for the research.

## II. Personnel

A. Psychologists should ensure that personnel involved in their research with animals be familiar with these guidelines.

B. Animal use procedures must conform with federal regulations regarding personnel, supervision, record keeping, and veterinary care.

C. Behavior is both the focus of study of many experiments as well as a primary source of information about an animal's health and well-being. It is therefore necessary that psychologists and their assistants be informed about the behavioral characteristics of their animal subjects, so as to be aware of normal, species-specific behaviors and unusual behaviors that could forewarn of health problems.

D. Psychologists should ensure that all individuals who use animals under their supervision receive explicit instruction in experimental methods and in the care, maintenance, and handling of the species being studied. Responsibilities and activities of all individuals dealing with animals should be consistent with their respective competencies, training, and experience in either the laboratory or the field setting.

## III. Care and Housing of Animals

The concept of "psychological well-being" of animals is of current concern and debate and is included in Federal Regulations (United States Department of Agriculture [USDA], 1991). As a scientific and professional organization, APA recognizes the complexities of defining psychological well-being. Procedures appropriate for a particular species may well be inappropriate for others. Hence, APA does not presently stipulate specific guidelines regarding the maintenance of psychological well-being of research animals. Psychologists familiar with the species should be best qualified professionally to judge measures such as enrichment to maintain or improve psychological well-being of those species.

A. The facilities housing animals should meet or exceed current regulations and guidelines (USDA, 1990, 1991) and are required to be inspected twice a year (USDA, 1989).

B. All procedures carried out on animals are to be reviewed by a local IACUC to ensure that the procedures are appropriate and humane. The committee should have representation from within the institution and from the local community. In the event that it is not possible to constitute an appropriate local IACUC, psychologists are encouraged to seek advice from a corresponding committee of a cooperative institution.

C. Responsibilities for the conditions under which animals are kept, both within and outside of the context of active experimentation or teaching, rests with the psychologist under the supervision of the IACUC (where required by federal regulations) and with individuals appointed by the institution to oversee animal care. Animals are to be provided with humane care and healthful conditions during their stay in the facility. In addition to the federal requirements to provide for the psychological well-being of non-human primates used in research, psychologists are encouraged to consider enriching the environments of their laboratory animals and should keep abreast of literature on well-being and enrichment for the species with which they work.

## IV. Acquisition of Animals

A. Animals not bred in the psychologist's facility are to be acquired lawfully. The USDA and local ordinances should be consulted for information regarding regulations and approved suppliers.

B. Psychologists should make every effort to ensure that those responsible for transporting the animals to the facility provide adequate food, water, ventilation, space, and impose no unnecessary stress on the animals.

C. Animals taken from the wild should be trapped in a humane manner and in accordance with applicable federal, state, and local regulations.

D. Endangered species or taxa should be used only with full attention to required permits and ethical concerns. Information and permit applications can be obtained from the Fish and Wildlife Service, Office of Management Authority, U.S. Dept. of the Interior, 4401 N. Fairfax Dr., Rm. 432, Arlington, VA 22043, 703-358-2104. Similar caution should be used in work with threatened species or taxa.

## V. Experimental Procedures

Humane consideration for the well-being of the animal should be incorporated into the design and conduct of all procedures involving animals, while keeping in mind the primary goal of experimental procedures—the acquisition of sound, replicable data. The conduct of all procedures is governed by Guideline I.

A. Behavioral studies that involve no aversive stimulation or overt sign of distress to the animal are acceptable. This includes observational and other noninvasive forms of data collection.

B. When alternative behavioral procedures are available, those that minimize discomfort to the animal should be used. When using aversive conditions, psychologists should adjust the parameters of stimulation to levels that appear minimal, though compatible with the aims of the research. Psychologists are encouraged to test painful stimuli on themselves, whenever reasonable. Whenever consistent with the goals of research, consideration should be given to providing the animals with control of the potentially aversive stimulation.

C. Procedures in which the animal is anesthetized and insensitive to pain throughout the procedure and is euthanized before regaining consciousness are generally acceptable.

D. Procedures involving more than momentary or slight aversive stimulation, which are not relieved by medication or other acceptable methods, should be undertaken only when the objectives of research cannot be achieved by other methods.

E. Experimental procedures that require prolonged aversive conditions or produce tissue damage or metabolic disturbances require greater justification and surveillance. This includes prolonged exposure to extreme environmental conditions, experimentally induced prey killing, or infliction of physical trauma or tissue damage. An animal observed to be in a state of severe distress or chronic pain that cannot be alleviated and is not essential to the purposes of the research should be euthanized immediately.

F. Procedures that use restraint must conform to federal regulations and guidelines.

G. Procedures involving the use of paralytic agents without reduction in pain sensation require particular prudence and humane concern. Use of muscle relaxants or paralytics alone during surgery, without general anesthesia, is unacceptable and shall not be used.

H. Surgical procedures, because of their invasive nature, require close supervision and attention to humane considerations by the psychologist. Aseptic (methods that minimize risks of infection) techniques must be used on laboratory animals whenever possible.

1. All surgical procedures and anesthetization should be conducted under the direct supervision of a person who is competent in the use of the procedures.

2. If the surgical procedure is likely to cause greater discomfort than that attending anesthetization, and unless there is specific justification for acting otherwise, animals should be maintained under anesthesia until the procedure is ended.

3. Sound postoperative monitoring and care, which may include the use of analgesics and antibiotics, should be provided to minimize discomfort and to prevent infection and other untoward consequences of the procedure.

4. Animals can not be subjected to successive surgical procedures unless these are required by the nature of the research, the nature of the surgery, or for the well-being of the animal. Multiple surgeries on the same animal must receive special approval from the IACUC.

I. When the use of an animal is no longer required by an experimental protocol or procedure, in order to minimize the number of animals used in research, alternatives to euthanasia should be considered. Such uses should be compatible with the goals of research and the welfare of the animal. Care should be taken that such an action does not expose the animal to multiple surgeries.

J. The return of wild-caught animals to the field can carry substantial risks, both to the formerly captive animals and to the ecosystem. Animals reared in the laboratory should not be released because, in most cases, they cannot survive or they may survive by disrupting the natural ecology.

K. When euthanasia appears to be the appropriate alternative, either as a requirement of the research or because it constitutes the most humane form of disposition of an animal at the conclusion of the research:

1. Euthanasia shall be accomplished in a humane manner, appropriate for the species, and in such a way as to ensure immediate death, and in accordance with procedures outlined in the latest version of the "American Veterinary Medical Association (AVMA) Panel on Euthanasia."

2. Disposal of euthanized animals should be accomplished in a manner that is in accordance with all relevant legislation, consistent with health, environmental, and aesthetic concerns, and approved by the IACUC. No animal shall be discarded until its death is verified.

## VI. Field Research

Field research, because of its potential to damage sensitive ecosystems and ethologies, should be subject to IACUC approval. Field research, if strictly observational, may not require IACUC approval (USDA, 1989, pg. 36126).

A. Psychologists conducting field research should disturb their populations as little as possible—consistent with the goals of the research. Every effort should be made to minimize potential harmful effects of the study on the population and on other plant and animal species in the area.

B. Research conducted in populated areas should be done with respect for the property and privacy of the inhabitants of the area.

C. Particular justification is required for the study of endangered species. Such research on endangered species should not be conducted unless IACUC approval has been obtained and all requisite permits are obtained (see above, III D).

## VII. Educational Use of Animals

APA has adopted separate guidelines for the educational use of animals in precollege education, including the use of animals in science fairs and demonstrations. For a copy of APA's "Ethical Guidelines for the Teaching of Psychology in the Secondary Schools," write to: High School Teacher Affiliate Program, Education Directorate, APA, 750 First St., NE, Washington, DC 20002-4242.

A. Psychologists are encouraged to include instruction and discussion of the ethics and values of animal research in all courses that involve or discuss the use of animals.

B. Animals may be used for educational purposes only after review by a committee appropriate to the institution.

C. Some procedures that can be justified for research purposes may not be justified for educational purposes. Consideration should always be given to the possibility of using nonanimal alternatives.

D. Classroom demonstrations involving live animals can be valuable as instructional aids in addition to videotapes, films, or other alternatives. Careful consideration should be given to the question of whether this type of demonstration is warranted by the anticipated instructional gains.

# PRINCIPLES AND GUIDELINES FOR THE USE OF ANIMALS IN PRECOLLEGE EDUCATION
### Institute of Laboratory Animal Resources (ILAR) National Research Council
1989

*The ILAR Principles and Guidelines provide guidance for improving the scientific integrity of precollege research and encouraging more humane study of animals in precollege education. They are designed to help schools implement changes in their use of animals in teaching programs to bring them more in line with current approaches to the use of animals in higher education and research.*

The humane study of animals in precollege education can provide important learning experiences in science and ethics and should be encouraged. Maintaining classroom pets in preschool and grade school can teach respect for other species, as well as proper animal husbandry practices. Introduction of secondary school students to animal studies in closely supervised settings can reinforce those early lessons and teach the principles of humane care and use of animals in scientific inquiry. The National Research Council recommends compliance with the following principles whenever animals are used in precollege education or in science fair projects.

## Principle 1

Observational and natural history studies that are not intrusive (that is, do not interfere with an animal's health or well-being or cause it discomfort) are encouraged for all classes of organisms. When an intrusive study of a living organism is deemed appropriate, consideration should be given first to using plants (including lower plants such as yeast and fungi) and invertebrates with no nervous systems or with primitive ones (including protozoa, planaria, and insects). Intrusive studies of invertebrates with advanced nervous systems (such as octopi) and vertebrates should be used only when lower invertebrates are not suitable and only under the conditions stated below in Principle 10.

## Principle 2

Supervision shall be provided by individuals who are knowledgeable about and experienced with the health, husbandry, care, and handling of the animal species used and who understand applicable laws, regulations, and policies.

## Principle 3

Appropriate care for animals must be provided daily, including weekends, holidays, and other times when school is not in session. This care must include
a. nutritious food and clean, fresh water;
b. clean housing with space and enrichment suitable for normal species behaviors; and
c. temperature and lighting appropriate for the species.

## Principle 4

Animals should be healthy and free of disease that can be transmitted to humans or to other animals. Veterinary care must be provided as needed.

## Principle 5

Students and teachers should report immediately to the school health authority all scratches, bites, and other injuries; allergies; or illnesses.

## Principle 6

Prior to obtaining animals for educational purposes, it is imperative that the school develop a plan for their procurement and ultimate disposition. Animals must not be captured from or released into the wild without the approval of the responsible wildlife and public health officials. When euthanasia is necessary, it should be performed in accordance with the most recent recommendations of the American Veterinary Medical Association's Panel Report on Euthanasia (*Journal of the American Veterinary Medical Association*, 188[3]:252–268, 1986, et seq.). It should be performed only by someone trained in the appropriate technique.

## Principle 7

Students shall not conduct experimental procedures on animals that
a. are likely to cause pain or discomfort or interfere with an animal's health or well-being;
b. induce nutritional deficiencies or toxicities; or
c. expose animals to microorganisms, ionizing radiation, cancer-producing agents, or any other harmful drugs or chemicals capable of causing disease, injury, or birth defects in humans or animals.
    In general, procedures that cause pain in humans are considered to cause pain in other vertebrates.

## Principle 8

Experiments on avian embryos that might result in abnormal chicks or in chicks that might experience pain or discomfort shall be terminated 72 hours prior to the expected date of hatching. The eggs shall be destroyed to prevent inadvertent hatching.

## Principle 9

Behavioral conditioning studies shall not involve aversive stimuli. In studies using positive reinforcement, animals should not be deprived of water; food deprivation intervals should be appropriate for the species but should not continue longer than 24 hours.

## Principle 10

A plan for conducting an experiment with living animals must be prepared in writing and approved prior to initiating the experiment or to obtaining the animals. Proper experimental design of projects and concern for animal welfare are important learning experiences and contribute to respect for and appropriate care of animals. The plan shall be reviewed by a committee composed of individuals who have the knowledge to understand and evaluate it and who have the authority to approve or disapprove it. The written plan should include the following:

a.  a statement of the specific hypotheses or principles to be tested, illustrated, or taught;

b.  a summary of what is known about the subject under study, including references;

c.  a justification for the use of the species selected and consideration of why a lower vertebrate or invertebrate cannot be used; and

d.  a detailed description of the methods and procedures to be used, including experimental design; data analysis; and all aspects of animal procurement, care, housing, use, and disposal.

## Exceptions

Exceptions to Principles 7–10 may be granted under special circumstances by a panel appointed by the school principal or his or her designee. This panel should consist of at least three individuals, including a science teacher, a teacher of a nonscience subject, and a scientist or veterinarian who has expertise in the subject matter involved. At least one panel member should not be affiliated with the school or science fair, and none should be a member of the student's family.

# SECTION VI

## Ethical Directives Pertaining to the Environment

*Bioethics refers not only to the ethics of health care but also to the ethics of the life sciences, which include ecology and environmental sciences. Enhancing the health of plants, animals, and the entire biosphere has inherent moral value; it is also crucial for the protection and promotion of human health and well-being, which depend upon a healthy environment. Whether the environment is perceived to have intrinsic value, instrumental value, or both, society increasingly recognizes moral duties to preserve and nurture it and to foster a health-promoting relationship between humans and their environment. Many countries have laws and regulations designed to protect the environment and its resources through limitations on the emissions of industrial pollutants, hazardous waste disposal, recycling programs, and conservation policy.*

*The documents in this section fall into two categories: policy and professional conduct. They are issued both by professional groups and by a nonprofessional body, the United Nations. The editors have not attempted to include any of the myriad national and international laws and regulations pertaining to the environment, opting instead for more general policy statements.*

# WORLD CHARTER FOR NATURE
## General Assembly of the United Nations
### 1982

*A multinational task force began drafting the World Charter for Nature in 1975. Sponsored by thirty-four developing nations, it was adopted by the General Assembly of the United Nations on October 29, 1982, by a vote of 111 to 1, with the United States casting the sole dissenting vote.*

*The General Assembly,*

*Reaffirming* the fundamental purposes of the United Nations, in particular the maintenance of international peace and security, the development of friendly relations among nations and the achievement of international co-operation in solving international problems of an economic, social, cultural, technical, intellectual or humanitarian character,

*Aware* that:

(*a*) Mankind is a part of nature and life depends on the uninterrupted functioning of natural systems which ensure the supply of energy and nutrients,

(*b*) Civilization is rooted in nature, which has shaped human culture and influenced all artistic and scientific achievement, and living in harmony with nature gives man the best opportunities for the development of his creativity, and for rest and recreation,

*Convinced* that:

(*a*) Every form of life is unique, warranting respect regardless of its worth to man, and, to accord other organisms such recognition, man must be guided by a moral code of action,

(*b*) Man can alter nature and exhaust natural resources by his action or its consequences and, therefore, must fully recognize the urgency of maintaining the stability and quality of nature and of conserving natural resources,

*Persuaded* that:

(*a*) Lasting benefits from nature depend upon the maintenance of essential ecological processes and life support systems, and upon the diversity of life forms, which are jeopardized through excessive exploitation and habitat destruction by man,

(*b*) The degradation of natural systems owing to excessive consumption and misuse of natural resources, as well as to failure to establish an appropriate economic order among peoples and among States, leads to the breakdown of the economic, social and political framework of civilization,

(*c*) Competition for scarce resources creates conflicts, whereas the conservation of nature and natural resources contributes to justice and the maintenance of peace and cannot be achieved until mankind learns to live in peace and to forsake war and armaments,

*Reaffirming* that man must acquire the knowledge to maintain and enhance his ability to use natural resources in a manner which ensures the preservation of the species and ecosystems for the benefit of present and future generations,

*Firmly convinced* of the need for appropriate measures, at the national and international, individual and collective, and private and public levels, to protect nature and promote international co-operation in this field,

*Adopts*, to these ends, the present World Charter for Nature, which proclaims the following principles of conservation by which all human conduct affecting nature is to be guided and judged.

## I. General Principles

1. Nature shall be respected and its essential processes shall not be impaired.

2. The genetic viability on the earth shall not be compromised; the population levels of all life forms, wild and domesticated, must be at least sufficient for their survival, and to this end necessary habitats shall be safeguarded.

3. All areas of the earth, both land and sea, shall be subject to these principles of conservation; special protection shall be given to unique areas, to representative samples of all the different types of ecosystems and to the habitats of rare or endangered species.

4. Ecosystems and organisms, as well as the land, marine and atmospheric resources that are utilized by man, shall be managed to achieve and maintain optimum sustainable productivity, but not in such a way as to endanger the integrity of those other ecosystems or species with which they coexist.

5. Nature shall be secured against degradation caused by warfare or other hostile activities.

## II. Functions

6. In the decision-making process it shall be recognized that man's needs can be met only by ensuring the proper functioning of natural systems and by respecting the principles set forth in the present Charter.

7. In the planning and implementation of social and economic development activities, due account shall be taken of the fact that the conservation of nature is an integral part of those activities.

8. In formulating long-term plans for economic development, population growth and the improvement of standards of living, due account shall be taken of the long-term capacity of natural systems to ensure the subsistence and settlement of the populations concerned, recognizing that this capacity may be enhanced through science and technology.

9. The allocation of areas of the earth to various uses shall be planned and due account shall be taken of the physical constraints, the biological productivity and diversity and the natural beauty of the areas concerned.

10. Natural resources shall not be wasted, but used with a restraint appropriate to the principles set forth in the present Charter, in accordance with the following rules:

(a) Living resources shall not be utilized in excess of their natural capacity for regeneration;

(b) The productivity of soils shall be maintained or enhanced through measures which safeguard their long-term fertility and the process of organic decomposition, and prevent erosion and all other forms of degradation;

(c) Resources, including water, which are not consumed as they are used shall be reused or recycled;

(d) Non-renewable resources which are consumed as they are used shall be exploited with restraint, taking into account their abundance, the rational possibilities of converting them for consumption, and the compatibility of their exploitation with the functioning of natural systems.

11. Activities which might have an impact on nature shall be controlled, and the best available technologies that minimize significant risks to nature or other adverse effects shall be used; in particular:

(a) Activities which are likely to cause irreversible damage to nature shall be avoided;

(b) Activities which are likely to pose a significant risk to nature shall be preceded by an exhaustive examination; their proponents shall demonstrate that expected benefits outweigh potential damage to nature, and where potential adverse effects are not fully understood, the activities should not proceed;

(c) Activities which may disturb nature shall be preceded by assessment of their consequences, and environmental impact studies of development projects shall be conducted sufficiently in advance, and if they are to be undertaken, such activities shall be planned and carried out so as to minimize potential adverse effects;

(d) Agriculture, grazing, forestry and fisheries practices shall be adapted to the natural characteristics and constraints of given areas;

(e) Areas degraded by human activities shall be rehabilitated for purposes in accord with their natural potential and compatible with the well-being of affected populations.

12. Discharge of pollutants into natural systems shall be avoided and:

(a) Where this is not feasible, such pollutants shall be treated at the source, using the best practicable means available;

(b) Special precautions shall be taken to prevent discharge of radioactive or toxic wastes.

13. Measures intended to prevent, control or limit natural disasters, infestations and diseases shall be specifically directed to the causes of these scourges and shall avoid adverse side-effects on nature.

## III. Implementation

14. The principles set forth in the present Charter shall be reflected in the law and practice of each State, as well as at the international level.

15. Knowledge of nature shall be broadly disseminated by all possible means, particularly by ecological education as an integral part of general education.

16. All planning shall include, among its essential elements, the formulation of strategies for the conservation of nature, the establishment of inventories of ecosystems and assessments of the effects on nature of proposed policies and activities; all of these elements shall be disclosed to the public by appropriate means in time to permit effective consultation and participation.

17. Funds, programmes and administrative structures necessary to achieve the objective of the conservation of nature shall be provided.

18. Constant efforts shall be made to increase knowledge of nature by scientific research and to disseminate such knowledge unimpeded by restrictions of any kind.

19. The status of natural processes, ecosystems and species shall be closely monitored to enable early detection of degradation or threat, ensure timely intervention and facilitate the evaluation of conservation policies and methods.

20. Military activities damaging to nature shall be avoided.

21. States and, to the extent they are able, other public authorities, international organizations, individuals, groups and corporations shall:

(a) Co-operate in the task of conserving nature through common activities and other relevant actions, including information exchange and consultations;

(b) Establish standards for products and manufacturing processes that may have adverse effects on nature, as well as agreed methodologies for assessing these effects;

(c) Implement the applicable international legal provisions for the conservation of nature and the protection of the environment;

(d) Ensure that activities within their jurisdictions or control do not cause damage to the natural systems located within other States or in the areas beyond the limits of national jurisdiction;

(e) Safeguard and conserve nature in areas beyond national jurisdiction.

22. Taking fully into account the sovereignty of States over their natural resources, each State shall give effect to the provisions of the present Charter through its competent organs and in co-operation with other States.

23. All persons, in accordance with their national legislation, shall have the opportunity to participate, individually or with others, in the formulation of decisions of direct concern to their environment, and shall have access to means of redress when their environment has suffered damage or degradation.

24. Each person has a duty to act in accordance with the provisions of the present Charter; acting individually, in association with others or through participation in the political process, each person shall strive to ensure that the objectives and requirements of the present Charter are met.

# RIO DECLARATION ON ENVIRONMENT AND DEVELOPMENT
### United Nations Conference on Environment and Development
### 1992

*The Rio Declaration on Environment and Development consists of twenty-seven principles for governing the economic and environmental behavior of individuals and states in the quest for global sustainability. The preamble to the declaration affirms the goal "of establishing a new and equitable global partnership" in the effort to develop international agreements that "respect the interests of all and protect the integrity of the global environmental and developmental system." It also recognizes "the integral and interdependent nature of the Earth, our home." The declaration was adopted by the United Nations Conference on Environment and Development at its meeting in Rio de Janeiro, June 3–14, 1992. The United States subscribes to the document. The text of the twenty-seven principles follows.*

1. Human beings are at the centre of concerns for sustainable development. They are entitled to a healthy and productive life in harmony with nature.

2. States have, in accordance with the Charter of the United Nations and the principles of international law, the sovereign right to exploit their own resources pursuant to their own environmental and developmental policies, and the responsibility to ensure that activities within their jurisdiction or control do not cause damage to the environment of other States or of areas beyond the limits of national jurisdiction.

3. The right to development must be fulfilled so as to equitably meet developmental and environmental needs of present and future generations.

4. In order to achieve sustainable development, environmental protection shall constitute an integral part of the development process and cannot be considered in isolation from it.

5. All States and all people shall cooperate in the essential task of eradicating poverty as an indispensable requirement for sustainable development, in order to decrease the disparities in standards of living and better meet the needs of the majority of the people of the world.

6. The special situation and needs of developing countries, particularly the least developed and those most environmentally vulnerable, shall be given special priority. International actions in the field of environment and development should also address the interests and needs of all countries.

7. States shall cooperate in a spirit of global partnership to conserve, protect and restore the health and integrity of the Earth's ecosystem. In view of the different contributions to global environmental degradation, States have common but differentiated responsibilities. The developed countries acknowledge the responsibility that they bear in the international pursuit of sustainable development in view of the pressures their societies place on the global environment and of the technologies and financial resources they command.

8. To achieve sustainable development and a higher quality of life for all people, States should reduce and eliminate unsustainable patterns of production and consumption and promote appropriate demographic policies.

9. States should cooperate to strengthen endogenous capacity-building for sustainable development by improving scientific understanding through exchanges of scientific and technological knowledge, and by enhancing the development, adaptation, diffusion and transfer of technologies, including new and innovative technologies.

10. Environmental issues are best handled with the participation of all concerned citizens, at the relevant level. At the national level, each individual shall have appropriate access to information concerning the environment that is held by public authorities, including information on hazardous materials and activities in their communities, and the opportunity to participate in decision-making processes. States shall facilitate and encourage public awareness and participation by making information widely available. Effective access to judicial and administrative proceedings, including redress and remedy, shall be provided.

11. States shall enact effective environmental legislation. Environmental standards, management objectives and priorities should reflect the environmental and developmental context to which they apply. Standards applied by some countries may be inappropriate and of unwarranted economic and social cost to other countries, in particular developing countries.

12. States should cooperate to promote a supportive and open international economic system that would lead to economic growth and sustainable development in all countries, to better address the problems of environmental degradation. Trade policy measures for environmental purposes should not constitute a means of arbitrary or unjustifiable discrimination or a disguised restriction on international trade. Unilateral actions to deal with environmental challenges outside the jurisdiction of the importing country should be avoided. Environmental measures addressing transboundary or global environmental problems should, as far as possible, be based on an international consensus.

13. States shall develop national law regarding liability and compensation for the victims of pollution and other environmental damage. States shall also cooperate in an expeditious and more determined manner to develop further international law regarding liability and compensation for adverse effects of environmental damage caused by activities within their jurisdiction or control to areas beyond their jurisdiction.

14. States should effectively cooperate to discourage or prevent the relocation and transfer to other States of any activities and substances that cause severe environmental degradation or are found to be harmful to human health.

15. In order to protect the environment, the precautionary approach shall be widely applied by States according to their capabilities. Where there are threats of serious or irreversible damage, lack of full scientific certainty shall not be used as a reason for postponing cost-effective measures to prevent environmental degradation.

16. National authorities should endeavour to promote the internalization of environmental costs and the use of economic instruments, taking into account the approach that the polluter should, in principle, bear the cost of pollution, with due regard to the public interest and without distorting international trade and investment.

17. Environmental impact assessment, as a national instrument, shall be undertaken for proposed activities that are likely to have a significant adverse impact on the environment and are subject to a decision of a competent national authority.

18. States shall immediately notify other States of any natural disasters or other emergencies that are likely to produce sudden harmful effects on the environment of those States. Every effort shall be made by the international community to help States so afflicted.

19. States shall provide prior and timely notification and relevant information to potentially affected States on activities that may have a significant adverse transboundary environmental effect and shall consult with those States at an early stage and in good faith.

20. Women have a vital role in environmental management and development. Their full participation is therefore essential to achieve sustainable development.

21. The creativity, ideals, and courage of the youth of the world should be mobilized to forge a global partnership in order to achieve sustainable development and ensure a better future for all.

22. Indigenous people and their communities and other local communities have a vital role in environmental management and development because of their knowledge and traditional practices. States should recognize and duly support their identity, culture and interests and enable their effective participation in the achievement of sustainable development.

23. The environment and natural resources of people under oppression, domination and occupation shall be protected.

24. Warfare is inherently destructive of sustainable development. States shall therefore respect international law providing protection for the environment in times of armed conflict and cooperate in its further development, as necessary.

25. Peace, development and environmental protection are interdependent and indivisible.

26. States shall resolve all their environmental disputes peacefully and by appropriate means in accordance with the Charter of the United Nations.

27. States and people shall cooperate in good faith and in a spirit of partnership in the fulfilment of the principles embodied in this Declaration and in the further development of international law in the field of sustainable development.

# CONSERVATION POLICIES
## OF THE WILDLIFE SOCIETY
**The Wildlife Society**
1988

*In addition to national and international bodies, professional organizations, such as the Wildlife Society, also issue environmental policies. Founded in 1937, the Wildlife Society is dedicated to the wise management and conservation of the world's wildlife resources. Excerpts from the society's Conservation Policies are printed below.*

### Human Populations

Burgeoning human populations continue to place an overwhelming and detrimental demand on many of the world's limited natural resources. Human degradation of terrestrial and aquatic communities is biologically unadvisable. Certain of these resources are irreplaceable, and others must be either preserved intact or managed carefully to ensure the integrity of the ecosystem and humanity. These resources will continue to decline or to sustain irreparable damage, despite scientific and technological advances, if the growth of the human population is not restrained.

The policy of The Wildlife Society, in regard to human populations is to:

1. Actively support an enlightened policy of population stabilization that will encourage the conservation of natural resources and enhance the quality of human existence.

2. Promote a better understanding of mankind's role in the world's ecosystems so as to minimize the contamination and harmful alteration of the global environment.

## Environmental Quality

The demands that human societies make upon the earth and its biota inevitably result in environmental change. Many ecosystems have been exploited for immediate monetary profit rather than managed for sustained biotic yields. Careless or excessive exploitation often leads to unnecessary degradation of the environment. The common aim of mankind should be to perfect processes for deriving support from the environment without destroying its stability, diversity, productivity, or aesthetic values.

The policy of The Wildlife Society, in regard to environmental quality, is to:

1. Stimulate and support educational programs that emphasize mankind's dependence on functional ecosystems, and, consequently, the necessity for living in harmony with the environment.

2. Foster research designed to elucidate the complex biotic relationships of ecosystems.

3. Encourage the development and use of methods designed to reduce environmental degradation and to reclaim and reconstitute degraded ecosystems.

4. Contribute to the development of technologies, social systems, and individual behaviors that will maintain the diversity and beauty of the environment.

## The Management of Living Natural Resources

Human population growth jeopardizes mankind's existence. The continued well-being of mankind, and earth's other living natural resources, is dependent upon a healthy environment maintained through the skilled management of resources. As human populations increase, wild plant and animal habitats usually decrease. Many people presume that all wild habitats are untouched by humanity. Actually, few natural areas have escaped the influence of mankind. Often these influences have disrupted natural areas, thus requiring the need for scientific management of these areas and their associated living resources.

A "hands-off," non-manipulative policy for plant and animal resources eventually could result in reestablishing naturally-functioning plant and animal communities as wild areas, if mankind's ever-present impacts could be eliminated. In such areas the actions of nature would dominate and low-priority would be given to material human wants. Such areas have been and are being established where practicable.

Only limited amounts of land can be devoted to wild areas because of the demands of our growing human population. Land is required for housing, crops, mineral and timber production, manufacture and sale of goods, intensive recreation, and other necessary and desirable purposes. Plant and animal communities associated with these more intensive land uses, although often highly productive, are usually unnatural in that they lack the diversity and stability of unaltered communities. Applying sound land and water management practices to these altered lands can assist natural processes in providing habitat suitable for plants and animals which are forced to live in close association with human activities. Plant and animal populations also may be enhanced and optimized at levels within the land's ability to support them through proven professional resource management practices.

The Wildlife Society recognizes the serious implications of mankind's ever-increasing worldwide demands for living space, food, shelter and other products. It also recognizes a need for a policy of continued, intensified and improved management for earth's living resources.

The policy of The Wildlife Society, in regard to management of living natural resources, is to:

1. Support and strengthen scientific management as the rational instrument for maintaining, restoring, and enhancing plant and animal resources for the continued use and appreciation by humanity.

2. Encourage the development and dissemination of information to improve public understanding of the need for, and the positive benefits from, scientific management.

3. Encourage the retention or enhancement of habitat for native plants and animals on public and private lands.

4. Seek support for ethical restraints in the use of living natural resources.

5. Reaffirm our view that scientific management includes both the regulated harvest of the surplus of those species in plentiful supply, as well as the protection of those plant or animal species which are rare, threatened, or in danger of extinction.

## Conservation Education

Worldwide growth of human populations is placing unprecedented demands and stresses on the world's finite natural resources. Satisfying human needs for energy, food, fibers, minerals, and wood products has the potential for further destruction of wildlife habitat and aesthetic resources. If these natural resources are to be given adequate consideration in the context of human needs, a sound program of conservation education is of paramount importance.

The educational process must contain four key elements if it is to be effective in enabling people to cope with resource problems. First, it must provide basic understanding of the properties and distribution of natural resources. Second, it must provide and encourage alternatives to current degrading resource uses and promote changes in life styles that can be accommodated by the existing resources base. Third, it must provide people with an understanding of the political, economic, and social processes by which changes in resource use can be effected. And last, it must lead to positive action in behalf of resource conservation.

The policy of The Wildlife Society, in regard to conservation education, is to:

1. Assist in the development and promotion of educational programs that will disseminate ecologically sound knowledge to advance wise management of wildlife and other natural resources.

2. Promote increased cooperation and communication among all agencies and groups concerned with conservation education and resource management.

3. Encourage members of the wildlife profession (a) to interpret and make readily available those results of wildlife research that citizens require for decision-making, and (b) to actively participate in the implementation of sound, publicly oriented programs in conservation education.

• • •

# CODE OF ETHICS FOR MEMBERS OF THE SOCIETY OF AMERICAN FORESTERS
### Society of American Foresters
### 1976, amended 1986, 1992

*In 1992 the Society of American Foresters adopted a new "land ethic canon" espousing "stewardship of" and "respect for the land." The new ethic is incorporated in the following 1992 revision of the society's Code of Ethics. Other society documents include an Ethics Guide, which discusses and elaborates upon the Code of Ethics, and the classic Forestry Handbook, which contains information for U.S. and Canadian forest practitioners.*

## Preamble

Stewardship of the land is the cornerstone of the forestry profession. The purpose of these canons is to govern the professional conduct of members of the Society of American Foresters in their relations with the public, their employers, including clients, and each other as provided in Article VIII of the Society's Constitution. Compliance with these canons demonstrates our respect for the land and our commitment to the wise management of ecosystems, and ensures just and honorable professional and human relationships, mutual confidence and respect, and competent service to society.

These canons have been adopted by the membership of the Society and can only be amended by the membership. Procedures for processing charges of violation of these canons are contained in Bylaws established by the Council. These canons and procedures apply to all membership categories in all forestry-related disciplines, except Honorary Members.

All members upon joining the Society agree to abide by this Code as a condition of membership.

## Canons

1. A member will advocate and practice land management consistent with ecologically sound principles.
2. A member's knowledge and skills will be utilized for the benefit of society. A member will strive for accurate, current and increasing knowledge of forestry, will commu-

nicate such knowledge when not confidential, and will challenge and correct untrue statements about forestry.

3. A member will advertise only in a dignified and truthful manner, stating the services the member is qualified and prepared to perform. Such advertisements may include references to fees charged.

4. A member will base public comment on forestry matters on accurate knowledge and will not distort or withhold pertinent information to substantiate a point of view. Prior to making public statements on forest policies and practices, a member will indicate on whose behalf the statements are made.

5. A member will perform services consistent with the highest standards of quality and with loyalty to the employer.

6. A member will perform only those services for which the member is qualified by education or experience.

7. A member who is asked to participate in forestry operations which deviate from accepted professional standards must advise the employer in advance of the consequences of such deviation.

8. A member will not voluntarily disclose information concerning the affairs of the member's employer without the employer's express permission.

9. A member must avoid conflicts of interest or even the appearance of such conflicts. If, despite such precaution, a conflict of interest is discovered, it must be promptly and fully disclosed to the member's employer and the member must be prepared to act immediately to resolve the conflict.

10. A member will not accept compensation or expenses from more than one employer for the same service, unless the parties involved are informed and consent.

11. A member will engage, or advise the member's employer to engage, other experts and specialists in forestry or related fields whenever the employer's interest would be best served by such action, and members will work cooperatively with other professionals.

12. A member will not by false statement or dishonest action injure the reputation or professional associations of another member.

13. A member will give credit for the methods, ideas, or assistance obtained from others.

14. A member in competition for supplying forestry services will encourage the prospective employer to base selection on comparison of qualifications and negotiation of fee or salary.

15. Information submitted by a member about a candidate for a prospective position, award, or elected office will be accurate, factual, and objective.

16. A member having evidence of violation of these canons by another member will present the information and charges to the Council in accordance with the Bylaws.

# CODE OF ETHICS AND STANDARDS OF PRACTICE FOR ENVIRONMENTAL PROFESSIONALS
## National Association of Environmental Professionals
### 1979, revised 1994

*The Code of the National Association of Environmental Professionals (NAEP) takes a broad view of environment, which includes physical, natural, and cultural systems. It is noteworthy that a New Jersey court ruled that the NAEP code of ethics be considered public policy in the state (Bowman v. Mobil Oil Corp., Civil Action No. 87-4093); as such, employees who abide by it cannot be fired for refusing to perform actions that directly contravene the code.*

The objectives of Environmental Professionals are to conduct their personal and professional lives and activities in an ethical manner. Honesty, justice and courtesy form moral philosophy which, associated with a mutual interest among people, constitute the foundation of ethics. Environmental Professionals should recognize such a standard, not in passive observance, but as a set of dynamic principles guiding their conduct and way of life. It is their duty to practice their profession according to this Code of Ethics.

As the keystone of professional conduct is integrity, Environmental Professionals will discharge their duties with fidelity to the public, their employers, clients, and with fairness and impartiality to all. It is their duty to interest themselves in public welfare, and to be ready to apply their special knowledge for the benefit of mankind and their environment.

## Creed

The objectives of an Environmental Professional are:

1. to recognize and attempt to reconcile societal and individual human needs with responsibility for physical, natural, and cultural systems.
2. to promote and develop policies, plans, activities and projects that achieve complementary and mutual support between natural and man-made, and present and future components of the physical, natural and cultural environment.

## Ethics

As an Environmental Professional I will:

1. be personally responsible for the validity of all data collected, analyses performed, or plans developed by me or under my direction. I will be responsible and ethical in my professional activities.
2. encourage reason, planning, design, management and review of activities in a scientifically and technically objective manner. I will incorporate the best principles of the environmental sciences for the mitigation of environmental harm and enhancement of environmental quality.
3. not condone misrepresentation of work I have performed or that was performed under my direction.
4. examine all of my relationships or actions which could be legitimately interpreted as a conflict of interest by clients, officials, the public or peers. In any instance where I have a financial or personal interest in the activities with which they are directly or indirectly involved, I will make a full disclosure of that interest to my employer, client, or other affected parties.
5. not engage in conduct involving dishonesty, fraud, deceit, or misrepresentation or discrimination.
6. not accept fees wholly or partially contingent on the client's desired result where that desired result conflicts with my professional judgement.

## Guidance for Practice as an Environmental Professional

As an Environmental Professional I will:

1. encourage environmental planning to begin in the earliest stages of project conceptualization.
2. recognize that total environmental management involves the consideration of all environmental factors including: technical, economic, ecological, and sociopolitical and their relationships.
3. incorporate the best principle of design and environmental planning when recommending measures to reduce environmental harm and enhance environmental quality.
4. conduct my analysis, planning, design and review my activities primarily in subject areas for which I am qualified, and shall encourage and recognize the participation of other professionals in subject areas where I am less experienced. I shall utilize and participate in interdisciplinary teams wherever practical to determine impacts, define and evaluate all reasonable alternatives to proposed actions, and assess short-term versus long-term productivity with and without the project or action.
5. seek common, adequate, and sound technical grounds for communication with and respect for the contributions of other professionals in developing and reviewing policies, plans, activities, and projects.
6. determine that the policies, plans, activities, or projects in which I am involved are consistent with all governing laws, ordinances, guidelines, plans, and policies, to the best of my knowledge and ability.
7. encourage public participation at the earliest feasible time in an open and productive atmosphere.
8. conduct my professional activities in a manner that ensures consideration of technically and economically feasible alternatives.

## Encourage Development of the Profession

As an Environmental Professional I will:

1. assist in maintaining the integrity and competence of my profession.
2. encourage education and research, and the development of useful technical information relating to the environmental field.

3. advertise and present my services in a manner that avoids the use of material and methods that may bring discredit to the profession.

# CODE OF ETHICS
### National Environmental Health Association
revised 1992

*The National Environmental Health Association's Code of Ethics explicitly states that the environment is not restricted by political boundaries; it must be viewed as a single entity. Health is recognized to be one of the fundamental rights of every human being, and those to whom the code applies have an obligation to work to provide a healthful environment for all. It is noteworthy that the code has a line for the member's signature, making it a personal pledge by the professional.*

As a member of the National Environmental Health Association, I acknowledge:

That I have an obligation to work to provide a healthful environment for all. I will uphold the standards of my profession, continually search for truths, and disseminate my findings. I will continually strive to keep myself fully informed on developments in the fields of public and environmental health and protection:

That I have an obligation to the public whose trust I hold and because of this, I will endeavor to the best of my ability to safeguard the public's health. I will be loyal to this trust in whatever governmental division, industry, or institution by which I am retained:

That the environment is not restricted by man-made political boundaries and therefore must be considered as a single entity;

That the enjoyment of the highest attainable standard of health is one of the fundamental rights of every human being without distinction of race, religion, cultural background, economic or social condition; and

That I will uphold the constitution and bylaws of the National Environmental Health Association and will at all times conduct myself in a manner worthy of my profession.

By my signature hereon, I acknowledge and affirm a realization of my personal responsibility to actively discharge these obligations.

# Bibliography

This bibliography provides references for additional codes, oaths, and directives related to bioethics to supplement the documents contained in this Appendix. The bibliography begins with a General References section, which includes several anthologies of codes and other bioethics directives, as well as three encyclopedias of organizations that contain extensive lists of pertinent associations and organizations, with their addresses and telephone/fax numbers. The remaining six sections of the bibliography represent and supplement the six sections of the Appendix.

Although intended as a useful resource, this bibliography in no way represents a complete list of bioethics directives. The anthologies listed in the General References section contain additional directives. In addition, interested readers can locate individual organizations through the encyclopedias of associations and contact them for information on their ethics publications. Further references also may be obtained by searching the BIOETHICSLINE database, accessed through the National Library of Medicine's MEDLARS system, or the CD-ROM versions of BIOETHICSLINE available from SilverPlatter Information, Inc., Norwood, Mass., and CD-Plus Technologies, New York, N.Y.; or by contacting the National Reference Center for Bioethics Literature, Kennedy Institute of Ethics, Georgetown University, Washington, D.C. 20057-1065; telephone 1-800-MED-ETHX (toll-free) or 1-202-687-3885.

*General References*

AMNESTY INTERNATIONAL, ed. 1984. *Ethical Codes and Declarations Relevant to the Medical Profession: An Amnesty International Compilation of Selected Ethical Texts for Health Professionals.* London: Author.

BAYLIS, FRANÇOISE, and JOCELYN DOWNIE, eds. 1992. *Codes of Ethics: Ethics Codes, Standards, and Guidelines for Professionals Working in a Health Care Setting in Canada.* Toronto: Department of Bioethics, Hospital for Sick Children.

BIRD, LEWIS PENHALL, and JAMES BARLOW, eds. 1989. *Codes of Medical Ethics, Oaths, and Prayers: An Anthology.* Richardson, Tex.: Christian Medical and Dental Society.

*Encyclopedia of Associations, 1993.* 1992. 27th ed. Edited by Deborah M. Burek. Detroit: Gale Research. (See Volume 1, Part II, Section 8, Health and Medical Organizations.)

*Encyclopedia of Medical Organizations and Agencies 1992–93.* 1992. 4th ed. Edited by Karen Backus. Detroit: Gale Research.

ETZIONY, M. B. 1973. *The Physician's Creed: An Anthology of Medical Prayers, Oaths, and Codes of Ethics Written and Recited by Medical Practitioners Through the Ages.* Springfield, Ill.: Charles C. Thomas.

GORLIN, RENA A., ed. 1990. *Codes of Professional Responsibility.* 2d ed. Washington, D.C.: Bureau of National Affairs. (See Section II. Health.)

HARRIS, NIGEL G. E. 1989. *Professional Codes of Conduct in the United Kingdom: A Directory.* New York: Mansell.

WORLD MEDICAL ASSOCIATION. 1993. *Handbook of Declarations.* Ferney-Voltaire, France: Author.

*Yearbook of International Organizations 1990/91.* 1990. 27th ed. Vol. 1. Edited by Union of International Associations. Munich: K. G. Saur.

*Section I. Directives on Health-Related Rights and Patient Responsibilities*

MINISTRY OF HEALTH. n.d. *Bill of Rights for the Residents of Ontario Nursing Homes.* Ontario, Canada: Ministry of Health.

NATIONAL ASSOCIATION OF PRIVATE PSYCHIATRIC HOSPITALS. 1990. *Patient Rights and Responsibilities Guidelines.* Washington, D.C.; Author.

NATIONAL COMMITTEE ON "THE DECLARATION OF PATIENTS' RIGHTS." 1984. *Kanja No Kenri Sengen* (The Declaration on Patients' Rights). Tokyo: Author.

NATIONAL CONSUMER COUNCIL (GREAT BRITAIN) AND THE ASSOCIATION OF COMMUNITY HEALTH COUNCILS FOR ENGLAND AND WALES. 1989. *Patients' Rights: A Summary of Your Rights and Responsibilities in the NHS.* London: Association of Community Health Councils for England and Wales.

SPAIN (BASQUE AUTONOMOUS COMMUNITY). 1989. "Decree No. 175/1989 of 18 July 1989 approving the Charter of the Rights and Obligations of Patients and Users of the Basque Health Service." *Boletín Oficial del Ministerio de Sanidad y Consumo* (July–Sept., No. 27):2023–2026. [Reprinted in *International Digest of Health Legislation* 43, no. 1:84–92.]

SWITZERLAND (BERNE). 1989. "Decree of 14 February 1989 on the Rights and Duties of Patients in Public Hospitals (The Decree on Patients)." [Reprinted in *International Digest of Health Legislation* 41, no. 1:98–101.]

UNITED STATES. 1990. Omnibus Budget Reconciliation Act of 1990 [Patient Self-Determination Act]. Public Law 101-508 (5 November 1990), Sections 4206, 4751. 104 Stat. 1388—115-117, 204-206.

*Section II. Ethical Directives for the Practice of Medicine*

AMERICAN ACADEMY OF CHILD AND ADOLESCENT PSYCHIATRY. 1980. *Code of Ethics and Clarification Notes on the Code of Ethics.* Washington, D.C.: Author.

AMERICAN ACADEMY OF OPHTHALMOLOGY. 1992. *Code of Ethics.* San Francisco: Author.

AMERICAN ACADEMY OF ORTHOPAEDIC SURGEONS. 1992. *Guide to the Ethical Practice of Orthopaedic Surgery.* 2d ed. Park Ridge, Ill.: Author.

AMERICAN ACADEMY OF PSYCHIATRY AND THE LAW. 1991. *Ethical Guidelines for the Practice of Forensic Psychiatry.* Baltimore: Author.

AMERICAN BOARD OF INTERNAL MEDICINE. 1986. *A Guide to the Awareness and Evaluation of Humanistic Qualities in the Internist.* Philadelphia: Author.

AMERICAN COLLEGE OF CHEST PHYSICIANS. 1990. "ACCP Guidelines for an Expert Witness." *Chest* 98:1006.

AMERICAN COLLEGE OF OBSTETRICIANS AND GYNECOLOGISTS. 1981. Ethical Considerations in the Practice of Obstetrics and Gynecology. In *Standards for Obstetric-Gynecologic Services,* 7th ed., 107–110. Washington, D.C.: Author.

AMERICAN COLLEGE OF PHYSICIANS. 1992. American College of Physicians Ethics Manual. 3d ed. [Position paper]. *Annals of Internal Medicine* 117:947–960.

———. 1993. "Guidelines for the Physician Expert Witness." *Annals of Internal Medicine* 113:789.

AMERICAN COLLEGE OF RADIOLOGY. 1991. Code of Ethics. In *The American College of Radiology 1991 Bylaws,* 15–16. Reston, Va.: Author.

AMERICAN COLLEGE OF SURGEONS. 1989. *Statements on Principles.* Chicago: Author.

AMERICAN MEDICAL ASSOCIATION. 1984– . *Reports of the Council on Ethical and Judicial Affairs.* Chicago: Author. [Published twice a year in January and July, the *Reports* contain in-depth analyses of the ethical questions considered by the council. Many past *Reports* have been published in the *Journal of the American Medical Association* and other peer-reviewed journals.]

AMERICAN PODIATRIC MEDICAL ASSOCIATION. n.d. *Code of Ethics.* Bethesda, Md.: Author.

AMERICAN PSYCHIATRIC ASSOCIATION. 1989. *Opinions of the Ethics Committee on the Principles of Medical Ethics.* Washington, D.C.: Author.

————. 1989. *Principles of Medical Ethics: With Annotations Especially Applicable to Psychiatry.* Washington, D.C.: Author.

AMERICAN PSYCHOANALYTIC ASSOCIATION. 1984. *Principles of Ethics for Psychoanalysis and Provisions for Implementation of the Principles of Ethics for Psychoanalysis.* New York: Author.

AMERICAN SOCIETY OF ANESTHESIOLOGISTS. 1987. *Guidelines for the Ethical Practice of Anesthesiology.* Park Ridge, Ill.: Author.

AMERICAN SOCIETY OF CLINICAL PATHOLOGISTS. n.d. *ASCP Guidelines for Ethical Behavior for Pathologists.* Chicago: Author.

AUSTRALIAN MEDICAL ASSOCIATION. 1975. *Code of Ethics.* Sydney: Author.

BELGIUM. CONSEIL NATIONAL DE L' ORDRE DES MÉDECINS. 1975. *Code de Déontologie Médicale.* Brussels: Conseil National.

BRITISH MEDICAL ASSOCIATION. 1992. *Rights and Responsibilities of Doctors.* 2d ed. London: Author.

————. 1993. *Medical Ethics Today: Its Practice and Philosophy.* London: Author.

CHRISTIAN MEDICAL & DENTAL SOCIETY. 1991. *Opinions on Ethical and Social Issues.* Richardson, Tex.: Author.

COSTA RICA. COLEGIO DE MÉDICOS Y CIRUJANOS DE COSTA RICA. 1981. *Código de Moral Médica.*

FRANÇOIS, JULES. INTERNATIONAL ACADEMY OF OPHTHALMOLOGY. 1978. Code of Ophthalmological Ethics. *Transactions of the Ophthalmological Society of the United Kingdom* 98:514–520.

HAITIAN MEDICAL ASSOCIATION. 1988. *Code de Déontologie de l'Association Médicale Haïtienne.* Haiti: Association Médicale Haïtienne.

*Hippocratic Oath—From the Oath According to Hippocrates Insofar as a Christian May Swear It.* n.d. In *Codes of Medical Ethics, Oaths, and Prayers: An Anthology.* Edited by Lewis Penhall Bird and James Barlow. Richardson, Tex.: Christian Medical & Dental Society, 1989.

ITALY. FEDERAZIONE NAZIONALE DEGLI ORDINI DEI MEDICI CHIRURGHI E DEGLI ODONTOIATRI. 1990. "Codice di Deontologia Medica." *Il Medico d' Italia,* suppl. to no. 44:1–30.

JAPAN HOSPITAL ASSOCIATION. 1983. *Kinmu Ishi Manual* (A Hospital Physician's Manual). Tokyo: Author.

JAPAN MEDICAL ASSOCIATION. 1956. *Physician's Code of Ethics* [1951]. Tokyo: Author.

MELLOR, CLIVE. 1980. "The Canadian Medical Association Code of Ethics Annotated for Psychiatrists." *Canadian Journal of Psychiatry* 25:432–438.

PERCIVAL, THOMAS. 1975. *Medical Ethics: A Code of Institutes and Precepts, Adapted to the Professional Conduct of Physicians and Surgeons.* Edited by Chauncey D. Leake. Huntington, N.Y.: R. E. Krieger. [Reprint of the 1927 edition published by Williams & Wilkins, Baltimore.]

POLAND. NATIONAL CONGRESS OF PHYSICIANS. 1992. "The Code of Medical Ethics [1991]." *Kennedy Institute of Ethics Journal* 2:371–384. [The 1991 Polish Code of Medical Ethics was updated in 1993.]

SWISS ACADEMY OF MEDICAL SCIENCES [ACADÉMIE SUISSE DES SCIENCES MÉDICALE]. 1989. *Directives et recommandations d'Éthique médicale de l'Académie Suisse des Sciences Médicales.* Basel: Author.

TUNISIA. 1993. "Decree No. 93-1155 of 17 May 1993 Promulgating the Code of Medical Ethics." *Journal Officiel de la République Tunisienne,* no. 40 (28 May and 1 June):764–770. [Excerpts reprinted in *International Digest of Health Legislation* 45(1):53–54.]

WORLD PSYCHIATRIC ASSOCIATION. GENERAL ASSEMBLY. 1977. "Declaration of Hawaii." *Psychiatric News* 12, no. 15:5, 15.

*Section III. Ethical Directives for Other Health-Care Professions*

AMERICAN ASSOCIATION FOR COUNSELING AND DEVELOPMENT. 1988. "Ethical Standards of the American Association for Counseling and Development." *Journal of Counseling and Development* 67 (Sept.):4–8.

AMERICAN ASSOCIATION FOR RESPIRATORY CARE. 1985. *Code of Ethics.* Dallas, Tex.: Author.

AMERICAN ASSOCIATION OF NURSE ANESTHETISTS. 1986. *Code of Ethics with Interpretive Statements for the Certified Registered Nurse Anesthetist.* Park Ridge, Ill.: Author.

AMERICAN ASSOCIATION OF OCCUPATIONAL HEALTH NURSES. 1991. "Code of Ethics with Interpretive Statements." *AAOHN Journal* 39 (10, Suppl. 470):S1–S4.

AMERICAN COLLEGE OF HEALTH CARE ADMINISTRATORS. n.d. *Code of Ethics.* Alexandria, Va.: Author.

AMERICAN COLLEGE OF NURSE-MIDWIVES. 1990. *Code of Ethics for Certified Nurse Midwives.* Washington, D.C.: Author.

AMERICAN DENTAL HYGIENIST'S ASSOCIATION. 1988. *Standards of Dental Hygiene Practice and Principles of Ethics.* Chicago: Author.

AMERICAN HOLISTIC NURSES ASSOCIATION. 1991. Code of Ethics for Holistic Nurses. *Beginnings* (American Holistic Nurses' Association) 11, no. 8:5.

AMERICAN HOSPITAL ASSOCIATION. 1994. *Values in Conflict: Resolving Ethical Issues in Health Care.* Chicago: Author.

AMERICAN MEDICAL RECORD ASSOCIATION. 1990. "Code of Ethics." In *AMRA Code of Ethics and Bylaws,* 2. Chicago: Author.

AMERICAN MEDICAL TECHNOLOGISTS. n.d. *Standards of Practice.* Park Ridge, Ill.: Author.

AMERICAN MENTAL HEALTH COUNSELOR'S ASSOCIATION. n.d. *Code of Ethics for Mental Health Counselors.* Alexandria, Va.: American Mental Health Counselor's Association, American Association for Counseling and Development.

AMERICAN NURSES' ASSOCIATION. 1988. *Ethics in Nursing: Position Statements and Guidelines.* Washington, D.C.: American Nurses Publishing.

AMERICAN OPTOMETRIC ASSOCIATION. 1976. *Code of Ethics and Standards of Conduct.* St. Louis, Mo.: Author.

AMERICAN SOCIETY FOR MEDICAL TECHNOLOGY. n.d. *Code of Ethics.* Washington, D.C.: Author.

AMERICAN SOCIETY OF CONSULTANT PHARMACISTS. n.d. *Code of Ethics.* Alexandria, Va.: Author.

AMERICAN SOCIETY OF RADIOLOGIC TECHNOLOGISTS. 1990. *Code of Ethics.* Albuquerque, N.M.: Author.

AMERICAN SPEECH-LANGUAGE-HEARING ASSOCIATION. 1992. "Code of Ethics." *ASHA: Journal of the American Speech and Hearing Association* 34 (Suppl. 9):1–2.

CANADIAN DENTAL HYGIENISTS' ASSOCIATION. 1989. "Code of Ethics of the Canadian Dental Hygienists' Association." *Probe* (Canadian Dental Hygienists' Association) 23:173.

CHRISTIAN ASSOCIATION FOR PSYCHOLOGICAL STUDIES. 1992. *Ethical Guidelines for the Christian Association for Psychological Studies.* Temecula, Cal.: Author.

CHRISTIAN MEDICAL DENTAL SOCIETY. 1991. *Opinions on Ethical and Social Issues.* Richardson, Tex.: Author.

COLLEGE OF CHAPLAINS. 1989. *Code of Ethics.* Schaumburg, Ill.: Author.

EMERGENCY NURSES ASSOCIATION. 1990. "Code of Ethics for Emergency Nurses with Interpretive Statements." *Journal of Emergency Nursing* 16, no. 6:22A–24A.

FRANCE. 1993. "Decree No. 93-221 of 16 February 1993 on the Professional Rules to Be Followed by Nurses." *Journal Officiel de la République Française,*

*Lois et Décrets* (18 February, No. 41):2646–2649. [Table of Contents reprinted in *International Digest of Health Legislation* 45, no. 1:53.]

INTERNATIONAL CHIROPRACTORS ASSOCIATION. 1991. *ICA Policy Handbook & Code of Ethics.* 2nd ed. Arlington, Va.: Author.

INTERNATIONAL COMMISSION ON OCCUPATIONAL HEALTH. 1992. "Occupational Health Code of Ethics." *Bulletin of Medical Ethics* (Oct., No. 82):7–11.

INTERNATIONAL COUNCIL OF NURSES. n.d. *ICN Guidelines.* Geneva, Switzerland: Author. [List of topics is available from the ICN.]

———. n.d. *ICN Position Statements.* Geneva, Switzerland: Author. [This is a collection of ICN position statements adopted by the Council of National Representatives, ICN's governing body. A list of statements in the set is available from the ICN.]

NATIONAL ASSOCIATION OF PRIVATE PSYCHIATRIC HOSPITALS. 1989. *Statement of Principles of Psychiatric Hospital Practice Ethics.* Washington, D.C.: Author.

NATIONAL FEDERATION OF SOCIETIES FOR CLINICAL SOCIAL WORK. 1987. "Code of Ethics." *Clinical Social Work Journal* 15:81–91.

NORWEGIAN NURSES ASSOCIATION. 1989. *Comments to Ethical Guidelines.* Norsk Sykepleierforbund.

NATIONAL SOCIETY OF GENETIC COUNSELORS. 1992. "Code of Ethics." *Journal of Genetic Counseling* 1:41–43.

PANAMERICAN FEDERATION OF NURSING PROFESSIONALS. 1991. *Codigo de Ethica.* Santiago, Chile: Federacion Panamericana de Profesionales de Enfermeria.

ROYAL COLLEGE OF NURSING SOCIETY OF OCCUPATIONAL HEALTH NURSING. 1987. *Code of Professional Practice in Occupational Health Nursing.* London: The Royal College of Nursing of the United Kingdom.

SOCIETY FOR CLINICAL AND EXPERIMENTAL HYPNOSIS. 1990. *Code of Ethics.* Liverpool, N.Y.: Author.

SOCIETY FOR PUBLIC HEALTH EDUCATION. 1983. *Code of Ethics.* San Francisco: Author.

SOCIETY OF DIAGNOSTIC MEDICAL SONOGRAPHERS. n.d. *Code of Professional Conduct for Diagnostic Medical Sonographers.* Dallas, Tex.: Author.

UNITED KINGDOM CENTRAL COUNCIL FOR NURSING, MIDWIFERY AND HEALTH VISITING. 1984. *UKCC Code of Professional Conduct for the Nurse, Midwife, and Health Visitor.* UKCC.

———. 1986. *A Midwife's Code of Practice for Midwives Practising in the United Kingdom.* UKCC.

*Section IV. Ethical Directives for Human Research*

AMERICAN COLLEGE OF NEUROPSYCHOPHARMACOLOGY. 1990. *Code of Ethics.* Nashville, Tenn.: Author. [The college is a scientific organization dedicated to research that will enhance treatment of brain and behavioral disorders; its code focuses on issues pertinent to research.]

———. 1985. *A Statement of Principle of Ethical Conduct for Neuropsychopharmacologic Research in Humans.* Nashville, Tenn.: Author.

AMERICAN FERTILITY SOCIETY. ETHICS COMMITTEE. 1990. "Ethical Considerations of the New Reproductive Technologies." *Fertility and Sterility* 53 (6, Suppl. 2):1S–109S.

AMERICAN MEDICAL ASSOCIATION. COUNCIL ON ETHICAL AND JUDICIAL AFFAIRS. 1994. *Code of Medical Ethics: Current Opinions with Annotations,* 12–15 [Clinical Investigation], 18–19 [Fetal Research Guidelines]. Chicago: Author.

AMERICAN OCCUPATIONAL THERAPY FOUNDATION. RESEARCH ADVISORY COUNCIL. 1988. "Ethical Considerations for Research in Occupational Therapy [Approved 1986]." *American Journal of Occupational Therapy* 42:129–130.

AMERICAN PSYCHOLOGICAL ASSOCIATION. 1992. *Ethical Principles of Psychologists and Code of Conduct.* Washington, D.C.: Author. [See Section III of this Appendix.]

AMERICAN SOCIETY OF HOSPITAL PHARMACISTS. 1983. "ASHP Guidelines for the Use of Investigational Drugs in Institutions." *American Journal of Hospital Pharmacy* 40:449–451.

AMERICAN SPEECH-LANGUAGE-HEARING ASSOCIATION. 1992. Ethics in Research and Professional Practice. *ASHA: Journal of the American Speech and Hearing Association* 34 (suppl. 9):11–12.

BEAUCHAMP, TOM L.; COOK, RALPH R.; FAYERWEATHER, WILLIAM E.; RAABE, GERHARD K.; et al. 1991. "Ethical Guidelines for Epidemiologists." *Journal of Clinical Epidemiology* 44 (suppl.):151S–169S.

BRITISH PAEDIATRIC ASSOCIATION. ETHICS ADVISORY COMMITTEE. 1992. *Guidelines for the Ethical Conduct of Medical Research Involving Children.* London: Author.

CANADIAN NURSES ASSOCIATION. 1983. *Ethical Guidelines for Nursing Research Involving Human Subjects.* Ottawa, Ontario: Author.

CANADIAN PSYCHOLOGICAL ASSOCIATION. 1986. *A Canadian Code of Ethics for Psychologists.* Ottawa, Ontario: Author.

COMMISSION OF THE EUROPEAN COMMUNITIES (CEC). WORKING GROUP ON THE ETHICAL, SOCIAL AND LEGAL ASPECTS OF HUMAN GENOME ANALYSIS. 1991. *Report of 31 December 1991.* Brussels: Author.

———. WORKING GROUP ON HUMAN EMBRYOS AND RESEARCH. 1992. *First Report, March 1992.* Brussels: Author.

COUNCIL FOR INTERNATIONAL ORGANIZATIONS OF MEDICAL SCIENCES (CIOMS). 1990. *Genetics, Ethics and Human Values: Human Genome Mapping, Genetic Screening and Gene Therapy* [The Declaration of Inuyama]. Geneva, Switzerland: Author.

———. 1991. *International Guidelines for Ethical Review of Epidemiological Studies.* Geneva, Switzerland: Author.

COUNCIL OF EUROPE. PARLIAMENTARY ASSEMBLY. 1982. *Recommendation 934 (1982) on Genetic Engineering.* Brussels: Author.

DENMARK. 1987. *Act on the Establishment of an Ethical Council and Regulation of Certain Forms of Biomedical Experiments.* Act No. 353 (3 June). Ministry of Health.

ETHICS ADVISORY BOARD. DEPARTMENT OF HEALTH, EDUCATION, AND WELFARE. 1979. *Report and Conclusions: HEW Support of Research Involving Human In Vitro Fertilization and Embryo Transfer.* Washington, D.C.: U.S. Government Printing Office.

EUROPEAN COMMISSION. WORKING PARTY. 1989. *Ethics of New Reproductive Technologies: The Glover Report to the European Commission.* DeKalb: Northern Illinois University Press.

FOOD AND DRUG ADMINISTRATION (U.S.). 1989. "FDA Regulations Which Relate to Institutional Review Board Activities." *FDA IRB Information Sheets* (February):53–55. [All of the final regulations can be found in Title 21 *Code of Federal Regulations,* which can be purchased from the Superintendent of Documents, U.S. Government Printing Office, Washington, D.C. 20402.]

———. 1989. "Treatment Use of Investigational New Drugs." *FDA Clinical Investigator Fact Sheets* (May):29–35. [See generally *FDA Clinical Investigator Fact Sheets,* Rockville, Md.: FDA.]

———. 1991. *Points to Consider in Human Somatic Cell Therapy and Gene Therapy.* Rockville, Md.: Center for Biologics Evaluation and Research.

———. 1992. "New Drug, Antibiotic, and Biological Drug Product Regulations; Accelerated Approval [Final Rule]." *Federal Register* 57:58942–58960.

FRANCE. 1991. "Protection of Persons Undergoing Biomedical Research: Code of Public Health; Book IIA [translated]." *Bulletin of Medical Ethics*, no. 66 (March):8–11.

GERMAN MEDICAL ASSOCIATION. FEDERAL MEDICAL BOARD. SCIENTIFIC ADVISORY BOARD. 1986. "Guidelines Concerning Research on Early Human Embryos [English translation]." *World Medical Journal* 33 (2/3):29–33.

IRELAND. NATIONAL DRUGS ADVISORY BOARD. 1985. "Guidelines Relevant to the Procedure for Conduct of Clinical Trials." *International Digest of Health Legislation* 38:376–383.

ISRAEL. 1980. "The Public Health (Medical Experiments Involving Human Subjects) Regulations." *Kovetz HaTakkanot* no. 4189:292. [Reprinted in *International Digest of Health Legislation* 38:270–272.]

MEDICAL RESEARCH COUNCIL OF CANADA. 1987. *Guidelines on Research Involving Human Subjects*. Ottawa, Ontario: Author. [Includes a selected bibliography of codes and guidelines for the protection of research subjects.]

———. 1990. *Guidelines for Research on Somatic Cell Gene Therapy in Humans*. Ottawa, Ontario: Author. [Includes a bibliography of government documents from eight countries and the Council of Europe.]

MEDICAL RESEARCH COUNCIL OF GREAT BRITAIN. 1992. "MRC Guidance on Research Ethics; Children, the Mentally Incapacitated." *Journal International de Bioéthique/International Journal of Bioethics* 3:185–186.

———. 1992. "New MRC Guidance on Research Ethics [Responsibility in Investigations on Human Participants and Material and on Personal Information]." *Bulletin of Medical Ethics* (December):18–23.

———. WORKING PARTY ON RESEARCH ON CHILDREN. 1991. *The Ethical Conduct of Research on Children*. MRC Ethics Series. London: Medical Research Council.

———. WORKING PARTY ON RESEARCH ON THE MENTALLY INCAPACITATED. 1991. *The Ethical Conduct of Research on the Mentally Incapacitated*. MRC Ethics Series. London: Medical Research Council.

MEXICO. 1986. Regulations of 23 December 1986 for the Implementation of the General Law on Health, in the Field of Health Research. *Diario Oficial*, no. 6 (6 January 1987):98–113. [Reprinted in *International Digest of Health Legislation* 38, no. 4:791–805.]

NATIONAL HEALTH AND MEDICAL RESEARCH COUNCIL. 1983. *Guidelines on Transplantation of Fetal Tissue and Fetal Research*. Canberra, Australia: Author.

———. 1987. *Ethical Aspects of Research on Human Gene Therapy*. Canberra, Australia: Author.

———. 1988. *NHMRC Statement on Human Experimentation and Supplementary Notes*. Canberra, Australia: Author. [Contains "1982 Statement on Human Experimentation" and seven supplementary notes on specific topics.]

———. 1992. *Guidelines for the Monitoring of Research by Institutional Ethics Committees*. Canberra, Australia: Author.

NATIONAL INSTITUTES OF HEALTH (NIH). 1986. *Guidelines for Research Involving Recombinant DNA Molecules*. Bethesda, Md.: Author. [Available from Office of Recombinant DNA Activities, National Institutes of Health, Bethesda, Md., USA.]

———. RECOMBINANT DNA ADVISORY COMMITTEE. 1985, rev. 1989. *Points to Consider in the Design and Submission of Protocols for the Transfer of Recombinant DNA into the Genome of Human Subjects*. Bethesda, Md.: Author. [Available from Office of Recombinant DNA Activities, National Institutes of Health, Bethesda, Md.: USA.]

NORDIC COUNCIL ON MEDICINES. 1989. *Good Clinical Trial Practice: Nordic Guidelines*. Uppsala, Sweden: Author.

APPENDIX

NORTHERN NURSES' FEDERATION. 1987. *Ethical Guidelines for Nursing Research in Nordic Countries.* Aurskog, Norway: Author. [The Northern Nurses' Federation is a regional body consisting of the nurses' associations of Denmark, Finland, Iceland, Norway, and Sweden.]

PRESIDENT'S COMMISSION FOR THE STUDY OF ETHICAL PROBLEMS IN MEDICINE AND BIOMEDICAL AND BEHAVIORAL RESEARCH. 1982. *Splicing Life: The Social and Ethical Issues of Genetic Engineering with Human Beings.* Washington, D.C.: U.S. Government Printing Office.

ROYAL COLLEGE OF NURSING. 1977. *Ethics Related to Research in Nursing.* London: Author.

ROYAL COLLEGE OF PHYSICIANS. 1986. *Research on Healthy Volunteers.* London: Author.

————. 1990. "Research Involving Patients: Summary and Recommendations of a Report of the Royal College of Physicians." *Journal of the Royal College of Physicians of London* 24, no. 1:10–14. [Text of the full report is available from the College.]

————. 1992. "Guidelines on the Practice of Ethics Committees in Medical Research Involving Human Subjects, 2nd ed." *Journal of the Royal College of Physicians of London* 26, no. 3:292.

WARNOCK, MARY. 1984. *Report of the Committee of Inquiry into Human Fertilization and Embryology.* London: Her Majesty's Stationery Office.

WORLD MEDICAL ASSOCIATION. 1987. *Statement on Genetic Counseling and Genetic Engineering.* Ferney-Voltaire, France: Author.

————. 1989. *World Medical Association Recommendations Guiding Physicians in Biomedical Research Involving Human Subjects.* Ferney-Voltaire, France: Author.

*Section V. Ethical Directives Pertaining to the Welfare and Use of Animals*

AMERICAN ASSOCIATION FOR THE ADVANCEMENT OF SCIENCE. 1990. "AAAS Resolution on the Use of Animals in Research, Testing, and Education." *Science* 248:611.

AMERICAN VETERINARY MEDICAL ASSOCIATION. 1993. "AVMA Policy Statements and Guidelines." In *1993 AVMA Membership Directory and Resource Manual,* 55–71. Schaumburg, Ill.: Author. [Includes "Guidelines on Alternate Therapies" (1988) and "Positions on Animal Welfare" (1990)—including the "AVMA Policy on Animal Welfare and Animal Rights."]

————. 1986. "1986 Report of the AVMA Panel on Euthanasia." *Journal of the American Veterinary Medical Association* 188:252–268.

Animal Welfare Act. 1966. 7 U.S.C. 2131 et seq.

ANIMAL WELFARE INSTITUTE. 1990. *Animals and Their Legal Rights.* 4th ed. Washington, D.C.: Author. [Includes an appendix with the principal laws affording animal welfare.]

BIOLOGICAL COUNCIL. 1987. *Guidelines on the Use of Living Animals in Scientific Investigations.* London: Author.

BRITISH ASSOCIATION FOR THE ADVANCEMENT OF SCIENCE. 1990. *Declaration on Animals in Medical Research.* London: Author.

BRITISH PSYCHOLOGICAL SOCIETY. SCIENTIFIC AFFAIRS BOARD. 1985. "Guidelines for the Use of Animals in Research." *Bulletin of the British Psychological Society* 38:289–291.

CANADIAN COUNCIL ON ANIMAL CARE. 1980–1984. *Guide to the Care and Use of Experimental Animals.* 2 vols. Ottawa, Ontario: Author.

COUNCIL OF THE EUROPEAN COMMUNITIES. 1986. Resolution Regarding the Protection of Animals Used for Experimental and Other Scientific Purposes (No. 86/C 331/2).

GREAT BRITAIN. 1986. *Animals (Scientific Procedures) Act 1986.* London: Her Majesty's Stationery Office.

Institute of Laboratory Animal Resources. National Research Council. n.d. *Education and Training in the Care and Use of Laboratory Animals: A Guide for Developing Institutional Programs.* Washington, D.C.: National Academy Press.

————. n.d. *Recognition and Alleviation of Pain and Distress in Laboratory Animals.* Washington, D.C.: National Academy Press.

National Academy of Sciences. 1988. *Use of Laboratory Animals in Biomedical and Behavioral Research.* Washington, D.C.: National Academy Press.

National Animal Ethics Advisory Committee. 1988. *Guidelines for Institutional Animal Ethics Committees.* New Zealand: National Animal Ethics Advisory Committee.

National Association of Biology Teachers. 1989. *The Responsible Use of Animals in Biology Classrooms, Including Alternatives to Dissection.* A NABT Policy Statement. Reston, Va.: Author.

National Institutes of Health. Public Health Service. 1985. *Guide for the Care and Use of Laboratory Animals.* NIH Publication No. 86-23. Washington, D.C.: U.S. Government Printing Office. [Prepared for NIH by the Institute of Laboratory Animal Resources, National Academy of Sciences, Washington, D.C.]

————. 1986. *Public Health Service Policy on Humane Care and Use of Laboratory Animals.* Bethesda, Md.: OPRR, National Institutes of Health.

National Society for Medical Research. n.d. *Principles of Laboratory Animal Care.* Washington, D.C.: Author.

New York Academy of Sciences. 1988. *Interdisciplinary Principles and Guidelines for the Use of Animals in Research, Testing, and Education.* New York: Author.

South African Veterinary Association. 1986. "Policy Statement on Laboratory Animals." *Journal of the South African Veterinary Association* 57:131–132.

Swiss Academy of Medical Sciences. Swiss Academy of Sciences. 1992. "Ethical Principles and Guidelines for Scientific Experiments on Animals." *Experientia* 48, no. 1:1–3.

United States Congress. Office of Technology Assessment. 1986. *Alternatives to Animal Use in Research, Testing, and Education.* Washington, D.C.: U.S. Government Printing Office.

United States Department of Agriculture Animal and Plant Inspection Service. n.d. *Code of Federal Regulations* (CFR), Title 9 (Animals and Animal Products), Subchapter A (Animal Welfare). [Regulations implementing the Animal Welfare Act.]

*Section VI. Ethical Directives Pertaining to the Environment*

Lubchenco, Jane; Olson, Annette M.; Brubaker, Lind B.; et al. 1991. "The Sustainable Biosphere Initiative: An Ecological Research Agenda. A Report from the Ecological Society of America." *Ecology* 72:371–412.

National Research Council. 1990. *Forestry Research: A Mandate for Change.* Washington, D.C.: National Academy Press.

Society of American Foresters. n.d. *Ethics Guide.* Bethesda, Md.: Society of American Foresters.

————. 1984. *Forestry Handbook.* New York: John Wiley & Sons.

United Nations World Commission on Environment and Development. 1987. *Our Common Future* (The Brundtland Report). New York: Oxford University Press.

United States Department of Agriculture Forest Service. 1990. *Strategy for the 90's for USDA Forest Service Research.* Washington, D.C.: United States Department of Agriculture.

# Credits

### Section I: Directives on Health-Related Rights and Patient Responsibilities

1. Constitution. World Health Organization. Reprinted by permission of the Organization.

2. Universal Declaration of Human Rights. *Yearbook of the United Nations 1948–49.* New York: Columbia University Press/United Nations, 1950, pp. 535–537. Reprinted by permission of the United Nations.

3. Rights of the Child. *Yearbook of the United Nations 1959.* New York: Columbia University Press/United Nations, 1960, pp. 198–199. Reprinted by permission of the United Nations.

4. Rights of Mentally Retarded Persons. *Yearbook of the United Nations 1971,* vol. 25. New York: United Nations, 1974, p. 368. Reprinted by permission of the United Nations.

5. A Patient's Bill of Rights. American Hospital Association. Reprinted by permission of the Association.

6. Declaration of Lisbon. World Medical Assocation. Reprinted by permission of the Association.

7. Declaration on Physician Independence. World Medical Association. Reprinted by permission of the Association.

8. Fundamental Elements. Council on Ethical and Judicial Affairs. *Code of Medical Ethics.* Chicago, Ill.: American Medical Association, 1994, pp. xxxiv–xxxv. Reprinted by permission of the Association.

9. Patient Responsibilities. Council on Ethical and Judicial Affairs. *Code of Medical Ethics.* Chicago, Ill.: American Medical Association, 1994, pp. xxxvi–xxxvii. Reprinted by permission of the Association.

10. Patient Rights. *Accreditation Manual for Hospitals, 1994.* Oakbrook Terrace, Ill.: Joint Commission on Accreditation of Healthcare Organizations, 1994, sec. 4. Reprinted by permission of the Joint Commission.

### Section II: Ethical Directives for the Practice of Medicine

1. Oath of Hippocrates. Ludwig Edelstein. "The Hippocratic Oath: Text, Translation and Interpretation." *Bulletin of the History of Medicine,* supplement 1 (1943): 1–64, p. 3. Reprinted by permission of the Johns Hopkins University Press.

2. Oath of Initiation. A. Menon and H. F. Haberman. "Oath of Initiation" (from the *Caraka Samhita*). *Medical History* 14 (1970): 295–296. Reprinted by permission of the BMJ Publishing Group, London.

3. Oath of Asaph. Translated by Dr. Suessman Munter for *Medical Ethics: A Compendium of Jewish Moral, Ethical and Religious Principles in Medical Practice.* Edited by M. D. Tendler. 5th ed. New York: Committee on Religious Affairs, Federation of Jewish Philanthropies, 1975, pp. 7–9. Reprinted by permission of the UJA-Federation of New York.

4. Advice to a Physician. Translated by Rahmatollah Eshraghi.

5. 17 Rules of Enjuin. Translated by William O. Reinhardt, John Z. Bowers. *Western Medical Pioneers in Feudal Japan.* Baltimore: Johns Hopkins University Press, 1970, pp. 8–10. Reprinted by permission of the publisher.

6. Five Commandments and Ten Requirements. Translated by T'ao Lee. "Medical Ethics in Ancient China." *Bulletin of the History of Medicine* 13 (1943): 268–277. Reprinted by permission of the Johns Hopkins University Press.

7. A Physician's Ethical Duties. Translated and condensed by Rahmatollah Eshraghi.

8. Daily Prayer of a Physician. Translated by Harry Friedenwald. *Bulletin of the Johns Hopkins Hospital* 28 (1917): 260–261. Reprinted by permission of the Johns Hopkins University Press.

9. Code of Ethics (1847). *Code of Ethics*. New York: H. Ludwig & Co., 1848. American Medical Association. Reprinted by permission of the Association.

10. Venezuelan Code. "Codigo Venezolano de Moral Medica." In Luis Razetti, *Obras Completas: I. Deontologia Medica.* Caracas: Ministerio de Sanidad y Asistencia Social, 1963, pp. 111–135. The excerpt translated here is found on pp. 124–127.

11. Declaration of Geneva. World Medical Association. Reprinted by permission of the Association.

12. International Code. World Medical Association. Reprinted by permission of the Association.

13. Principles (1957). American Medical Association. Reprinted by permission of the Association.

14. Principles (1980). Council on Ethical and Judicial Affairs. *Code of Medical Ethics.* Chicago: American Medical Association, 1994, p. xiv. Reprinted by permission of the Association.

15. Current Opinions. Council on Ethical and Judicial Affairs. *Code of Medical Ethics.* Chicago, Ill.: American Medical Association, 1994. Reprinted by permission of the Association.

16. Moral and Technical Competence. American Academy of Ophthalmology. Reprinted by permission of the Academy.

17. Code of Ethics. American Osteopathic Association. Reprinted by permission of the Association.

18. Code of Ethics and Guide. Canadian Medical Association. Reprinted by permission of the Association.

19. Code of Ethics and Guide. New Zealand Medical Association. Reprinted by permission of the Association.

20. Code of Ethics. Translated by Glenn A. Wilson. "Codigo de Etica del Colegio Medico de Chile." *Revista Medica de Chile* 112 (1984):516–522. Reprinted by permission of the Revista Medica de Chile.

21. Code of Medical Ethics. Translated by Hilde Bremmer Novaes. "Codigo de Etica Medica, Brasil." Conselho Federal de Medicina, Brasil. Reprinted by permission of the Council.

22. European Code. *World Medical Journal* 34, no. 5 (September/October 1987):66–69. Deutscher Aerzte-Verlag GmbH.

23. Code of Ethics for Doctors. Norske Laegeforening (Norwegian Medical Association). Reprinted by permission of the Association.

24. Final Report on Brain Death and Organ Transplantation. Japan Medical Association. Reprinted by permission of the Association.

25. Summary of the Report on Information. Japan Medical Association. Reprinted by permission of the Association.

26. Oath of Soviet Physicians. Translated by Zenonas Danilevicius. *Journal of the American Medical Association* 217 (1971):834. Reprinted by permission of the American Medical Association.

27. Solemn Oath. Translated by Larisa Yurievna Podovalenko and Chris Speckhardt. *Kennedy Institute of Ethics Journal* 3, no. 4 (1993):419. The Russian text of the oath was originally published in *Meditsinskaya Gazeta* (no. 44, 5

June 1992). Reprinted by permission of the Johns Hopkins University Press.

28. Regulations on Criteria for Medical Ethics. Translated by Shi Da-pu. *Kennedy Institute of Ethics Newsletter* 3, no. 4 (October 1989):3. Reprinted by permission of the Johns Hopkins University Press.

29. Ethical and Religious Directives. United States Catholic Conference. Reprinted by permission of the Conference.

30. Health Care Ethics Guide. Catholic Health Association of Canada. Reprinted by permission of the Association.

31. Oath of a Muslim Physician. Islamic Medical Association of North America. Reprinted by permission of the Islamic Medical Association.

32. Islamic Code. Islamic Organization for Medical Sciences. Reprinted by permission of the Islamic Organization.

### Section III: Ethical Directives for Other Health-Care Professions

1. Code for Nurses. International Council of Nurses. Reprinted by permission of the Council.

2. Code for Nurses. American Nurses' Association. Reprinted by permission of the Association.

3. Code of Ethics for Nursing. Canadian Nurses Association. Reprinted by permission of the Association.

4. Code of Ethics. American Chiropractic Association. Reprinted by permission of the Association.

5. Principles of Ethics. American Dental Association. Reprinted by permission of the Association.

6. Code of Ethics for the Profession of Dietetics. American Dietetic Association. Reprinted by permission of the Association.

7. Code of Ethics. American Association of Pastoral Counselors. Reprinted by permission of the Association.

8. Guidelines for the Chaplain's Role in Bioethics. College of Chaplains, Inc., American Protestant Health Association. Reprinted by permission of the Association.

9. Code of Ethics. American Pharmaceutical Association. Reprinted by permission of the Association.

10. Guidelines for Codes of Ethics. Fédération Internationale Pharmaceutique. Reprinted by permission of the Federation.

11. Code of Ethics and Guide. American Physical Therapy Association. Reprinted by permission of the Association.

12. Occupational Therapy Code. *American Journal of Occupational Therapy* 42, no. 12:795–796. American Occupational Therapy Association. Reprinted by permission of the Association.

13. Code of Ethics. American Academy of Physician Assistants. Reprinted by permission of the Academy.

14. Ethical Principles of Psychologists. *American Psychologist* (December 1992). American Psychological Association. Reprinted by permission of the Association.

15. Code of Ethics. National Association of Social Workers. Reprinted by permission of the Association.

16. Code of Ethics. American College of Healthcare Executives. Reprinted by permission of the College.

17. Ethical Conduct. American Hospital Association. Reprinted by permission of the Association.

### Section IV: Ethical Directives for Human Research

1. German Guidelines (1931). *International Digest of Health Legislation* 31, no. 2 (1980):408–411.

2. Nuremberg Code. "Permissible Medical Experiments." *Trials of War Criminals Before the Nuernberg Military Tribunals Under Control Council Law No. 10: Nuernberg, October 1946–April 1949.* Washington, D.C.: U.S. Government Printing Office (n.d.), vol. 2, pp. 181–182.

3. Principles. *World Medical Journal* 2 (1955):14–15.

4. Article Seven. *Yearbook of the United Nations 1958.* New York: Columbia University Press, p. 205. Reprinted by permission of the United Nations.

5. Declaration of Helsinki. World Medical Association. Reprinted by permission of the Association.

6. The Belmont Report. OPRR Reports. Washington, D.C.: U.S. Government Printing Office (1988) 201-778/80319.

7. DHHS Regulations. OPRR Reports. Washington, D.C.: U.S. Government Printing Office (1992) 0-307-551.

8. Summary Report. *Towards an International Ethic for Research with Human Beings: Proceedings of the International Summit Conference on Bioethics, April 5–10, 1987, Ottawa, Canada,* pp. 60–66. Ottawa, Ontario: Medical Research Council of Canada (1988). Reprinted by permission of the Council.

9. Recommendation No. R (90) 3. Council of Europe.

10. International Ethical Guidelines. Council for International Organizations of Medical Sciences. Reprinted by permission of the Council.

### Section V: Ethical Directives Pertaining to the Welfare and Use of Animals

1. Veterinarian's Oath. American Veterinary Medical Association. Reprinted by permission of the Association.

2. Principles of Veterinary Medicine. American Veterinary Medical Association. Reprinted by permission of the Association.

3. International Guiding Principles. Council for International Organizations of Medical Sciences. Reprinted by permission of the Council.

4. Principles for the Utilization and Care. NIH Guide Supplement for Grants and Contracts 14, no. 8 (June 25, 1985). Special Edition: Laboratory Animal Welfare, pp. 82–83. Washington, D.C.: U.S. Government Printing Office (1985) 527-967/30595.

5. Ethics of Animal Investigation. Canadian Council on Animal Care. Reprinted by permission of the Council.

6. Australian Code of Practice. National Health and Medical Research Council, Canberra, ACT. Reprinted by permission of the Council.

7. World Medical Association Statement. World Medical Association. Reprinted by permission of the Association.

8. Guidelines for Ethical Conduct. American Psychological Association. Reprinted by permission of the Association.

9. Principles and Guidelines. Institute of Laboratory Animal Resources, National Research Council. Reprinted by permission of the Council.

### Section VI: Ethical Directives Pertaining to the Environment

1. World Charter. *Yearbook of the United Nations 1982,* vol. 36. New York: United Nations, pp. 1024–1026. Reprinted by permission of the United Nations.

2. Rio Declaration. *Yearbook of the United Nations 1992*, vol. 46. Dordrecht, The Netherlands: Martinus Nijhoff Publishers, pp. 670–672. Reprinted by permission of the United Nations.

3. Code of Ethics for Members. Society of American Foresters. Reprinted by permission of the Society.

4. Conservation Policies. The Wildlife Society. Reprinted by permission of the Society.

5. Code of Ethics and Standards of Practice. National Association of Environmental Professionals. Reprinted by permission of the Association.

6. Code of Ethics. National Environmental Health Association. Reprinted by permission of the Association.

# Additional Resources
## in Bioethics

In the intervening years since the first edition of this Encyclopedia in 1978, the diversity and wealth of bioethics resources has increased enormously. The explosion of interest in this field is readily observable in the growth of the literature in all kinds of journals, the establishment of many new periodicals devoted exclusively to bioethics along with increasing attention to bioethics by both general journals and speciality journals covering related disciplines, and the development of various organizational entities in bioethics, many of which have begun to collect literature in bioethics. Lists of all these types of resources are provided below.

### Information Services of the Kennedy Institute of Ethics

Since the early 1970s the Kennedy Institute of Ethics has made a sustained effort to foster research and education in bioethics by collecting, analyzing, and disseminating bioethics information through various means. Its information services programs have grown significantly since the first edition of this work. The two primary information projects are: (1) the operation of a comprehensive bioethics library (the National Reference Center for Bioethics Literature), and (2) the ongoing development of an automated, bibliographic database (BIOETHICSLINE).

An ethics library was established in 1973 with funding from the Joseph P. Kennedy, Jr., Foundation; in 1985, it became the National Reference Center for Bioethics Literature (NRC), supported primarily by the U.S. National Library of Medicine. The NRC now subscribes to more than 240 periodicals and contains 20,000 books, a file of approximately 100,000 cataloged, article-length documents, extensive archival materials pertaining to government organizations, more than 200 audiovisuals, and a collection of more than 300 course syllabi. Open to the public, the NRC serves both on-site researchers and remote users through its reference desk service, through its toll-free number (1-800-MED-ETHX, in the United States and Canada) and via electronic mail (medethx@guvm.ccf.georgetown.edu). Services include reference service, BIOETHICSLINE searches, a multifaceted publications program, document delivery, and a syllabus exchange clearinghouse for educators.

The Bioethics Information Retrieval Project, begun in 1975 with a grant from the National Library of Medicine, makes English-language literature accessible via the production of the online database BIOETHICSLINE (updated bimonthly) and through the publication of its print counterpart, the annual *Bibliography of Bioethics*. At present, 3,600 documents are added to the database annually; about 20 percent of them include abstracts. The Project has developed an indexing language, the Bioethics Thesaurus, which affords very precise retrieval of bioethics literature. Among the nine different publication types indexed are: journal articles (69%); analytics, that is, chapters in books (12%); books and monographic reports (7%); newspaper articles (6%). Court decisions, bills, laws, audiovisuals, and unpublished documents comprise the remaining publication types.

One of the major reasons for developing a bibliographic database such as BIOETHICSLINE is to pull together the literature of a highly interdisciplinary field of study. In spite of the fact that specialty journals now exist, and that the major weeklies, such as *The Lancet* and *Science,* cover bioethical issues routinely, the literature is still widely dispersed. An examination of the source journals represented in BIOETHICSLINE reveals that citations from the thirty-two publications listed in the Periodical Literature section below published only 25 percent of the journal articles cited in the entire database. The remaining 75 percent of journal articles (18,387 citations) appeared in 2,666 different journals! It is precisely because bioethics information is so widely scattered that it is important to rely on a bibliography or bibliographic database for adequate coverage of the literature.

Access to BIOETHICSLINE is available directly from the U.S. National Library of Medicine and the following MEDLARS-affiliated centers outside the United States: Australia, Canada, Egypt, France, Germany, India, Israel, Italy, Korea, Kuwait, Mexico, PAHO/Brazil, South Africa, Sweden, Switzerland, Taiwan, and the United Kingdom. (A current list of the addresses of these centers can be obtained from the Bioethics Information Retrieval Project.) The National Library of Medicine also makes access codes available to individuals with their own computers and modems.

Other commercial or governmental distributors of databases have brought BIOETH-ICSLINE to institutional and individual users. Two examples are the Minitel system in France and Data Star, now a part of Dialog Information Services, Inc., 3460 Hillview Ave., P.O. Box 10010, Palo Alto, CA 94303-0993, USA.

Another distribution method for bibliographic databases is via a subscription to a CD-ROM version of BIOETHICSLINE. Speed and storage enhancements of personal computers have made it possible for libraries and researchers to enjoy unlimited use of entire bibliographic databases on a personal or networked computer. At the present time, both SilverPlatter Information, Inc., 100 River Ridge Drive, Norwood, MA 02062-5026, USA, and CD-Plus Technologies, 333 Seventh Avenue, New York, NY 10001, USA, lease the BIOETHICSLINE database from the National Library of Medicine and provide searching software for their subscribers. Updates are currently provided every four months; the subscription price may vary depending upon the number of users anticipated.

The data prepared for BIOETHICSLINE is also available in print form as the annual *Bibliography of Bioethics*, which has been published directly by the Project, at the Kennedy Institute of Ethics, since the appearance of Volume 10 in 1984. Volume 20, to be published in the fall of 1994, will be more than 800 pages in length. Citations, approximately 20 percent of which are accompanied by abstracts, are arranged by subject and include source information and indexing terms chosen from the *Bioethics Thesaurus*, the controlled vocabulary (also published annually every February).

The *Bioethics Thesaurus* has been translated into several languages and modified by bibliographers in other countries in order to reflect concepts of importance in their respective regions. The documentation centers associated with the European Association of Centres of Medical Ethics have adapted the *Bioethics Thesaurus* for their use in English and further translated it into Dutch and French. The Akademie für Ethik in der Medizin, Göttingen University, is working on a German translation, and the Centro de Bioética, Fundación Dr. José María Mainetti, Buenos Aires (La Plata), Argentina, a Spanish translation.

## Periodical Literature

Given the growth of interest in the field, it is not surprising that specialty journals have emerged that are devoted primarily to bioethical issues. A few have been published for a decade or more, while others first appeared more recently. Some are affiliated with research organizations or professional societies. Publication information for several such periodicals is provided below in the section on Bioethics and Health Law Journals. This is not a comprehensive list, but it is representative of English-language sources. For information regarding foreign-language sources, readers may wish to contact the documentation centers mentioned above who are analyzing bioethics literature in other languages.

Since bioethical topics continue to receive a great deal of attention, the periodicals of contributing disciplines likewise continue to devote considerable space to pertinent issues. Medical, scientific, and philosophical journals that have consistently covered bioethics are also listed under General Philosophical, Scientific, and Medical Journals, below.

### Bioethics and Health Law Journals

*American Journal of Law and Medicine*, quarterly, published by: American Society of Law, Medicine & Ethics, 765 Commonwealth Ave., 16th Floor, Boston, MA 02215, ISSN: 0098-8588.

*Bioethics* (official journal of the International Association of Bioethics), quarterly, published by: Basil Blackwell Journals, c/o Marston Book Services Limited, P.O. Box 87, Oxford OX2 ODT, England, ISSN: 0269-9702.

*Biolaw*, monthly, published by: University Publications of America, P.O. Box 64292, Baltimore, MD 21264, ISSN: none.

*Cambridge Quarterly of Healthcare Ethics*, quarterly, published by: Cambridge University Press, 40 West 20th Street, New York, NY 10011-4211, ISSN: 0963-1801.

*Hastings Center Report*, six times per year, published by: The Hastings Center, 255 Elm Road, Briarcliff Manor, NY 10510, ISSN: 0093-0334.

*Health Matrix: The Journal of Law-Medicine,* twice per year, published by: Case Western Reserve University, School of Law, 11075 East Boulevard, Cleveland, OH 44106, ISSN: none.

*HEC Forum (Healthcare Ethics Committee Forum),* six times per year, published by: Kluwer Academic Publishers Group, P.O. Box 322, 3300 AH Dordrecht, The Netherlands, or P.O. Box 358, Accord Station, Hingham, MA 02018-0358, ISSN: 0956-2737.

*International Journal of Bioethics/Journal International de Bioéthique,* three times per year, published by: Editions Alexandre Lacassagne, 162, avenue Lacassagne, 69003 Lyon, France, ISSN: 1145-0762.

*Journal of Clinical Ethics,* quarterly, published by: Journal of Clinical Ethics, 107 East Church Street, Frederick, MD 21701, ISSN: 1046-7890.

*The Journal of Law, Medicine & Ethics,* quarterly, published by: American Society of Law, Medicine & Ethics, 765 Commonwealth Avenue, 16th Floor, Boston, MA 02215, ISSN: none.

*Journal of Medical Ethics,* quarterly, published by: BMJ Publishing Group (on behalf of the British Medical Association and the Institute of Medical Ethics), Box 560B, Kennebunkport, ME 04046, ISSN: 0306-6800.

*Journal of Medical Humanities,* quarterly, published by: Human Sciences Press, 233 Spring Street, New York, NY 10013-1578, ISSN: 1041-3545.

*The Journal of Medicine and Philosophy,* six times per year, published by: Kluwer Academic Publishers Group, P.O. Box 322, 3300 AH Dordrecht, The Netherlands, or P.O. Box 358, Accord Station, Hingham, MA 02018-0358, ISSN: 0360-5310.

*Kennedy Institute of Ethics Journal,* quarterly, published by: Johns Hopkins University Press, 701 W. 40th Street, Baltimore, MD 21211-2190, ISSN: 1054-6863.

*Second Opinion: Health, Faith & Ethics,* quarterly, published by: Park Ridge Center, 221 E. Ontario, Suite 800, Chicago, IL 60611-3215, ISSN: 0890-1570.

*Theoretical Medicine,* quarterly, published by: Kluwer Academic Publishers Group, P.O. Box 322, 3300 AH Dordrecht, The Netherlands, or P.O. Box 358, Accord Station, Hingham, MA 02018-9990, ISSN: 0167-9902.

### General Philosophical, Scientific, and Medical Journals

*American Journal of Public Health,* monthly, published by: American Public Health Association, 1015 15th St., NW, Washington, DC 20005, ISSN: 0090-0036.

*Annals of Internal Medicine,* twice per month, published by: Annals of Internal Medicine (on behalf of the American College of Physicians), P.O. Box 7777-R-0320, Philadelphia, PA 19175, ISSN: 0003-4819.

*Archives of Internal Medicine,* twice per month, published by: American Medical Association, Subscription Department, P.O. Box 5826, Carol Stream, IL 60197-9877, ISSN: 0003-9926.

*British Medical Journal (BMJ),* weekly, published by: British Medical Journal, P.O. Box 560B, Kennebunkport, ME 04046, ISSN: 0959-8146.

*Ethics,* quarterly, published by: University of Chicago Press, P.O. Box 37005, Chicago, IL 60637, ISSN: 0014-1704.

*Journal of Health Politics, Policy and Law,* quarterly, published by: Duke University Press, Journals Dept., P.O. Box 90660, Durham, NC 27708, ISSN: 0361-6878.

*Journal of the American Medical Association,* weekly, published by: American Medical Association, Subscription Department, 515 North State Street, Chicago, IL 60610-9986, ISSN: 0098-7484.

*The Lancet,* weekly, published by: Williams & Wilkins, 428 East Preston Street, Baltimore, MD 21202, ISSN: 0140-6736.

*Milbank Quarterly,* quarterly, published by: Cambridge University Press (for the Milbank Memorial Fund), 40 West 20th Street, New York, NY 10011, ISSN: 0887-378X.

*Nature,* weekly, published by: Nature, P.O. Box 1733, Riverton, NJ 08077-9733, ISSN: 0028-0836.

*New England Journal of Medicine,* weekly, published by: New England Journal of Medicine, 1440 Main Street, Waltham, MA 02154-1649, ISSN: 0028-4793.

*Philosophy & Public Affairs*, quarterly, published by: Johns Hopkins University Press, 701 W. 40th Street, Baltimore, MD 21211-2190, ISSN: 0048-3915.

*Science*, weekly, published by: American Association for the Advancement of Science, P.O. Box 2032, Marion, OH 43305-0001, ISSN: 0036-8075.

## Bioethics Organizations

If the emergence of organizational entities in a new field of endeavor signifies a maturing of a discipline, bioethics is well on its way to adulthood. In 1993, the NRC published the *International Directory of Bioethics Organizations*, listing over 340 organizations in 41 countries. The approach of the compilers was inclusionary in an attempt to facilitate communication between centers, regardless of size.

Diverse types of programs were identified: degree-granting, academic programs; clinical and medical center-affiliated programs; professional societies; government-sponsored bodies; international associations; and grass-roots organizations. Persons requiring detailed information are encouraged to contact the NRC, which maintains a database of organizations interested in bioethics in general as well as corporate bodies dedicated to specialty areas, such as euthanasia, reproductive rights, animal experimentation, and genetic intervention.

A few of the many organizations listed in the Directory are briefly identified here in order to provide the reader with a very general overview of the types of organizations coming into being. Due to space limitations and the inconstant nature of such information as telephone and fax numbers, only addresses are provided.

Bioethics literature draws upon many disciplines, and the contributions of the relevant literatures are available, often piecemeal, in large medical, academic, law, theology, special and public libraries. As the bioethics literature grows, however, specialized collections that concentrate on bioethics are emerging. Many organizations listed here are establishing special collections of bioethics literature. If an organization makes its collection available to persons outside its immediate staff, that information is listed. Although many of these collections are small, they nevertheless constitute a valuable resource for researchers in these regions. In spite of the fact that the data provided here will become dated over time, they give an indication of an organizational commitment to the development of library resources. Many graduate programs in bioethics that may not have established their own libraries nevertheless are associated with larger university libraries that may have extensive bioethics holdings. Those have not been included here.

The following list is certainly not comprehensive; it is intended to direct researchers to regional, specialized resources. Updated information and data regarding other library collections should be sent to the NRC for inclusion in its database.

Persons doing research in Italy would want to consult *Centri di Bioetica in Italia: Orientamenti a Confronto* published by the Fondazione Lanza and the Gregoriana Libreria Editrice in 1993. In addition, a new European directory of bioethics edited by Nicole Lery is to be published by the Association Descartes in Paris, in 1994.

ARGENTINA (Buenos Aires)
Centro de Bioética
Fundación Dr. Jose María Mainetti
Calle 508 e/16 y 18
1897 M.B. Gonnet, Buenos Aires 1897
Books and journals; computerized database; open to scholars
and researchers.

AUSTRALIA (Glendalough)
L. J. Goody Bioethics Centre
39 Jugan Street
Glendalough, Western Australia 6016
Books, journals, and audiovisual materials; open to the public.

AUSTRALIA (South Brisbane)
Provincial Bioethics Centre
P.O. Box 3343
South Brisbane, Queensland 4101
Books (4,000), periodicals (70); open to the public.

AUSTRALIA (Victoria)
Centre for Human Bioethics
Monash University
Clayton, Melbourne, Victoria 3168

BELGIUM (Brussels)
Centre de Recherches Interdisciplinaires en Bioéthique
(CRIB)
Université Libre de Bruxelles
145, avenue Adolphe Buyl (CP 188)
B-1050 Bruxelles
Books (500), periodicals (10); open to the public.

BELGIUM (Leuven)
Centrum voor Bio-Medische Ethiek en Recht
Katholieke Universiteit Leuven
Faculteit der Geneeskunde
Kapucijnenvoer 35
3000 Leuven
Books (4,000), periodicals (44); open to the public.

CANADA (Edmonton)
Canadian Bioethics Society (CBS)
A.N.R. 222, 8220 - 114 St.
Edmonton, Alberta, T6G 2J3

CANADA (Edmonton)
St. Joseph's College Catholic Bioethics Centre
University of Alberta
8409 - 112 Street, Suite 520
Edmonton, Alberta T6G 1K6
Books (600), periodicals (45), audiovisual materials; open to
the public.

CANADA (London)
Westminster Institute for Ethics and Human Values
Westminster College
361 Windermere Road
London, Ontario N6G 2K3
Books (3,000), periodicals (40); open to the public.

CANADA (Montreal)
Center for Bioethics
Clinical Research Institute of Montreal
110 Pine Avenue West
Montreal, Quebec H2W 1R7
An extensive collection of articles, reports, and Canadian cur-
riculum materials; open to the public.

CANADA (Montreal)
McGill Centre for Medicine, Ethics and Law
McGill University
3690 Peel Street
Montreal, Quebec, H3A 1W9

CANADA (Ottawa)
Catholic Health Association of Canada
1247 Kilborn
Ottawa, Ontario K1H 6K9
Books (2,000), periodicals (108); open to the public by ap-
pointment.

CANADA (Toronto)
Centre for Bioethics
University of Toronto
88 College Street
Toronto, Ontario M5G 1L4
Books (300), periodicals (8); open to students and to members
of the center.

COLOMBIA (Bogotá)
Centro de Etica Medica de Ascofame
Asociación Colombiana de Facultades de Medicina "ASCO-
FAME" [Colombian Association of Medical Schools]
Calle 39A No. 28–63
Santa Fe de Bogotá D.C.

ASCOFAME library: books (3,000), periodicals (200); open to the public by request.

DENMARK (Copenhagen)
Danish Council on Ethics
Ravnsborggade, 2–4
DK-2200 Copenhagen N

ENGLAND (London)
Centre of Medical Law and Ethics
King's College London (KCL)
Strand
London, WC2R 2LS
Books (1,000), periodicals (26).

ENGLAND (London)
Linacre Centre for Health Care Ethics
60 Grove End Road St. John's Wood
London NW8 9NH
Books (4,000), periodicals (50); open to students of bioethics.

ENGLAND (London)
Nuffield Council on Bioethics
28 Bedford Square
London, WC1B 3EG

FRANCE (Lille)
Centre d'Éthique Médicale Fédération Universitaire et Polytechnique de Lille
Institut Catholique de Lille
60, boulevard Vauban
BP 109 59 016 Lille Cedex
Books (2,500), periodicals (42), newsletters (12), reprints (1,500), proceedings and other materials; computerized database; open to the public.

FRANCE (Paris)
Centre de Documentation et d'Information en Éthique des Sciences de la Vie et de la Santé
Institut National de la Senté et de la Recherche Médicale (INSERM)
101 rue de Tolbiac, 75654 Paris Cedex 13
Books, laws, theses, government reports, and periodicals, including reports and works of the Comité Consultatif National d'Éthique pour les Sciences de la Vie et de la Santé; open to the public.

FRANCE (Paris)
Départment d'Éthique Biomédicale
Centre Sèvres
12, rue d'Assas
F-75006 Paris
Books (1,800), periodicals (43); open to the public.

FRANCE (Paris)
International Committee on Bioethics
UNESCO
7, Place de Fontenoy
75700 Paris

FRANCE (Strasbourg)
International Association of Law, Ethics and Science (The Milazzo Group)
6, boulevard Gambetta
67000 Strasbourg

FRANCE (Strasbourg)
Steering Committee for Bioethics (CDBI, formerly CAHBI)
Council of Europe
Pièce 2004
67006 Strasbourg

GERMANY (Bochum)
Zentrum für medizinische Ethik
Ruhr Universität-Bochum
Gebäude GA 3/53

Postfach 102148
Universitätsstrasse 150
4630 Bochum 1

GERMANY (Göttingen)
Akademie für Ethik in der Medizin
Institut für Geschichte der Medizin
Humboldtallee 36
D-3400 Göttingen
Medical ethics database in development in cooperation with the Deutsches Institut für medizinische Dokumentation und Information (DIMDI) in Cologne and the Kennedy Institute of Ethics.

ITALY (Genoa)
Consiglio Nazionale delle Ricerche
Università di Genova Centro di Studi Sulla Filosofia
Contemporanea
Via Lomellini, 8/8
Genoa 16124
Books (3,200), periodicals (4); open to the public.

ITALY (Padua)
Fondazione Lanza
Via Dante, 55
Padova 35139
Books (2,000), periodicals (80); open to the public.

ITALY (Palermo)
Istituto Siciliano di Bioetica
Facoltà Teologica di Sicilia
Corso Vittorio Emanuele 463
Palermo 90134
Materials on bioethics; housed within the Central Library for the Churches of Sicily.

ITALY (Rome)
Centro di Bioetica/Istituto di Bioetica
Università Cattolica del Sacro Cuore, Facoltà di Medicina e Chirurgia "A. Gemelli"
Largo Francesco Vito, 1
Roma 00168
Books (2,000), periodicals (70); open to the public.

ITALY (Rome)
Comitato Nazionale per la Bioetica
Via dei Villini 16
Roma

JAPAN (Tokyo)
Bioethics Research Project
Waseda University Advanced Research Center for Human Sciences
1-6-1, Nishiwaseda Shinjuky-ku
Tokyo 169-50
Books (3,000), periodicals (78); housed in the Waseda University Library.

THE NETHERLANDS (Ede)
Prof. Dr. G. A. Lindeboom Instituut
Centrum voor Medische Ethiek (Center for Medical Ethics)
Galvanistraat 7, P.O. Box 224
6710 BE Ede
Books (1,000), periodicals (50), reprints (2,500); not open to the public, but will accept outside requests for information.

THE NETHERLANDS (Nijmegen)
Department of Ethics, Philosophy, and History of Medicine
Catholic University of Nijmegen
P.O. Box 9101
6500 HB Nijmegen
Books (1,000), periodicals (5); open to the public.

THE NETHERLANDS (Utrecht)
Centrum voor Bio-Ethiek en Gezondheidsrecht
Utrecht University
Heidelberglaan 2, Postbus 80.105
3508-TC Utrecht
Books (300), periodicals (30), reprints (2,500); open to the public.

NEW ZEALAND (Dunedin)
Bioethics Research Centre
University of Otago
P.O. Box 913
Dunedin
Books, periodicals (11), reports; open to "Friends of the Centre" and to others by arrangement.

NORWAY (Oslo)
Center for Medical Ethics
University of Oslo
(also: National Committee for Medical Research Ethics
Norwegian Research Council for Science and the Humanities)
Gaustadalleen 21
0371 Oslo 3
Books (900), periodicals (40).

THE PHILIPPINES (Manila)
South East Asian Center for Bioethics
St. Martin de Porres Building, Room 226
UST, España Manila
Books (140), periodicals (3); open to the public.

SOUTH AFRICA (Cape Town)
Bioethics Centre
Department of Medicine
Cape Town Observatory, 7925

SPAIN (Barcelona)
Instituto Borja de Bioetica
Llaseres 30
08190 Sant Cugat del Valles
Barcelona
Books (10,000), periodicals (200), reprints.

SWEDEN (Lund)
Department of Medical Ethics
Lund University
Solvegatan 9
S-223 62 Lund
Periodicals (15); open to the public.

SWEDEN (Stockholm)
Ersta Institute for Health Care Ethics (Ersta Diakonisällskap)
Box 4619
S-116 91 Stockholm
Books (300), periodicals (30).

UNITED STATES (California: Davis)
American Institute of Medical Ethics
409 Encina Avenue
Davis, CA 95616
Books (1,000), periodicals (12); open to the public upon request.

UNITED STATES (California: Los Angeles)
Pacific Center for Health Policy and Ethics
University of Southern California
Los Angeles, CA 90089-0071

UNITED STATES (California: Orange)
Center for Healthcare Ethics
St. Joseph Health System
440 South Batavia Street
Orange, CA 92668-3995
Audiovisual materials.

UNITED STATES (California: San Diego)
Center for Medical Ethics and Mediation
1081 Camino del Rio South, Suite 217
San Diego, CA 92108-3545
Books (550), periodicals (15); open to professionals, students, and community groups upon request.

UNITED STATES (District of Columbia: Washington)
Kennedy Institute of Ethics
Washington, DC 20057-1065
National Reference Center for Bioethics Literature. Books (20,000), periodicals (240), audiovisuals (200), reprint collection (100,000), curriculum collection (333), Shriver Collection of Christian Ethics, Kampelman Collection of Jewish Ethics, archival materials; computerized databases; open to the public.

UNITED STATES (Illinois: Chicago)
Center for Clinical Medical Ethics
University of Chicago
Department of Medicine, MC-6098
5841 South Maryland Ave.
Chicago, IL 60637-1470

UNITED STATES (Illinois: Chicago)
Department of Medical Humanities
University of Illinois at Chicago
Department of Medical Education (M/C 591)
986 College of Medicine East
808 South Wood St.
Chicago, IL 60612

UNITED STATES (Illinois: Chicago)
Park Ridge Center for the Study of Health, Faith, and Ethics
211 E. Ontario, Suite 800
Chicago, IL 60611-3215

UNITED STATES (Illinois: Maywood)
Medical Humanities Program
Loyola University of Chicago
Medical Center
2160 South First Avenue
Maywood, IL 60153

UNITED STATES (Illinois: Park Ridge)
Center for Clinical Ethics
Lutheran General Hospital
1775 Dempster Street, 8 South
Park Ridge, IL 60068
Books (300), periodicals (20), audiovisual materials; open to the public.

UNITED STATES (Massachusetts: Boston)
American Society of Law, Medicine and Ethics
765 Commonwealth Avenue, 16th Floor
Boston, MA 02215
The Segall Library of Law, Medicine and Ethics; open to Society members.

UNITED STATES (Massachusetts: Boston)
Public Responsibility in Medicine and Research (PRIM&R)
132 Boylston Street, 4th floor
Boston, MA 02116

UNITED STATES (Massachusetts: Braintree)
Pope John XXIII Medical-Moral Research and Education Center
186 Forbes Road
Braintree, MA 02184
Books (800), periodicals (60); open to members of the Center and students.

UNITED STATES (Minnesota: Minneapolis)
Center for Biomedical Ethics
University of Minnesota
University Office Plaza
2221 University Avenue, S.E., Suite 110
Minneapolis, MN 55414-3074

UNITED STATES (New York: Briarcliff Manor)
The Hastings Center
255 Elm Road
Briarcliff Manor, NY 10510-9974
Books (6,500), periodicals (120); provides information services to members of the Hastings Center but is not open to the public.

UNITED STATES (Ohio: Cleveland)
Department of Bioethics
Cleveland Clinic Foundation
Desk P31 9500 Euclid Avenue
Cleveland, OH 44195
Books (500), journals (30); open to the public by appointment only.

UNITED STATES (Pennsylvania: Pittsburgh)
Center for Medical Ethics
3400 Forbes Avenue
Pittsburgh, PA 15213

UNITED STATES (Tennessee: Memphis)
Department of Human Values and Ethics
University of Tennessee, Memphis College of Medicine
956 Court Street, Room B324 Coleman Bldg.
Memphis, TN 38163
Books (2,000), periodicals (16); collection is housed in the Health Sciences Center Library.

UNITED STATES (Texas: Galveston)
Institute for the Medical Humanities
University of Texas Medical Branch
Room 2.208
Ashbel Smith Building, M-11
Galveston, TX 77555-1311

UNITED STATES (Texas: Houston)
Center for Ethics, Medicine and Public Issues
Baylor College of Medicine
Texas Medical Center
One Baylor Plaza
Houston, TX 77030

UNITED STATES (Virginia: Charlottesville)
Center for Biomedical Ethics
University of Virginia
Health Sciences Center
Box 348
Charlottesville, VA 22908

UNITED STATES (Virginia: McLean)
Society for Health and Human Values
6728 Old McLean Village Drive
McLean, VA 22101

UNITED STATES (Washington: Seattle)
Department of Medical History and Ethics
University of Washington
School of Medicine
A-204 Health Sciences, SB-20
Seattle, WA 98195

UNITED STATES (Washington: Seattle)
Northwest Ethics Institute
1411 Fourth Avenue Building, Suite 625
Seattle, WA 98101-2216
Library available for members and the interested public.

UNITED STATES (Wisconsin: Madison)
Program in Medical Ethics
University of Wisconsin
Department of History of Medicine
1420 Medical Sciences Center

1300 University Ave.
Madison, WI 53706

URUGUAY (Montevideo)
Servicio de Bioética
Universidad Católica del Uruguay "Damaso Antonio Larranago"
Institute of Philosophy and Ethics
Av. 8 de Octubre No. 2738
Montevideo 11600
Books (300), reprints (3,000); open to the public.


Prepared by:
Doris Mueller Goldstein, M.L.S., M.A.
Director, Library and Information Services
Kennedy Institute of Ethics
Georgetown University
June 1994

# ACKNOWLEDGMENTS BY CONTRIBUTORS

The following contributors wish to extend their thanks for the special assistance they received in the preparation of their articles:

Robert M. Arnold and Charles W. Lidz, to Paul S. Appelbaum, Randall Barker, Neil Farber, Lachlan Forrow, and Alan Meisel for many of the ideas found in "Informed Consent: Clinical Aspects of Consent in Health Care."

John P. Bunker, to Bryan Jennett of the University of Glasgow and Myer Rosenthal of Stanford University, for assistance in preparing the entry on "Artificial Organs and Life-Support Systems."

Nancy E. Gin and Howard Waitzkin, for grants received from the Poverty and Race Research Action Council, Washington, D.C.; the Pacific Rim Program of the University of California; the National Institute on Aging (1-F32-AG 05438); and the Division of Medicine of the U.S. Public Health Service (PE-19154), in support of the work that led to "Health Policy: Politics and Health Care."

Clifford Grobstein, to Howard W. Jones, Jr., for his assistance in bringing the article on "Fetus: Human Development from Fertilization to Birth" to completion.

Richard P. Haynes, to Jeffrey Burkhard, Katherine Clancy, and Jennie Elliott for their comments on various drafts of the entry on "Agriculture."

Carol C. Nadelson, to the John D. and Catherine T. MacArthur Foundation for financial support while preparing "Women: Health-Care Issues."

Nanette Newell, to Robert Alder, Andrew Balber, Susan Clymer, and Scott Shore for useful comments on early drafts of "Biotechnology."

Warren Thomas Reich, to Frank Chessa, Lauren Deichman, Markus Ege, Mary B. Evans, Jesse Mann, Laurence B. McCullough, Timothy Miller, Maria Murray, Leanne Pierce, Josef Priller, Susan Stark, Isabel Winter, and Matthias Winter for suggestions and research efforts for the articles on "Care: History of the Notion of Care," and "Care: Historical Dimensions of an Ethic of Care in Health Care."

Bettina Schöne-Seifert, Hans-Martin Sass, Laura Jane Bishop, and Alberto Bondolfi, to Franz Illhardt, Hans-Georg Koch, and Klaus-Peter Rippe for information supplied in the preparation of "Medical Ethics, History of: Europe: Contemporary Period: German-Speaking Countries and Switzerland."

Victor W. Sidel, to E. A. Vastyan and Mark Sidel for supplying material, and to Stephen Amis, Jr., Tod Ensign, and H. Jack Geiger for their comments in the preparation of "Warfare: Medicine and War," and to Gordon Burck, Leonard Cole, Robert Cook-Deegan, Paul Epstein, Naomi Franklin, Jack

Geiger, Erhard Geissler, Robert Goldwyn, Ira Helfand, Jay Jacobson, Jonathan King, Meryl Nass, Richard Novick, Theodor Rosebury, Barbara Hatch Rosenberg, William Sayres, Nachama Wilker, Susan Wright, and Raymond Zilinskas for their help in preparing "Warfare: Chemical and Biological Weapons."

Calvin Stiller, to Cate Abbott for editorial assistance in preparing "Organ and Tissue Transplants: Medical Overview."

# Index

Numbers in **boldface** *refer to the main entry on the subject.*

China
abortion issues, 17, 21, 785, 840,
1481–1482, 2024, 2025, 2041
AIDS policy, 1489
animal welfare in, 177
bioethics education, 267
Buddhism, 314, 316, 493, 494, 1470, 1472,
1477, 1478, 1487, 1490
chemical and biological weapons, 2544
compassion perspective, 442
Confucianism, **465–468**, 1477, 1478,
1487, 1490
cosmic-unity belief, 759
culture-specific psychiatric disorders,
1745
death perspectives, 479, 480, 493, 494,
495–497, 1486–1487
environmental issues, 708
eugenics laws, 767
fertility-control program, 21, 1487–1488,
1955, 1970–1971, 2009, 2010,
2011–2012, 2018–2019, 2021, 2023,
2024–2026, 2041; see also subhead
sterilization policy below
gender-related mortality rates, 2000
genome project, 1015
health-care delivery, 1488–1490
health and disease concepts, 1086
infanticide practice, 1207
information-disclosure practices, 1230
international weapons trade, 2550
kidney dialysis, 1323
medical codes and oaths, 1422, 1428,
1432, 1482–1483, 1484–1485
medical practice and ethics, contemporary,
1483–1490
medical practice and ethics, prerepublican,
1469, 1470, 1471, 1472, 1477–1483,
1492, 1494
nuclear weapons, 2542
organ donation and transplants, 1893
prostitution, 2113
psychiatry, 1745
public health, 446–447, 1483–1484, 1485
religion and morality, 759, 761, 762
sex-selection practices, 785
sexual beliefs, 2389
sterilization policy, 968, 1471, 1970, 2024,
2041
Taoism, 140, 1477, **2463–2469**
women physicians, 2577, 2583
Chinese Medical Association, 1486, 1488
Chinese Society for Medical Ethics, 1486
Chiropractic medicine, 66, 131–132, 140,
2507, 2508
Chisholm, Roderick, 57
Chlamydia, 941
Chlorpromazine (Thorazine), 2139, 2143,
2147, 3522
Chodorow, Nancy, 810
Choice
as woman's reproductive right, 6–7,
813–814, 881, 886, 982, 1408

see also Decision making; Freedom and
coercion; Informed consent
Cholera, 716, 717, 2158, 2160
Cholesterol, 944, 1366
Chomsky, Noam, 235, 1178
Chorionic villus sampling (CVS)
for fetal assessment, 862, 1403
for genetic testing, 988, 989
Irish restrictions, 1578
for sex selection, 2213
Chren, M. M., 1943
Christianity
abortion position, 8, 27, 30–37,
1529–1530, 1535
on abuse, interpersonal, 48
on action, 59
African religion and, 80
on aging and aged, 92, 98, 99
on animal research, 149
on animal welfare, 161, 174
bioethics education and, 267
blood symbolism in, 1346
on body, 305, 307
on cadaveric integrity, 1863
care tradition, in, 321, 332, 341
casuistric-based morality, 344–350
children's issues and, 372
circumcision and, 385–386, 388
civil disobedience and, 391, 392
on compassion, 442
on concubinage, 1400
conscience and, 470
contraception views, 833, 834, 839–840
death perspective, 501, 503, 506–512,
514–515, 516–517, 544, 549–551, 556,
561, 563, 588–589, 1174, 1521, 1535
disability views, 609, 610–611
disease interpretation, 1283
early historical antiprocreative stance,
1962, 1983
early hospitals, 1088, 1160–1162, 1519,
2322
early philosophy. See Aquinas, Thomas
early somatic view of madness, 1699
environmental views, 708, 709–711
ethics of, 720, 721, 723, 724, 725, 739,
758, 759, 761, 862
ethics and law relationship, 1558–1559
eugenics issues, 779–781
evolution theory and, 277, 792–793, 1176
fidelity and loyalty ethic, 865, 866
on freedom, 882
friendship model, 889–890
fundamentalism. See Fundamentalist
Christians
on genetics, 915
God and personhood in, 1934–1935
healing tradition, 1037, 1087–1088, 1908,
2322
historical medical ethics, 1446,
1516–1536, 1610, 1611, 1612, 2322; see
also Roman Catholicism; specific countries,
eras, and geographical regions

infanticide condemnation, 1201–1202
informed-consent tradition, 1242
interpretation theory, 1283
life valuation, 563, 1346
love concept, 865, 1392, 1393, 1519, 1558
marriage laws, 779–781
on marriage and procreation, 1398, 1399,
1400
medieval. See Aquinas, Thomas;
Scholasticism
natural-law foundation, 759, 1806–1807
pastoral care, 1905, 1907, 1908
physicians' prayers and oaths, 1419,
1420–1421
Platonism and, 1813–1814
"playing God" metaphor, 1769
on prostitution, 2113
Renaissance. See Renaissance
resurrection beliefs, 506–507, 515
sexual ethics, 1148, 2366–2371, 2372, 2389
suffering perspective, 1088, 1901, 1903,
2322
on suicide, 1088, 1520, 1521, 2446, 2447
and therapeutic relationship, 2078–2080,
2081
on tragedy, 2493, 2495
utilitarian morality, 2509
vegetarianism and, 174
virtue and character in, 739, 2526, 2527,
2529, 2530, 2531
and women's health-care role, 2578
and women's historical role, 2556
see also Bible; Eastern Orthodox
Christianity; Jesus Christ; Protestantism;
Religion; Roman Catholicism; specific sects
Christian Science, 1701, 2119
and abuse, interpersonal, 43, 138
alternative therapies, 130–131, 137–138
body perspective, 305
children and, 43, 137–138, 359
treatment refusal by, 43, 137–138, 305,
359
Chromosomes
abnormalities, 773, 952, 985, 989, 996
gender assignment, 902
genome mapping and sequencing,
**1011–1018**
markers, 1013
sex-linked traits, 950–951
see also Genetic headings; Human Genome
Project; Medical genetics
Chronic care, **378–381**
by allied health professionals, 124
for children, 359
disability and, 603
economic issues, 652
electrical stimulation of the brain, 659
euthanasia issues, 555–556, 572–573
kidney dialysis and, 1317–1323
quality of life and, 1352
see also Commitment to mental
institutions; Institutionalization and
deinstitutionalization; Long-term care

abortion views, 7, 10, 11, 15, 32, 37, 1334, 2000
on abuse, interpersonal, 48
bioethics and, 253, 1627
on bioethics education, 262, 271
birth-control issues, 828–829, 835, 836, 1625, 2006
body perspectives, 302, 304, 307
care perspective, 335–336, 338–339, 811, 814, 866, 1228, 1353, 1820, 1825, 2586
on childhood sexual abuse, 2360
civil rights influence on, 884
compassion and, 445
confidentiality issues and, 454
criticism of biological sciences, 278
defining, 2557–2558
ecofeminism, 168, 683–684, 690–693, 811–812, 2458
ethics of, 338–339, 724, 749, 803, 810–812, 866
family perspectives, 803
feminist vs. feminine ethics, 338–339
gene-therapy issues, 920
health-care issues, 1071, 1104, 2339
on health-care teams, 2470
on historical women's "disorders," 1700
history of, 750–751, 808–810, 2554, 2557
on hunting, 188–189
individualistic vs. relational forms of, 2558
on information disclosure, 1226, 1228
Judaic, 1307
on justice, 1312–1313
on life and personhood, 1349
marital inequalities and, 1399, 1400
medical ethics and, 1036, 1553, 2329
medical genetics and, 1650, 1652
and moral-development model, 246, 319, 336–337, 1036, 2586
and nursing identity, 1818–1819, 1820
objectivity critique by, 733
on paternalism, 1919
on prostitution issues, 2114, 2115–2116
on psychiatric stereotyping of women, 2127, 2135–2136
quality-of-life views, 1353
on reproductive technologies, 767, 1571, 1637, 2226, 2227, 2233–2234
rights theories, 2309–2310
Roman Catholic medical ethics and, 2329
on romantic love, 1393–1394
on sexism, 808–810, 812, **2344–2347**
sexual ethics and, 2353, 2371, 2373, 2377, 2386
on sexual identity, 2378–2379
social and political theories, 750–751
surrogacy pro and con arguments, 813, 2226, 2227, 2234
on technology, 2482
on transgender therapy, 904
on trust relationships, 2502–2503
types of, 808
Feral animals, 179
Ferré, Frederick, 2480

Fertility control, **818–845**, 2023–2027
abortion as, 838, 839, 840, 843, 1606, 2029
adolescent, 65, 66, 819, 829, 830, 836, 1947, 1949, 2393
adoption affected by, 71–72
African issues, 1462–1463
behavior control and, 225
Benelux countries, 1564, 1565, 1566
bioethics and, 250
Buddhist position, 784–787, 2003
Chinese programs, 1487–1488, 1955, 1970–1971, 2009, 2010, 2011–2012, 2018–2019, 2021, 2023, 2024–2026, 2041
civil disobedience and, 390
coerced, 829–830, 837, 842, 956, 983, 1970–1971, 2023–2027, 2040–2042; see also subhead population policies and ethics of below
conscience in prescribing, 471, 1947, 1949
decisional privacy basis, 2067, 2069, 2070, 2396
donor-agency strategies, 1281–1282, **2038–2042**
early Christian condemnation of, 1520, 1521
Eastern Orthodox position, 1991–1994
ethical issues, **832–838**, 1947, 1949, 1971–1972; see also subhead population policies and ethics of below
as eugenics policy, 766, 773
health effects and risks, 819, 821, 823–824, 1947–1949, 1971–1972, 2028–2031
Hindu position, 784–787, 835, 1134–1135, 1474, 1975, 1999–2000
historical views of, 833–834, 2363
impact on families, 801
incentive- and disincentive-based, 2011–2016, 2023, 2040
in India, 1474, 1955, 1965, 1969, 1971, 1972, 2000, 2008, 2011, 2012–2013, 2018, 2024, 2025, 2026, 2030
infanticide as, 351–352
infant-mortality decrease and, 1196, 1281–1282
international programs. See subhead donor-agency strategies above
Islamic beliefs, 1296, 1456–1457, 1975, 1977–1981, 2009
Judaic position, 833, 835, 839, 1975, 1981–1984
Latin American policy, 1641
legal and regulatory issues, 18, **839–845**, 1336, 1339, 2392–2393
in marriage, 1398, 1810
medical aspects, **818–827**; see also subhead health effects and risks above
minorities as unwitting research subjects, 1778
natural-law perspective, 1809, 1810–1811

persuasion-based, 2017–2022
philosophy of biology and, 277, 278
population policies and ethics of, **1954–1973**, **2004–2027**, 2039–2043, 2314
pronatalist strategies, 2021–2022, 2023, 2024, 2395
Protestant position, 833, 834, 840, 1975, 1995–100, 2369
as public-health policy vs. personal needs, 1115
quality of life and, 1352
religious traditions and, **1974–2004;** see also subheads for specific religions
research ethics, 2263, 2563
Roman Catholic opposition, 766, 832, 833, 834–835, 836, 837, 848, 1463, 1564, 1641, 1809, 1975, 1976, 1985–1990, 2006, 2007, 2021, 2323, 2326, 2327, 2329, 2369
and sex as pleasure, 2382
social issues, **828–831**
technology of, 2488
types of, 818
U.S. issues, 1625, 1810–1811, 2242, 2392, 2393
veterinary ethics and, 2522
women's issues, 813–814, 2006–2007, 2563–2564
see also Abortion; Animal breeding; Rights, reproductive; Sterilization
Fertility problems. See Reproductive technologies
Fertilization, 847–851
Fetal alcohol syndrome, 1405, 1411, 2428
Fetal-protection policies
analysis of, 1851, 2558
see also Maternal–fetal relationship
Fetal reduction, 856
Fetal testing. See Prenatal technologies
Fetal tissue
analysis and research issues, 853–854, **857–863**, 988–989
Arab transplantation regulations, 1456
French regulations, 1560–1561
German regulations, 1586, 2245
for Parkinson's disease treatment, 856
personal-identity issue, 1940
postabortion use of, 1862–1863, 1868, 1879, 2238
U.S. regulations, 853, 1626, 2186, 2288
Feticide, 26–27
female, 1471, 1474, 1970, 2000
see also Abortion headings
Fetus, **847–863**
abortion issues, 1–5, 7, 15, 20, 23–24, 26, 29, 30, 31, 606, 613, 767, 773–774, 961, 1181, 1454, 1456, 1459, 1520, 1529, 1577, 1584, 1592, 1625, 1637, 1937, 2238
abuse of, 982
AIDS transmitted to, 119
definition of, 851

Quebec Medical Society, 1632
Quesnay, François, 1962
QUICK MEDICAL REFERENCE (QMR) (medical expert system), 1660
Quimby, Phineas, 130, 2119
Quinlan case (1976)
  advance directives and, 573, 575
  family role in proxy consent, 805
  legal aspects, 583, 1331, 1332
  protected liberty interests, 583
  right-to-die issues, 404, 409, 435, 438, 1169, 1621, 1625, 2183
Quinlan, Karen Ann. *See* Quinlan case
Qur'an (Islamic scripture), 345, 1290, 1292, 1295
  on community and family, 1977, 1978
  on health and medical practices, 1452, 1453, 1454, 1455, 1457

**R**
Rabbis. *See* Clergy; Judaism; Pastoral care
Rabies, 144–145, 2249
Rabkin, Eric, 1372
Race and racism, **2189–2199**
  adoption issues, 72
  AIDS issues, 110, 119
  anti-Semitism, 715, 961, 1647, 1795, 1796, 1966
  contractarianism and, 163
  crime and violence issues, 947, 951, 1140, 1141–1142
  dentistry and, 600
  environmental health issues, 695–696, 697
  erroneous views, 2194
  as eugenics basis, 767, 770–772, 978, 1176, 1647
  feminist views on, 809
  gene therapy and, 912
  genetics and, 944–945, 947, 951, **976–983**, 1006, 1010
  as health and disease variable, 1093
  historical constructions, 2189–2191
  Nazi ideology, 961, 1176, 1647, 1746, 1794, 1795, 1797, 1966, 2191
  pharmacological dosages and, 1178–1779, 1748–1749, 2196
  prostitution and, 2115
  psychiatric diagnoses and, 1747, 1753
  sociobiological view of, 278, 1176
  South African apartheid, 1466, 1467, 1468, 2127, 2195
  sterilization and, 845
  *see also* African Americans; Minorities as research subjects
Rachels, James, 58
"Racial hygiene," 1647, 1794, 1795, 2191
Racketeer Influences and Corrupt Organizations (RICO) statute, 25
Radiation
  animal research on, 148
  cancer link, 694, 695
  environmental health risks, 694, 695, 698
  genetic changes caused by, 775, 941

nuclear, 2542
  unethical studies, 2258–2259
Radiation therapy, 121
Radical behaviorism, 236, 240
Radical feminists
  beliefs, 808
  on sexual ethics, 2373
  on surrogacy, 2227
Radioactive wastes. *See* Hazardous wastes and toxic substances
Radon, 695
Rahit (Sikh code), 2398–2399
Rahner, Karl, 915
Ramadan (Islamic month), 1292
Ramazzini, Bernardino, 1839–1840, 2400
Ramsey, Paul
  embodiment theme, 2122, 2123, 2125
  fidelity-based theory, 865–866
  on human genetic intervention, 915
  on informed consent, 1243, 1246–1247
  on medical ethics, 1620, 2121, 2255
  on metaphors in health care, 1769, 1771
  model of professional–patient relationship, 2095–2096, 2100, 2122, 2124
  on patient-as-person focus, 2528–2529
  on situation ethics, 2123
  on sovereignty of God, 2122
Rand Health Insurance Study (1979), 1044
Randomized controlled trial, 2275, 2276, 2279
Ranjit Singh, 2398
Rape
  as abortion criterion, 11, 17, 29, 37
  African religion on, 83
  DNA typing as conviction tool, 634–635, 973–974, 1017
  feminist critiques of, 809
  legal perspective, 2392, 2393–2394
  marital, 46, 2392, 2394
  social perspective, 2388, 2389, 2390, 2391
  as woman issue, 2567–2568
Rascher, Sigmund, 2259
Rashi, 1305
*Rassenhygiene* (racial hygiene), 1647, 1794, 1795, 2191
*Rassenkunde* (race science), 1966
Rational emotive therapy, 239
Rationalism, 730–731, 1557, 1935
Rationality
  autonomy and, 216
  body views, 293–294
  environmental ethics and, 689
  ethics and, 721
  as unique to humans, 1176, 1808–1809, 1935, 2325, 2326
Rationing of biomedical technology. *See* Triage; *specific technology, e.g.,* Kidney dialysis
Rationing of health care. *See* Health-care resources, allocation of; Triage
Ratzinger, Joseph Cardinal, 1809–1810
Rauschenbusch, Walter, 2124

Rawls, John, 979, 1835, 2175, 2308, 2309
  on contracts, 162, 163, 904
  ethical theory, 723, 731
  on family, 803
  on justice, 366, 396–397, 731, 979, 1310–1311, 1312, 1313
Raynaud, Théophile, 2323
Raz, Joseph, 1835, 2306
Razetti, Luis, 1640
RCT. *See* Randomized controlled trial
RDNA. *See* Recombinant DNA
Reagan, Ronald, 1059, 1996
  abortion counseling policies, 829
  "Baby Doe" regulations, 360, 1215
  contraceptives policies, 829, 830
  environmental policies, 703–704
Realism, 731–732
Reasoning
  analogical, 1770–1772
  authority and, 210
  medical, 1682
  moral. *See* Moral reasoning
  as personhood manifestation, 1174, 1938, 2325, 2326
  scientific method, 2337
Rebirth beliefs. *See* Afterlife
Rebirth metaphor, 1766
REC. *See* Research ethics committees
Recessive genetic traits, 949–950
Reche, Otto, 1797
Reciprocal determinism, 240
Reciprocity, 1392
Recombinant DNA
  bioethical issues, 1625
  biotechnology of, 283, 286, 287
  eugenic applications, 957
  gene therapy and, 907, 974
  philosophy of biology and, 275–276
  regulation of, 972–973
  technology of, 2481, 2485
Recombinant DNA Advisory Committee, 2289
Records, medical. *See* Medical information systems
Recreational drug use. *See* Substance abuse
Rectal cancer, 172
Red blood cells, 997
Red Cross, 2045, 2534, 2540, 2551
Redman, John, 1610
Reductionism, 273, 1176
Reed, Walter, 1234, 1774, 2250
Reemtsma, Keith, 2594
Reformation
  abortion perspective, 35
  aging perspective, 99
  authority and, 210
  background, 2117–2118
  death perspective, 515
  disability perspective, 611
  fertility-control perspective, 833
  married vs. celibate clergy issue, 1398
  scientific revolution, 2118
  sexual ethics, 2368–2369

2006, 2007, 2021, 2323, 2326, 2327, 2329, 2369
on fetal ensoulment, 1181
on gene therapy, 916
on genetic defects, 994
on genetic engineering, 932
on genetic screening, 977, 1599
in Germany, 1580
hierarchical authoritative teachings, 2325–2326, 2329
on homosexuality, 1148, 1149, 2330
in Ireland, 1576, 1577, 1578
legal and ethical intertwinement, 1336, 1559, 2325; *see also* Canon law; Double effect; Natural law
marriage views, 779–780, 1398, 2327
medical ethics codes, 1025, 1046, 1426, 1430, 1431, 1529–1530, 1564, 1573–1574, 1578, 1580, 1595, 1618–1621, 1633, 1639, 2321–2330
medical missionaries, 1493
medieval European medical ethics and practice, 1161–1162, 1522, 1528–1536 1699, 2323
mental-health concepts, 1699
moral theological basis of, **636–640**, 758, 2322–2330; *see also* Casuistry; Double effect
natural-law belief, 1148–1149, 1620, 1639, 1806–1807, 1809–1810, 2007, 2323–2330, 2329
on natural and revealed truths, 1814, 2326–2328
on organ donation, 1863, 1888, 2223, 2328
pastoral care, 1905, 1907, 1908, 2324
on personhood, 1935
in Poland, 1595, 1599
population policy, 1985–1986; *see also* *subheads* abortion position; fertility-control position *above*; *subhead* sterilization position *below*
proportionality principle, 2510
Protestant counterarguments, 2117, 2124
reproductive-technology position, 1571, 1586, 1641, 2219, 2223, 2233, 2235
revisionist ethicists, 2329–2330
scholasticism. *See* Aquinas, Thomas; Scholasticism
sexual ethics, 1148–1149, 2327, 2360, 2367, 2369
sterilization position, 836, 837, 1426, 1987, 2326, 2327
supererogation theology, 1834
*see also* Double effect
Romanell, Patrick, 1620
Roman Empire. *See* Rome, ancient; Byzantine Empire
Romanes, George, 230
Roman Hospital of the Holy Spirit, 1162
Romania
abortion issues, 12, 840, 1599, 2021, 2022, 2023

infanticide practice, 1208
medical ethics, 1595–1600
Romanticism, 1089, 1815, 2446
phenomenology and, 1284
technology and, 2480
Romantic love, 1393, 2352, 2383
Romberg, Ernst, 1102
Rome, ancient
abortion views, 1087, 1514, 1515, 2364
abuse, interpersonal, practices, 48
adoption practices, 71
animal research, 143–144
authority, 207
care tradition, 319–320
casuistic thought, 344–345
chemical and biological warfare, 2545
childhood in, 351, 352
contraception views, 833, 840
death perspective, 501, 555–556
epidemics, 714, 715
ethics, 740, 759
eugenics, 780
expert testimony, 796
female circumcision, 384
friendship in, 889
health and disease concepts, 1698
hospital origins, 1160
infanticide practices, 1200
insanity law, 1734
law and morality, 1336
legal sexism, 2345
medical ethics, 1509–1515, 1516–1519, 1639
population theory, 1962
public-health measures, 2157
public vs. private sphere, 2067
religion and morality, 759
sexual ethics, 1148, 2363–2365, 2372–2373
Stoic legal influence, 1558
women physicians, 2577
zoos, 184
*see also* Byzantine Empire
Roosevelt, Franklin D., 626–627, 2201, 2251
Rorty, Richard, 732–733
Rose, Gerhard, 1797
Rose, James, 1691
Rosebury, Theodore, 2546, 2547
Rosenberg, Alfred, 961
Rosenhan, David, 1737
Rosner, Fred, 1620
Ross, W. D., 721, 727, 1226
Roth, Julius A., 2089
Rothman, Barbara Katz, 814
Rothman, David, 1629, 1734, 1736, 1775
Rousel Uclaf, Inc., 843
Rousseau, Jean-Jacques
on child rearing, 353
on freedom, 882–883
on marriage, 2370
on political ethics, 748
rights emphasis, 1429, 2014

on social improvement, 1089, 2157
on woman's role, 2557
Roussignan, Nahabed, 1451
Rowland, Robyn, 1645
Royal Australian and New Zealand College of Psychiatrists, 2130, 2131
Royal College of Physicians (U.K.)
founding charter (1518), 1691
human-research guidelines, 1570, 1761, 1763
jurisdiction, 1550
medical practitioner code, 1422–1423
smoking-risks report, 2422
Royal Women's Hospital (Australia), 1644
Royce, Josiah, 865
RU-486 (abortion pill), 3, 12–14, 18, 838, 843, 1474, 1561, 2287, 2393
Ruddick, Sara, 338, 339, 810–811
Rule consequentialism, 740
Rule of St. Benedict, 1039
"Rule of thumb" (wife beating), 48
Rush, Benjamin, 1232–1233, 1423, 1612, 1692
anti-alcohol stance, 2440, 2441
mental-illness treatment invention, 1733, 1741
Rusk, Howard, 2201
Russia
abortion issue, 1606
chemical and biological weapons, 2544, 2546, 2547
euthanasia, 1607
feminism, 2557
genome project, 1015, 1016
health-care delivery, 1606
international weapons trade, 2550
medical ethics, 1425–1426, 1427, 1428, 1431, 1432
organ and tissue transplantation, 1608
women physicians, 2581, 2583
*see also* Soviet Union (former)
Russia, prerevolutionary
abortion issue, 1606
medical practice and ethics, 1601–1603, 2083
Russian Academy of Sciences, 1609
Russian National Committee on Bioethics, 1609
Russian Orthodox Church, 1606
Russian Society of Psychiatrists, 1608
Russo–Turkish War, 2583
Rustam (Persian hero), 1445
*Rust v. Sullivan* (1991), 23, 886
Ryle, Gilbert, 234
Ryle, John A., 2400–2401, 2537
Rzepkowski, Neal, 2312

**S**
Sabshin, Melvin, 1701
Sacred culture, 478–480
Sacrifice. *See* Obligation and supererogation
Sadistic personality disorder, 1745

and children and infants, 360, 1214–1215, 1217, 1218
conflict of interest, 461
death criteria and, 524, 529
DNA typing, **633–635**
Eastern Orthodox perspective, 646
electrical stimulation of the brain, 659
and environmental issues, 703, 704, 705
and eugenics practices, 766
and euthanasia, 560
of fertility control, 838, 841–843
and food supply, 870–871
genetics-related. *See* Gene therapy; Genetic engineering; Genetic testing and screening; Genome mapping and sequencing
genetic testing, 991–992
history of medical, **2472–2477**
hospital ethical issues, 1169–1170
Islamic perspective, 1296–1297
Jainist perspective, 1300
life-processes modification, 1345, 1350, 1359
media coverage of, 425, 436
medical information systems, **1656–1661**
microallocation decisions, 1076
nature in relationship with, 1815–1816
nuclear weapons, 2541–2543
philosophy of, **2477–2483**
and physician–patient relationship, 890
prenatal. *See* Prenatal technologies
Protestant perspective, 2121
reproductive. *See* Reproductive technologies
and scientific publishing, 433
surgical innovations, 2452
testing of medical devices, 941
tragic aspects, 2494
trust issues, 2501
value and valuation in, 2516
Teenagers. *See* Adolescents
Tegh Behadur, Guru, 2398
Teleology, 273–274, 1174
*see also* Ethics, normative theories
Television, 436–437
Temkin, Owsei, 1441, 1681, 1701
Temperance movements, 2440, 2441
Ten Commandments, 721
Tendler, Moses, 1620
Tenon, James René, 2081
Teresa, Mother, 1393
Terminal illness. *See* Death and dying: euthanasia and sustaining life; Hospice and end-of-life care; Truth
Terry, Randall E., 390
Testing and screening. *See* Animal research; Genetic testing and screening; Health screening and testing in the public-health context; Laboratory testing
Testosterone, 2409
"Test-tube baby," first, 435–436, 438, 858, 1571, 2233

Texas Medical Center, bioethical studies, 1628
Thackrah, Turner, 2083, 2158
Thailand
  Buddhism, 314, 494–495, 1470, 1506, 2002–2004
  death perspective, 494–495
  family-planning support, 2003, 2004, 2012
  medical practice and ethics, 1506, 1507, 1508–1509
Thalassemia. *See* Beta-thalassemia
Thalidomide, 1123, 1187, 1624, 1943, 2573
Thanatology. *See* Death education
Thatcher, Margaret, 1569
Theft. *See* Fraud, theft, and plagiarism
Theodosian Code, 1401
Theodosius I, Roman emperor, 1517
Theology. *See* Ethics, religion and morality; Religion; *specific religions*
Theoretical bioethics, 250
*Theory of Justice, A* (Rawls), 1310
*Theory of Medical Ethics* (Veatch), 1627
Theory of the mind. *See* Psychoanalysis and dynamic therapies
Therapeutic privilege, 1248, 1918
Therapeutic relationship. *See* Professional–patient relationship
Theravada Buddhism, 315, 2002–2004
Third-party assisted reproduction. *See* Reproductive technologies
Third-party consent. *See* Proxy consent
Third-party disclosure
  ethical guidelines, 1578, 1758–1759
  population problem, 1958–1959
  untested pharmaceutical use, 1123
  *see also* Confidentiality
Third Reich. *See* National Socialism
Third World
  abortion issues, 12
  aging and aged in, 91
  agriculture, 192
  AIDS cases, 112, 831
  animal welfare, 192
  arms sales to, 2550
  chemical weapons, 2548
  ecofeminism, 691
  environmental ethics, 687, 691, 934
  environmental health, 696
  epidemics, 718
  feminism, 2559
  fertility control, 2005, 2038–2042
  food-supply problems, 870
  genetically linked infant mortality, 1652
  hazardous substances and toxic wastes, 1028
  lactose intolerance, 944
  live-donor organ sales, 1869
  medical-research subjects, 1780, 1781–1782, 1972
  population ethics and policy, 1971–1972, 2005, 2006, 2008–2014, 2038–2042
  prenatal-diagnosis limitations, 1653

prenatal diagnosis for sex selection, 2214–2215
public-health initiatives, 1123
research subjects' risk-benefits distribution, 2298
schizophrenia outcomes, 1747
technology, 2485
tobacco sales, 2426
*see also specific countries*
Thomas, Clarence, 2393, 2394
Thomas Aquinas. *See* Aquinas, Thomas
Thomasius, Christian, 1543
Thomasma, David, 245, 1923, 1924, 2098, 2099
Thomism. *See* Aquinas, Thomas; Scholasticism
Thomson, Judith Jarvis, 813, 1771, 1772
Thomson, Samuel, 128, 2506
Thomsonian movement. *See* Thomson, Samuel
Thorazine. *See* Chlorpromazine
Thoreau, Henry David, 726
*Thornburgh v. American College of Obstetricians and Gynecologists* (1986), 23
Thymidine, 212
Tibet, 177, 314, 1472
Tiger, Lionel, 1176
Tipping (Soviet-bloc health-care custom), 1597–1598
Tisdale, William, 334
Tissue procurement. *See* Organ and tissue procurement
Tissue targeting, 910
Tissue transplants. *See* Organ and tissue procurement; Organ and tissue transplants
Title X, 828, 829, 830
Titmuss, Richard, 290, 1837
Tobacco industry. *See* Smoking
Tocqueville, Alexis de, 754
Tokugawa Ieyasu, 1493
Tokushima University Medical School, 1502
Tokyo declarations, 1555
Tolerance, governmental, 2067
Tolman, E. C., 232–233
Tolstoy, Leo, 1110, 1901
Tong, Rosemarie, 338
Tooley, Michael, 1937, 1938
Topographic theory, 2132
Torah (Judaic scripture), 1301, 1442, 1443, 1444, 1983, 2123
*see also* Bible; Talmudic ethics
Tort law
  artificial-insemination disclosure, 2218
  contraceptive safety and effectiveness, 842–843
  medical malpractice, 1662–1663, 1665, 2453
  privacy rights, 2069
Torture
  medical codes and, 1640, 2052–2057
  physician-assisted, 2540